Frailty in Older Adults with Cancer

Fabio Gomes
Editor

Frailty in Older Adults with Cancer

Springer

Editor
Fabio Gomes
Medical Oncology Department
The Christie NHS Foundation Trust
Manchester, UK

ISBN 978-3-030-89164-0 ISBN 978-3-030-89162-6 (eBook)
https://doi.org/10.1007/978-3-030-89162-6

This Springer imprint is published by the registered company Springer Nature Switzerland AG
The registered company address is: Gewerbestrasse 11, 6330 Cham, Switzerland

Preface

Cancer care and treatment decision-making is often challenging and must be personalised. But as I started my career in Oncology, I recognised that a considerable number of patients attending clinics were not being represented in the studies or trials that guide our treatment decisions and many aspects of our daily clinical practice. Although Oncology is an inquisitive and research-oriented field, the sub-group of older adults like those aged 70+ years has not been routinely considered as an integral part of research. This is particularly obvious for those older adults with frailty where there is a complex interplay between ageing, cancer, and other conditions. But as the world population is ageing, this means that older adults with cancer are no longer a small sub-group, in fact, in many practices around the world they already represent the majority.

In this context, a persistent question in the back of my mind became increasingly hard to dismiss in clinic: "how confident am I regarding this treatment being the best strategy for this patient?" This question turned into a passion for the field of geriatric oncology particularly after joining the Senior Adult Oncology Programme at the Moffitt Cancer Centre (Tampa, Florida, United States of America) under the leadership of Dr Martine Extermann and Dr Lodovico Balducci. Following that experience, my interest and dedication to the field continued to grow, not just as I developed my clinical practice and research in Manchester (United Kingdom), but also through my participation within the International Society of Geriatric Oncology (SIOG). In this society, I found a group of like-minded colleagues from all over the world, aligned with a single purpose, to improve our knowledge and the care of older adults with cancer.

This led to the opportunity to develop this educational book addressing not just the significance of ageing in the management of patients with cancer but more importantly, the impact of one's frailty in this context. Frailty is the most problematic expression of ageing, where individuals experience increased vulnerability related to decline in function and reserve across multiple organ systems. Hence the need to look beyond chronological age on its own and it is paramount to incorporate frailty in the decision-making process. This is intended to influence the anti-cancer treatment decision and to implement a holistic strategy, from dietary interventions to tailored physical exercise, psychological support, and optimisation of other medical conditions. In fact, this is the key focus of this book as there is a significant unmet need regarding evidence for the sub-group of older adults who have cancer and frailty.

This ambitious project resulted in 27 chapters through a collaboration of about 100 co-authors across 16 countries in 5 continents. The co-authors, all health care professionals, from medical doctors to nurses and allied health professionals, represent the multidisciplinary care required by this group of patients. As the Editor and a co-author myself, this book is a testament to the dedication of so many colleagues who contributed to this project even throughout the COVID-19 pandemic, which was such a challenging period, particularly for health care systems around the world.

The book consists of 27 chapters: Chaps. 1–2 set the scene by introducing the topic and providing an overview of the significance and challenges of ageing and frailty in patients with cancer, as well as key worldwide actions and policies; Chap. 3 covers how clinical teams may assess their patients for frailty through screening tools and subsequent in-depth assessments through a comprehensive geriatric assessment; Chaps. 4–8 provide a deep dive on the different components of a comprehensive geriatric assessment which play a key role in one's frailty (e.g. polypharmacy, cognitive impairment, etc.). This includes not just how to assess and intervene to support/optimise these patients but also a review of the evidence specific to older adults with cancer; Chaps. 9–12 reflect on the concepts of pre- and re-habilitation of these older adults with frailty, the different models by which multidisciplinary care may be integrated for these patients, and how to optimise the decision-making process and consider advance care planning; Chaps. 13–15 provide considerations for this group of patients according to the type of anti-cancer treatment (e.g. surgery, radiotherapy, chemotherapy, immunotherapy…) and also in the setting of palliative care; Chap. 16 provides an insightful perspective of the present areas of frailty research and key areas leading the future research in this field; and finally, the last section consists of Chaps. 17–27 which provide detailed reviews of the evidence in this field according to the cancer sub-type to inform treatment decisions from early to advanced/metastatic stages (e.g. the management of breast cancer in older adults with frailty, etc.).

Ultimately, this book aims to educate and empower clinical teams to manage this complex and heterogeneous group of patients who are often underrepresented in research. But I also hope that this valuable resource will fuel a passion for this field, raising even more questions and the need for change and research to improve the care of these patients.

Manchester, UK Fabio Gomes

Contents

Part I
Frailty in Context, Assessment and its Management

Chapter 1
Introduction to Frailty in Older Adults with Cancer

Kristen Haase, Ines B. Menjak, and Martine Puts

Introduction

The world's population is aging, with an anticipated 16% of the global population predicted to be aged 65 years or older by 2050 [1]. Older adults enrich societies through their great wealth of knowledge and life experience, however older adults are vulnerable to several health conditions [2]. Frailty is a condition which disproportionally impacts older adults and has been called the "most problematic expression of aging" [3]. Frailty is defined as a condition of diminished functional and physiological reserve capacity [4] which creates a state where the individual is vulnerable to acute and everyday stressors [5, 6]. This is an important consideration in older populations because it exposes older adults to subsequent vulnerabilities and health decline from which it may be difficult to recover leading to significant disability or death [7].

This chapter will introduce definitions, mechanisms, and screening methods of frailty, followed by an overview of how it relates to the treatment and management of older adults with cancer. Lastly, this chapter will cover the future directions in this field in terms of clinical practice, education, and research.

K. Haase (✉)
Faculty of Applied Science, School of Nursing, University of British Columbia, Vancouver, BC, Canada
e-mail: kristen.haase@ubc.ca

I. B. Menjak
Sunnybrook Health Sciences Centre, Toronto, ON, Canada
e-mail: Ines.Menjak@sunnybrook.ca

M. Puts
University of Toronto, Toronto, ON, Canada
e-mail: martine.puts@utoronto.ca

F. Gomes (ed.), *Frailty in Older Adults with Cancer*,
https://doi.org/10.1007/978-3-030-89162-6_1

Frailty

Frailty is best understood as a state [8, 9] wherein older people experience increased vulnerability related to decline in function and reserve across multiple organ systems [10]. A consensus statement specifically on physical frailty characterizes it as: "a medical syndrome with multiple causes and contributors characterized by diminished strength, endurance, and reduced physiologic function that increases an individual's vulnerability for developing increased dependency and/or death" [11]. Two complementary definitions with accompanying assessments include: the (1) the frailty phenotype; and (2) the frailty index (Fig. 1.1). First, Fried's frailty phenotype classifies frailty as a biologically driven syndrome of accumulated declines across multiple systems. This characterization of frailty includes several symptoms, such as weakness, low energy, slow walking speed, low physical activity, and weight loss [12]. Second, Rockwood and colleagues define frailty as a deficit-driven state [13–15]. This is operationalized through the frailty index wherein the greater the number and nature of aggregate health deficits an individual has, the greater the level of frailty [16, 17]. These conceptualizations see frailty as both an etiology and an outcome of accumulated deficits, respectively.

While frailty has been categorized as "all or none," others argue it is a dynamic process [18]. Although it is important to identify and categorize those who are frail, identifying those at risk of becoming frail [19] is equally important. A person in a pre-frail state is characterized as having a health state that is not robust, and not yet frail, but predisposed to becoming frail [8]. Pre-frailty is therefore a critical period, as interventions implemented during the pre-frail period have been shown to postpone decline into a frail state [20, 21]. Thus, a continuum exists with those who are robust, pre-frail, and those who are experiencing frailty at different levels of severity causing varying levels of dependence [22].

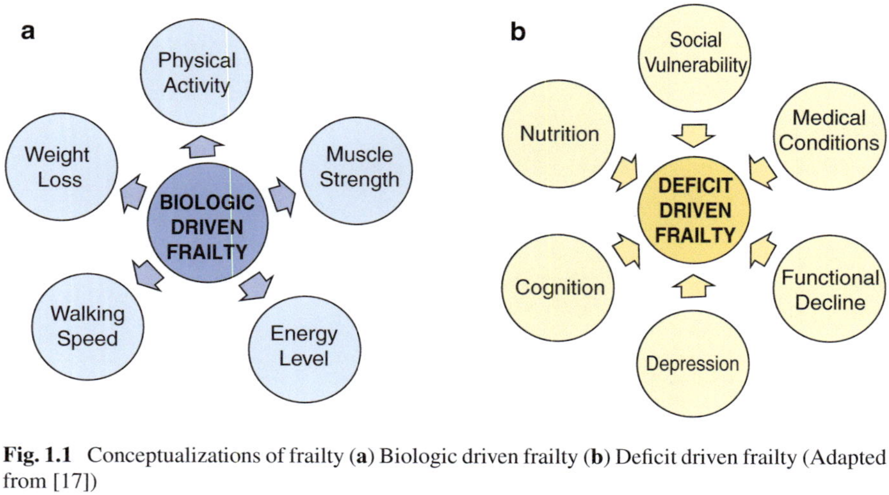

Fig. 1.1 Conceptualizations of frailty (**a**) Biologic driven frailty (**b**) Deficit driven frailty (Adapted from [17])

Prevalence

A recent systematic review [23] of 46 observational studies including pooled data from more than 120,000 older adults from 28 countries found that one in six community-dwelling adults aged 60 years or older experience frailty. This same systematic review found frailty and pre-frailty were higher amongst women than men and noted methodological challenges related to variation in frailty measurement and level of country income. A prior systematic review [24] including 61,500 community-dwelling adults from 21 studies found frailty prevalence rates ranged from 4 to 59%. When these findings were limited to those using Fried's phenotype model, prevalence rate was 10% (95% CI 9.6–10.2) for frailty and 44% (44.2–44.7) for pre-frailty. Frailty rates were also shown to increase with age, ranging from 4% for those aged 65–69 up to 26% for those >85 years.

Mechanisms of Frailty

Much like aging, the mechanisms of frailty are multifactorial [25] and include an accumulation of physiological changes over time within the context of an individual's environmental exposure [26, 27]. A growing body of literature supports that frailty is caused by aging-related biologic changes, dysregulation and dysfunction in multiple physiological pathways, and chronic disease (Fig. 1.2).

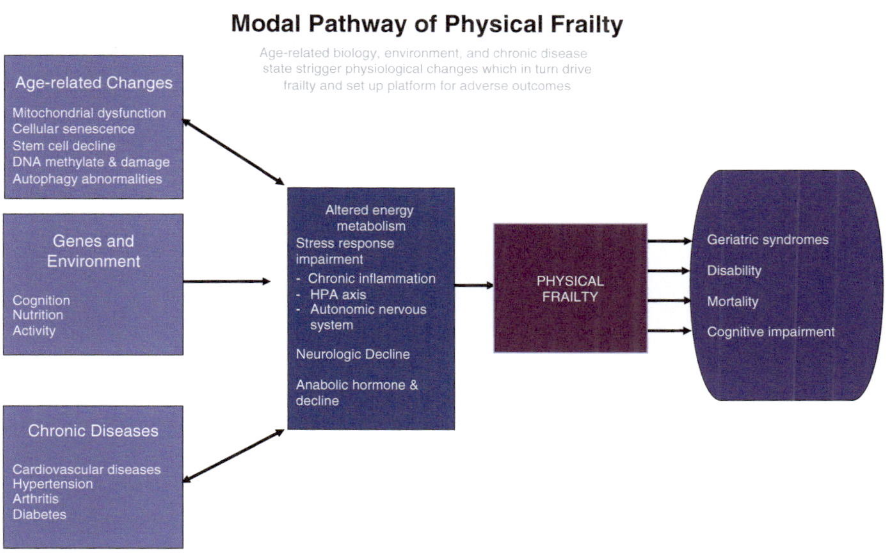

Fig. 1.2 Modal pathway of physical frailty (Adapted from [16])

Frailty develops as a result of gradual decline in physiological reserve across systems associated with aging, but this process is accelerated due to the failure of homeostasis which occurs in frailty [3, 28, 29]. This decrease in homeostasis leaves older adults vulnerable to subsequent stressors. Aging mechanisms are determined by both genetic and environmental factors, combined with epigenetic mechanisms regulating gene expression [30]. As a result of biological changes and decline, older adults are also predisposed to chronic disease which further deplete physiological reserve, and ultimately, these combined physiological changes drive the development of frailty, and predispose older adults to geriatric syndromes (such as delirium, falls, and incontinence [31]), disability, cognitive impairment, and mortality [30].

There is also growing awareness of the role of mediating factors in the development of frailty [32, 33], which include environmental exposures [26], social support and isolation [34, 35], exercise [36, 37], and nutrition [38, 39]. A recent study by Welsted et al. [40] on frailty trajectories found that despite the heterogeneity of the literature, the progression of frailty is the result of numerous risk and protective factors, with important influence from brain pathology, social demographics, and comorbidities. There is also growing evidence of the role of inequities predisposing certain populations to greater risk for frailty than others [41].

Types of Frailty

Most definitions of frailty emphasize the physical component of frailty, such as the Fried's frailty phenotype model, describing it as a set of symptoms like weakness, low energy, slow walking speed, low physical activity, and weight loss [12]. Therefore, the term "frailty" in the literature more often concerns physical frailty. Whilst one may argue that the physical domain is the main component of frailty, the concept of frailty also includes other domains, such as the cognitive, psychological, and the social domains, which are often interlinked. For example, it is widely recognized that a cognitive impairment may result in physical impairments, and this largely relies on neurodegenerative disorders (such as Alzheimer's disease). In that regard, the definition by Rockwood on the Frailty index, previously described, is more encompassing.

However, some recent concepts of frailty refer to this condition as "physical frailty," "psychological frailty," "cognitive frailty," and "social frailty," based on its dominant domain for a given individual. In the absence of any generally accepted criteria, these definitions must be used cautiously.

Other emerging definitions, for example regarding the cognitive domain, distinguish cognitive frailty as a concept where the cognitive impairment is caused by physical factors related to frailty and pre-frailty (instead of the other way around, therefore excluding neurodegenerative diseases). The key factors defining such a condition include: (1) presence of physical frailty and cognitive impairment; and (2) exclusion of concurrent dementia [42]. Another key aspect in this concept is that this cognitive impairment has a potential of reversibility [42].

Moreover, a concept of social frailty has emerged as a multidimensional concept where social resources (or restrictions), behaviors, and activities make people more vulnerable [43]. In this setting it is important to consider how the social determinants of health (SDOH) may play a central role in preventing or predicting deterioration into a physically frail state [44]. SDOH include education; health care; neighborhood and environment; social and community context; and economic stability, and have been shown to play a critical role in health [45] and aging [46, 47]. Woo et al. [48] identified that for older men, increasing frailty was observed for those from non-white collar occupations, with limited social support, and low socioeconomic status. For older women, little contact with relatives and absence of participation in religious and community activities were also risk factors. Therefore, social frailty also warrants close consideration by cancer clinicians.

Frailty in Older Cancer Patients

Older adults are more likely to experience both cancer and frailty as age is the most important risk factor for both conditions [49]. Globally, older adults account for nearly half of all cancer cases [50]. Approximately 40% of older adults with cancer are frail, and as age increases, the risk of frailty increases [51]. Those older adults who are frail, are more vulnerable to functional impairments, declining health status [3], and are also more likely to experience a deterioration in overall physical function than non-frail older adults [52]. Moreover, they are also at greater risk than their younger counterparts of developing toxicity with anti-cancer treatments, such as chemotherapy [53]. Hence the importance of understanding the role frailty plays in oncology decision-making and how best to support older adults with cancer, their families, and caregivers.

Frailty Screening

Numerous tools and measures have been developed to identify frailty, all of which try to capture frailty as previously defined by the two predominant conceptualizations of frailty [30]. A detailed review of frailty assessment tools is presented in Chap. 3.

Several screening questionnaires exist to measure frailty in oncology and combine the multidimensional concepts of frailty, through questionnaires, rather than physical measurements. Two commonly used screening tools in oncology include: the Geriatric 8 (G8) and the Vulnerable Elders Survey (VES-13). The G8 includes 8-items: patient age, appetite changes, weight loss, mobility, body mass, neuropsychological problems, medications, and self-rated health. The G8 has been found concise and feasible with good sensitivity [54]. The VES-13 assesses the level of frailty in older persons through 13 items, assessing: age, self-rated health, functional disability and physical function limitations [55, 56]. Cognitive decline measures are often included in frailty assessments, as cognition has been shown to be an important leading/aggravating aspect of frailty [5]. Both the G8 and the VES-13 are easy and quick to deliver and are recommended by the American Society of Clinical Oncology *(ASCO) Guideline for Geriatric Oncology* [57].

Single item physical measures of frailty include gait speed and the timed up and go (TUG). The TUG is a simple method to assess mobility and physical reserve through the assessment of balance [58, 59]. The patient is timed while they raise from an armed chair, walk three meters, turn around, walk back, and sit down in the chair. In a gait speed assessment, the older adult is timed while walking four meters, unassisted. For both gait speed and TUG, those below the 25% mark for their age-matched cohort are considered frail [30]. These tools lack sensitivity but are useful for those looking for quick and easy in-office assessments that indicate the need for further investigation.

Geriatric Assessment

The comprehensive geriatric assessment (CGA) originates from geriatric medicine and takes a holistic view of aging and health by broadly assessing all domains including physical and psychological health, functional status, and wellbeing [60, 61]. A detailed review of CGA and its different domains is presented in Chaps. 3–8.

Guidelines from the International Society of Geriatric Oncology (SIOG) indicate that a CGA is the best approach to tailor care, treatment, and intervene to prevent further decline amongst older adults with cancer [62]. This includes assessment of functional status, fatigue, cognition, social support, mental health, geriatric syndromes, comorbidity, and nutrition. CGA has been shown to influence cancer treatment decision-making in 20–47% of cases, predominantly toward less intensive treatment but sometimes preventing under-treatment [63–69]. By virtue of identifying frailty and vulnerability, patients and clinicians can make more informed decisions about risks and benefits of treatments, interventions can be undertaken to address deficits in preparation for treatment, and more tailored support can be delivered during cancer treatments. Frailty alone is not the determining factor for decision-making, but it should be considered as a key factor, alongside comorbidity, etc. The CGA equips clinicians and older adults with all of that information. A systematic review of frailty screening methods by Hamaker et al. concluded that all older adults with cancer would be better supported if they underwent a CGA, due to the limited discriminative power of frailty screening methods [56]. Therefore, CGA is the ideal approach, whilst screening methods are alternatives, following by a CGA for those screened positive for frailty. Ultimately, CGA is of great value and international guidelines advocate its use for older adults with cancer [57].

Impact on Decision Making

There is mounting supporting evidence that cancer treatment decisions for older adults should be based on CGA to ensure treatment considers both an older person's health and frailty [70]. A detailed review of the decision-making process in this context is presented in Chap. 12.

Using CGA as a guiding tool for older adults is particularly important given the exclusion of frail older adults from clinical trials [57, 62], which has led to patterns of both over- and under-treatment [71–92]. Frailty impacts cancer treatment decision making in numerous ways [68]. There is also a need to consider the role of the caregiver and available supports in the decision-making process. However, the most critical piece is for the older adult to have comprehensive information about their state of health, and potential vulnerabilities, all of which are best determined through CGA.

Attending to Frailty in Cancer Screening and Diagnosis

Early detection of cancers via screening is designed to provide patients with the best outcomes by virtue of diagnosing cancer at its earliest stages. However, there is limited data regarding early diagnosis amongst frail older adults. One population-based study of almost 4000 patients aged ≥65 years found that cancer incidence was lower for frail patients (OR 0.64; 95% CI 0.46–0.89) [93]. Although data is limited for frail older adults related to early diagnosis, there is data available on older adults with comorbidities, and multimorbidity can be linked to frailty [12, 15, 16]. There is also data indicating that older adults with comorbidity do receive cancer screening and, in some cases, are even more likely to be diagnosed with early-stage cancer than their healthier counterparts. Women with comorbid conditions limiting their function were more likely to be diagnosed with breast cancer at an earlier stage than their healthier counterparts [94]. A SEER-Medicare study indicated that older men with chronic conditions were also more likely to be diagnosed with prostate cancer at an earlier stage than their healthier counterparts [95]. These data suggest that older frail adults with multiple comorbidities are receiving more medical monitoring that results in increased opportunities for cancer screening and early cancer diagnosis. However, studies involving colon cancer screening have shown conflicting results on the association of comorbidity and screening [96–98]. When examining cognitive decline specifically, reports show those with cognitive decline are less likely to receive cancer screening and are more likely to be diagnosed with later stage disease or receive a noninvasive diagnosis rather than a histological diagnosis [99–101].

There is population-level data regarding older women with breast, colorectal, lung, and prostate cancer having invasive diagnostic procedures, however, this research did not analyze frailty as a factor. Data from SEER-Medicare indicated that 92% of patients had an invasive procedure during the diagnostic phase or their care, while 62% had invasive procedures during continuing care and 25% had a procedure in their last month of life [102]. This data was also examined the use of diagnostic imaging, such as computed tomography (CT), magnetic resonance imaging (MRI), and positron emission tomography (PET) and found that in patients with stage IV cancer, 90% had one of these procedures in the diagnostic phase, while another 75% were scanned during continuing care [103]. Therefore, there is a need for research which interrogates the role of frailty in aiding the decision-making for cancer screening and diagnosis.

Attending to Frailty in Cancer Treatment

Surgery

Preoperative assessments focus on determining a patient's fitness for surgery. A detailed review of perioperative care in this context is presented in Chap. 13.

Frailty has been shown to be a better predictor of postoperative outcomes when compared to other surgical risk-assessment tools [104–106] and has been associated with higher rates of complications, mortality, and poor treatment tolerance [107–110]. The modified Frailty Index (mFI) was shown to predict post-operative complications and mortality in several population-based studies in cancer populations through the National Surgical Quality improvement Project (NSQIP) Participant Use File, including head and neck, bladder, pancreas, urologic and in a large single center study involving gastro-intestinal (GI) malignancies [111–116].

The first prospective study to evaluate quality of life (QOL) and functional recovery as primary outcomes after oncologic surgery is still underway [117]. In the GOSAFE study, data are being collected at baseline to complete multidimensional evaluation before major elective surgery in patients (≥70 years) from 26 international units with short-, mid-, and long-term surgical outcomes. An early analysis showed that frailty was present in a large proportion of these patients, reaching 68% when using the G8 screening tool, but rates varied based on the tool used [117]. The final results of this study will be instructive in managing the surgical approach to older adults living with both frailty and cancer.

Two scoring systems based on frailty and geriatric parameters have been developed to predict postsurgical outcomes in older oncology patients. The PREOP (Preoperative risk estimation for onco-geriatric patients) score predicts 30-day major post-operative complications [118]. The Memorial Sloan Kettering Frailty Index (MSK FI) was associated with longer hospital length of stay, higher odds of intensive care unit admission and lower overall survival [119]. However, it was not significantly associated with major complications or readmissions. The authors postulated this may be due to compensatory care offered to frail patients, as all were co-managed by the geriatrics service during the post-operative period.

Chemotherapy

Frailty is associated with chemotherapy tolerance and has been shown to help guide appropriate treatment decisions for systemic therapy in patients with various tumors [120]. A detailed review on treatment-specific considerations in the context of frailty is presented in Chap. 14.

The ASCO has published guidelines for the assessment of older patients being considered for chemotherapy, and the assessment of frailty is a central component, with a recommendation that all adults over age 65 being considered for chemotherapy have a geriatric assessment [57]. Aspects of frailty and CGA parameters, along with other factors were validated in a group of 500 patients and developed into a prediction tool for grade 3–5 toxicity with chemotherapy by Dr Hurria and the Cancer and Aging Research Group (CARG) [121, 122]. Similarly, the Chemotherapy Risk Assessment Scale for High-age patients (CRASH) similarly predicts for increased toxicity with systemic therapy and accounts for factors related to frailty and CGA in a variety of tumor types [123]. Hamaker et al. reported the association of frailty and chemotherapy-related toxicity as well as survival in a smaller group of breast cancer patients [120]. European investigators also determined that a combination of mini nutritional assessment (MNA), advanced cancer, age, and TUG were predictive of higher risk of early death in patients treated with first-line chemotherapy [124].

The Elderly Selection on Geriatric Index Assessment (ESOGIA) trial was a landmark phase III randomized controlled study which assigned patients with metastatic non-small cell lung cancer (NSCLC) to treatment based on a CGA in the experimental arm or based on a standard assessment with performance status and age [125]. The primary outcome of overall survival was not different between the groups, however, patients in the CGA group experienced less toxicity and had fewer treatment failures due to toxicity. This study is valuable in indicating that CGA can be used to identify the most appropriate treatment to minimize toxicity and attain similar survival to standard care. The MRC FOCUS2 trial investigated chemotherapy options on patients with metastatic colorectal cancer considered unfit for full dose chemotherapy due to advanced age, frailty, or both [126]. These patients were randomized to one of four treatment options. Patients treated with the more aggressive oxaliplatin-doublet regimens had a higher response rate and trend toward better survival, however a detrimental impact on QOL was observed. The recent GO2 phase III trial evaluated the optimum dosing of oxaliplatin and capecitabine in 514 frail older patients (median age of 76) with gastro-esophageal cancer who were unfit for full dose triplet chemotherapy [127]. The study found that the lowest dose level of 60%, versus 80% and standard dose was non-inferior for progression free survival (lowest dose versus standard HR 1.10, 95% CI 0.90–1.33). Patients experienced less toxicity and better overall treatment utility. Therefore, this study demonstrated that lower dose of treatment does not compromise disease control on survival or negatively impact quality of life.

Radiotherapy

Radiation is often used in frail older adults with cancer who are not candidates for other modalities of treatment or to palliate symptoms. A detailed review on treatment-specific considerations in the context of frailty is presented in Chap. 14.

As a result, shorter course radiation regimens have been evaluated for use in older or frail patients. In the field of glioblastoma multiforme, a study randomized frail and/or older patients to receive a short course of radiotherapy versus a standard longer course. This study showed similar survival outcomes in both arms [128] and improved cost-effectiveness [129]. Moreover, in the field of NSCLC, older adults who are frail or have comorbidities do tolerate and receive benefit from Stereotactic Body Radiation Therapy (SBRT) [130–132].

There has been conflicting evidence on the impact of frailty on radiation toxicity and outcomes. A systematic review of the use of CGA in radiation oncology identified 12 non-randomized studies in small populations [133]. CGA "vulnerability" showed a non-statistically significant association with treatment tolerance and a significant association with mortality. A prospective study in 402 patients with various cancers examined two frailty screening assessments, the G8 and the TUG, for association with acute toxicity and non-compliance with curative radiation [134]. No clear relationship was found between the frailty scores and treatment tolerability. But multivariable analysis showed that the type of cancer, older age (>80 years), worse performance status, and chemoradiotherapy were all associated with more toxicity. Also, the type of tumor and older age (>85 years) were associated with non-compliance with treatment. Another study of 230 older patients with different cancers who received radical or palliative radiotherapy showed that frailty determined by the VES-13 screening tool had an independent association with non-completion radiotherapy (adjusted for age, comorbidity, type of RT, and side effects) [135]. However, Keenan et al. did not find a correlation between frailty determined by the Edmonton Frail Scale and toxicity, breaks in treatment or hospitalization in patients receiving radical radiation [136]. Lastly, in a group of older patients being treated with radiation or chemoradiotherapy for head and neck or lung cancer, Vanderwalde et al. found that patients who had dysfunction in instrumental activities of daily living (IADLs) at baseline had worse health-related QOL scores after radiotherapy [137].

Approaches to Care

Due to the multidimensional nature of frailty [138], care provision in the inpatient, outpatient, and community setting should engage diverse members of the available multidisciplinary teams. However, teams vary by region, country, health system design, and available resources. A detailed review on the role of multidisciplinary teams and models of care for older cancer patients with frailty is presented in Chaps. 10 and 11.

Engaging the multidisciplinary team is a logical outcome of geriatric assessments, whenever deficits are identified. Typically, registered nurses specialized in either oncology or geriatrics (or both) lead to coordination, assessment, and navigation of patients and their caregivers as they connect with other members of the multidisciplinary team [139]. Collaboration with rehabilitation specialists, including occupational- and physio-therapists are essential to manage and assess functional status, mobility, fall risk, and exercise/activity guidelines. Given the importance of nutrition, dieticians play an essential role in determining nutrition needs and developing interventions to address potential shortfalls. Due to the prevalence of polypharmacy amongst older adults with cancer [140], the involvement of a pharmacist is also critical. To support older adults as they transition to, or remain in their home, connection with community supports and home support workers is an essential aspect of ensuring frail older adults with cancer are able to maintain their health and independence. Finally, while the role of unpaid or informal caregivers for older adults with cancer is acknowledged there are few supports for them. Understanding the challenges and stresses faced by caregivers is an important role for all members of the multidisciplinary team; if caregivers become unwell and are unable to provide care, this will have a negative impact on the frail older adult with cancer.

Future Directions

While significant advances have occurred in understanding the needs of older adults with cancer experiencing frailty, important gaps in clinical practice, education, and research remain.

Practice

As frailty is prevalent in older adults with cancer [51] and the global population is ageing with increasing numbers of cancer diagnosis [141], it is important to assess for frailty and identify it early to prevent or postpone further decline. However, the implementation of frailty screening in clinical practice is hampered by the aforementioned lack of a clear consensus definition, a lack of a gold standard for its diagnosis and issues around timing and feasibility [22, 142]. While there are many different frailty screening tools developed, there is less evidence which tool is best in which setting and different tools identify different groups of people [142]. However, despite which tool is best to use, it is important to identify frailty so that interventions can be selected to prevent and manage frailty. Several reviews on the management of frailty have been published [21, 143–146]. The most recent network meta-analyses showed that physical activity interventions and physical activity plus nutritional supplementation are the most effective interventions but the authors of the network analyses reported that the quality of the evidence was low and more robust studies of higher quality are needed [147]. However, these intervention studies did not focus on older adults with cancer. In this context there is even less evidence [148] but the little evidence there is suggests that older adults with cancer can benefit from exercise and nutrition interventions during cancer treatment.

Many new electronic health (eHealth) interventions are currently being developed to identify and assess frailty. Examples include computer-guided geriatric assessments and interventions which can support health care providers in seeing more older adults, while identifying those who are frail and need more support [149–155]. Technology could be used to connect with older adults and their caregivers to monitor treatment side effects, remind them of their treatments, and also to alert health care providers if the older adults' health worsens significantly [156]. However, technology use and comfort amongst frail older adults is critical. A study of virtual care for older adults during the COVID-19 pandemic highlighted barriers due to sensory impairment, cognitive impairment, and limited access to such devices [157].

Another important consideration is the role of caregivers, as many older adults with cancer who are frail may or may not be supported by a caregiver. It is important to assess the caregiver if they have enough support as many of the caregivers may have chronic conditions and caregiving itself may also negatively impact the caregiver's health and wellbeing [158–160].

Lastly, it is important to consider the use of the term frailty in practice. Prior research demonstrates that referring to someone as "frail," rather than someone experiencing the condition of frailty, stigmatizes older adults [143, 161, 162]. Older adults and their caregivers prefer this term is used to refer to their condition and not to them, therefore it should be used cautiously [143, 161, 162].

Education

Studies with different health care providers and trainees regarding their knowledge of geriatric oncology showed several significant gaps [163–166] and experts have advocated for further geriatric oncology education for health care providers [141, 167, 168]. The European Commission has prioritized frailty within the health policy agenda of the majority of the European Union member states through its "Joint Action on Frailty Prevention" (ADVANTAGE JA) [169]. Their systematic review reported that there were no relevant publications addressing the evidence and sustainability of educational or training programs for frailty prevention or frailty management [170]. ADVANTAGE JA together with the European Geriatric Medicine Society (EuGMS) developed a European Collaborative and Interprofessional Capability Framework for Prevention and Management of Frailty [169]. This interprofessional framework covers competencies related to the understanding about frailty, skills for screening and assessment, as well as management procedures for every profession involved. The majority of items focus on interprofessional collaboration, communication, and person-centered care planning. Currently, there are no identified geriatric oncology competencies available and the development of an interprofessional framework based on this frailty framework may help the development of a robust training program for all health care providers involved. Furthermore, the Institute of Medicine report entitled Delivering High Quality Cancer Care [171] identified a need to prepare the workforce for an aging population and having a competency framework would help establish the expectations for such workforce.

Research

There are many research opportunities for addressing frailty in older adults with cancer and a detailed review on this topic is presented in Chap. 16.

Older adults with frailty have been underrepresented in clinical studies [172] leading to a lack of evidence on how best to treat frail older adults with cancer with possible harmful consequences due to over- and under-treatment [173, 174]. Several recommendations have been published to develop studies that are more inclusive of frail older adults and to ensure that relevant outcomes for older adults are included, such as loss of function, independence, institutionalization, and cognitive impairment in addition to the usual outcomes such as progression free survival and mortality [175–178]. However, to date, few studies which include these patient-reported outcomes have been published. In addition, a minimum geriatric dataset has been developed [179] so that in future clinical studies a measure of frailty can be included to promote a better representation of older adults with frailty, as well as having comparable study populations. However, this dataset needs to be validated.

While there are some randomized studies demonstrating the effectiveness of CGA-guided interventions to improve clinical outcomes [180–182], more studies are needed to evaluate this implementation in daily practice. Specifically, more information is required to identify what method of intervention delivery works best and in which setting. Further research advancing an equity perspective and aiming to understand the experiences of those who are impacted by intersecting health and social inequities is also needed [183]. For example, older adults experiencing social isolation, those who only speak English as a second language (or not at all), have lower education levels, and are from a lower socioeconomic background. Whilst research in community-dwelling older adults showed that social isolation and loneliness have negative impacts on the development and progression of frailty, this relationship has not been studied in older adults with cancer [35, 43, 184]. Furthermore, more robust studies are needed to examine interventions to prevent and reduce the level of frailty in older adults with cancer which have shown to be effective in community-dwelling older adults [21, 22, 142, 147, 148].

Conclusion

Older adults with cancer are a growing population, of whom many are living with some form of frailty. As such, it is important to understand the implications for delivering multidisciplinary cancer care that can proactively manage their needs. Recognizing the different types of frailty and how these are affected by an individual's environment, such as social determinants of health is an important consideration when caring for frail older adults with cancer and their caregivers. There are important gaps in clinical practice, education and research regarding frailty, which need to be addressed. Particularly, more research is needed to understand and optimize the clinical management and supportive interventions tailored to these older adults living with both cancer and frailty.

References

1. United Nations Department of Economic and Social Affairs/Population Division. World Population Prospects: The 2008 Revision. 2010. Internet: http://esa.un.org/unpp (gelesen am 16).
2. Yoshikawa TT. Epidemiology and unique aspects of aging and infectious diseases. Clin Infect Dis. 2000;30(6):931–3.
3. Clegg A, Young J, Iliffe S, Rikkert MO, Rockwood K. Frailty in elderly people. Lancet. 2013;381(9868):752–62.
4. Fedarko NS. The biology of aging and frailty. Clin Geriatr Med. 2011;27(1):27–37.
5. Rodríguez-Mañas L, Féart C, Mann G, Viña J, Chatterji S, Chodzko-Zajko W, et al. Searching for an operational definition of frailty: a Delphi method based consensus statement. The frailty operative definition-consensus conference project. J Gerontol Ser A Biomed Sci Med Sci. 2013;68(1):62–7.
6. Cesari M, Calvani R, Marzetti E. Frailty in older persons. Clin Geriatr Med. 2017;33(3):293–303.
7. Vermeiren S, Vella-Azzopardi R, Beckwee D, Habbig A-K, Scafoglieri A, Jansen B, et al. Frailty and the prediction of negative health outcomes: a meta-analysis. J Am Med Dir Assoc. 2016;17(12):1163.e1–17.
8. Xue Q-L. The frailty syndrome: definition and natural history. Clin Geriatr Med. 2011;27(1):1–15.
9. Sourdet S, Rouge-Bugat M, Vellas B, Forette F. Frailty and aging. J Nutr Health Aging. 2012;16(4):283–4.
10. World Health Organization. WHO Clinical Consortium on Healthy Ageing. Geneva, Switzerland: World Health Organization; 2016. Contract No.: (WHO/FWC/ALC/17.2). Licence: CCBY-NC-SA3.0IGO.
11. Morley JE, Vellas B, van Kan GA, Anker SD, Bauer JM, Bernabei R, et al. Frailty consensus: a call to action. J Am Med Dir Assoc. 2013;14(6):392–7.
12. Fried LP, Tangen CM, Walston J, Newman AB, Hirsch C, Gottdiener J, et al. Frailty in older adults: evidence for a phenotype. J Gerontol A Biol Sci Med Sci. 2001;56(3):M146–56.
13. Rockwood K, Mitnitski A. Frailty in relation to the accumulation of deficits. J Gerontol A Biol Sci Med Sci. 2007;62(7):722–7.
14. Searle SD, Mitnitski A, Gahbauer EA, Gill TM, Rockwood K. A standard procedure for creating a frailty index. BMC Geriatr. 2008;8(1):24.

15. Jones DM, Song X, Rockwood K. Operationalizing a frailty index from a standardized comprehensive geriatric assessment. J Am Geriatr Soc. 2004;52(11):1929–33.
16. Michel J-P, Walston JD. Oxford textbook of geriatric medicine. Oxford: Oxford University Press; 2018.
17. Robinson TN, Walston JD, Brummel NE, Deiner S, Brown CH, Kennedy M, et al. Frailty for surgeons: review of a national institute on aging conference on frailty for specialists. J Am Coll Surg. 2015;221(6):1083–92.
18. Cesari M, Theou O. Frailty: the broad view. In: Fillit HM, Rockwood K, Young JB, editors. Brocklehurst's textbook of geriatric medicine and gerontology. 8th ed. Philadelphia: Elsevier; 2017. p. 84–7.
19. Rasiah J, Cummings GG, Gruneir A, Oelke ND, Estabrooks C, Holroyd-Leduc J. Prefrailty in older adults: a concept analysis. Int J Nurs Stud. 2020;108:103618.
20. Serra-Prat M, Sist X, Domenich R, Jurado L, Saiz A, Roces A, et al. Effectiveness of an intervention to prevent frailty in pre-frail community-dwelling older people consulting in primary care: a randomised controlled trial. Age Ageing. 2017;46(3):401–7.
21. Apóstolo J, Cooke R, Bobrowicz-Campos E, Santana S, Marcucci M, Cano A, et al. Effectiveness of interventions to prevent pre-frailty and frailty progression in older adults: a systematic review. JBI Database System Rev Implement Rep. 2018;16(1):140–232.
22. Dent E, Martin FC, Bergman H, Woo J, Romero-Ortuno R, Walston JD. Management of frailty: opportunities, challenges, and future directions. Lancet. 2019;394(10206): 1376–86.
23. Ofori-Asenso R, Chin KL, Mazidi M, Zomer E, Ilomaki J, Zullo AR, et al. Global incidence of frailty and prefrailty among community-dwelling older adults: a systematic review and meta-analysis. JAMA Netw Open. 2019;2(8):e198398-e.
24. Collard RM, Boter H, Schoevers RA, Oude Voshaar RC. Prevalence of frailty in community-dwelling older persons: a systematic review. J Am Geriatr Soc. 2012;60(8):1487–92.
25. Bisset ES, Howlett SE. The biology of frailty in humans and animals: understanding frailty and promoting translation. Aging Med. 2019;2(1):27–34.
26. Geller AM, Zenick H. Aging and the environment: a research framework. Environ Health Perspect. 2005;113(9):1257–62.
27. Kuh D. A life course approach to healthy aging, frailty, and capability. J Gerontol Ser A Biol Sci Med Sci. 2007;62(7):717–21.
28. Ferrucci L, Cavazzini C, Corsi A, Bartali B, Russo C, Lauretani F, et al. Biomarkers of frailty in older persons. J Endocrinol Invest. 2002;25(10 Suppl):10–5.
29. Taffett GE. Physiology of aging. In: Geriatric medicine. New York: Springer; 2003. p. 27–35.
30. Watson J. Frailty in older adults In: Michel J-P, Walston JD, editors. Oxford textbook of geriatric medicine. New York: Oxford University Press; 2018.
31. Inouye SK, Studenski S, Tinetti ME, Kuchel GA. Geriatric syndromes: clinical, research, and policy implications of a core geriatric concept. J Am Geriatr Soc. 2007;55(5):780–91.
32. Gobbens RJ, van Assen MA, Luijkx KG, Schols JM. Testing an integral conceptual model of frailty. J Adv Nurs. 2012;68(9):2047–60.
33. Solfrizzi V, Scafato E, Lozupone M, Seripa D, Schilardi A, Custodero C, et al. Biopsychosocial frailty and the risk of incident dementia: the Italian longitudinal study on aging. Alzheimers Dement. 2019;15(8):1019–28.
34. Gale CR, Westbury L, Cooper C. Social isolation and loneliness as risk factors for the progression of frailty: the English Longitudinal Study of Ageing. Age Ageing. 2018;47(3):392–7.
35. Maltby J, Hunt SA, Ohinata A, Palmer E, Conroy S. Frailty and social isolation: comparing the relationship between frailty and unidimensional and multifactorial models of social isolation. J Aging Health. 2020;32(10):1297–308.
36. Kojima G. Frailty as a predictor of nursing home placement among community-dwelling older adults: a systematic review and meta-analysis. J Geriatr Phys Ther. 2018;41(1):42–8.
37. Liu CJ, Latham NK. Progressive resistance strength training for improving physical function in older adults. Cochrane Database Syst Rev. 2009;2009(3):Cd002759.

38. Martone AM, Onder G, Vetrano DL, Ortolani E, Tosato M, Marzetti E, et al. Anorexia of aging: a modifiable risk factor for frailty. Nutrients. 2013;5(10):4126–33.
39. Gabrovec B, Veninšek G, Samaniego LL, Carriazo AM, Antoniadou E, Jelenc M. The role of nutrition in ageing: a narrative review from the perspective of the European joint action on frailty—advantage JA. Eur J Intern Med. 2018;56:26–32.
40. Welstead M, Jenkins ND, Russ T, Luciano M, Muniz-Terrera G. A systematic review of frailty trajectories: their shape and influencing factors. Gerontologist. 2020. https://doi.org/10.1093/geront/gnaa061.
41. Hale M, Shah S, Clegg A. Frailty, inequality and resilience. Clin Med. 2019;19(3):219.
42. Kelaiditi E, Cesari M, Canevelli M, Van Kan GA, Ousset P-J, Gillette-Guyonnet S, et al. Cognitive frailty: rational and definition from an (IANA/IAGG) international consensus group. J Nutr Health Aging. 2013;17(9):726–34.
43. Bunt S, Steverink N, Olthof J, van der Schans C, Hobbelen J. Social frailty in older adults: a scoping review. Eur J Ageing. 2017;14(3):323–34.
44. World Health Organization. WHO Commission on Social Determinants of Health: closing the gap in a generation: health equity through action on the social determinants of health: Commission on Social Determinants of Health final report. World Health Organization; 2008. Report No.: 9241563702.
45. Kirby M. The health of Canadians-The federal role: final report on the state of the health care system in Canada, volume six: recommendations for reform. Ottawa, Canada: Health Canada/Santé Canada; 2002.
46. Northwood M, Ploeg J, Markle-Reid M, Sherifali D. Integrative review of the social determinants of health in older adults with multimorbidity. J Adv Nurs. 2018;74(1):45–60.
47. McMunn A, Breeze E, Goodman A, Nazroo J, Oldfield Z. Social determinants of health in older age. Soc Determinant Health. 2006;2:267–98.
48. Woo J, Goggins W, Sham A, Ho S. Social determinants of frailty. Gerontology. 2005;51(6):402–8.
49. Smith BD, Smith GL, Hurria A, Hortobagyi GN, Buchholz TA. Future of cancer incidence in the United States: burdens upon an aging, changing nation. J Clin Oncol. 2009;27(17):2758–65.
50. Pilleron S, Sarfati D, Janssen-Heijnen M, Vignat J, Ferlay J, Bray F, et al. Global cancer incidence in older adults, 2012 and 2035: a population-based study. Int J Cancer. 2019;144(1):49–58.
51. Handforth C, Clegg A, Young C, Simpkins S, Seymour MT, Selby PJ, et al. The prevalence and outcomes of frailty in older cancer patients: a systematic review. Ann Oncol. 2015;26(6):1091–101.
52. Kirkhus L, Saltyte Benth J, Rostoft S, Gronberg BH, Hjermstad MJ, Selbaek G, et al. Geriatric assessment is superior to oncologists' clinical judgement in identifying frailty. Br J Cancer. 2017;117(4):470–7.
53. Muss HB, Berry DA, Cirrincione C, Budman DR, Henderson IC, Citron ML, et al. Toxicity of older and younger patients treated with adjuvant chemotherapy for node-positive breast cancer: the Cancer and Leukemia Group B Experience. J Clin Oncol. 2007;25(24):3699–704.
54. Soubeyran P, Bellera C, Goyard J, Heitz D, Curé H, Rousselot H, et al. Screening for vulnerability in older cancer patients: the ONCODAGE Prospective Multicenter Cohort Study. PLoS One. 2014;9(12):e115060.
55. Saliba D, Elliott M, Rubenstein LZ, Solomon DH, Young RT, Kamberg CJ, et al. The Vulnerable Elders Survey: a tool for identifying vulnerable older people in the community. J Am Geriatr Soc. 2001;49(12):1691–9.
56. Hamaker ME, Jonker JM, de Rooij SE, Vos AG, Smorenburg CH, van Munster BC. Frailty screening methods for predicting outcome of a comprehensive geriatric assessment in elderly patients with cancer: a systematic review. Lancet Oncol. 2012;13(10):e437–e44.

57. Mohile SG, Dale W, Somerfield MR, Hurria A. Practical assessment and management of vulnerabilities in older patients receiving chemotherapy: ASCO guideline for geriatric oncology summary. J Oncol Pract. 2018;14(7):442–6.
58. Podsiadlo D, Richardson S. The timed "Up & Go": a test of basic functional mobility for frail elderly persons. J Am Geriatr Soc. 1991;39(2):6.
59. Pondal M, del Ser T. Normative data and determinants for the timed "Up and Go" test in a population-based sample of elderly individuals without gait disturbances. J Geriatr Phys Ther. 2008;31(2):6.
60. DuMontier C, Sedrak MS, Soo WK, Kenis C, Williams GR, Haase K, et al. Arti Hurria and the progress in integrating the geriatric assessment into oncology: Young International Society of Geriatric Oncology review paper. J Geriatr Oncol. 2020;11(2):203–11.
61. Rubenstein LZ, Joseph T. Freeman award lecture: comprehensive geriatric assessment: from miracle to reality. J Gerontol A Biol Sci Med Sci. 2004;59(5):M473–M7.
62. Wildiers H, Heeren P, Puts M, Topinkova E, Janssen-Heijnen ML, Extermann M, et al. International Society of Geriatric Oncology consensus on geriatric assessment in older patients with cancer. J Clin Oncol. 2014;32(24):2595–603.
63. Kenis C, Bron D, Libert Y, Decoster L, Van Puyvelde K, Scalliet P, et al. Relevance of a systematic geriatric screening and assessment in older patients with cancer: results of a prospective multicentric study. Ann Oncol. 2013;24(5):1306–12.
64. Hamaker ME, Schiphorst AH, ten Bokkel HD, Schaar C, van Munster BC. The effect of a geriatric evaluation on treatment decisions for older cancer patients—a systematic review. Acta Oncol. 2014;53(3):289–96.
65. Chaibi P, Magne N, Breton S, Chebib A, Watson S, Duron JJ, et al. Influence of geriatric consultation with comprehensive geriatric assessment on final therapeutic decision in elderly cancer patients. Crit Rev Oncol Hematol. 2011;79(3):302–7.
66. Decoster L, Kenis C, Van Puyvelde K, Flamaing J, Conings G, De Greve J, et al. The influence of clinical assessment (including age) and geriatric assessment on treatment decisions in older patients with cancer. J Geriatr Oncol. 2013;4(3):235–41.
67. Caillet P, Canoui-Poitrine F, Vouriot J, Berle M, Reinald N, Krypciak S, et al. Comprehensive geriatric assessment in the decision-making process in elderly patients with cancer: ELCAPA study. J Clin Oncol. 2011;29(27):3636–42.
68. Farcet A, De Decker L, Pauly V, Rousseau F, Bergman H, Molines C, et al. Frailty markers and treatment decisions in patients seen in oncogeriatric clinics: results from the ASRO pilot study. PLoS One. 2016;11(2):e0149732.
69. Marenco D, Marinello R, Berruti A, Gaspari F, Stasi MF, Rosato R, et al. Multidimensional geriatric assessment in treatment decision in elderly cancer patients: 6-year experience in an outpatient geriatric oncology service. Crit Rev Oncol Hematol. 2008;68(2):157–64.
70. Giri S, Chakiba C, Shih Y-Y, Chan W-L, Krok-Schoen JL, Presley CJ, et al. Integration of geriatric assessment into routine oncologic care and advances in geriatric oncology: a young International Society of Geriatric Oncology Report of the 2020 American Society of Clinical Oncology (ASCO) annual meeting. J Geriatr Oncol. 2020;11(8):1324–8.
71. DuMontier C, Loh KP, Bain PA, Silliman RA, Hshieh T, Abel GA, et al. Defining undertreatment and overtreatment in older adults with cancer: a scoping literature review. J Clin Oncol. 2020. https://doi.org/10.1200/JCO.19.02809.
72. Bagegni NA, Peterson LL. Age-related disparities in older women with breast cancer. Adv Cancer Res. 2020;146:23–56.
73. Liu N, Molena D, Stem M, Blackford AL, Sewell DB, Lidor AO. Underutilization of treatment for regional gastric cancer among the elderly in the USA. J Gastrointest Surg. 2018;22(6):955–63.
74. Vyas AM, Aroke H, Kogut S. Guideline-concordant treatment among elderly women with HER2-positive metastatic breast cancer in the United States. J Natl Compr Canc Netw. 2020;18(4):405–13.

75. Baban CK, Devane L, Geraghty J. Change of paradigm in treating elderly with breast cancer: are we undertreating elderly patients? Ir J Med Sci. 2019;188(2):379–88.
76. Biskup E, Vetter M, Wedding U. Fighting diagnostic and therapeutic nihilism in the elderly with cancer. Ann Palliat Med. 2020;9(3):1324–32.
77. Derks MGM, Bastiaannet E, Kiderlen M, Hilling DE, Boelens PG, Walsh PM, et al. Variation in treatment and survival of older patients with non-metastatic breast cancer in five European countries: a population-based cohort study from the EURECCA Breast Cancer Group. Br J Cancer. 2018;119(1):121–9.
78. Dragun AE, Huang B, Tucker TC, Spanos WJ. Disparities in the application of adjuvant radiotherapy after breast-conserving surgery for early stage breast cancer: impact on overall survival. Cancer. 2011;117(12):2590–8.
79. Enewold L, Harlan LC, Tucker T, McKenzie S. Pancreatic cancer in the USA: persistence of undertreatment and poor outcome. J Gastrointest Cancer. 2015;46(1):9–20.
80. Fakhri B, Fiala MA, Tuchman SA, Wildes TM. Undertreatment of older patients with newly diagnosed multiple myeloma in the era of novel therapies. Clin Lymphoma Myeloma Leuk. 2018;18(3):219–24.
81. Kuper-Hommel MJ, van de Schans SA, Vreugdenhil G, van Krieken JH, Coebergh JW. Undertreatment of patients with localized extranodal compared with nodal diffuse large B-cell lymphoma. Leuk Lymphoma. 2013;54(8):1698–705.
82. Lunardi P, Ploussard G, Grosclaude P, Roumiguie M, Soulie M, Beauval JB, et al. Current impact of age and comorbidity assessment on prostate cancer treatment choice and over/undertreatment risk. World J Urol. 2017;35(4):587–93.
83. Lycken M, Drevin L, Garmo H, Larsson A, Andren O, Holmberg L, et al. Adherence to guidelines for androgen deprivation therapy after radical prostatectomy: Swedish population-based study. Scand J Urol. 2020:1–7.
84. Malik MK, Tartter PI, Belfer R. Undertreated breast cancer in the elderly. J Cancer Epidemiol. 2013;2013:893104.
85. Narayan V, Jiang S, Warlick CA. Early stage cancer in older adults: prostate-avoiding overtreatment and undertreatment. Cancer J. 2017;23(4):238–41.
86. Rocco N, Rispoli C, Pagano G, Ascione S, Compagna R, Danzi M, et al. Undertreatment of breast cancer in the elderly. BMC Surg. 2013;13 Suppl 2:S26.
87. Shumway DA, Hamstra DA. Ageism in the undertreatment of high-risk prostate cancer: how long will clinical practice patterns resist the weight of evidence? J Clin Oncol. 2015;33(7):676–8.
88. Ugurlu MU, Gulluoglu BM. Impact of older age on local treatment decisions. Breast. 2019;48(Suppl 1):S57–s61.
89. Walter J, Tufman A, Holle R, Schwarzkopf L. "Age matters"-German claims data indicate disparities in lung cancer care between elderly and young patients. PLoS One. 2019;14(6):e0217434.
90. Walter V, Boakye D, Weberpals J, Jansen L, Haefeli WE, Martens UM, et al. Decreasing use of chemotherapy in older patients with stage III colon cancer irrespective of comorbidities. J Natl Compr Canc Netw. 2019;17(9):1089–99.
91. Weiss A, Noorbakhsh A, Tokin C, Chang D, Blair SL. Hormone receptor-negative breast cancer: undertreatment of patients over 80. Ann Surg Oncol. 2013;20(10):3274–8.
92. Williams CP, Kenzik KM, Azuero A, Williams GR, Pisu M, Halilova KI, et al. Impact of guideline-discordant treatment on cost and health care utilization in older adults with early-stage breast cancer. Oncologist. 2019;24(1):31–7.
93. Kanapuru B, Simonsick EM, Ershler WB. Is cancer incidence decreased in the frail elderly? Evidence from a prospective cohort study. J Geriatr Oncol. 2013;4(1):19–25.
94. Vaeth PA, Satariano WA, Ragland DR. Limiting comorbid conditions and breast cancer stage at diagnosis. J Gerontol A Biol Sci Med Sci. 2000;55(10):M593–600.
95. Raval AD, Madhavan S, Mattes MD, Sambamoorthi U. Association between types of chronic conditions and cancer stage at diagnosis among elderly medicare beneficiaries with prostate cancer. Popul Health Manag. 2016;19(6):445–53.

96. Sewitch MJ, Fournier C, Dawes M, Yaffe M, Snell L, Roper M, et al. Do physician recommendations for colorectal cancer screening differ by patient age? Can J Gastroenterol. 2007;21(7):435–8.
97. Fisher DA, Galanko J, Dudley TK, Shaheen NJ. Impact of comorbidity on colorectal cancer screening in the veterans healthcare system. Clin Gastroenterol Hepatol. 2007;5(8):991–6.
98. Garman KS, Jeffreys A, Coffman C, Fisher DA. Colorectal cancer screening, comorbidity, and follow-up in elderly patients. Am J Med Sci. 2006;332(4):159–63.
99. Legg JS, Clement DG, White KR. Are women with self-reported cognitive limitations at risk for underutilization of mammography? J Health Care Poor Underserved. 2004;15(4):688–702.
100. Gorin SS, Heck JE, Albert S, Hershman D. Treatment for breast cancer in patients with Alzheimer's disease. J Am Geriatr Soc. 2005;53(11):1897–904.
101. Gupta SK, Lamont EB. Patterns of presentation, diagnosis, and treatment in older patients with colon cancer and comorbid dementia. J Am Geriatr Soc. 2004;52(10):1681–7.
102. Kwok AC, Hu YY, Dodgion CM, Jiang W, Ting GV, Taback N, et al. Invasive procedures in the elderly after stage IV cancer diagnosis. J Surg Res. 2015;193(2):754–63.
103. Hu YY, Kwok AC, Jiang W, Taback N, Loggers ET, Ting GV, et al. High-cost imaging in elderly patients with stage IV cancer. J Natl Cancer Inst. 2012;104(15):1164–72.
104. Makary MA, Segev DL, Pronovost PJ, Syin D, Bandeen-Roche K, Patel P, et al. Frailty as a predictor of surgical outcomes in older patients. J Am Coll Surg. 2010;210(6):901–8.
105. Revenig LM, Canter DJ, Taylor MD, Tai C, Sweeney JF, Sarmiento JM, et al. Too frail for surgery? Initial results of a large multidisciplinary prospective study examining preoperative variables predictive of poor surgical outcomes. J Am Coll Surg. 2013;217(4):665–70. e1
106. Arya S, Kim SI, Duwayri Y, Brewster LP, Veeraswamy R, Salam A, et al. Frailty increases the risk of 30-day mortality, morbidity, and failure to rescue after elective abdominal aortic aneurysm repair independent of age and comorbidities. J Vasc Surg. 2015;61(2):324–31.
107. Kristjansson SR, Nesbakken A, Jordhoy MS, Skovlund E, Audisio RA, Johannessen HO, et al. Comprehensive geriatric assessment can predict complications in elderly patients after elective surgery for colorectal cancer: a prospective observational cohort study. Crit Rev Oncol Hematol. 2010;76(3):208–17.
108. Clough-Gorr KM, Stuck AE, Thwin SS, Silliman RA. Older breast cancer survivors: geriatric assessment domains are associated with poor tolerance of treatment adverse effects and predict mortality over 7 years of follow-up. J Clin Oncol. 2010;28(3):380–6.
109. Clough-Gorr KM, Thwin SS, Stuck AE, Silliman RA. Examining five- and ten-year survival in older women with breast cancer using cancer-specific geriatric assessment. Eur J Cancer. 2012;48(6):805–12.
110. PACE Participants, Audisio RA, Pope D, Ramesh HS, Gennari R, van Leeuwen BL, et al. Shall we operate? Preoperative assessment in elderly cancer patients (PACE) can help. A SIOG surgical task force prospective study. Crit Rev Oncol Hematol. 2008;65(2):156–63.
111. Adams P, Ghanem T, Stachler R, Hall F, Velanovich V, Rubinfeld I. Frailty as a predictor of morbidity and mortality in inpatient head and neck surgery. JAMA Otolaryngol Head Neck Surg. 2013;139(8):783–9.
112. Lascano D, Pak JS, Kates M, Finkelstein JB, Silva M, Hagen E, et al. Validation of a frailty index in patients undergoing curative surgery for urologic malignancy and comparison with other risk stratification tools. Urol Oncol. 2015;33(10):426 e1–12.
113. Abt NB, Richmon JD, Koch WM, Eisele DW, Agrawal N. Assessment of the predictive value of the modified frailty index for Clavien-Dindo grade IV critical care complications in major head and neck cancer operations. JAMA Otolaryngol Head Neck Surg. 2016;142(7):658–64.
114. Chappidi MR, Kates M, Patel HD, Tosoian JJ, Kaye DR, Sopko NA, et al. Frailty as a marker of adverse outcomes in patients with bladder cancer undergoing radical cystectomy. Urol Oncol. 2016;34(6):256 e1–6.
115. Mogal H, Vermilion SA, Dodson R, Hsu FC, Howerton R, Shen P, et al. Modified frailty index predicts morbidity and mortality after pancreaticoduodenectomy. Ann Surg Oncol. 2017;24(6):1714–21.

116. Buettner S, Wagner D, Kim Y, Margonis GA, Makary MA, Wilson A, et al. Inclusion of sarcopenia outperforms the modified frailty index in predicting 1-year mortality among 1,326 patients undergoing gastrointestinal surgery for a malignant indication. J Am Coll Surg. 2016;222(4):397–407. e2
117. Montroni I, Rostoft S, Spinelli A, Van Leeuwen BL, Ercolani G, Saur NM, et al. GOSAFE—Geriatric Oncology Surgical Assessment and Functional rEcovery after surgery: early analysis on 977 patients. J Geriatr Oncol. 2020;11(2):244–55.
118. Huisman MG, Audisio RA, Ugolini G, Montroni I, Vigano A, Spiliotis J, et al. Screening for predictors of adverse outcome in onco-geriatric surgical patients: a multicenter prospective cohort study. Eur J Surg Oncol. 2015;41(7):844–51.
119. Shahrokni A, Tin A, Alexander K, Sarraf S, Afonso A, Filippova O, et al. Development and evaluation of a new frailty index for older surgical patients with cancer. JAMA Netw Open. 2019;2(5):e193545.
120. Hamaker ME, Seynaeve C, Wymenga AN, van Tinteren H, Nortier JW, Maartense E, et al. Baseline comprehensive geriatric assessment is associated with toxicity and survival in elderly metastatic breast cancer patients receiving single-agent chemotherapy: results from the OMEGA study of the Dutch breast cancer trialists' group. Breast. 2014;23(1):81–7.
121. Hurria A, Togawa K, Mohile SG, Owusu C, Klepin HD, Gross CP, et al. Predicting chemotherapy toxicity in older adults with cancer: a prospective multicenter study. J Clin Oncol. 2011;29(25):3457–65.
122. Hurria A, Mohile S, Gajra A, Klepin H, Muss H, Chapman A, et al. Validation of a prediction tool for chemotherapy toxicity in older adults with cancer. J Clin Oncol. 2016;34(20):2366–71.
123. Extermann M, Boler I, Reich RR, Lyman GH, Brown RH, DeFelice J, et al. Predicting the risk of chemotherapy toxicity in older patients: the Chemotherapy Risk Assessment Scale for High-Age Patients (CRASH) score. Cancer. 2012;118(13):3377–86.
124. Soubeyran P, Fonck M, Blanc-Bisson C, Blanc JF, Ceccaldi J, Mertens C, et al. Predictors of early death risk in older patients treated with first-line chemotherapy for cancer. J Clin Oncol. 2012;30(15):1829–34.
125. Corre R, Greillier L, Le Caer H, Audigier-Valette C, Baize N, Berard H, et al. Use of a comprehensive geriatric assessment for the management of elderly patients with advanced non-small-cell lung cancer: the phase III randomized ESOGIA-GFPC-GECP 08-02 study. J Clin Oncol. 2016;34(13):1476–83.
126. Seymour MT, Thompson LC, Wasan HS, Middleton G, Brewster AE, Shepherd SF, et al. Chemotherapy options in elderly and frail patients with metastatic colorectal cancer (MRC FOCUS2): an open-label, randomised factorial trial. Lancet. 2011;377(9779):1749–59.
127. Hall PS, Swinson D, Waters JS, Wadsley J, Falk S, Roy R, et al. Optimizing chemotherapy for frail and elderly patients (pts) with advanced gastroesophageal cancer (aGOAC): the GO2 phase III trial. J Clin Oncol. 2019;37(15_suppl):4006. American Society of Clinical Oncology.
128. Roa W, Kepka L, Kumar N, Sinaika V, Matiello J, Lomidze D, et al. International atomic energy agency randomized phase III study of radiation therapy in elderly and/or frail patients with newly diagnosed glioblastoma multiforme. J Clin Oncol. 2015;33(35):4145–50.
129. Ghosh S, Baker S, de Castro DG, Kepka L, Kumar N, Sinaika V, et al. Improved cost-effectiveness of short-course radiotherapy in elderly and/or frail patients with glioblastoma. Radiother Oncol. 2018;127(1):114–20.
130. Shinde A, Li R, Kim J, Salgia R, Hurria A, Amini A. Stereotactic body radiation therapy (SBRT) for early-stage lung cancer in the elderly. Semin Oncol. 2018;45(4):210–9.
131. Kreinbrink P, Blumenfeld P, Tolekidis G, Sen N, Sher D, Marwaha G. Lung stereotactic body radiation therapy (SBRT) for early-stage non-small cell lung cancer in the very elderly (>/=80years old): extremely safe and effective. J Geriatr Oncol. 2017;8(5):351–5.
132. Franco I, Chen YH, Chipidza F, Agrawal V, Romano J, Baldini E, et al. Use of frailty to predict survival in elderly patients with early stage non-small-cell lung cancer treated with stereotactic body radiation therapy. J Geriatr Oncol. 2018;9(2):130–7.

133. Szumacher E, Sattar S, Neve M, Do K, Ayala AP, Gray M, et al. Use of comprehensive geriatric assessment and geriatric screening for older adults in the radiation oncology setting: a systematic review. Clin Oncol (R Coll Radiol). 2018;30(9):578–88.
134. Middelburg JG, Mast ME, de Kroon M, Jobsen JJ, Rozema T, Maas H, et al. Timed get up and go test and geriatric 8 scores and the association with (chemo-)radiation therapy noncompliance and acute toxicity in elderly cancer patients. Int J Radiat Oncol Biol Phys. 2017;98(4):843–9.
135. Spyropoulou D, Pallis AG, Leotsinidis M, Kardamakis D. Completion of radiotherapy is associated with the Vulnerable Elders Survey-13 score in elderly patients with cancer. J Geriatr Oncol. 2014;5(1):20–5.
136. Keenan LG, O'Brien M, Ryan T, Dunne M, McArdle O. Assessment of older patients with cancer: Edmonton Frail Scale (EFS) as a predictor of adverse outcomes in older patients undergoing radiotherapy. J Geriatr Oncol. 2017;8(3):206–10.
137. VanderWalde NA, Deal AM, Comitz E, Stravers L, Muss H, Reeve BB, et al. Geriatric assessment as a predictor of tolerance, quality of life, and outcomes in older patients with head and neck cancers and lung cancers receiving radiation therapy. Int J Radiat Oncol Biol Phys. 2017;98(4):850–7.
138. Pilotto A, Custodero C, Maggi S, Polidori MC, Veronese N, Ferrucci L. A multidimensional approach to frailty in older people. Ageing Res Rev. 2020;60:101047.
139. Nightingale G, Haase KR, Sattar S, Burhenn P, Puts M, Stolz-Baskett P, et al. Integrating Nurses and Allied Health Professionals in the care of older patients with cancer: a report from the SIOG Nursing and Allied Health Interest Group. J Geriatr Oncol. 2020;11(2):187–90.
140. Sharma M, Loh KP, Nightingale G, Mohile SG, Holmes HM. Polypharmacy and potentially inappropriate medication use in geriatric oncology. J Geriatr Oncol. 2016;7(5):346–53.
141. Soto-Perez-de-Celis E, de Glas NA, Hsu T, Kanesvaran R, Steer C, Navarrete-Reyes AP, et al. Global geriatric oncology: achievements and challenges. J Geriatr Oncol. 2017;8(5):374–86.
142. Hoogendijk EO, Afilalo J, Ensrud KE, Kowal P, Onder G, Fried LP. Frailty: implications for clinical practice and public health. Lancet. 2019;394(10206):1365–75.
143. Puts MTE, Toubasi S, Andrew MK, Ashe MC, Ploeg J, Atkinson E, et al. Interventions to prevent or reduce the level of frailty in community-dwelling older adults: a scoping review of the literature and international policies. Age Ageing. 2017;46(3):383–92.
144. Gielen E, Beckwée D, Delaere A, De Breucker S, Vandewoude M, Bautmans I. Nutritional interventions to improve muscle mass, muscle strength, and physical performance in older people: an umbrella review of systematic reviews and meta-analyses. Nutr Rev. 2021;79(2):121–47.
145. Lim SER, Cox NJ, Tan QY, Ibrahim K, Roberts HC. Volunteer-led physical activity interventions to improve health outcomes for community-dwelling older people: a systematic review. Aging Clin Exp Res. 2021;33(4):843–53.
146. Travers J, Romero-Ortuno R, Bailey J, Cooney MT. Delaying and reversing frailty: a systematic review of primary care interventions. Br J Gen Pract. 2019;69(678):e61–e9.
147. Negm AM, Kennedy CC, Thabane L, Veroniki AA, Adachi JD, Richardson J, et al. Management of frailty: a systematic review and network meta-analysis of randomized controlled trials. J Am Med Dir Assoc. 2019;20(10):1190–8.
148. Guida JL, Agurs-Collins T, Ahles TA, Campisi J, Dale W, Demark-Wahnefried W, et al. Strategies to prevent or remediate cancer and treatment-related aging. J Natl Cancer Inst. 2021;113(2):112–22.
149. Shahrokni A, Alexander K. What will perioperative geriatric assessment for older cancer patients look like in 2025? Advantages and limitations of new technologies in geriatric assessment. Eur J Surg Oncol. 2020;46(3):305–9.
150. Shahrokni A, Loh KP, Wood WA. Toward modernization of geriatric oncology by digital health technologies. Am Soc Clin Oncol Educ Book. 2020;40:1–7.
151. Shahrokni A, Maggiore RJ, Ghassemzadeh H. New technologies in geriatric oncology care. J Geriatr Oncol. 2018;9(6):687–9.

152. Shahrokni A, Tin A, Downey RJ, Strong V, Mahmoudzadeh S, Boparai MK, et al. Electronic rapid fitness assessment: a novel tool for preoperative evaluation of the geriatric oncology patient. J Natl Compr Canc Netw. 2017;15(2):172–9.
153. Shahrokni A, Vishnevsky BM, Jang B, Sarraf S, Alexander K, Kim SJ, et al. Geriatric assessment, not ASA physical status, is associated with 6-month postoperative survival in patients with cancer aged >/=75 years. J Natl Compr Canc Netw. 2019;17(6):687–94.
154. Loh KP, Ramsdale E, Culakova E, Mendler JH, Liesveld JL, O'Dwyer KM, et al. Novel mHealth app to deliver geriatric assessment-driven interventions for older adults with cancer: pilot feasibility and usability study. JMIR Cancer. 2018;4(2):e10296.
155. Haase KR, Drury A, Puts M. Supportive care and eHealth: a narrative review of technologies, interventions, and opportunities for optimizing care in patients with cancer. Clin J Oncol Nurs. 2020;24(3):32–41.
156. Soto-Perez-De-Celis E, Kim H, Rojo-Castillo MP, Sun CL, Chavarri-Guerra Y, Navarrete-Reyes AP, et al. A pilot study of an accelerometer-equipped smartphone to monitor older adults with cancer receiving chemotherapy in Mexico. J Geriatr Oncol. 2018;9(2):145–51.
157. Lam K, Lu AD, Shi Y, Covinsky KE. Assessing telemedicine unreadiness among older adults in the united states during the COVID-19 pandemic. JAMA Intern Med. 2020;180(10):1389–91.
158. Hsu T, Loscalzo M, Ramani R, Forman S, Popplewell L, Clark K, et al. Are disagreements in caregiver and patient assessment of patient health associated with increased caregiver burden in caregivers of older adults with cancer? Oncologist. 2017;22(11):1383–91.
159. Hsu T, Nathwani N, Loscalzo M, Chung V, Chao J, Karanes C, et al. Understanding caregiver quality of life in caregivers of hospitalized older adults with cancer. J Am Geriatr Soc. 2019;67(5):978–86.
160. Kehoe LA, Xu H, Duberstein P, Loh KP, Culakova E, Canin B, et al. Quality of life of caregivers of older patients with advanced cancer. J Am Geriatr Soc. 2019;67(5):969–77.
161. Warmoth K, Lang IA, Phoenix C, Abraham C, Andrew MK, Hubbard RE, et al. 'Thinking you're old and frail': a qualitative study of frailty in older adults. Ageing Soc. 2016;36:1483–500.
162. Schoenborn NL, Van Pilsum Rasmussen SE, Xue QL, Walston JD, McAdams-Demarco MA, Segev DL, et al. Older adults' perceptions and informational needs regarding frailty. BMC Geriatr. 2018;18(1):46.
163. Maggiore RJ, Dale W, Hurria A, Klepin HD, Chapman A, Dotan E, et al. Hematology-oncology fellows' training in geriatrics and geriatric oncology: findings from an American Society of Clinical Oncology-Sponsored National Survey. J Oncol Pract. 2017;13(11):e900–e8.
164. Maggiore RJ, Gorawara-Bhat R, Levine SK, Dale W. Perceptions, attitudes, and experiences of hematology/oncology fellows toward incorporating geriatrics in their training. J Geriatr Oncol. 2014;5(1):106–15.
165. Leifer R, Bristow B, Puts M, Alibhai S, Cao X, Millar BA, et al. National survey among radiation oncology residents related to their needs in geriatric oncology. J Cancer Educ. 2019;34(1):9–13.
166. Rittberg R, Sutherland J, Huynh E, Green S, Wiens A, Stirling M, et al. Assessing the learning needs of the multidisciplinary team on geriatric oncology and frailty. J Geriatr Oncol. 2019;10(5):829–31.
167. Hsu T. Educational initiatives in geriatric oncology—who, why, and how? J Geriatr Oncol. 2016;7(5):390–6.
168. Goldberg JI, Burhenn PS, Ginex PK. Nursing education: review of assessment, clinical care, and implications for practice regarding older adult patients with cancer. Clin J Oncol Nurs. 2018;22(6):19–25.
169. Roller-Wirnsberger R, Lindner S, Liew A, O'Caoimh R, Koula ML, Moody D, et al. European Collaborative and Interprofessional Capability Framework for Prevention and Management of Frailty—a consensus process supported by the Joint Action for Frailty Prevention (ADVANTAGE) and the European Geriatric Medicine Society (EuGMS). Aging Clin Exp Res. 2020;32(4):561–70.

170. Windhaber T, Koula ML, Ntzani E, Velivasi A, Rizos E, Doumas MT, et al. Educational strategies to train health care professionals across the education continuum on the process of frailty prevention and frailty management: a systematic review. Aging Clin Exp Res. 2018;30(12):1409–15.
171. Ganz PA, Balogh E. Delivering high-quality cancer care: charting a new course for a system in crisis. Washington, DC: Inst Med Natl Acad; 2013.
172. Scher KS, Hurria A. Under-representation of older adults in cancer registration trials: known problem, little progress. J Clin Oncol. 2012;30(17):2036–8.
173. DuMontier C, Loh KP, Bain PA, Silliman RA, Hshieh T, Abel GA, et al. Defining undertreatment and overtreatment in older adults with cancer: a scoping literature review. J Clin Oncol. 2020;38(22):2558–69.
174. Outlaw D, Williams GR. Is the lack of evidence in older adults with cancer compromising safety? Expert Opin Drug Saf. 2020:1–3.
175. Levit LA, Singh H, Klepin HD, Hurria A. Expanding the evidence base in geriatric oncology: action items from an FDA-ASCO workshop. J Natl Cancer Inst. 2018;110(11):1163–70.
176. Singh H, Hurria A, Klepin HD. Progress through collaboration: an ASCO and U.S. Food and Drug Administration workshop to improve the evidence base for treating older adults with cancer. Am Soc Clin Oncol Educ Book. 2018;38:392–9.
177. Wildiers H, Mauer M, Pallis A, Hurria A, Mohile SG, Luciani A, et al. End points and trial design in geriatric oncology research: a Joint European Organisation for Research and Treatment of Cancer—Alliance for Clinical Trials in Oncology—International Society of Geriatric Oncology position article. J Clin Oncol. 2013;31(29):3711–8.
178. Pallis AG, Ring A, Fortpied C, Penninckx B, Van Nes MC, Wedding U, et al. EORTC workshop on clinical trial methodology in older individuals with a diagnosis of solid tumors. Ann Oncol. 2011;22(8):1922–6.
179. Paillaud E, Soubeyran P, Caillet P, Cudennec T, Brain E, Terret C, et al. Multidisciplinary development of the Geriatric Core Dataset for clinical research in older patients with cancer: a French initiative with international survey. Eur J Cancer. 2018;103:61–8.
180. Soo W-K, King M, Pope A, Parente P, Darzins P, Davis ID. Integrated geriatric assessment and treatment (INTEGERATE) in older people with cancer planned for systemic anticancer therapy. J Clin Oncol. 2020;38:12011a. American Society of Clinical Oncology.
181. Li D, Sun C-L, Kim H, Chung V, Koczywas M, Fakih M, et al. Geriatric assessment-driven intervention (GAIN) on chemotherapy toxicity in older adults with cancer: a randomized controlled trial. J Clin Oncol. 2020;38(15_suppl):12010. American Society of Clinical Oncology.
182. Mohile SG, Mohamed MR, Culakova E, Xu H, Loh KP, Magnuson A, et al. A geriatric assessment (GA) intervention to reduce treatment toxicity in older patients with advanced cancer: a University of Rochester Cancer Center NCI community oncology research program cluster randomized clinical trial (CRCT). J Clin Oncol. 2020; 38(15_suppl):12009. American Society of Clinical Oncology.
183. Ashing KT, Soto-Perez-de-Celis E. Disparities within a disparity: global health and health equity in geriatric oncology. J Geriatr Oncol. 2020;11(2):200–2.
184. Mehrabi F, Béland F. Effects of social isolation, loneliness and frailty on health outcomes and their possible mediators and moderators in community-dwelling older adults: a scoping review. Arch Gerontol Geriatr. 2020;90:104119.

Chapter 2
Global Action and Policies in Older Adults with Cancer and Frailty

Najia Musolino, Nicolò Matteo Luca Battisti, and Martine Extermann

Introduction

Traditionally, researchers and the United Nations define an older person as an individual who is over 60–65 years of age [1]. However this definition of an older person has been changing with the ageing population. The World Health Organization (WHO) reports that the pace of population ageing is much faster than in the past with older people over 60 years estimated at two billion by 2020 [2]. A key implication of this is the increase in the incidence of patients with cancer alongside multimorbidities and geriatric syndromes. In this context, frailty is a key consideration that may substantially influence the management of cancer and increase the risk of complications and adverse outcomes of anti-cancer treatments. Frailty has become increasingly recognized as an important component of the call for global action by the International Society of Geriatric Oncology (SIOG) for the care of older adults with cancer. It clearly has an impact on the treatment of cancer in older adults and needs to be addressed and integrated in policies for cancer in ageing.

It is well established and documented that routine clinical evaluations are not adequate for older cancer patients, particularly with frailty, as these do not address

N. Musolino (✉)
International Soceity of Geriatric Oncology, Châtelaine, Geneva, Switzerland
e-mail: najia.musolino@siog.org

N. M. L. Battisti
Breast Unit, Department of Medicine, The Royal Marsden NHS Foundation Trust & Breast Cancer Division, The Institute of Cancer Research, London, UK
e-mail: Nicolo.Battisti@rmh.nhs.uk

M. Extermann
International Society of Geriatric Oncology (SIOG), Châtelaine, Switzerland

Senior Adult Oncology Program, University of Florida, Gainesville, FL, USA
e-mail: martine.extermann@moffitt.org

F. Gomes (ed.), *Frailty in Older Adults with Cancer*,
https://doi.org/10.1007/978-3-030-89162-6_2

the complexity of this population [3, 4]. Frailty is a clinical state of vulnerability with an increased risk of adverse health outcomes, including functional decline and mortality. Although a number of frailty measures have been included in many population-based studies of frailty, this is estimated to affect 42% of older adults with cancer [5]. Older individuals with frailty are less prone to tolerate and adapt to stressors such as acute illness, surgical or medical interventions or trauma compared with younger or non-frail older adults [6]. These factors increase the risk of complications, falls, institutionalization, disability and mortality in this population [7].

Ageist stereotypes assume older people to be dependent and a burden to society [8]. Moreover, solutions for the adequate identification and prioritization of the health needs of older individuals are often not made explicit. It is, therefore, essential to ensure that older cancer patients with frailty are not disadvantaged. Acknowledging these challenges, this chapter illustrates the key guiding principles for the provision of patient-centric care for older cancer patients with frailty, with the intention to advocate for the strenghtening of education and training regarding cancer in ageing. This chapter also invites readers to join the efforts led by SIOG within a global platform of multidisciplinary collaborations at all levels of the health sector for the benefit of older cancer patients, particularly those with frailty.

International Society of Geriatric Oncology (SIOG)

When in the year 2000, the founding members of SIOG hosted the first Annual Conference in New York, geriatric oncology was a completely new field and only a few researchers had highlighted the need to address the unique needs of older patients with cancer [9]. At that time, these founding members were the first group of oncologists to initiate a collaborative international society to rethink practices for an ageing population increasingly burdened by cancer [10–12]. Geriatric oncology has since been the focus of SIOG for the past two decades, enhancing good clinical practices for better outcomes for older cancer patients through education and training. The SIOG experts further set out to establish an interdisciplinary process to determine the medical, psychosocial and functional capabilities in older adults with the aim of optimizing their overall health and well-being. These actions have been instrumental to improve outcomes also for the most vulnerable segment of the older cancer patient population: those individuals living with both cancer and frailty.

For more than two decades after the creation of SIOG, the resolve of its members to advocate for the needs of the older cancer patients has never been stronger. In 2020, as the society celebrated 20 years of active engagement at all levels for cancer in ageing, it acknowledged the contributions of the past presidents of the society who forged and helped establishing extensive research whilst also providing health care professionals the education and training to treat older cancer patients, particularly those more complex also living with frailty.

As a result, SIOG has gained a central role in advocating for the value of multidisciplinary collaborations to drive research, training and influencing treatment decisions for older patients with cancer. Geriatric oncology is, therefore, no longer considered a niche field with only a few dedicated research clusters. For example, geriatric assessments are acknowledged as standard of care for the management of older adults with cancer [13, 14].

Moreover, a number of dedicated clinical groups and programmes across the world are leading the way and these include the Senior Adult Oncology Program of the Moffitt Cancer Center in the United States of America (USA) (https://moffitt.org/), the Canadian Network on Ageing and Cancer (https://www.cancerandaging.ca/) and the newly developed country-specific SIOG United Kingdom group (https://www.siog.org/content/siog-country-group-uk) amongst many others [15–17]. Additionally, collaborative research groups such as the Cancer and Aging Research Group (CARG) (https://www.mycarg.org/) and the European Organisation for Research and Treatment of Cancer (EORTC) in Elderly Task Force (https://www.eortc.org/research_field/cancer-in-elderly/) are conducting a number of clinical trials that are expanding the evidence base for the management of cancer in older individuals [18, 19].

Comprehensive geriatric assessment (CGA) is now widely accepted as a holistic, diagnostic process in routine oncology practice, with clear therapeutic implications for the care for older patients with cancer, aimed particularly at those with significant vulnerabilities and frailty. The integration of patient-centric information on overall health and fitness gathered from the implementation of geriatric assessments in routine clinical practice along with disease-related factors is, therefore, a key aspect of precision medicine allowing to maximize benefits and minimize complications of anti-cancer treatments in this population. Recently, at the American Society of Clinical Oncology (ASCO) 2020 Annual meeting, four randomized clinical trials reported to have demonstrated a significant impact of integrated oncogeriatric care on key endpoints including risk of severe toxicities, hospitalizations and quality of life for older patients receiving systemic anti-cancer treatments or undergoing surgery, along with increased completion of advanced directives in this population. These clinical trials represent a major breakthrough for the field of geriatric oncology [20–23] and provide a compelling rationale for the implementation of SIOG's Top Priorities for the Global Development of Geriatric Oncology [24].

The success of SIOG's activities is reflected in meeting the specific needs and interests of patients, following the highest scientific and ethical standards of care and treatment—all aligned with national contexts and priorities including recommendations for cancer and ageing proposed by the member states of the WHO [25–27]. On Nov 14th 2020, at the opening of the Global Policy Dialogue on Cancer in Ageing Populations at the United Nations in Geneva, SIOG was congratulated by the WHO for bringing together stakeholders to address the challenges related to the issues of cancer in the ageing. In recognition of the importance of community input on the topic of cancer in ageing, the WHO has also acknowledged the multisectoral dialogues of the educational events led by the SIOG COVID-19 Working Group, during this tragic pandemic where patient perspectives have mattered the most [28].

Building on the experience of its network, SIOG has been encouraged by the WHO's Ageing and Life Course Programme to pursue its collaboration plans on capacity building of health and social care workers in primary care in order to respond to diverse needs of older adults with cancer. And finally, in the context of the COVID-19 pandemic, WHO has acknowledged SIOG in the care and support for cancer patients, to ensure that the care for the most vulnerable patients continue in spite of the challenges related to the pandemic [29]. These achievements are significant steps for SIOG in supporting countries to improve the training and education of health care professionals treating older and frail cancer patients.

The Global Ageing Population

The global population is ageing, which is also the driver of frailty and increasing cancer incidence [1, 7]. Globally, there are geographic and economic factors that affect the number of older people living with and surviving cancer, but data show a common trend for large proportions of people with cancer being older [30]. In fact, in high-income countries, half of cancers occur in patients aged 70 and older. In booming nations, the ageing trend is particularly striking. By 2050, the world population will comprise approximately 2 billion people aged over 65 years, of which the majority will live in low- and middle-income countries [1, 31, 32]. According to the United Nations Population Fund (UNFPA) and non-governmental organizations such as the International Federation on Ageing (IFA) and Help Age International, the support for older people particularly those with frailty is a growing priority [33–35]. The WHO's Guidelines on Integrated Care for Older People (ICOPE) proposing evidence-based recommendations for health care professionals is an important achievement for all countries placing the needs and preferences of older adults at the centre to coordinate care [36]. The Global Strategy and Action Plan on Ageing and Health in accordance with the World Health Assembly Resolution (67/13) is another successful global consultative initiative building on existing activities to address the priority areas for action in Ageing and Health [2]. Furthermore, The European Collaborative and Interprofessional Capability Framework for Prevention and Management of Frailty recently produced a consensus process supported by the Joint Action for Frailty Prevention (ADVANTAGE) and the European Geriatric Medicine Society (EuGMS) [37]. In light of the issues of cancer in the ageing, this important framework regarding frailty may pave the way for application to oncology in the near future. Moreover, the Political Declaration of the Madrid International Plan of Action on Ageing of the Second World Assembly in 2002 offered a remarkable framework for handling this rising challenge of the twenty-first century [38]. Ever since, renewed international commitment and increased investments in initiatives to improve health services for the treatment and care of older cancer patients have resulted in positive outcomes in many countries [39].

Indeed, these global efforts complement concrete actions taken by some countries that have recognized the challenges and opportunities of the ongoing demographic changes. For example, in France, the National Cancer Institute has supported the creation of geriatric oncology units throughout the country since 2006 [40]. These national cancer policy efforts in France are also paired by the work of a national scientific society, the *Societé Francophone d'Onco-Gériatrie* (SoFOG) [41] and the *Dialogue intergroupe pour la personnalisation de la prise en charge en oncogériatrie* (DIALOG) [42]. Another example, in the Philippines, includes the 2019 National Integrated Cancer Control Act (Republic Act No. 11215) and the Universal Health Care Act (RA No. 11223), proposing a blueprint of the health sector plans and commitments for the medium-term in response to Filipinos living longer thus facing age-old illnesses such as cancer. The Philippine Cancer Society is extensively working towards putting this law into action by building capacity on knowledge and expertise in geriatric oncology. In Latin America and the Caribbean, the Pan American Health Organization/WHO representation for Trinidad and Tobago, Aruba, Curacao, Sint Maarten, Bonaire, Saba and Sint Eustatius is part of the Madrid International Plan of Action on Ageing and the San José Charter on the Rights of Older Persons. In this region, a recent review by the United Nations Publication reported on the equitable access to comprehensive services and the creation of formal graduation and post-graduation degree programmes in geriatric and gerontologic services as well as policies to address non-communicable diseases [43]. Furthermore, the high-level meeting on Universal Health Coverage held in September 2019 at the United Nations General Assembly in New York offered an important opportunity for the global community to ensure better serving the health needs of older adults with frailty [44]. And more recently, in August 2020, the Member States of the 73rd World Health Assembly endorsed the Decade of Healthy Ageing up to 2030 and called countries for 10 years of concerted action to foster healthy ageing [45].

However, in many parts of the world, older patients with cancer and frailty still continue to face many barriers to accessing quality health care [46]. Due to the side effects of treatments in this age group, they are still under-represented in clinical trials for cancer treatment. In fact, research tailored for older and frail patients is particularly scarce. Geriatric medicine, for example, may be offered as a speciality in many parts of the world, but in other parts, it is overlooked in traditionally structured health services as well as in epidemiological research [2]. One major issue is also the mismatch of available services to the health needs of this population. For example, in some low- and middle-income countries there may be an oncologist in a district hospital but the hospital may not have an oncology service, or in other cases, a hospital may have a doctor but not an oncologist or a geriatrician, providing only some cancer services to older patients. In other settings there is a lack of referral health system which is crucial for cancer services.

Whilst education and formal training are offered in some countries, this is more fragmented in many regions of the world. Cancer professionals in many regions do not get formal training in geriatrics [47, 48]. Designing education so as to improve the training of oncologists, surgeons, geriatricians as well as nursing and allied health professionals for older cancer adults with frailty is, therefore, particularly relevant for shaping patient-centred treatment and care. Training and education in geriatric oncology is key to accelerating advances in precision medicine, tailored to the specific clinical needs, preferences and available resources. It will also play an important role in empowering cancer professionals for the better assessment of patient's biological age, frailty and functional status, geriatric syndromes, unmet needs and potential for pre-habilitation and rehabilitation.

And last but not least, there is a critical gap in medical education and medical curricula on gender dimensions in clinical research. Women and men suffer from different co-morbidities. There are important differences between men and women, both in terms of biology (e.g. susceptibility and risk, pattern and profile of cancer, survival, co-morbidities) and socioeconomic factors (e.g. experience of health care, access to and affordability of health services, health insurance and social protection, etc.) that merit in-depth assessment [49].

With the shift in demographics worldwide and its related complexities, management of older cancer patients clearly requires multidisciplinary and holistic care. Despite developments in the health sector, there are still wide disparities, reported not only within continents but also within countries, rural and urban populations, ethnicities and in some parts of the world even between genders. It is known that the implementation of geriatric oncology in itself is different in various parts of the world [24]. Furthermore, cancer care, research and clinical trials for the older patients with cancer as a whole, but particularly for those with frailty, remain a low priority. Therefore, for nearly two decades now, equity in care and quality of life for older patients with cancer has remained one of the main priorities for SIOG.

Adequate resources need to be deployed to address such knowledge gaps, design appropriate solutions and support their implementation to ensure equitable treatment and care. Governments, health agencies, civil societies, international and non-governmental organizations, academic institutions and the medical community at large have acknowledged this most pressing issue. In many parts of the world, much still needs to be done for better treatment outcomes and quality of life of older cancer patients.

Mapping the Current Needs

Very early on, SIOG's approach focused on collecting evidence for the need to train health professionals in geriatric oncology as well as the existing resources and national frameworks in place, for better coordination of efforts. Between 2009 and 2010, SIOG launched a global consultation to identify ten priorities for progress and development in geriatric oncology. Guided by the feedback from the multiple SIOG National Representatives, these priorities were detailed in a monograph in 2011 [50, 51]. The report formulated the outcomes of the consultation and was structured to give an overview of the scope of those ten top priorities in Geriatric Oncology, as well as the potential translation of these priorities into tangible recommendations for uptake by health institutions. For a decade, the impacts of

SIOG's 10 Priorities continued to play a significant role in reaching a wide network of medical professionals and in improving patient care. Ever since the publication of The SIOG 10 Priorities in 2011, significant scientific, clinical and educational progress has been made worldwide. Furthermore, the priorities of the international health agenda have been reviewed and adopted by countries within the framework of the post-2015 Sustainable Development Goals of the United Nations [52].

In light of these international developments, during the year 2018 and using an international, multidisciplinary and multisectoral consultative process, a review of this report was undertaken for a new edition of the work through a wider global consultation. SIOG sets up a working committee and gathered new input through regional consultations. The data and recommendations were used to define trends likely to impact the direction of healthcare in the next two decades for older cancer patients. In 2020, the outputs of these consultations found expression in The SIOG Priorities Initiative. In comparison to the publication of 2011, the new edition of the recommendations focused on four priority domains, namely Education, Clinical Practice, Research and Collaborations/Partnerships (Fig. 2.1). This is a composite of key messages aligned with the priorities of the health goals for the member states of the WHO. Moreover, it is addressed to policy makers, health professionals and to the wider international community for contextualized, improved health systems and strengthened human resources for cancer in the ageing [24]. This knowledge aims at supporting and building on the existing geriatric oncology initiatives in different regions, as well as in addressing appropriate training of community health care workers to enable quality care across the health systems [6]. It is also intended to stimulate and guide action, for larger and better trained health care professionals treating older cancer patients.

Supporting Country Actions and Plans

Education and Training

Efficient treatment of older patients with cancer requires well-trained geriatric oncologists. Geriatric oncology is rapidly expected to come to the foreground of oncology practice, and therefore an increased international cooperation guided by a code of ethics that is sensitive to national and regional issues for healthy ageing is important for implementing an impactful change in this area. Building on the success of the educational initiatives of SIOG, such as the SIOG Advanced Courses in Geriatric Oncology, the society is working with country partners to develop cost-effective delivery of tailored courses and workshops in geriatric oncology. This is aligned with SIOG's strategic activity plan for the preparation of the next generation of clinicians, nurses and allied health workers to address the combined challenges of cancer, ageing and frailty.

Education

- Priority 1: integrate geriatric oncology into medical, nursing, and allied health professionals schools and residency training programmes, and promote involvement of trainees in research
- Priority 2: provide educational material and organise formal educational activities focused on geriatric oncology for practising health-care professionals
- Priority 3: educate the general public about the relevance of providing age-appropriate care for older adults with cancer

Clinical practice

- Priority 4: develop and implement models to provide optimal care for older adults with cancer
- Priority 5: develop guidelines for the optimal treatment of older adults with cancer
- Priority 6: establish centres of excellence in geriatric oncology for delivering clinical care, conducting clinical and translational research, and providing educational opportunities

Research

- Priority 7: improve the relevance of clinical trials to older adults with cancer
- Priority 8: evaluate the benefits of geriatric assessment-allocated treatments and geriatric comnanagement in improving treatment outcomes for older adults with cancer
- Priority 9: use personalised medicine technologies to enhance cancer understanding and management of older adults

Collaborations and partnerships

- Priority 10: develop and strengthen links between SIOG and the geriatric oncology workforce, international specialised agencies, global and regional professional organisations, policy makers, and patient advocacy groups
- Priority 11: promote the inclusion of specific provisions for delivering high-quality evidence-based care for older adults in national cancer control plans
- Priority 12: create global funding mechanisms aimed at fostering professional development of the geriatric oncology workforce and promoting research on the interface of cancer and ageing

Fig. 2.1 SIOG Top Priorities for the global advancement of care for older adults with cancer (reprinted from [24] with permission from Elsevier)

Guidelines and Recommendations

With the intention of capturing the full complexity of capacity building in cancer in the ageing, SIOG provides evidence-based guidelines and clinical recommendations for the best standards of cancer care for older patients. The key recommendations of SIOG guidelines have benefited a large community of health care professionals treating older cancer patients. These clinical guidelines have in turn been developed into training and advanced courses in geriatric oncology. In the context of developing countries or low resource settings, where there is chronic under investment in human resources for health, SIOG ensures to provide affordable access to these trainings at the community level through capacity strengthening of primary health care workers and caregivers [53].

Tools for Primary Care Providers

The integration of effective geriatric assessment tools in clinical practice is a key component of a tailored approach in care and treatment, which can consequently have benefits in terms of health and economy. Based on this, SIOG supports both individuals and health institutions in providing technical assistance for the uptake and implementation of CGA tools in the routine care of older cancer patients for well-trained primary care specialists, including the relevant expertise across the spectrum of healthcare professionals [24].

International Network

Combined with targeted advocacy on the strengthening of human resources for health planning, resource mobilization and implementation across different institutions, SIOG's mission has been designed to capitalize on global synergies. For this, SIOG has created an international network for promoting and participating in collective initiatives ensuring that multidisciplinary and international cooperation is enhanced at all levels without redundancy or duplication of efforts. SIOG boasts a wide international membership of health professionals (nurses, general practitioners, clinical oncologists, geriatricians, surgeons, radiation oncologists, anesthesiologists and allied health professionals) including health economists, patient advocates and experts in sex and gender dimension of health programmes. It also offers a representation for the highly demanded health workforce, i.e. nurses, community health workers and informal caregivers, thereby ensuring that there is a level of awareness and recognition for nurses and allied health professionals who are at the core of older cancer patient care, especially in low- and middle-income countries and other low resource settings.

Global Partnerships and Convening

In undertaking an approach grounded in advocacy, SIOG has established international collaborations for transferring skills to institutions in order to ensure tailored training where and when needed. SIOG's advocacy programme under the SIOG Top Priorities Initiative has succeeded in garnering private and public partner support and commitments for improving the quality of care of older cancer patients [51].

In 2021, countries are channelling efforts towards the achievement of the goals of Universal Health Coverage through the health priority areas of the Sustainable Development Goals in the regions of the Member States of the WHO [44]. SIOG has initiated several areas of partnership dedicated to leading continuous and diversified actions for stronger education, clinical practice and research in geriatric oncology. SIOG and its partners continue to identify strategies to support local efforts in countries developing such linkages and guidelines. In line with the policy objectives of the United Nations Sustainable Development Goals, SIOG partnerships in advocacy aims to enhance education investments for international and innovative approaches for improved health care of older cancer patients, increase regional commitments to coordinate training, as well as support and further enforce local policies.

Recognizing the importance of health services responsive to older cancer patients' needs, SIOG has already facilitated and contributed to a conducive environment for the progress of the principles of geriatric oncology through education in many institutions [54]. The SIOG network will continue in this direction, by generating evidence to influence health policy, working closely with existing stakeholders including governments, and civil society organizations—to advocate for improved investments and funding in human resources for health, thereby ensuring quality healthcare in many more regions of the globe for older cancer patients and specifically those with frailty.

Conclusion

Older adults with cancer are heterogeneous and in the context of the challenges, these have an increased risk of adverse outcomes. Those with frailty are a key target for action to improve clinical practice, foster education, expand the evidence base and inform cancer policy at national and international level. The recognized need for enhancing clinical practice, research and education for the older population with cancer, particularly those with frailty, represents a new shift in thinking, with the objective being to provide all countries the resources to monitor, prioritize and maintain, locally relevant, clinical practices for the ageing population. Since the first publication of the SIOG Ten Priorities Initiative, SIOG has used the recommendations from countries as building blocks for assessing and mapping of what capacity is currently in place and what needs further strengthening and development [50].

Geriatric oncology must become mainstream for all health care workers in oncology. In other words, it should be integrated within oncology training in order that all health professionals in this area are appropriately trained. This can be achieved by improving the training and education in this field, and by facilitating the implementation of the principles of general geriatrics for the wider oncology community. Since the challenges for optimally treating older cancer patients are similar for all oncology disciplines (medical oncology, surgery, radiotherapy, nursing and allied health), we believe that international and transdisciplinary collaborations need to continue to stay on the forefront.

It is not possible to propose a 'one size fits all' system for all countries and regions. SIOG's ambition is, therefore, to catalyze collaborations with stakeholders and policy makers towards integrating research, awareness and education on frailty for older cancer patients. In doing so, it aims to amplify the impacts of such actions as it continues in this much needed endeavour aligning its mission to the WHO's 10 Priorities for a decade of healthy ageing and Universal Health Coverage 2030 [55].

Acknowledgements The authors acknowledge Dr Meena Nathan Cherian MBBS, MD (Anaesthesia), for her advice in the 2019 global consultation process of the SIOG Top Priorities Initiative and for reviewing this manuscript.

References

1. World Population Ageing 2019. 2020.
2. Ageing and health. 2018. [05/02/2018 25/03/2021]. Available from: https://www.who.int/news-room/fact-sheets/detail/ageing-and-health.
3. Wildiers H, et al. International Society of Geriatric Oncology consensus on geriatric assessment in older patients with cancer. J Clin Oncol. 2014;32(24):2595–603.
4. Dzau VJ, et al. Enabling healthful aging for all—the national academy of medicine grand challenge in healthy longevity. N Engl J Med. 2019;381(18):1699–701.
5. Handforth C, et al. The prevalence and outcomes of frailty in older cancer patients: a systematic review. Ann Oncol. 2015;26(6):1091–101.
6. Coker JF, et al. Frailty: an in-depth qualitative study exploring the views of community care staff. BMC Geriatr. 2019;19(1):47.
7. Clegg A, et al. Frailty in elderly people. Lancet. 2013;381(9868):752–62.
8. Mikton C, et al. Ageism: a social determinant of health that has come of age. Lancet. 2021;397(10282):1333–4.
9. Balducci L, et al. Issues in treatment. Cancer. 1991;68(S11):2527–9.
10. Monfardini S, et al. Cancer in older adults: the history of geriatric oncology, 1980–2015. 2020. [25/03/2021]. Available from: https://ascopost.com/issues/october-10-2020/the-history-of-geriatric-oncology-1980-2015/.
11. Monfardini S, et al. Cancer in older adults: the history of geriatric oncology, part 2: 1990–2020. 2020 [06/04/2021]. Available from: https://ascopost.com/issues/october-25-2020/cancer-in-older-adults-the-history-of-geriatric-oncology-part-2-1990-2020/.
12. Monfardini S, et al. Cancer in older adults: the history of geriatric oncology, part 3. Geriatric oncology nurses in the care of elderly patients with cancer. 2020 [06/04/2021]. Available from: https://ascopost.com/issues/november-10-2020/cancer-in-older-adults-the-history-of-geriatric-oncology-part-3/.
13. Lichtman SM. Polypharmacy: geriatric oncology evaluation should become mainstream. J Clin Oncol. 2015;33(13):1422–3.
14. Mohile SG, et al. Practical assessment and management of vulnerabilities in older patients receiving chemotherapy: ASCO guideline for geriatric oncology. J Clin Oncol. 2018;36(22):2326–47.
15. Moffitt Cancer Center: Senior Adult Oncology Program. [25/03/2021]. Available from: https://moffitt.org/for-healthcare-professionals/clinical-programs-and-services/senior-adult-oncology-program/.

16. SIOG Country Group - UK. [25/03/2021]. Available from: https://siog.org/content/siog-country-group-uk.
17. Canadian Network Ion Aging and Cancer. [25/03/2021]. Available from: https://www.cancerandaging.ca/.
18. Cancer and Aging Research Group. 2020 [25/03/2021]. Available from: https://www.mycarg.org/.
19. European Organisation for Research and Treatment of Cancer—Cancer in the Elderly Task Force. [25/03/2021]. Available from: https://www.eortc.org/research_field/cancer-in-elderly/.
20. Li D, et al. Geriatric assessment-driven intervention (GAIN) on chemotherapy toxicity in older adults with cancer: a randomized controlled trial. J Clin Oncol. 2020;38(15_suppl):12010–12010.
21. Mohile SG, et al. A geriatric assessment (GA) intervention to reduce treatment toxicity in older patients with advanced cancer: a University of Rochester Cancer Center NCI community oncology research program cluster randomized clinical trial (CRCT). J Clin Oncol. 2020;38(15_suppl):12009.
22. Qian CL, et al. Randomized trial of a perioperative geriatric intervention for older adults with cancer. J Clin Oncol. 2020;38(15_suppl):12012.
23. Soo W-K, et al. Integrated geriatric assessment and treatment (INTEGERATE) in older people with cancer planned for systemic anticancer therapy. J Clin Oncol. 2020;38(15_suppl):12011.
24. Extermann M. Top priorities for the global advancement of cancer care in older adults: an update of the International Society of Geriatric Oncology (SIOG) Priorities Initiative. Lancet Oncol. 2021;22(1):e29–36.
25. Political declaration approved by the high-level meeting on universal health coverage on September 2019. United Nations General Assembly. 2019.
26. Integrated care for older people: realigning primary health care to respond to population ageing, in Technical series on primary health care. World Health Organization. 2018.
27. Health workforce for ageing populations. World Health Organization. 2016.
28. Battisti NML, et al. Adapting care for older cancer patients during the COVID-19 pandemic: recommendations from the International Society of Geriatric Oncology (SIOG) COVID-19 Working Group. J Geriatr Oncol. 2020;11(8):1190–8.
29. Pre-SIOG 2020 Policy Webinar. 2020 [25/03/2021]. Available from: https://www.siog.org/content/siog-2020-annual-meeting-online#presiog-2020-policy-webinar.
30. Silver economy: seizing opportunities. 2018 [26/09/2020]. Available from: https://www.credit-suisse.com/nl/en/private-banking/learn-more-about-market-trends/supertrends-silver-economy.html.
31. Gibson C, Jung K. Population Division. Washington, DC: US Census Bureau; 2006.
32. Kinsella K, Phillips D. Global aging: the challenge of success. Popul Bull. 2005;60
33. Meeting the needs of older people through solidarity, empowerment and data. [26/09/2020]. Available from: https://www.unfpa.org/news/meeting-needs-older-people-through-solidarity-empowerment-and-data.
34. Addressing Inequalities. [26/09/2020]. Available from: https://ifa.ngo/positions/addressing-inequalities/.
35. HelpAge International. [26/09/2020]. Available from: https://www.helpage.org/.
36. WHO guidelines on integrated care for older people (ICOPE). World Health Organization. 2017.
37. Roller-Wirnsberger R, et al. European Collaborative and Interprofessional Capability Framework for Prevention and Management of Frailty—a consensus process supported by the Joint Action for Frailty Prevention (ADVANTAGE) and the European Geriatric Medicine Society (EuGMS). Aging Clin Exp Res. 2020;32(4):561–70.
38. Report of the second world assembly on ageing. In Second world assembly on ageing 2002. Madrid: United Nations.
39. Lichtman SM. Geriatric assessment: what are you waiting for? 2020 [26/09/2020]. Available from: https://ascopost.com/issues/july-10-2020/geriatric-assessment-what-are-you-waiting-for/.

40. Hauchecorne M, et al. Perspectives on cancer care in older patients in France. Ecancermedicalscience. 2020;14:1103.
41. Société Francophone d'Onco-Gériatrie. [25/03/2021]. Available from: https://sofog.org/.
42. DIALOG - GERICO-UCOG. [25/03/2021]. Available from: https://dialog-oncogeriatrie.fr/.
43. Caribbean synthesis report on the Madrid International Plan of Action on Ageing and the San José Charter on the Rights of Older Persons in Latin America and the Caribbean. Santiago: United Nations; 2018.
44. Universal Health Coverage. [25/03/2021]. Available from: https://www.who.int/health-topics/universal-health-coverage#tab=tab_1.
45. 73rd World Health Assembly Decisions. 2020 [25/03/2021]. Available from: https://www.who.int/news-room/feature-stories/detail/73rd-world-health-assembly-decisions.
46. Soto-Perez-de-Celis E, et al. Global geriatric oncology: achievements and challenges. J Geriatr Oncol. 2017;8(5):374–86.
47. Hsu T. Educational initiatives in geriatric oncology—who, why, and how? J Geriatr Oncol. 2016;7(5):390–6.
48. Puts M, et al. Position statement on oncology and cancer nursing care for older adults with cancer and their caregivers of the International Society of Geriatric Oncology Nursing and Allied Health Interest Group, the Canadian Association of Nurses in Oncology Oncology & Aging Special Interest Group, and the European Oncology Nursing Society. J Geriatr Oncol. 2021;12(7):1000–4.
49. Heidari S, et al. Sex and gender equity in research: rationale for the SAGER guidelines and recommended use. Res Integrity Peer Rev. 2016;1(1):2.
50. Extermann M, et al. Main priorities for the development of geriatric oncology: a worldwide expert perspective. J Geriatr Oncol. 2011;2(4):270–3.
51. SIOG Top Priorities Initiative. [25/03/2021]. Available from: https://www.siog.org/content/siog-top-priorities-initiative.
52. Post-2015 Development Agenda. [25/03/2021]. Available from: https://www.unodc.org/unodc/en/about-unodc/post-2015-development-agenda.html.
53. Red Cross joins partnership to boost healthcare for elderly cancer patients. 2019 [26/09/2020]. Available from: https://redcross.org.ph/2019/04/10/red-cross-joins-partnership-to-boost-healthcare-for-elderly-cancer-patients/.
54. SIOG Advanced Course in GO. [25/03/2021]. Available from: https://www.siog.org/content/siog-advanced-course-go.
55. 10 Priorities towards a decade of healthy ageing. World Health Organization.

Chapter 3
Frailty Screening and Comprehensive Geriatric Assessment

Lore Decoster, Gabor Liposits, and Clark Dumontier

Introduction

Treatment decisions for older patients with cancer are often challenging because of the heterogeneity of the population and a lack of data from randomized clinical trials [1, 2]. As a consequence, a personalized care plan should be proposed, not based on chronological age but rather on a person's functional age and frailty [2].

Frailty is a state of reduced physiologic reserve characterized by an increased vulnerability to external stressors [3]. A consensus conference in 2013 defined frailty as a "medical syndrome with multiple causes and contributors that is characterized by diminished strength, endurance and reduced physiologic function that increases an individual's vulnerability for developing increased dependency and/or death" [3]. Frailty is strongly linked to adverse outcomes, such as, including mortality, nursing home admission, and falls [4, 5].

L. Decoster (✉)
Department of Medical Oncology, Vrije Universiteit Brussel (VUB), Universitair Ziekenhuis Brussel (UZ Brussel), Brussels, Belgium
e-mail: lore.decoster@uzbrussel.be

G. Liposits
Department of Oncology, Odense University Hospital, Odense, Denmark

Department of Clinical Research, University of Southern Denmark, Odense, Denmark

Academy of Geriatric Cancer Research (AgeCare), Odense, Denmark
e-mail: Gabor.Istvan.Liposits@rsyd.dk

C. Dumontier
Division of Aging, Brigham and Women's Hospital and Harvard Medical School, Boston, MA, USA

Marcus Institute for Aging Research, Boston, MA, USA
e-mail: cdumontier@partners.org

F. Gomes (ed.), *Frailty in Older Adults with Cancer*,
https://doi.org/10.1007/978-3-030-89162-6_3

Both cancer and its treatment are significant stressors that challenge the physiological reserve of an older patient. Many tools and assessments have been developed to distinguish those older patients who are fit, vulnerable, or frail. A Comprehensive Geriatric Assessment (CGA) is considered the gold standard to identify geriatric syndromes and frailty [6, 7]. However, CGA may be time consuming and not always feasible in oncology clinics without a geriatric service. For this reason, both in geriatric medicine and in oncology, short screening tools have been developed to identify patients at high risk of frailty that would benefit the most from a CGA [8, 9]. The commonly used performance scores in oncology such as Eastern Cooperative Oncology Group (ECOG) performance status (PS) or Karnofsky PS as well as the standard clinical approach (including past medical history and physical examination) are often insufficient to adequately identify frailty [10]. This chapter will review and discuss the value of frailty/geriatric screening for older cancer patients and the different tools available, as well as review the principles and challenges of implementing a CGA.

Frailty Screening Tools in Older Patients with Cancer

Many frailty/geriatric screening tools have been developed and reported in the literature, including in the subpopulation of older patients with cancer [8, 9, 11]. Such screening tools should be simple and take only a few minutes while demonstrating a high sensitivity and negative predictive value for identification of frailty/vulnerabilities from CGA. A task force of the International Society of Geriatric Oncology (SIOG) systematically reviewed all evidence on the use of screening tools in older patients with cancer with regard to sensitivity and specificity as well as their predictive value for different outcomes [8]. Here we describe some commonly used screening tools (Table 3.1).

Fried's Frailty Phenotype

The Fried's frailty phenotype considers frailty by its physical characteristics or "phenotype" based on the presence of unintentional weight loss (4.5 kg or more in the last year), weakness by low grip strength using a handheld dynamometer, slow gait speed, self-reported exhaustion, and low physical activity [12]. Patients with a score of three or more are considered frail, while those with a score of 1–2 are pre-frail. In the general population this tool is associated with risk of falls, disability, and fracture as well as death [13]. It has also been associated with survival in older patients with colorectal cancer and older patients with multiple myeloma [14, 15]. A limitation of this tool is the inclusion of measurements not routinely used for patient assessment, such as grip strength. It also does not include psychosocial components of frailty or the presence of comorbidities.

Table 3.1 Summary of screening tools [8, 11]

Screening tool	Origin	Age group for whom it was developed	Validation in cancer patients	Number of items	Cutoff for abnormal	Sensitivity in geriatric oncology (%)	Specificity in geriatric oncology (%)
Fried's frailty phenotype	Geriatrics	≥65	Yes	5	≥3/5	37–87	49–86%
Frailty Index Based on Deficit Accumulation (DA-FI)	Geriatrics	≥65	Yes	≥30	–	NR	NR
Rockwood CFS	Geriatrics	≥65	No	–	–	–	–
SOF	Geriatrics	≥65	Yes	3	>1	89	81
VES-13	Geriatrics	≥65	Yes	13	≥3/13	20–88	62–100
GFI	Geriatrics	≥65	Yes	15	≥4/15	39–76	73–87
G8	Geriatric Oncology	≥70	Yes	8	≤14/17	45–97	3–100
SAOP-2	Geriatric Oncology	≥65	Yes	15	≥1	100	40

DA-FI, Deficit accumulation-Frailty Index; CFS, Clinical Frailty Scale; SOF, Study of Osteoporotic Fractures Index; VES-13, Vulnerable Elders Survey-13; GFI, Groningen Frailty indicator; G8, Geriatric 8; SAOP-2, Senior Adult Oncology Profram-2 screening; NR, not reported

Frailty Index Based on Deficit Accumulation (DA-FI)

The DA-FI was first proposed by Rockwood and Mitniski, and it grades frailty as the accumulation of 30 or more age-related indicators of health covering different CGA domains, including comorbidities, symptoms, diseases, disabilities, or any deficiency in health [16]. These parameters are combined into a single index, thereby "quantifying" the frailty. The index is scored cumulatively such that the higher the number of health deficits, the higher the frailty score [17]. Comprehensive guidelines for creating a DA-FI have been provided by Searle et al. [17]. The variables can be used to calculate a Frailty Index (FI) score, which is a simple calculation of the presence or absence of each variable as a proportion of the total. Several studies have found that DA-FI is highly predictive of adverse clinical events, including in patients with cancer [18, 19]. However, in-person DA-FIs can be time consuming to calculate. Since the DA-FI does not require the same deficits as the original index, electronic DA-FIs have been constructed and validated in order to measure frailty more rapidly from readily available data in administrative claims and electronic health records (EHRs) [20]. An example is the electronic DA-FI currently being used by the United Kingdom's National Health Service to assist general practitioners with identification of older patients with frailty in primary care [21]. Embedded in the EHR, the NHS electronic FI is made up of 36 health deficits measured from around 2000 clinical codes. This electronic FI automatically screens patients age ≥65 years old, identifying those estimated to be severely frail (around 3%) and moderately frail (around 12%). Older patients who screen positive on the electronic FI are recommended to undergo an in-person frailty assessment, using validated tools such as the Rockwood Clinical Frailty Scale.

Rockwood Clinical Frailty Scale (CFS)

The CFS was originally developed by Rockwood and colleagues for the Canadian Study of Health and Aging as a tool to summarize the results of a CGA performed by an experienced clinician [22]. It has since evolved into a "judgement-based" frailty assessment tool used by multiple specialties to broadly classify frailty using information derived from a clinical encounter [23]. The clinician assigns a score of 1 through 9 (originally 1 through 7) based on increasing limitations on the activities of daily living. These limitations can be driven by symptoms related to comorbidities or geriatric syndromes such as cognitive impairment. The discrete levels of frailty as defined by the CFS have been shown to stratify survival in multiple studies, confirming their predictive validity [24]. Given the inherent subjectivity in a clinician-reported tool, a classification tree was recently developed to improve the validity and reliability of CFS scoring [25]. This tool was developed primarily for a community-dwelling population and was designed to reflect the patients' health status/function 2 weeks before, in order to understand their baseline status prior to an acute event (e.g., fall or infection), which may have caused an acute deterioration.

Study of Osteoporotic Fractures Index (SOF)

The SOF frailty index is a short 3-item tool based on the presence or absence of: weight loss (>5% in the last year), exhaustion, and low mobility based on the capability to perform a chair rise five times [13]. Patients presenting with one of these items are considered to be in a "pre-frailty" status and patients with more than one item are considered frail. The SOF has also been shown to be an independent predictor of adverse outcomes in the community-dwelling population [13].

Vulnerable Elders Survey-13 (VES-13)

The VES-13 is a 13-item self-administered screening tool, developed to identify older patients at increased risk of health deterioration in the community [26]. A score of three or more identifies individuals as frail [26]. In older persons in the community, an abnormal VES-13 was associated with functional decline, survival, and health outcomes [27]. In older patients with cancer, VES-13 was predictive for the occurrence of severe chemotherapy toxicity and survival [28] but not for post-operative morbidity and mortality [29]. This is one of the most frequently studied tools in older patients with cancer [8, 9]. Limitations of VES-13 are that self-completion may often be troublesome [30] and that patients older than 85 years are already at the cut off value solely because of age.

The Groningen Frailty Indicator (GFI)

The GFI is a tool composed of 15 dichotomous self-reported items, comprising: physical factors (independence in shopping, walking, dressing, toileting physical fitness, vision, hearing, weight loss, and polypharmacy), a cognitive component (memory issues), social factors (emptiness, missing others, feeling abandoned), and psychological components (feeling downhearted or sad, feeling nervous or anxious) [31]. A score of four or more indicates frailty. In community-dwelling older adults, an abnormal GFI correlated more strongly with decline in self-management abilities than chronological age [32]. In older patients with cancer treated with chemotherapy, the GFI was correlated with toxicity and survival [33, 34].

Geriatric 8 (G8)

The G8 is an 8-item screening tool developed specifically for older patients with cancer [35]. It includes nutritional items such as loss of appetite, weight loss and body mass index, mobility, neuropsychological problems such as dementia and depression, polypharmacy, self-assessed health status, and age. A score of 14 or less out of 17 is considered abnormal. In older patients with cancer the G8 is associated with functional decline, chemotherapy-related toxicity and survival [28, 36]. Together with the VES-13, it is one of the most studied and widely used tools in older patients with cancer [8, 9]. In a direct comparison with the VES-13, the G8 was more sensitive at identifying vulnerabilities in two studies, yet less specific [8].

Senior Adult Oncology Program (SAOP)-2 Screening

The SAOP2 screening tool was developed for older patients with cancer and consists of 11 items with respect to functional status, psychological status, nutritional status, and self-evaluated quality of life and overall health [37]. In a direct comparison with the G8, the SAOP2 had a better sensitivity for identifying vulnerabilities on CGA than the G8 ($p < 0.032$), with higher performance in breast cancer and in patients aged 70–80 years [38].

Selecting a Screening Tool

Many different screening tools to identify vulnerabilities in older patients with cancer are available for clinicians and researchers. The majority have demonstrated acceptable sensitivity and predictive value to identify vulnerabilities on CGA in the geriatric oncology setting [8, 9], however none of them are perfect and subsequently these are unable to replace a CGA completely. In a busy clinical practice, the use of a screening tool is recommended by SIOG and the American Society of Clinical Oncology (ASCO) to identify patients in need of further evaluation by CGA [8, 39]. In this case, the choice of screening tool should be based on (1) the feasibility and intention of implementing it into clinical practice, (2) the specific clinical or research needs while also considering the limitations of available data, and (3) local experience [40]. The G8 and VES-13 currently have the most evidence to support their use in geriatric oncology. The G8 is more sensitive and will, therefore, identify more patients who may benefit from CGA where the VES-13 is more specific, therefore the latter may be an option in case of limited resources for CGA. Although an abnormal screening tool should ideally be followed by CGA, the screening tools on itself may also give information on survival, toxicity, and risk of functional decline [8].

Principles of a Comprehensive Geriatric Assessment (CGA)

Definition and Domains of CGA

A CGA is a multidimensional evaluation of domains necessary for older adult health and well-being [41]. This domain-based approach stands in contrast to the disease-based approach that is traditionally applied in medicine. Instead of focusing on individual diagnoses such as heart disease or cancer, the CGA views multiple diagnoses in the context of an older individual's entire medical history. The CGA additionally examines beyond one's medical history to assess physical health (including mobility, senses, and nutrition), psychological health (including cognition and mood), social well-being, and functional status. Taken together, these five domains constitute the core of a geriatric assessment (Fig. 3.1) [42, 43].

Individually, each domain of the CGA carries vital, distinct information regarding an older adult's health status. The medical domain consists of ensuring that each comorbidity is optimized and there are no unnecessary or interacting medications (minimizing inappropriate polypharmacy). The physical domain entails assessing for motor and sensory impairments that may limit an older individual's ability to mobilize throughout their home and their community. The psychological domain requires investigating the status of one's executive functioning, visuospatial ability, memory, and mood—all humanistic properties that emerge from the structural neuroanatomy of the brain. Social well-being and support encompass an older

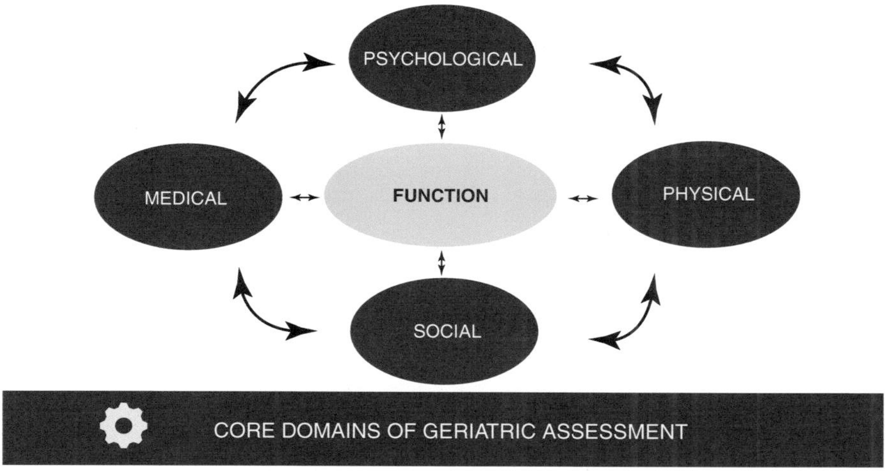

Fig. 3.1 Core geriatric assessment (GA) domains and their interdependency

individual's connection to others, either family, friends, or hired caregivers. Lastly, the functional domain consists of determining an older adult's ability to complete basic (e.g., transferring), instrumental (e.g., financial management), and advanced activities of daily living (e.g., occupation and hobbies). Validated screening and assessment tools for each of these domains are listed in both the previously highlighted SIOG and ASCO guidelines [39, 44].

Collectively, the domains of the CGA are interdependent. Older adults with cognitive impairment can continue to thrive in their community as long as they have a strong social support network. However, if socially isolated, they will be at high risk for institutionalization. An older patient with multiple chronic conditions can avoid physical frailty by remaining physically active. However, if one condition compromises their mobility, the decline of activity may result in a progression into a frail status.

Indeed, an older adult's functional status is dependent on the integration of the other geriatric domains. With an increasing number of deficits within and across domains correlating with an increasing risk of functional dependency. For this reason, functional status is a powerful predictor of outcomes as well as an outcome in itself. Many older adults value preservation of functional status just as much, if not more, than survival benefit [45, 46]. Another distinction between the CGA and disease-based approaches—particularly traditional oncology assessments of performance status (e.g., ECOG)—is its emphasis on function as primary endpoint in contrast to disease response rates or surrogate endpoints of survival. This prioritization of function as an outcome aligns with older adult values in preserving independence and quality of life [45, 46].

A natural conclusion that extends from the interdependency of CGA domains is that the more domains that are assessed, the more comprehensive the evaluation and the greater the ability to detect and manage age-related vulnerabilities. Similarly, having an interdisciplinary team, rather than a single provider, may help provide more efficient and effective implementation of interventions aimed at reversing these vulnerabilities. In this context, some leaders in the geriatric oncology field have advocated for a strict use of the term CGA to be reserved for evaluations that are interdisciplinary (vs. individual), led by a geriatrician, cover all core domains of the geriatric assessment (vs. only a few), and include interventions with longitudinal follow-up (vs. baseline assessment only) [47]. Although ideal, this degree of thoroughness may not be widely feasible, based on the limited resources and time constraints of oncology practices. Nonetheless, if an older patient screens positive on one of the previously described screening tools, a CGA should be performed to identify the drivers and interacting domains contributing to the patient's frailty. The exact number of domains assessed, and tools used to assess them, should be determined by local clinical resources and experience.

Challenges of CGA

CGA is often difficult to systematically implement for all older patients in oncology with different barriers frequently reported [48, 49]. Two frequently cited challenges are scarce resources, regarding time and work force. Indeed, performing a CGA requires time, often approximately 60 min, as well as trained staff who may not always be available. Geriatricians in particular are a scarce resource in many countries. In the United States, only 5% of community oncology practices have access to a geriatrician to provide consultation or co-management within the oncology clinic [50]. A possible solution here is the development of a protocolized organizational structure in order to outsource the CGA to other trained health care providers. In addition, having patient self-reported assessment of some domains can save time from the clinical team.

Another cited barrier is the cost–benefit of systematic CGA. For this reason, authorities, insurers, and payers should be convinced of the broader value of such a multidimensional approach. Importantly, the relative cost of CGA is small compared to the cost of currently used diagnostic procedures and treatments routinely used in oncology [51].

Finally, the last barriers are practical concerns such as lack of awareness about tools, uncertainty about their use, and overall lack of training. No consensus exists regarding the optimal number and type of CGA domains that should be included. In addition, cutoff values directing concrete treatment decisions and changes in anticancer treatments are also lacking, making the interpretation difficult in a clinical situation where specific and straightforward direction is desired. Therefore, training for oncologists, geriatricians as well as nursing and allied health care professionals is one of the main aims of SIOG.

Importantly, a balance must be struck between the comprehensiveness of a CGA and the practicality of delivering its essence, which is taking a more holistic, domain-based approach to older adult health instead of a limited, disease-based approach. Although many forms of modified CGA are currently being tested and implemented, which may not be a CGA in the strict sense, integrating some elements of the CGA into oncology care is better than integrating none; and accepting nothing less than that may also adversely affect its widespread implementation [52]. Moreover, although there are ethical considerations regarding the implementation of frailty screening or other geriatric assessment without explicit follow-up interventions for uncovered vulnerabilities, treating older patients with intensive cancer therapies without first assessing for age-related vulnerabilities poses a greater concern. At the very least, simply providing oncologists with the results of a geriatric/frailty assessment improves communication and patient and caregiver satisfaction, regardless of implementation of interventions and impact on treatment outcomes [53].

Advantages of CGA

As previously described, CGA may reveal deficits that go undetected by routine past medical history or physical examination in older patients with cancer [39, 44, 54].

The comprehensive and multi-professional management of older adults with cancer needs to involve a broad spectrum of healthcare providers and caregivers from different professions, including oncologists, geriatricians, nurses, dietitians, physiotherapists, occupational therapists, psychologists, and pharmacists. Identifying impairments through CGA makes the implementation of personalized interventions possible, resulting in several substantial benefits and improved outcomes.

Advantages in Surgical Oncology

In the last decade, increasing attention was paid to frailty assessment in the preoperative evaluation of older patients with cancer, showing that CGA also provides several benefits in the surgical setting: less post-operative complications, shorter length of hospital stay, and decreased mortality rates [55–57]. Based on CGA, reversible conditions like functional status, malnutrition, comorbidities, and polypharmacy can be optimized by tailored interventions before surgery. This concept is called pre-habilitation and is defined as the care between the time of cancer diagnosis and the beginning of cancer treatment, typically lasting about 4 weeks [58, 59]. This multimodal approach, incorporating both physical and psychological interventions, leads to the patient being in a better condition when surgery is performed, and it may also include the period of neo-adjuvant medical treatment and/or radiotherapy, if necessary.

Involving geriatricians not only in the pre-operative evaluation and care but also in the post-operative process showed significant benefit. A recently conducted observational study by Shahrokni and colleagues demonstrated a significant advantage of geriatric co-management, a concept including both pre-operative evaluation and post-operative inpatient care involving geriatric expertise [60]. Geriatric co-management was compared to surgical management (without either pre-operative CGA or post-operative geriatric management) in 1855 patients aged 75 years or older who underwent elective surgery for cancer between 2015 and 2018 at Memorial Sloan Kettering Cancer Center. The results suggest that geriatric co-management decreased 90-day mortality from 9.2 to 4.3%, elucidating the importance of the comprehensive approach where CGA and interventions are cornerstones.

Furthermore, several studies showed that CGA is a predictor for all-cause and post-operative mortality, post-operative complications, duration of hospital stay and costs, but data regarding quality of life and functional recovery after surgery are still lacking [61–63].

The multicenter GOSAFE study is prospectively evaluating 977 older patients (aged 70+) with cancer who underwent major elective cancer surgery preceded by geriatric and frailty assessments. This study aims to evaluate the patients' quality of life after cancer surgery; assess baseline frailty indicators in unselected patients; and clarify the most relevant tools in predicting functional recovery and clinical outcomes [64]. The final results of this study are awaited.

Advantages in Non-surgical Oncology

In daily oncology practice, CGA and CGA-driven interventions showed benefits in several areas of the complex management of older patients with cancer.

CGA outperforms routinely used performance scores (ECOG, Karnofsky) in oncology in terms of describing physical performance [65–68]. It also showed being superior to oncologists' clinical judgement in identifying frailty [69], and at estimating survival [70].

Moreover, CGA is able to guide decision-making processes and modify treatment plans tailored to the individual patient [71, 72]. Regarding cancer treatments, it also predicts treatment-related complications and toxicities, treatment completion, admission to long-term care, and mortality [44, 71, 72]. In this context, several efforts were made to develop tools being able to accurately predict toxicity of systemic anti-cancer treatment in older patients with cancer. The ASCO guideline for geriatric oncology recommends either the use of Cancer and Aging Research Group (CARG) or the Chemotherapy Risk Assessment Scale for High-Age Patients (CRASH) tools [39, 73, 74].

Therefore, implementing CGA minimizes over- and under-treatment [75], identifies when patients are declining in function throughout the treatment course, guides supportive care interventions (e.g., social support, nutrition, physical therapy) and rehabilitation needs [76, 77], and offers an opportunity to optimize medication use by identification of potential inappropriate medications and deprescribing [78].

Randomized Clinical Trials Incorporating CGA in Oncology

In a landmark randomized phase 3 trial, a CGA-based treatment allocation in older patients with advanced non-small cell lung cancer treated with chemotherapy resulted in significant less all grade toxicity (85.6% vs. 93.4% respectively; $p = 0.015$), non-significant higher quality of life scores and less treatment failures because of toxicity (4.8% vs. 11.8% respectively; $p = 0.07$) versus standard of care [79]. Although there was no improvement in progression free survival or overall survival for the CGA-based treatment allocation arm, one can consider this as a positive trial because of the beneficial effects on the other above-mentioned outcomes, particularly relevant to older patients.

In addition, a second randomized trial demonstrated that giving oncologists a tailored CGA summary with recommendations for older patients with cancer significantly increases patient satisfaction with communication about age-related concerns and with overall care when compared with standard practice [53].

More recently, at the ASCO 2020 annual meeting, the publication of four prospective randomized trials provided high-level evidence in oncology regarding the benefit of implementing a CGA (geriatric assessments with tailored interventions) or geriatric assessments-only [80–83]. In the GAIN study, a multidisciplinary team implemented CGA for cancer patients undergoing systemic anti-cancer treatment in the intervention arm, versus a standard of care arm where the treating oncologists received only a summary of the geriatric assessments to use at their discretion [80]. This study resulted in less toxicity (9.9% reduction in incidence of grade 3–5 toxicities) and improved completion of prescribed therapy for the intervention arm (24.1% vs. 10.4% respectively; $p < 0.001$). A second randomized controlled trial in a similar setting also focused primarily on high-grade toxicity and compared the effects of providing a summary of the geriatric assessments (with recommendations to the treating oncologist), versus a standard of care arm without any geriatric assessments [81]. This trial demonstrated less grade 3–5 toxicities for the intervention arm (50% vs. 71%) with no changes in survival at 6 months between the arms (71% vs. 74% respectively; $p = 0.3$). In the INTEGRATE-study, a randomized trial primarily focused on health-related QoL, the important role of CGA in patients aged >70 years receiving systemic anti-cancer treatment was further confirmed [82]. Patients in the intervention arm with CGA had significantly higher QoL, versus a standard of care arm without any geriatric assessments. Furthermore, significant differences were seen in favor of the intervention arm regarding unplanned hospital admissions, early treatment discontinuation, and in several QoL domains; physical function, role and social functioning; mobility, burden of illness, and future worries. Lastly, a fourth study investigated the effect of peri-operative geriatric intervention in older patients undergoing elective surgery for gastrointestinal cancers [83]. No significant differences were found regarding post-operative length of stay, critical care use, and readmission rates within 90 days after surgery between the two arms. However, patients in the intervention arm reported lower depression symptoms and fewer moderate-severe symptom burden post-operatively.

Conclusion

As the world's population ages, health care workers involved in the care of cancer are confronted with an increasing number of older patients, and many of those present with multiple deficits in geriatric domains resulting in frailty-syndrome. This will often lead to difficult and complex cancer treatment decisions and challenging cancer management. Although chronological age often still guides treatment decisions, it is clear that this is a poor indicator of a patient's global health status. Functional age, on the other hand, reflects the cumulative effects of different stressors on the aging process and may differ significantly between patients with the same chronological age [2]. The integration of frailty/geriatric screening and CGA into clinical practice has shown to provide information on all domains of an older adult's health, including their medical, psychological, social, physical, and functional domains, identifying the need for CGA-driven interventions. Moreover, there is now high-level evidence available confirming the benefits of implementing such assessments and strategies for older cancer patients with the significant potential of improving patient outcomes.

Conflicts of Interest The authors have no relevant conflicts of interest related to the manuscript. Lore Decoster is a recipient of a grant from the non-profit organization "Kom op tegen Kanker" for research in geriatric oncology.
C DuMontier was supported by the Harvard Translational Research in Aging Training Program (NIH/NIA: T32AG023480).

References

1. Singh H, Kanapuru B, Smith C, Pashoyin-Aje LA, Myers A, Kim G, et al. FDA analysis of enrolment of older adults in clinical trials for cancer dug registration: a 10-year experience by the US Food and Drug Administration. J Clin Oncol. 2017;35(suppl):abstr 10009.
2. Soto-Perez E, Li D, Yuan Y, Ming Kau Y, Hurria A. Functional versus chronological age: geriatric assessments to guide decision making in older patients with cancer. Lancet Oncol. 2018;19:e305–16.
3. Morley JE, Vellas B, van Kan GA, Anker SD, Bauer JM, Bernabei R, et al. Frailty consensus: a call to action. J Am Med Dir Assoc. 2013;14:392–7.
4. Kane RL, Shamliyan T, Talley K, Pacala J. The association between geriatric syndromes and survival. J Am Geriatr Soc. 2012;60:896–904.
5. Clegg A, Young J, Iliffe S, Rikkert MO, Rockwood K. Frailty in elderly people. Lancet. 2013;381:752–62.
6. Solomon D, Brown AS, Brummel-Smith K, et al. National Institutes of Health Consensus Development Conference Statement: geriatric assessment methods for clinical decision-making. J Am Geriatr Soc. 2003;51(10):1490–4.
7. Rubenstein LZ, Stuck AE, Siu AL, Wieland D. Impacts of geriatric evaluation and management programs on defined outcomes: overview of the evidence. J Am Geriatr Soc. 1991;39:8S–16S.
8. Decoster L, Van Puyvelde K, Mohile S, et al. Screening tools for multidimensional health problems warranting a geriatric assessment in older cancer patients: an update on SIOG recommendations. Ann Oncol. 2015;26:288–300.

9. Garcia MJ, Agar MR, Soo WK, et al. Screening tools for identifying older adults with cancer who may benefit from a geriatric assessment: a systematic review. JAMA Oncol. 2021; https://doi.org/10.1001/jamaoncol.2020.6736.
10. Wedding U, Kodding D, Pientka L, et al. Physicians' judgment and comprehensive geriatric assessment (CGA) select different patients as fit for chemotherapy. Crit Rev Oncol Hematol. 2007;64:1–9.
11. Dent E, Kowal P, Hoogendijk EO. Frailty measurement in research and clinical practice: a review. Eur J Intern Med. 2016;31:3–10.
12. Fried LP, Tangen CM, Walston J, et al. Frailty in older adults: evidence for a phenotype. J Gerontol A Biol Sci Med Sci. 2001;56:M146–56.
13. Ensrud KE, Ewing SK, Taylor BC, et al. Comparison of two frailty indexed for prediction of falls, disability fractures and death in older women. Arch Intern Med. 2008;168:382–9.
14. Kristjansson SR, Ronning B, Hurria A, et al. A comparison of two pre-operative frailty measures in older surgical cancer patients. J Geriatr Oncol. 2012;3:1–7.
15. Murillo A, Cronin AM, Laubach JP, et al. Performance of the International Myeloma Working Group myeloma frailty score among patients 75 and older. J Geriatr Oncol. 2019;10(3):486–9.
16. Mitniski AB, Mogilner AJ, Rockwood K. Accumulation of deficits as a proxy measure of aging. ScientificWorldJournal. 2001;1:323–36.
17. Searle SD, Mitnitski A, Gahbauer EA, Gill TM, Rockwood K. A standard procedure for creating a frailty index. BMC Geriatr. 2008;8:24.
18. Dent E, Perez-Zepeda M. Comparison of five indices for prediction of adverse outcomes in hospitalized Mexican older adults: a cohort study. Arch Gerontol Geriatr. 2015;60:89–95.
19. Cohen HJ, Smith D, Sun CL, et al. Frailty as determined by a comprehensive geriatric assessment - derived deficit - accumulation index in older patients with cancer who receive chemotherapy. Cancer. 2016;122:3865–72.
20. Kim DH, Schneeweiss S, Glynn RJ, et al. Measuring frailty in medicare data: development and validation of a claims-based frailty index. J Gerontol Ser A. 2018;73(7):980–7.
21. Clegg A, Bates C, Young J, et al. Development and validation of an electronic frailty index using routine primary care electronic health record data. Age Ageing. 2018;47(2):319.
22. Rockwood K, Song X, MacKnight C, et al. A global clinical measure of fitness and frailty in elderly people. CMAJ. 2005;173:489–95.
23. Church S, Rogers E, Rockwood K, et al. A scoping review of the clinical frailty scale. BMC Geriatr. 2020;20:393.
24. Pulok MH, Theou O, van der Valk AM, Rockwood K. The role of illness acuity on the association between frailty and mortality in emergency department patients referred to internal medicine. Age Ageing. 2020;49(6):1071–9.
25. Theou O, Pérez-Zepeda MU, van der Valk AM, Searle SD, Howlett SE, Rockwood K. A classification tree to assist with routine scoring of the Clinical Frailty Scale. Age Ageing. 2021. https://doi.org/10.1093/ageing/afab006.
26. Saliba D, Elliott M, Rubenstein LZ, et al. The vulnerable elders-13 survey: a tool for identifying vulnerable older people in the community. JAGS. 2001;49:1691–9.
27. Min L, Yoon W, Mariano J, et al. The vulnerable elders-13 survey predicts 5-year functional decline and mortality outcomes in older ambulatory care patients. J Am Geriatr Soc. 2009;57:2070–6.
28. Stokoe JM, Pearce J, Sinha R, et al. G8 and VES-13 scores predict chemotherapy toxicity in older patients with cancer. J Geriatr Oncol. 2012;3:S81.
29. Papis D, Lembo R, O'Reilly D, et al. The predictive ability of timed "up & go", VES-13 and GFI in hepato-pancreato-biliary onco-geriatric surgical patients. J Geriatr Oncol. 2012;3:S100–1 (abstr P75).
30. Monfardini S, Basso U, Fiduccia P, et al. Can the short screening test vulnerable elders survey 13 (VES-13) substitute for the time-consuming comprehensive geriatric assessment (CGA) to identify vulnerable/frail elderly breast cancer patients. J Clin Oncol. 2010;28(15 suppl):abstr 9114.

31. Steverink N, Slaets JPJ, Schuurmans H, et al. Measuring frailty: developing and testing the GFI (Groningen Frailty Indicator). Gerontologist. 2001;41(special issue 1):236.
32. Schuurmans H, Steverink N, Lindenberg S, et al. Old or frail: what tells us more? J Gerontol A Biol Sci Med Sci. 2004;59:962–5.
33. Van Frayenhove F, Baitar A, De Vos M, et al. Prediction of chemotherapy toxicity by the Groningen Frailty Index (GFI) and the comprehensive geriatric assessment (CGA) in elderly cancer patients (pts): an interim analysis. Ann Oncol. 2010;21 (suppl 8):viii185 (abstr 568 PD).
34. Aaldriks AA, Maartense E, le Cessie S, et al. Predictive value of geriatric assessment for older patients older than 70 years, treated with chemotherapy. Crit Rev Oncol Hematol. 2011;79:205–12.
35. Bellera CA, Rainfray M, Mathoulin-Pélissier S, Mertens C, Delva F, Fonck M, et al. Screening older cancer patients: first evaluation of the G-8 geriatric screening tool. Ann Oncol. 2012;23:2166–72.
36. Kenis C, Decoster L, Van Puyvelde K, et al. Performance of two geriatric screening tools in older cancer patients. J Clin Oncol. 2014;32:19–26.
37. Extermann M, Green T, Tiffenberg G, et al. Validation of the Senior Adult Oncology Program (SAOP) 2 screening questionnaire. Crit Rev Oncol Hematol. 2009;69:185.
38. Russo C, Giannotti C, Signori A, Cea M, Murialdo R, Ballestrero A, et al. Predictive values of two frailty screening tools in older patients with solid cancer: a comparison of SAOP2 and G8. Oncotarget. 2018;9:35056–68.
39. Mohile SG, Dale W, Somerfield M, et al. Practical assessment and management of vulnerabilities in older patients receiving chemotherapy: ASCO guideline for geriatric oncology. J Clin Oncol. 2018;36:2326–47.
40. Huisingh-Scheetz M, Walston J. How should older adults with cancer be evaluated for frailty? J Geriatr Oncol. 2017;8:8–15.
41. Reuben DB, Rosen S, Schickedanz HB. Principles of geriatric assessment. In: Halter JB, Ouslander JG, Studenski S, High KP, Asthana S, Supiano MA, Ritchie C, editors. Hazzard's geriatric medicine and gerontology, 7e. New York: McGraw-Hill. Accessed 25 July 2020. https://accessmedicine-mhmedical-com.ezp-prod1.hul.harvard.edu/content.aspx?bookid=1923&sectionid=144517796.
42. DuMontier C, Sedrak MS, Soo WK, et al. Arti Hurria and the progress in integrating the geriatric assessment into oncology: Young International Society of Geriatric Oncology review paper. J Geriatr Oncol. 2020;11(2):203–11.
43. Rubenstein LZ, Joseph T. Freeman award lecture: comprehensive geriatric assessment: from miracle to reality. J Gerontol A Biol Sci Med Sci. 2004;59(5):473–7.
44. Wildiers H, Heeren P, Puts M, et al. International Society of Geriatric Oncology Consensus on Geriatric Assessment in older patients with cancer. J Clin Oncol. 2014;32:2595–603.
45. Fried TR, Bradley EH, Twole VR, et al. Understanding the treatment preferences of seriously ill patients. N Eng J Med. 2002;346:1061–6.
46. Pinquart M, Duberstein PR. Information needs and decision-making process in older patients with cancer. Crit Rev Oncol Hematol. 2004;51:69–80.
47. Puts MTE, Alibhai SMH. Fighting back against the dilution of the Comprehensive Geriatric Assessment. J Geriatr Oncol. 2018;9(1):3–5. https://doi.org/10.1016/j.jgo.2017.08.009.
48. McKenzie GAG, Bullock AF, Greenley SL, et al. Implementation of geriatric assessment in oncology settings: a systematic realist review. J Geriatr Oncol. 2021;12:22–33.
49. Dale W, Williams GR, MacKenzie AR, et al. How is geriatric assessment used in clinical practice for older adults with cancer, A survey of cancer providers by the American Society of Clinical Oncology. JCO Oncol Pract. 2020; https://doi.org/10.1200/OP.20.00442.
50. Williams GR, Weaver KE, Lesser GJ, et al. Capacity to provide geriatric specialty care for older adults in community oncology practices. Oncologist. 2020;25:1032–8.
51. Hamaker M, Wildes TM, Rostoft S. Time to stop saying geriatric assessment is too time consuming. J Clin Oncol. 2017;35:2871–4.

52. Klepin HD, Wildes TM. Fighting for the integration of geriatric principles into oncology. J Geriatr Oncol. 2018;9(6):705–6. https://doi.org/10.1016/j.jgo.2018.05.013.
53. Mohile SG, Epstein RM, Hurria A, et al. Communication with older patients with cancer using geriatric assessment: a cluster - randomized clinical trial from the National Cancer Institute Community Oncology Research Program. JAMA Oncol. 2019;6:196–204.
54. Paillaud E, Soubeyran P, Caillet P, et al. Multidisciplinary development of the Geriatric Core Dataset for clinical research in older patients with cancer: a French initiative with international survey. Eur J Cancer. 2018;103:61–8. https://doi.org/10.1016/j.ejca.2018.07.137.
55. Rostoft S, Audisio RA. Recent advances in cancer surgery in older patients. F1000Res. 2017;6:1242. Published 2017 July 27. https://doi.org/10.12688/f1000research.10683.1
56. Fagard K, Casaer J, Wolthuis A, et al. Value of geriatric screening and assessment in predicting postoperative complications in patients older than 70 years undergoing surgery for colorectal cancer. J Geriatr Oncol. 2017;8(5):320–7. https://doi.org/10.1016/j.jgo.2017.07.008.
57. Ommundsen N, Wyller TB, Nesbakken A, et al. Preoperative geriatric assessment and tailored interventions in frail older patients with colorectal cancer: a randomized controlled trial. Colorectal Dis. 2018;20(1):16–25. https://doi.org/10.1111/codi.13785.
58. Silver JK, Baima J. Cancer prehabilitation: an opportunity to decrease treatment-related morbidity, increase cancer treatment options, and improve physical and psychological health outcomes. Am J Phys Med Rehabil. 2013;92(8):715–27. https://doi.org/10.1097/PHM.0b013e31829b4afe.
59. Silver JK. Cancer rehabilitation and prehabilitation may reduce disability and early retirement. Cancer. 2014;120(14):2072–6. https://doi.org/10.1002/cncr.28713.
60. Shahrokni A, Tin A, Sarraf A, et al. Reduced 90-day postoperative mortality through geriatric comanagement after cancer surgery. J Clin Oncol. 2019;37(15_suppl):11512.
61. Kristjansson SR, Nesbakken A, Jordhøy MS, et al. Comprehensive geriatric assessment can predict complications in elderly patients after elective surgery for colorectal cancer: a prospective observational cohort study. Crit Rev Oncol Hematol. 2010;76(3):208–17. https://doi.org/10.1016/j.critrevonc.2009.11.002.
62. Ommundsen N, Wyller TB, Nesbakken A, et al. Frailty is an independent predictor of survival in older patients with colorectal cancer. Oncologist. 2014;19(12):1268–75. https://doi.org/10.1634/theoncologist.2014-0237.
63. Handforth C, Clegg A, Young C, et al. The prevalence and outcomes of frailty in older cancer patients: a systematic review. Ann Oncol. 2015;26(6):1091–101. https://doi.org/10.1093/annonc/mdu540.
64. Montroni I, Rostoft S, Spinelli A, et al. GOSAFE—Geriatric Oncology Surgical Assessment and Functional rEcovery after Surgery: early analysis on 977 patients. J Geriatr Oncol. 2020;11(2):244–55. https://doi.org/10.1016/j.jgo.2019.06.017.
65. Ghosn M, Ibrahim T, El Rassy E, et al. Abridged geriatric assessment is a better predictor of overall survival than the Karnofsky Performance Scale and Physical Performance Test in elderly patients with cancer. J Geriatr Oncol. 2017;8(2):128–32.
66. Jolly TA, Deal AM, Nyrop KA, et al. Geriatric assessment-identified deficits in older cancer patients with normal performance status. Oncologist. 2015;20(4):379–85. https://doi.org/10.1634/theoncologist.2014-0247.
67. Kirkhus L, Harneshaug M, Šaltytė Benth J, et al. Modifiable factors affecting older patients' quality of life and physical function during cancer treatment. J Geriatr Oncol. 2019;10(6):904–12. https://doi.org/10.1016/j.jgo.2019.08.001.
68. Repetto L, Fratino L, Audisio RA, et al. Comprehensive geriatric assessment adds information to Eastern Cooperative Oncology Group performance status in elderly cancer patients: an Italian Group for Geriatric Oncology Study. J Clin Oncol. 2002;20(2):494–502. https://doi.org/10.1200/JCO.2002.20.2.494.
69. Kirkhus L, Šaltytė Benth J, Rostoft S, et al. Geriatric assessment is superior to oncologists' clinical judgement in identifying frailty. Br J Cancer. 2017;117(4):470–7. https://doi.org/10.1038/bjc.2017.202.

70. Klepin HD, Geiger AM, Tooze JA, et al. Geriatric assessment predicts survival for older adults receiving induction chemotherapy for acute myelogenous leukemia. Blood. 2013;121(21):4287–94. https://doi.org/10.1182/blood-2012-12-471680.
71. Hamaker ME, Schiphorst AH, ten Bokkel HD, Schaar C, van Munster BC. The effect of a geriatric evaluation on treatment decisions for older cancer patients—a systematic review. Acta Oncol. 2014;53(3):289–96. https://doi.org/10.3109/0284186X.2013.840741.
72. Decoster L, Kenis C, Van Puyvelde K, et al. The influence of clinical assessment (including age) and geriatric assessment on treatment decisions in older patients with cancer. J Geriatr Oncol. 2013;4(3):235–41. https://doi.org/10.1016/j.jgo.2013.04.010.
73. Extermann M, Boler I, Reich RR, et al. Predicting the risk of chemotherapy toxicity in older patients: the Chemotherapy Risk Assessment Scale for High-Age Patients (CRASH) score. Cancer. 2012;118(13):3377–86. https://doi.org/10.1002/cncr.26646.
74. Hurria A, Mohile S, Gajra A, et al. Validation of a prediction tool for chemotherapy toxicity in older adults with cancer. J Clin Oncol. 2016;34(20):2366–71. https://doi.org/10.1200/JCO.2015.65.4327.
75. DuMontier C, Loh KP, Bain PA, et al. Defining undertreatment and overtreatment in older adults with cancer: a scoping literature review. J Clin Oncol. 2020; https://doi.org/10.1200/JCO.19.02809.
76. Pergolotti M, Lyons KD, Williams GR. Moving beyond symptom management towards cancer rehabilitation for older adults: answering the 5W's. J Geriatr Oncol. 2018;9(6):543–9. https://doi.org/10.1016/j.jgo.2017.11.009.
77. Pergolotti M, Deal AM, Williams GR, et al. Older adults with cancer: a randomized controlled trial of occupational and physical therapy. J Am Geriatr Soc. 2019;67(5):953–60. https://doi.org/10.1111/jgs.15930.
78. Ramsdale E, Lemelman T, Loh KP, et al. Geriatric assessment-driven polypharmacy discussions between oncologists, older patients, and their caregivers. J Geriatr Oncol. 2018;9(5):534–9. https://doi.org/10.1016/j.jgo.2018.02.007.
79. Corre R, Greillier L, Le Caër H, et al. Use of a comprehensive geriatric assessment for the management of elderly patients with advanced non-small cell lung cancer: the phase III randomized ESOGIA-GFPC-GECP 08-02 study. J Clin Oncol. 2016;34:1476–83.
80. Li D, Sun CL, Kim H, et al. Geriatric assessment-driven intervention (GAIN) on chemotherapy toxicity in older adults with cancer: a randomized controlled trial. J Clin Oncol. 2020;38(15_suppl):12010.
81. Mohile SG, Mohamed MR, Culakova R, et al. A geriatric assessment (GA) intervention to reduce treatment toxicity in older patients with advanced cancer: a University of Rochester Cancer Center NCI community oncology research program cluster randomized clinical trial (CRCT). J Clin Oncol. 2020;38(15_suppl):12009.
82. Soo W-K, King M, Pope A, et al. Integrated geriatric assessment and treatment (INTEGERATE) in older people with cancer planned for systemic anticancer therapy. J Clin Oncol. 2020;38(15_suppl):12011.
83. Qian CL, Knight HP, Ferrone CR, et al. Randomized trial of a perioperative geriatric intervention for older adults with cancer. J Clin Oncol. 2020;38(15_suppl):12012.

Chapter 4
Cognitive Impairment in Older Adults with Cancer and Frailty

Lorraine Burgess, Cindy Kenis, and Daniel Anderson

Introduction

Cognitive impairment is not caused by any one disease or condition, nor is it limited to a specific age group. Whilst age is the primary risk factor, there are several others, such as family history, education level, brain injury, exposure to pesticides or toxins, physical inactivity, and chronic conditions such as Parkinson's disease, heart disease, stroke, and diabetes [1]. Ageing affects all systems in the body differently, and normal changes due to the physiology of ageing can affect function, such as cognition, impacting individuals in varying degrees [2]. The prevalence rates of cognitive impairment in older adults in the general population vary between 5 and 29% [3]. Its most common causes are delirium and dementia, but their interrelation remains poorly understood [4].

The intermediate stage between normal ageing and early dementia is called Mild Cognitive Impairment (MCI) [5, 6]. MCI is therefore common in older populations, and its prevalence increases with age and lower educational level. Dementia requires substantial cognitive impairment in one or more cognitive domains that interfere with independence in daily activities, whereas MCI does not. In the latest edition (5th edition) of the Diagnostic and Statistical Manual of Mental Disorders (DSM-5), the term MCI was updated to the term 'mild neurocognitive disorder' and the term

L. Burgess (✉) · D. Anderson
The Christie NHS Foundation Trust, Manchester, UK
e-mail: Lorraine.burgess8@nhs.net; daniel.anderson16@nhs.net

C. Kenis
Department of General Medical Oncology and Geriatric Medicine, University Hospitals Leuven, Leuven, Belgium

Department of Public Health and Primary Care, Academic Centre for Nursing and Midwifery, KU Leuven - University of Leuven, Leuven, Belgium
e-mail: cindy.kenis@uzleuven.be

F. Gomes (ed.), *Frailty in Older Adults with Cancer*,
https://doi.org/10.1007/978-3-030-89162-6_4

dementia was updated to 'major neurocognitive disorder' [6, 7]. There are several subtypes of dementia of which Alzheimer's dementia and vascular dementia are the most common. Less common causes of dementia include dementia with Lewy bodies, fronto-temporal dementia or other causes like neurological diseases (e.g. Huntington's disease) or long-term heavy alcohol consumption (Korsokoff's dementia). The prevalence of dementia is 13.9% in patients older than 70 years and it increases exponentially with age, doubling every 5 years after the age of 65 [6, 8, 9].

Delirium is defined as an acute change in mental status with a fluctuating course of attention and alertness, accompanied by delusions and/or perceptual disturbances. This can occur secondary to medications or underlying medical aetiologies. Older age and pre-existing cognitive impairment are well-documented risk factors for delirium. Delirium is characterised by three subtypes based on the patient's level of psychomotor activity; hyperactive, hypoactive or mixed [10–12].

Cognitive impairment and frailty have been shown to be often linked and multiple studies implicated the co-occurrence of both [13]. Frailty is often described as a clinically recognised state of limited reserve based on the accumulation of comorbidities and functional limitations [14]. Physical impairments due to cognitive decline are well established and largely rely on neurodegenerative disorders. However, when the cognitive impairment is caused by physical factors related to frailty and pre-frailty, this has been defined as cognitive frailty. The key factors defining such a condition include: (1) presence of physical frailty and cognitive impairment; and (2) exclusion of concurrent dementia. Important to mention is that cognitive impairment caused by physical frailty has the potential of reversibility [15].

This chapter will address cognitive impairment in older adults with frailty affected by cancer and it will provide an overview of the available assessment tools and interventions to support these patients. Lastly, a composite case study taken from an anonymised patient will be utilised to apply these to a real-world case highlighting the key challenges and the importance of a multidisciplinary team.

Cognitive Impairment in Oncology

The incidence of cancer is increasing annually, with 50% of new cancer diagnoses found in people aged over 70 [16]. As both cancer and cognitive impairment in all its forms become more common as people get older, it is not surprising that cancer and cognitive impairment are frequently co-occurring in the older population [17]. However, it is still unclear how these three entities—ageing, cognition and cancer—are interacting with each other [18].

After a diagnosis of cancer and/or cancer treatment initiation, subjective and objective changes can occur in cognitive function. This is called cancer-related cognitive decline (CRCD) and includes problems with memory, attention, executive function, and speed of processing information [13]. Patients' functional abilities and quality of life can be affected by these problems, although they are generally more subtle than those that occur in other disorders, like MCI and dementia [19]. The prevalence of CRCD varies from 10 to 50% depending on the setting, population, measurement, cancer type and treatment (e.g., chemotherapy, endocrine therapies, and radiation) [13]. The majority of studies evaluating the impact of cancer and cancer treatment on cognition have focused on short-term effects (i.e., less than 1 year post treatment). Some data suggests, however, that a diagnosis of cancer places an individual at increased risk for cognitive impairment later in life [18].

Cancer treatment, chemotherapy, in particular, has been shown to negatively impact cognition for some patients and it is likely that older patients with pre-existing cognitive impairment are the most vulnerable, which in turn increases the risk of adverse events whilst on treatment [18]. Moreover, patients with frailty before cancer treatment appear most susceptible to cognitive decline under treatment [20]. Since being recognised as a risk factor for chemotherapy toxicity, cognitive impairment has been incorporated as a key factor in several toxicity prediction tools, such as the CARG and CRASH tools [21, 22]. Importantly, cognitive impairment can also affect the reporting of symptoms, such as the treatment toxicity itself.

Cognitive impairment is, therefore, an important consideration during treatment decision-making in oncology, particularly for older patients with frailty as this leads to a heightened risk for CRCD and other adverse cancer outcomes [23]. Moreover, oncology teams need to consider a range of additional issues, in particular the impact it could have on the person's daily life [18]. Another key aspect is that cognitive impairment may affect a patient's ability to participate in some aspects of the treatment decision-making process for cancer, which can be particularly challenging in an older patient with cancer and frailty [13, 24, 25]. Recognising that the older patient may have communication issues is also vital to appropriately discuss their cancer and related decisions. This was highlighted in a recent qualitative study on patient and carer experiences of those people living with dementia receiving cancer treatment [26]. The likely consequences of such communication issues mean that patients with dementia and cancer can be both under-treated and over-treated. Therefore, performing a holistic assessment and discussing in detail, with the patients and their families, the risks prior to cancer treatment is not only good practice but also essential.

Ultimately, the problematic of cognitive impairment in oncology needs highlighting for several reasons: (1) it is common particularly in the older population with cancer and frailty; (2) it can cause significant impairments in the patient functional capabilities with complex health and social care needs; (3) it is often missed by the treating oncology team; and (4) it can negatively impact an appropriate cancer treatment decision-making process leading to poor cancer outcomes [25]. Therefore, this is increasingly recognised as a key challenge for clinicians with the need to develop dedicated research [18, 27].

Cognitive Impairment Assessment

An important step in managing cognitive impairment in the older patient with cancer is the identification of pre-existing cognitive changes prior to cancer diagnosis and treatment [18]. The assessment of a patient suspected of having a cognitive impairment should start with a detailed history with input from a reliable caregiver focusing on the patient's previous level of functioning, the temporal course and the degree of cognitive decline [28]. An even more in-depth assessment comprises a full drug history, including recent cessation or increase in medication, alcohol history, nutritional status, bowel and bladder function, sleep deprivation, pain and any sensory deficits. Apart from history taking, a full physical examination should be carried out, particularly neurological examination, alongside focusing on signs of infection, dehydration and alcohol/drug abuse. Lastly, brain imaging with a CT or MRI scan is indicated if an intracranial lesion is suspected, particularly when managing patients with some cancers.

However, a cognitive impairment can be missed during standard oncological assessments and the implementation of short cognitive screening/assessment tools can play a very useful role in a busy oncology practice at identifying patients and monitoring them over time such as, throughout the cancer treatment pathway. A variety of cognitive screening tools is well known in oncology practice, and can be used to evaluate cognitive status in older patients with cancer [18, 29, 30]. Examples of these cognitive screening tools are the Clock Drawing test (CDT) [31], the Mini-Cog [32], the Mini-Mental State Examination (MMSE) [33], the Montreal Cognitive Assessment (MoCA) [34] and the Blessed Orientation-Memory-Concentration (BOMC) test [35].

The CDT is used for screening of cognitive impairment and dementia and as a measure of spatial dysfunction and neglect [31]. When this test is combined with a delayed recall three item test for memory, it is called the Mini-Cog which takes approximately 3 min to administer [32]. The MMSE is a brief screening tool to screen for cognitive impairment, to estimate its severity at a specific time point, to follow the course of cognitive changes over time, and to document a person's response to treatment. It includes evaluation of orientation (in time and place), registration, attention, and calculation, three item recall, language, and copying and takes approximately 10–15 min to administer [33]. The MoCA is a brief screening tool that evaluates multiple cognitive domains including short-term memory, visuospatial abilities, executive function, and attention and takes approximately 10 min to administer. The MoCA is not only known for the detection of mild cognitive impairment (MCI) but has also the ability to detect mild dementia [34]. The BOMC test is a short cognitive screen that takes approximately 5 min to administer and is comprised of six questions focusing on orientation, memory and concentration. It has been shown to discriminate among mild, moderate, and severe cognitive impairments [35].

Despite the implementation of these screening tools, a full neuropsychological evaluation remains the gold standard to diagnose a cognitive disorder like dementia.

So when a short cognitive screening tool detects an abnormality, referral for a full neuropsychological evaluation is recommended [18]. Moreover, it remains difficult to state which tool is superior to another since they all have advantages and disadvantages in clinical practice. Choice of cognitive screening tool might rely on local preference, the aim of the tool, or resources present [29].

Lastly, given the complexity of decisions that patients with cancer are faced with, and the under-recognition of cognitive impairment in older adults, clinicians should be familiar with the assessment of treatment decision-making capacity. A diagnosis of cognitive impairment does not determine a lack of treatment decision-making capacity. Capacity assessments are specific to the decision being questioned and to the time of evaluation (Table 4.1). The four pillars of decision-making capacity are

Table 4.1 Mental capacity assessment (A) and best interest meeting (B)

(A) Mental capacity assessment	
Decision, consultation and support	• The decision to be made • People consulted as part of the decision (list all and whether they were physically present) • Support given to make the decision/maximise capacity meeting • External factors affecting the patient's decision-making (e.g., environmental, cultural or social pressures)
Diagnostic test of capacity	• Yes, the patient has an impairment • No, the patient does not have an impairment
Functional test of capacity	• Can the patient understand the information relevant to the decision being assessed? • Can the patient retain the information relevant to the decision being assessed? • Can the patient use or weigh up information relevant to the decision being assessed? • Can the patient communicate their decision?
Summary and conclusions	• Summarise and conclude
Patient capacity	• Yes, I consider that the patient has the capacity to make the decision • No, I do not consider that the patient has the capacity to make the decision • Delay, I consider it appropriate to delay the decision until the patient is better able to demonstrate their capacity If decision reached and the person *does not have capacity*, consider a best interest meeting
(B) Best interest meeting	
The decision to be made	• The decision to be made
People consulted as part of the decision	• List all and whether they were physically present • Is an independent mental capacity advocate (IMCA) involved in the decision? • A referral must be made if friends and family cannot advocate
Options available to discuss	• List options and their risks and benefits; the first option listed should be the option of doing nothing
Decision reached and agreed upon	• What is the decision reached in the patient's best interests? • Should the decision be reviewed? • Any further information

as follows: (1) understanding the relevant information; (2) appreciating the current situation and its consequences; (3) manipulating the information rationally; and (4) communicating a consistent choice [36].

Cognitive Impairment Management

A multidisciplinary team (MDT) is important for the care of older patients with cognitive impairment and frailty, since these are often complex cases with multiple comorbidities and functional impairments. The goal of this MDT is to establish the person's needs, plan support and aid in treatment decision-making particularly in the context of cancer care. The MDT can include any healthcare professionals involved in that person's care such as nursing staff, consultant oncologists, physical therapists, social workers, occupational therapists, general practitioners and psychologists.

There are different models of care within oncology to support these patients, in particular those with dementia. In the person-centred oncology liaison model of care, a nurse consultant with expertise in dementia and the psycho-oncology team can support the oncology team to deliver most of the care, instead of the typical model of care delivered exclusively the oncology team [37, 38]. The fundamental principle of liaison is the importance of establishing and maintaining collaborative working relationships between healthcare professionals, services, and organisation. A component of a liaison model of care; is mental health assessment and delivery of psychotherapeutic interventions by the trained liaison practitioners themselves. However, the emphasis within the person-centred liaison oncology model of care is on the development and maintenance of working relationships with interdisciplinary oncology staff as this has the greatest impact on the delivery of holistic care. This enables the promotion of personhood of the patients for whom they are caring.

Some causes of cognitive impairment may be treatable and reversible, like when related to medication side effects, vitamin B12, thyroid or thiamine deficiency, and depression [3]. It is therefore essential to identify and evaluate older patients who are showing signs of cognitive impairment for treatable causes or aggravating factors.

Dementia however is more challenging to manage and not curable. However, there are medicines and other interventions that can reduce symptoms [39]. There is also evidence that more can be done to delay the onset of dementia by reducing risk factors and living a healthier lifestyle. Regarding non-pharmacological options, the cognitive symptoms may be ameliorated using psychological interventions with cognitive stimulation and pharmacological strategies. Cognitive stimulation is used particularly in milder stages of dementia. This entails exposure to and engagement with activities and materials involving some degree of thinking, challenge, and stimulation. The emphasis should be on social activities that participants enjoy. Sometimes these activities might focus on problem-solving, education, the practical management of forgetfulness, or reminiscence. Regarding pharmacological options, for example, acetylcholinesterase inhibitors are often used to delay the progression of Alzheimer's dementia [40, 41]. Treatment should be initiated only by a specialist in dementia care—in most cases, this would be a psychiatrist, neurologist, or general practitioner with a special interest in dementia care.

Lastly, for the management of CRCD, behavioural interventions, such as cognitive rehabilitation approaches and physical activity, have been the primary area of investigation [13]. Cognitive rehabilitation programmes broadly include two treatment types—strategy or educational programmes (typically a cognitive behavioural therapy-based approach) and computer-based cognitive training programmes—or a combination of the two types. In general, a growing body of evidence suggests that physical activity and exercise programmes may also play a role in managing CRCD [42, 43]. Research on pharmacologic interventions for CRCD has been limited, and results to date have shown that there are no established pharmacologic interventions for CRCD [44].

Conclusion

Cognitive impairment can add significantly to the complexity of caring for an older person with cancer and frailty. Moreover, these complex cases are on the rise with an ageing population. This highlights the importance of oncology teams identifying patients with cognitive impairment, particularly as cancer treatments can often precipitate deterioration of cognitive symptoms. Oncology teams should also exclude potentially reversible causes or aggravating factors of cognitive impairment. Ultimately, cognitive impairment affects every aspect of a person's life and in this context, it can also negatively affect the outcomes of cancer management. Therefore, a person-centred care needs to be the bedrock underpinning any collaborative model of care for the management of these complex older patients with cancer [45].

Case Study

Cancer Presentation and Assessment at the Specialist Oncology Centre

Rosie, an 84-year-old widowed lady who lives alone in her own private accommodation, is financially sound and relatively independent but has no relatives or friends. Her medical history includes hypertension, diabetes mellitus type 2 and a previous right mastectomy for cancer of the breast. She was also recently diagnosed with Alzheimer's type dementia but declined further interventions and was discharged from the memory clinic.

Rosie has a community matron that visits regularly to check on her health. She noticed that Rosie was less compliant with her medication and was losing weight. However, it was only when she started walking strangely, which when questioned was due to pain (down below around her vulva area) that triggered a referral. She was then diagnosed with a stage 3b squamous cell carcinoma of the vulva. She was referred to the local Specialist Oncology Centre for further treatment, but Rosie failed to attend despite several appointments until the dementia nurse consultant at the cancer centre intervened by contacting her community matron who felt it was not her responsibility to take Rosie for her appointments.

The dementia nurse consultant went to Rosie's home to assess her and support her attendance to the hospital appointment. Whilst Rosie's home was overall well kept, she did not question who the nurse was by letting her in and she was also willing to go with her to the hospital appointment, which was of concern. Moreover, it soon became obvious Rosie required prompts, like instructing her to get find her the coat, and she had lost her dentures. She also needed assistance to put her shoes on as she could not bend down due to pain (related to her cancer). On leaving the home, an anxious gentleman suddenly appeared in the hallway who stated he was Rosie's friend and seemed upset asking where she was going. Rosie completely ignored his presence and when questioned later on clarified he was her husband's friend who lived down the road and she was not bothered with him. She also expressed she had no other family or friends, and felt she was old and wanted to join her deceased husband but denied any intention to take her own life. The dementia nurse consultant contacted the community team and was told she previously had a social worker due to safeguarding concerns of a gentleman friend asking her for money. However, when the social worker was contacted due to growing concerns regarding her vulnerability, the team was informed she had been discharged from his caseload as felt there were no concerns. This however had not been communicated to anyone and it further indicated significant gaps in her community support.

Rosie was assessed by the consultant oncologist and was found to be in significant pain, which prevented a complete examination. Nonetheless, she was also found to have some bleeding and a smelly discharge from her tumour. It was discussed with her that she did have advanced cancer that could not be cured. The consultant proposed to treat the pain and bleeding by offering her palliative radiotherapy which would mean she would need to come in daily for treatment. The consultant feared that a more intense curative-intent treatment was less likely in her best interest considering the tumour stage and her frailty. It was explained to her that she would need to be in a room on her own whilst having treatment and she replied this could make her anxious. After the risks and benefits of radiotherapy were explained to her, she agreed to have treatment. However, it was uncertain how much information she retained, since she also did not wish to attend daily for the treatment. She also asked the Consultant oncologist if she could give her some medication to end her life.

Several concerns were raised at this point: (1) Does Rosie have the mental capacity to understand her cancer diagnosis and the implications of treatment? (2) Would Rosie be compliant with treatment? (3) Would Rosie be able to cope and alert the medical team with any potential side effects? (4) Could the cancer-related symptoms be optimised soon? (5) Having no family or friends, who could support her? (6) What support was she getting in the community regarding her dementia? (7) Could the treatment aggravate her mental health considering her low mood? (8) Could the treatment aggravate her cognitive status? (9) Considering her vulnerability, was the gentleman in Rosie's home taking advantage of her financially.

Cancer Treatment Decision

Rosie recalled that she had been to the oncology centre regarding her previous breast cancer. She was also able to share information that she was Austrian and had moved to England to get married 40 years ago, but her husband had since passed away although could not remember exactly when. She was also able to state who the gentleman was but was not very forthcoming regarding details about him other than he was her late husband's friend. Once her general practitioner was contacted, he clarified that he was called "Bill" and has also been diagnosed with dementia and self-discharged from the memory clinic. He was unclear if Bill actually lived with Rosie or just stayed there as he had his own property down the road, but the general practitioner did state there were concerns at some point that he was asking her for money, hence the initial involvement of a social worker. Moreover, it later on transpired that he apparently was the one turning the hospital transport away when they came to pick Rosie up for her oncology appointments.

Rosie was explained she could have a trial run in the radiotherapy room to see how she coped with this, as there were concerns that if she got distressed it may put her at risk, particularly if she moved or fell off the treatment table. This was trialled with her and everything went well, but since she did not wish to attend daily and due to her complex needs, it was felt the best thing for Rosie would be to admit her to a ward to address her pain, assess her mood and her cognition, and monitor her nutrition. Rosie initially did not wish to be admitted but when the nursing team suggested it could be nice for her to have someone to care for her for a whilst and help aid her pain; she accepted the suggestion and was admitted.

After a mental capacity was performed to establish if Rosie had the mental capacity to understand the implications of the treatment being offered, it was determined Rosie lacked the mental capacity due to her inability to retain the information long enough or weigh up the risks and benefits to make such decision. Therefore, a best interest meeting was agreed to be necessary (Table 4.1).

As Rosie had no family or friends and as it was still unclear who the gentleman friend was, an urgent referral was made to an Independent Mental Capacity Advocate (IMCA) and once one was allocated, a best interest meeting was then held with the IMCA, a newly assigned Social worker, her community matron, her Consultant oncologist, oncology specialist nurse, dementia nurse consultant and a radiotherapist within the oncology centre to establish if they thought it was in Rosie's best interest to have treatment. Moreover, if it would be in Rosie's best interest to have palliative radiotherapy rather than aiming for a more intense curative-intent treatment, considering her advanced stage and complex needs. Rosie herself was in favour of this multidisciplinary meeting and the community nurse also liaised with the general practitioner to seek his views. The best interest meeting agreed that the palliative intent treatment was in Rosie's best interest.

Holistic Management

During the first few days in the ward, Rosie was extremely disorientated and confused talking about her home in Austria and believing she still lived there. She would often walk around the ward and at times attempt to leave the ward. Therefore, she was commenced on a Deprivation of Liberty Order as she was unable to leave the ward of her own accord due to staff fear of her getting lost or falling.

Rosie completed cognitive assessments by the dementia nurse consultant and an occupational therapist on the ward also performed a functional assessment to determine her functioning capabilities. She proved relatively independent in activities of daily living but getting herself dressed proved difficult due to her pain and she required prompts on how to perform activities that required sequencing or planning. A physiotherapist was also involved in her care to assess her mobility. She did not initiate conversation but would answer questions when asked and her retention of what had been asked and recall was poor. Rosie was also assessed by a Consultant Psychiatrist regarding her mood. During that assessment, Rosie spoke about her home in Austria and smiled a lot. She stated she enjoyed being cared for but did not admit to wanting to her end her life or feeling depressed; therefore, it was decided to monitor her.

Rosie was not eating well, complained about feeling sick at times and her diabetes also became unstable. A referral to a dietician to address and monitor her nutritional needs and weight loss was crucial to improving Rosie's physical health. Rosie had a very sweet tooth which can be a common occurrence in dementia and therefore adding sweet foods and supplement drinks to her diet proved beneficial, alongside adequate control of her diabetes.

Her pain was also monitored, and opiates commenced. She tended to not admit having pain when asked, but her body language and her reluctance to mobilise suggested otherwise so she was commenced on the PAINAD assessment tool where body language is observed and recorded regularly rather than reliance on her verbal communication [46]. She was also referred to the supportive care team.

The various MDT professionals all collaborated and played their part in Rosie's treatment to ensure she got the correct holistic care. Even the hospital chaplain would visit Rosie daily as he was aware that she had no visitors. Rosie did not identify with a particular religion, but she did enjoy his company and interaction.

When Bill came to visit her, a nurse observed him asking her for taxi money which Rosie gave him. Rosie then became upset as he was asking her to go home with him. The nurse later asked Rosie if she could keep her bag safe for her whilst she was in the hospital (£1000 in cash was recorded as being in it). This once again highlighted her vulnerability.

Rosie on occasion would get irritated if she were stopped from doing certain things like leaving the ward. Therefore, the dementia nurse consultant worked with the ward staff to get them to complete an ABC chart (antecedents, behaviours, and consequences) to monitor any distress or behavioural issues, and a behavioural and functional analysis was undertaken in conjunction with the nursing staff. This would examine a specific behaviour in relation to antecedent events (A), the actual subsequent behaviour (B) and the consequences of that behaviour for the person and carers (C). These were recorded in Rosie's daily nursing notes and a care plan developed and acted on, and then reviewed regularly. One of the care plans involved staff taking Rosie out for a short walk to enable her to get away from the ward environment for a short period of time. Another involved the Social worker bringing in Rosie's crocheting which she enjoyed and reduced her agitation.

Cancer Treatment and Planning for Future Needs

A mental capacity assessment and best interest meeting took place involving an Independent Mental Capacity Assessor (IMCA) and Rosie was admitted to the ward. Despite becoming sore where her radiotherapy was given, Rosie tolerated her radiotherapy well. She did become less mobile due to pain at some point and was commenced on increased opiates which may have caused her to develop delirium presenting with symptoms of visual hallucinations which both distressed her and caused agitation. Rosie was reviewed by a Consultant Psychiatrist and was commenced on a minimal amount of haloperidol to help reduce her distressing hallucinations. This was discontinued when the delirium resolved. Antipsychotic medications are not recommended for patients with dementia and should not be prescribed lightly for these patients. Although delirium is a more common occurrence in patients with dementia, particularly under a stressor event like a hospital admission and cancer treatment. Other causes were also investigated, and she was found to have abnormal renal function, unstable diabetes and a urinary tract infection. As this was corrected and the delirium resolved, Rosie became much more oriented, alert, cheerful, and even more mobile. She was still not completely medically fit and required some prompts to eat and drink but, in general, appeared brighter and no longer complained of pain or even spoke of wanting to die.

As Rosie was regarded as vulnerable in relation to her relationship with the gentleman friend Bill, The Safeguarding Team became involved to monitor the situation with Bill whilst she was on the ward. Regarding Bill, an urgent referral to a social worker was made for him and his general practitioner was informed in order to assist them in supporting him.

Regarding her discharge from the ward, although Rosie enjoyed being cared for, she did state she wished to return to her own house. As she was becoming more mobile and bored with lack of stimulation, the nurses on the ward considered what resources they could use to help stimulate her. Rosie cognitively whilst discharge plans were being made for her. As Rosie was feeling brighter an occupational therapist was also involved in her care and worked alongside the dementia nurse consultant to assess her functional capacity which would give some indication of her needs and support if and when she was to return home.

Rosie did not fully understand her poor prognosis regarding her cancer and once radiotherapy was complete, discharge plans commenced. The MDT felt there were still concerns around Rosie and she was still a little sore from her radiotherapy which was affecting her mobility. Despite Rosie saying she wanted to return to her local home, there were still anxieties she may at risk due to vulnerability, poor dietary intake, falls and pain. Whilst many people with dementia do live in their own homes independently with the assistance of care packages and technology, as Rosie's condition was palliative, monitoring of her symptoms was the cause for real concern. Another mental capacity test was performed; this time to establish if Rosie understood the risks of returning home and a best interest meeting was held to plan the next steps of care. It was agreed for her to go into intermediate care and then re-evaluate plans later down the line. As Rosie indicated she enjoyed being cared for this was felt to be the best option. Although her mood had also lifted and she no longer mentioned she wanted to die, a request to her general practitioner was made to refer her to the local later life mental health team to monitor her cognition and mental health.

References

1. Cognitive impairment: a call for action NOW!: Center for Disease Control and Prevention; 2011. Available from: https://www.cdc.gov/aging/pdf/cognitive_impairment/cogimp_poilicy_final.pdf.
2. Harada CN, Natelson Love MC, Triebel KL. Normal cognitive aging. Clin Geriatr Med. 2013;29(4):737–52.
3. Dementia: assessment, management and support for people living with dementia and their carers: National Institute for Health and Care Excellence; 2018. Available from: https://www.nice.org.uk/guidance/ng97.
4. Fong TG, Davis D, Growdon ME, Albuquerque A, Inouye SK. The interface between delirium and dementia in elderly adults. Lancet Neurol. 2015;14(8):823–32.
5. Brodaty H, Aerts L, Crawford JD, Heffernan M, Kochan NA, Reppermund S, et al. Operationalizing the diagnostic criteria for mild cognitive impairment: the salience of objective measures in predicting incident dementia. Am J Geriatr Psychiatry. 2017;25(5):485–97.
6. Hugo J, Ganguli M. Dementia and cognitive impairment: epidemiology, diagnosis, and treatment. Clin Geriatr Med. 2014;30(3):421–42.
7. Petersen RC, Lopez O, Armstrong MJ, Getchius TSD, Ganguli M, Gloss D, et al. Practice guideline update summary: mild cognitive impairment. Report of the Guideline Development, Dissemination, and Implementation Subcommittee of the American Academy of Neurology. Neurology. 2018;90(3):126–35.
8. Livingston G, Sommerlad A, Orgeta V, Costafreda SG, Huntley J, Ames D, et al. Dementia prevention, intervention, and care. Lancet. 2017;390(10113):2673–734.

9. Plassman BL, Langa KM, Fisher GG, Heeringa SG, Weir DR, Ofstedal MB, et al. Prevalence of dementia in the United States: the aging, demographics, and memory study. Neuroepidemiology. 2007;29(1-2):125–32.
10. Breitbart W, Alici Y. Evidence-based treatment of delirium in patients with cancer. J Clin Oncol. 2012;30(11):1206–14.
11. Bush SH, Lawlor PG, Ryan K, Centeno C, Lucchesi M, Kanji S, et al. Delirium in adult cancer patients: ESMO clinical practice guidelines. Ann Oncol. 2018;29(suppl 4):iv143–65.
12. Guthrie PF, Rayborn S, Butcher HK. Evidence-based practice guideline: delirium. J Gerontol Nurs. 2018;44(2):14–24.
13. Magnuson A, Ahles T, Chen BT, Mandelblatt J, Janelsins MC. Cognitive function in older adults with cancer: assessment, management, and research opportunities. J Clin Oncol. 2021. https://doi.org/10.1200/JCO.21.00239.
14. Rockwood K, Mitnitski A. Frailty defined by deficit accumulation and geriatric medicine defined by frailty. Clin Geriatr Med. 2011;27(1):17–26.
15. Kelaiditi E, Cesari M, Canevelli M, van Kan GA, Ousset PJ, Gillette-Guyonnet S, et al. Cognitive frailty: rational and definition from an (I.A.N.A./I.A.G.G.) international consensus group. J Nutr Health Aging. 2013;17(9):726–34.
16. Cancer Statistics: Cancer Research UK. 2017. Available from: https://www.cancerresearchuk.org/health-professional/cancer-statistics/risk.
17. Lloyd-Williams M, Mogan C, Harrison Dening K. Cognitive impairment in older adults with cancer. Curr Opin Support Palliat Care. 2021;15(1):11–5.
18. Magnuson A, Mohile S, Janelsins M. Cognition and cognitive impairment in older adults with cancer. Curr Geriatr Rep. 2016;5(3):213–9.
19. Selamat MH, Loh SY, Mackenzie L, Vardy J. Chemobrain experienced by breast cancer survivors: a meta-ethnography study investigating research and care implications. PLoS One. 2014;9(9):e108002.
20. Mandelblatt JS, Zhou X, Small BJ, Ahn J, Zhai W, Ahles T, et al. Deficit accumulation frailty trajectories of older breast cancer survivors and non-cancer controls: the thinking and living with cancer study. J Natl Cancer Inst. 2021;113(8):1053–64.
21. Extermann M, Boler I, Reich RR, Lyman GH, Brown RH, DeFelice J, et al. Predicting the risk of chemotherapy toxicity in older patients: the Chemotherapy Risk Assessment Scale for High-Age Patients (CRASH) score. Cancer. 2012;118(13):3377–86.
22. Hurria A, Mohile S, Gajra A, Klepin H, Muss H, Chapman A, et al. Validation of a prediction tool for chemotherapy toxicity in older adults with cancer. J Clin Oncol. 2016;34(20):2366–71.
23. Mandelblatt JS, Stern RA, Luta G, McGuckin M, Clapp JD, Hurria A, et al. Cognitive impairment in older patients with breast cancer before systemic therapy: is there an interaction between cancer and comorbidity? J Clin Oncol. 2014;32(18):1909–18.
24. Bridges J, Hughes J, Farrington N, Richardson A. Cancer treatment decision-making processes for older patients with complex needs: a qualitative study. BMJ Open. 2015;5(12):e009674.
25. Surr CA, Kelley R, Griffiths AW, Ashley L, Cowdell F, Henry A, et al. Enabling people with dementia to access and receive cancer treatment and care: the crucial role of supportive networks. J Geriatr Oncol. 2020;11(7):1125–31.
26. McWilliams L, Farrell C, Keady J, Swarbrick C, Burgess L, Grande G, et al. Cancer-related information needs and treatment decision-making experiences of people with dementia in England: a multiple perspective qualitative study. BMJ Open. 2018;8(4):e020250.
27. Lange M, Rigal O, Clarisse B, Giffard B, Sevin E, Barillet M, et al. Cognitive dysfunctions in elderly cancer patients: a new challenge for oncologists. Cancer Treat Rev. 2014;40(6):810–7.
28. Magnuson A, Sattar S, Nightingale G, Saracino R, Skonecki E, Trevino KM. A practical guide to geriatric syndromes in older adults with cancer: a focus on falls, cognition, polypharmacy, and depression. Am Soc Clin Oncol Educ Book. 2019;39:e96–e109.
29. Wildiers H, Heeren P, Puts M, Topinkova E, Janssen-Heijnen ML, Extermann M, et al. International Society of Geriatric Oncology consensus on geriatric assessment in older patients with cancer. J Clin Oncol. 2014;32(24):2595–603.

30. Burhenn PS, McCarthy AL, Begue A, Nightingale G, Cheng K, Kenis C. Geriatric assessment in daily oncology practice for nurses and allied health care professionals: opinion paper of the Nursing and Allied Health Interest Group of the International Society of Geriatric Oncology (SIOG). J Geriatr Oncol. 2016;7(5):315–24.
31. Agrell B, Dehlin O. The clock-drawing test. 1998. Age Ageing. 2012;41 Suppl 3:iii41–5.
32. Borson S, Scanlan JM, Chen P, Ganguli M. The Mini-Cog as a screen for dementia: validation in a population-based sample. J Am Geriatr Soc. 2003;51(10):1451–4.
33. Folstein MF, Folstein SE, McHugh PR. "Mini-mental state". A practical method for grading the cognitive state of patients for the clinician. J Psychiatr Res. 1975;12(3):189–98.
34. Nasreddine ZS, Phillips NA, Bédirian V, Charbonneau S, Whitehead V, Collin I, et al. The Montreal Cognitive Assessment, MoCA: a brief screening tool for mild cognitive impairment. J Am Geriatr Soc. 2005;53(4):695–9.
35. Kawas C, Karagiozis H, Resau L, Corrada M, Brookmeyer R. Reliability of the blessed telephone information-memory-concentration test. J Geriatr Psychiatry Neurol. 1995;8(4):238–42.
36. Marron JM, Kyi K, Appelbaum PS, Magnuson A. Medical decision-making in oncology for patients lacking capacity. Am Soc Clin Oncol Educ Book. 2020;40:1–11.
37. Sharrock J, Grigg M, Happell B, Keeble-Devlin B, Jennings S. The mental health nurse: a valuable addition to the consultation-liaison team. Int J Ment Health Nurs. 2006;15(1):35–43.
38. Roberts D. Working models in practice. In: Regel S, Roberts D, editors. Liaison mental health—a handbook for nurses and healthcare. London: Baillière Tindall; 2002.
39. Ngo J, Holroyd-Leduc JM. Systematic review of recent dementia practice guidelines. Age Ageing. 2015;44(1):25–33.
40. Renn BN, Asghar-Ali AA, Thielke S, Catic A, Martini SR, Mitchell BG, et al. A systematic review of practice guidelines and recommendations for discontinuation of cholinesterase inhibitors in dementia. Am J Geriatr Psychiatry. 2018;26(2):134–47.
41. Frederiksen KS, Cooper C, Frisoni GB, Frölich L, Georges J, Kramberger MG, et al. A European Academy of Neurology guideline on medical management issues in dementia. Eur J Neurol. 2020;27(10):1805–20.
42. Campbell KL, Zadravec K, Bland KA, Chesley E, Wolf F, Janelsins MC. The effect of exercise on cancer-related cognitive impairment and applications for physical therapy: systematic review of randomized controlled trials. Phys Ther. 2020;100(3):523–42.
43. Treanor CJ, McMenamin UC, O'Neill RF, Cardwell CR, Clarke MJ, Cantwell M, et al. Non-pharmacological interventions for cognitive impairment due to systemic cancer treatment. Cochrane Database Syst Rev. 2016;(8):Cd011325.
44. Magnuson A, Ahles T, Chen BT, Mandelblatt J, Janelsins MC. Cognitive function in older adults with cancer: assessment, management, and research opportunities. J Clin Oncol. 2021;39(19):2138–49.
45. Lockwood G, Henderson C, Thornicroft G. The Equality Act 2010 and mental health. Br J Psychiatry. 2012;200(3):182–3.
46. Warden V, Hurley AC, Volicer L. Development and psychometric evaluation of the Pain Assessment in Advanced Dementia (PAINAD) scale. J Am Med Dir Assoc. 2003;4(1):9–15.

Chapter 5
Psychosocial Dimension in Older Adults with Cancer and Frailty

Christian Bjerre-Real, Nikita Shah, and Yesne Alici

Introduction

Older adults comprise more than half of the cancer diagnoses and even a greater percentage of cancer survivors [1]. But chronological age alone is a poor predictor of cancer outcomes; therefore, the assessment of older cancer patients requires a comprehensive assessment, including frailty, to guide individualized treatment decisions. Frailty affects about half of older cancer patients, and this should lead to considerations regarding their increased risk of treatment side effects, postsurgical complications, and mortality [2]. Comprehensive Geriatric Assessment (CGA), a multidimensional, multidisciplinary assessment process, is the most commonly used clinical tool for identification of frailty in cancer settings [3]. Frequently, older cancer patients experience impairments in multiple domains, increasing their risk of adverse outcomes [3]. Assessment of the psychosocial domain such as the assessment of psychological well-being, social support systems, and cognition are integral elements of a CGA.

Cancer has psychosocial implications for patients. These may include the stigma and demoralization related to cancer and its treatments, loss of independence, loss of dignity, as well as the existential distress of facing mortality. It is also common for the older adult with frailty to feel guilty about the added burden to the family.

C. Bjerre-Real (✉) · N. Shah
Department of Psychiatry and Behavioral Sciences, Memorial Sloan Kettering Cancer Center, New York, NY, USA
e-mail: bjerrerc@mskcc.org; ShahN8@mskcc.org

Y. Alici
Department of Psychiatry and Behavioral Sciences, Memorial Sloan Kettering Cancer Center, New York, NY, USA

Weill Cornell Medical College, New York, NY, USA
e-mail: aliciy@mskcc.org

F. Gomes (ed.), *Frailty in Older Adults with Cancer*,
https://doi.org/10.1007/978-3-030-89162-6_5

Moreover, the growing number of cancer survivors, majority of which aged 65 and older [4], often experience late effects of cancer, most commonly depression, pain, and fatigue. But sometimes it is difficult to differentiate between the effects of cancer and the effects of aging [5]. Furthermore, many survivors experience psychological distress after active treatment. Distress can result from the fear of recurrence, death, or secondary to physical, social, or practical problems such as employment, finances, etc. In fact, about 20% of survivors meet criteria for post traumatic disorder [6]. Therefore, it is essential that survivorship care plans are also tailored to individuals' psychosocial needs and preferences, and enhance their self-efficacy [7].

Psychosocial impairments include primarily, anxiety, depression, impaired cognition, and poor social support. Although commonly encountered, these are underreported and often poorly managed among older cancer adults [1]. Psychosocial distress is a risk factor for poor adherence to cancer treatments, impacts decision making, results in extra visits to emergency rooms, and increases the amount of time spent by the oncology teams [8]. Therefore, screening, timely recognition, assessment and management of psychosocial distress improve medical outcomes [8]. This is particularly important in the setting of older cancer patients with frailty where interventions should be tailored to their complex needs. Ultimately, psychosocial impairments may lead or aggravate frailty in older cancer patients.

This chapter will provide an overview of the commonly encountered psychosocial issues in older adults with cancer and frailty. It will review the assessment and management of common problematics such as anxiety, depression, suicide ideation, fatigue, sleep disturbances, substance-use disorders, and deficient social support. The problematic of cognitive impairment is presented on a separate chapter.

Anxiety

Anxiety is common in cancer patients from early diagnosis to survivorship, with highest rates seen at the end of life [8]. Over 40% of older adults with cancer report clinically significant anxiety [1]. The prevalence estimates among older adults with cancer can be misleading. In fact, the detection of anxiety disorders in late life is complicated by a number of factors that make it different from assessment in younger adults, such as differential symptom presentation, high comorbidity with medical and mental disorders, the aging process, and newly emergent changes in life circumstances. There are reports of similar rates of anxiety in older adults with hematologic cancers and healthy community-dwelling adults [9]. The prevalence of anxiety increases with advancing cancer, decline in the patient's physical status, and worsening frailty [10]. Increased social isolation, comorbid medical conditions, financial burden, fear of worsening physical and cognitive functioning, and limited access to care in older adults with frailty can increase the risk of anxiety symptoms.

Anxiety disorders include specific phobias, social anxiety disorder, panic disorder with or without agoraphobia, generalized anxiety disorder, and obsessive-compulsive disorder. Although anxiety can play an adaptive role for cancer patients, encouraging a more active approach to their health. When the anxiety is severely disproportionate to the threat, it can be maladaptive [3]. A Norwegian study revealed that the severity of anxiety symptoms was associated with the severity of depression and suicidality in older adults [11], highlighting the importance of thorough psychiatric evaluation in older adults presenting with severe anxiety symptoms.

Assessment

The assessment of anxiety can be challenging as symptoms may overlap with the comorbidities of aging, cancer, and the side effects of cancer treatments. Pain, dyspnea, and nausea are common triggers of anxiety. Adverse effects of medications such as glucocorticosteroids may contribute to anxiety symptoms. Withdrawal from alcohol, benzodiazepines, and opioids may present with anxiety [12]. Consideration of multiple factors including description of the timing of onset of symptoms, as well as the quality, frequency, duration, and triggers of symptoms, will help the clinician determine the etiology of the anxiety syndrome (preexisting or secondary to cancer diagnosis or treatment) and to create a viable treatment plan. A comprehensive medical history and physical evaluation are also important to assess cardiovascular, neurological, gastrointestinal, and respiratory systems whose syndromes may mimic or exacerbate anxiety. Delirium, dementia, and other cognitive syndromes should be considered in the differential given high rates of comorbid anxiety syndromes in these patients [13]. If the symptoms of anxiety are found to be an exacerbation of a preexisting anxiety disorder, aggravated in the context of a cancer diagnosis or recurrence, treatment of the primary underlying disorder may be the most effective way to alleviate the symptoms of anxiety.

Screening for anxiety in the older cancer patient with frailty allows for early identification of symptoms and timely management. The American Society of Clinical Oncology (ASCO) recommends for screening to be done at the initial visit, at points of change in disease trajectory, as well as the point of transition to end of life [14]. It is recommended that patients be assessed for generalized anxiety disorder, as it is the most prevalent of all anxiety disorders and it is commonly comorbid with other anxiety and mood disorders [14]. Using scales such as the Generalized Anxiety Disorder 7 (GAD-7), the Beck Anxiety Inventory (BAI), Hospital Anxiety Depression Scale (HADS), and the Geriatric Anxiety Inventory has proven to be effective in screening for anxiety [15–19]. The HADS is a well-known emotional distress self-report questionnaire. It is one of the most frequently used in cancer patients as well as in other medical settings. HADS excludes somatic symptoms of emotional distress (e.g., headache, weight loss, insomnia) that could be caused by the illness itself (including its treatments) rather than being emotional distress expressions [17, 18]. The GAI consists of 20 "Agree/Disagree" items designed to assess typical common anxiety symptoms [20]. The measurements of somatic symptoms with the instrument are limited in order to minimize confusion between symptoms common to anxiety and general medical conditions. Despite its use in anxiety screening in patients with other medical conditions, it has not been specifically validated in older adults with cancer. The BAI is a 21-question multiple-choice self-report inventory that is used for measuring the severity of anxiety. In older adults, the main limitation of the BAI is its inability to dedifferentiate between anxiety and depression, and the somatic subset that can overlap with symptoms of medical illness [21, 22]. The GAD-7 [23] contains seven items assessing core symptoms of generalized anxiety disorder. Patients rate their frequency of symptoms within the last 2 weeks on a 4-point scale ranging from "not at all" to "almost every day." Scores can take values from 0 to 21, with higher scores indicating higher GAD symptomatology. The American Society for Clinical Oncology [24] recommends the GAD-7 with a cut-off ≥10 indicating the need for intervention. Despite shortcomings of many screening tools listed here, using screening tools is helpful in identifying patients who require assessment by a mental health clinician. When moderate to severe or severe symptomatology is detected through screening, individuals should have a diagnostic assessment to identify the nature and extent of the anxiety symptoms and the presence or absence of an anxiety disorder or disorders.

Concerns for risk of harm to self and/or others, severe anxiety or agitation, or the presence of psychosis or delirium require referral to a psycho-oncologist. Given the multifactorial nature of anxiety in older adults with cancer and frailty, a multimodal biopsychosocial assessment is recommended with attention to biological, psychological, and psychosocial triggers of anxiety.

Management

Management of anxiety in cancer patients with frailty improves functioning, adherence to treatments, and overall quality of life. Untreated anxiety leads to social isolation, further worsening of symptoms and it may also interfere with decision-making capacity in older cancer patients with frailty facing complex decisions. Research in older adults with generalized anxiety disorders have shown increased risk of cerebrovascular and cardiovascular events, as well as an increased risk of conversion from mild cognitive impairment to dementia [25–27]. A retrospective cohort analysis of 13,426 cancer patients revealed that compared to patients with neither anxiety nor depression, those with anxiety alone, depression alone, or comorbid anxiety and depression were more likely to need an emergency room visit and be hospitalized. Length of hospital stays were also longer and annual healthcare costs were significantly higher in all three clinical groups [28]. Although data specific to older adults with cancer and frailty is limited, the burden of anxiety on patients and health care systems is notable and supports the need to vigilantly assess and manage anxiety in this patient population.

Treatment of anxiety varies depending on the severity of symptoms, including both psychotherapeutic approaches and pharmacological treatment. In older adults with cancer and frailty, non-pharmacological interventions may be preferred to minimize polypharmacy and reduce risk of aggravating comorbidities and geriatric syndromes. Psychotherapy modalities, such as cognitive behavioral therapy and problem-solving therapy are found to be effective for older adults in treating the symptoms of anxiety and are feasible to deliver in this population [15, 29]. Therapies like meaning-centered psychotherapy are particularly effective when an existential distress component is underlying [30]. The pharmacological treatment of anxiety in older adults with cancer primarily includes benzodiazepines, antidepressants, and low dose antipsychotics [31]. Although there is clinical evidence for using these medications for anxiety in older patients with cancer, there is scarce evidence on risks and benefits in the population with frailty [3]. According to a meta-analysis of 32 studies, pharmacotherapy is more effective than psychotherapy for late-life anxiety in community-dwelling older adults [32]. Often, benzodiazepines are used to address immediate and severe symptoms of anxiety and can provide benefits. They, however, carry the risk of excessive sedation, as well as cognitive impairment. The use of such sedating medications can lead to falls and delirium. Benzodiazepines additionally carry an increased risk of abuse and dependence. Given the increased risk of medication side effects among the older cancer patients with frailty, benzodiazepines should be judiciously used. Low dose antipsychotics may provide significant relief of anxiety symptoms; however, adverse effects should be closely monitored for. Antidepressants, specifically selective serotonin reuptake inhibitors (SSRIs) and serotonin-norepinephrine reuptake inhibitors (SNRIs) are considered the first-line treatment for late-life anxiety disorders [33]. While they may provide benefit in the long-term treatment of anxiety, they often take several weeks to reach optimal response. In older cancer patients with frailty, it is especially important to monitor for drug–drug interactions, syndrome of inappropriate antidiuretic hormone secretion, bleeding risk, and gastrointestinal side effects among others.

Depression

The prevalence of depression in older cancer patients ranges from 17 to 26% [34–36]. The severity of depressive symptoms in the context of cancer ranges from low mood to a full blown major depressive episode, commonly presenting with comorbid anxiety. Depression is typically characterized by anhedonia, depressed mood, low energy, sleep disturbances, loss of appetite, weight loss, inability to concentrate, feelings of guilt, and recurrent thoughts of death or suicide [37]. Depressive symptoms are often associated with negative outcomes including social isolation, poor quality of life, and treatment non-adherence [37]. In a prospective study of older cancer patients, geriatric assessment findings such as impaired mobility, impaired functional for activities of daily living, as well as inadequate social support, cognitive impairment, polypharmacy, multimorbidity, and cancer-related pain were all independently associated with depressive syndromes [38]. A study examining the impact of frailty on physical, mental, and social health among older women with breast cancer patients found that patients identified as pre-frail/frail reported worse depression compared to robust patients at follow-up. This study also showed that frailty in older women with breast cancer was associated with not only depression but also worse long-term quality of life [39]. A study focusing on older adults with gastrointestinal malignancies revealed that more than one out of eight older adults reported moderate/severe depression prior to chemotherapy, which was associated with impairments in several geriatric assessment domains and quality of life [40].

Assessment

Identifying depression in older adults with cancer and frailty presents challenges. While collateral information is helpful in providing details of functioning, level of activity, and changes from baseline, it is not always available. Many symptoms of depression may overlap with symptoms of frailty, symptoms of cancer, and cancer-treatment side effects. Patients who are non-compliant with cancer treatments or indecisive around treatment options should be screened for depression. Moreover, the assessment of depression should always include review of underlying medical etiologies such as hypothyroidism or brain metastasis, or medications such as corticosteroids, that may present with depressive symptoms.

When assessing for depression, it is also important to rule out any cognitive impairments. For example, it is not uncommon for hospitalized cancer patients with hypoactive subtype of delirium to be misdiagnosed as having depression [41]. Often, depressive symptoms are wrongfully considered to be a normal part of aging, both by patients and providers [42]. Commonly used depression diagnostic scales are not sensitive or specific enough to older people with cancer and may "miss" as many as 33–83% of older patients with clinically significant depressive symptoms [43]. Thus, it is likely that depression is underestimated in this population. The Diagnostic and Statistical Manual for Mental Disorders (DSM) criteria [44] consist of anhedonia, concentration difficulties, sleep disturbances, psychomotor retardation/agitation, and loss of energy. Loss of purpose, loneliness, irritability, and anxiety may also be indicative of depressive syndromes in older adults [43].

Screening for depression is a helpful and recommended strategy and some validated tools are available [45]. However, identifying depression in older patients with cancer and frailty is more complex [45, 46]. Nelson and colleagues examined eight commonly used depression measures to assess their utility with older cancer patients. A symptom profile analysis was conducted to determine if the screening measures addressed symptoms specific to older adults with depression including generalized aches and pains, diffuse somatic complaints, insomnia, malaise, hopelessness, mood variation, and change in sexual interest. None of the eight measures were deemed to adequately address these constructs [46]. Thus, the authors concluded that further validation and measure development with older cancer patient samples are needed. Saracino and colleagues examined the ability of three popular self-report measures of depression to assess depression in geriatric cancer patients. For this study, cancer patients aged 70 years or older completed the Geriatric

Depression Scale-Short Form, the Hospital Anxiety and Depression Scale, and the Center for Epidemiological Studies Depression Scale—Revised (CES-D). They were also interviewed using the depression module of the Structured Clinical Interview for DSM disorders (SCID) as the "gold standard." Although these measures produced good internal consistency and were better than chance at predicting depression in a geriatric cancer sample, the published cutoff scores for these measures did not perform well in predicting major depression or minor depression. Of the three measures, the CES-D appeared to have the most utility. This data suggested that these popular screening measures may be inadequate for reliably identifying depression in an older cancer population [45]. A French study looking at the diagnostic performance of the self-report 4-item version of the Geriatric Depression Scale has revealed the tool to be clinically relevant, easy to use for routine depression screening in older patients with cancer. The authors concluded that asking four questions might enable physicians to screen older patients with cancer for depression and guide them toward further clinical evaluation and appropriate care if required [38].

Management

Treatment of depression in older adults with cancer and frailty includes assessment and management of underlying medical etiologies that contribute to depressive symptoms, psychotherapy, and pharmacological interventions targeting depressive symptoms. Depression in patients with cancer is associated with worse physical symptoms, poor quality of life, longer hospitalizations, increased risk of emergency department visits, overnight hospitalization, and 30-day readmission, and shorter survival [47–51]. Furthermore, older adults with cancer are at increased risk for suicide relative to peers in the general population and those with other medical illnesses [51–53]. Therefore, older adults with cancer and depression are likely at heightened risk for suicide.

Despite the availability of efficacious treatments for depression in older adults with cancer, implementation of these interventions into clinical care settings has been poor [54, 55]. Approximately one-half of distressed patients with cancer do not receive mental health care, and only 5% receive evidence-based psychological care. Furthermore, older adults with cancer who screen positive for elevated distress are more likely than younger adults to decline a mental health referral [51, 56]. Barriers to mental health treatment in older adults with cancer include but are not limited to lack of knowledge about mental health treatments in patients and providers, stigma regarding receipt of mental health services, the number of competing appointments, and physical and financial hardships associated with aging [57]. Inadequate staffing can also reduce patient access to mental health services. The cost of providing mental health services and limited resources in health care settings are often cited as barriers to providing psychosocial care. However, research suggests that health care costs for patients with cancer and depression are much higher than for patients with cancer only [50, 58]. In a study of older adults with multiple myeloma, the cost of care in the first 6 months following the diagnosis was higher in patients with depression ($19,500) than in patients without depression ($12,300 [59]). Therefore, multiple studies suggest that untreated depression in patients with cancer may increase health care costs that can be reduced with mental health treatment [60]. Moreover, provision of mental health services to older adults with cancer and depression is likely to also improve quality of life [51]. Although these studies did not focus on frail older adults with cancer and depression, they certainly support management of depression in this patient population.

Regarding non-pharmacological interventions, evidence shows that structured modalities such as Cognitive Behavioral Therapy and Problem-Solving Therapy are more effective for older adults than less directive approaches such as psychodynamic psychotherapy [15]. In the older cancer patient with frailty, it is most beneficial to use a combination of various therapies as well as styles adapted to fit the complex needs of this patient population. Emphasizing psychosocial issues in treatment by encouraging social engagement and working with a social worker to address environmental and financial concerns may help alleviate distress for patients. Increasing social engagement is especially important to mitigate social isolation that interferes with treatment of depression and engagement of patients' in cancer care [61]. Exercise, behavioral activation, relaxation techniques, mindfulness-based stress reduction have all been studied, and found effective in management of depression in the medically ill [62–64]. The CARE Intervention (Cancer and Aging: Reflections of Elders) is one of the interventions that is specifically geared toward reducing depression, isolation, and despair related to the "double whammy" of aging and cancer [65]. The goal of CARE is to foster relatedness, acceptance of illness, and a sense of meaningful integration. It is a cognitive based, six-session intervention. CARE is grounded in an integration of Susan Folkman's cognitive coping paradigm, which utilizes reappraisal, and Erik Erikson's eighth and final psychosocial developmental life stage, in which the task is to achieve ego integrity. A pilot randomized controlled trial from our center suggests the CARE Intervention is feasible and effective in reducing depression, anxiety demoralization, and loneliness among older adults with cancer [65]. This pilot randomized controlled trial tested the feasibility and initial efficacy of CARE, drawing from age-appropriate developmental themes and well-established coping theory. Fifty-nine participants were randomized to either the CARE arm ($n = 31$) or the enhanced Social Work Control arm ($n = 28$). The intervention was feasible and tolerable, meeting a priori criteria for rates of eligibility, acceptance, retention, assessment, and treatment fidelity. Upon completion of the intervention, participants in the CARE arm demonstrated lower mean depression scores ($d = 0.58$ [CI: 0.04–1.12], $P = 0.01$). Promising trends in anxiety ($d = 0.41$ [CI: −0.17 to 0.98], $P = 0.10$) emerged at 2 months post-intervention; effects for coping-planning dissipated.

Regarding pharmacological interventions, antidepressants are the mainstay of pharmacological treatment in depression in cancer patients [66]. Antidepressants include selective serotonin reuptake inhibitors (SSRIs) such as sertraline, fluoxetine, escitalopram, and citalopram; serotonin and norepinephrine reuptake inhibitors (SNRIs) like venlafaxine and duloxetine; and the dopamine reuptake inhibitor bupropion. While these medications are generally well tolerated by older cancer patients, caution should be utilized when administering antidepressants with anticholinergic side effects such as tricyclic antidepressants or SSRI's like paroxetine [3]. Anticholinergic burden has been associated with increased risk of falls, fractures, cognitive impairment, and mortality in older adults, hence should be prevented [67, 68]. When initiating new medications, potential drug–drug interactions should be thoroughly reviewed. Starting low, going slow is the best strategy when using antidepressants in older adults with cancer, particularly those with frailty and polypharmacy. Medications like mirtazapine can be preferred in patients with insomnia or appetite loss, given its side effects of increased sleep and appetite. Common side effects of antidepressants may include gastrointestinal symptoms such as discomfort, nausea, diarrhea as well as drowsiness and sexual problems [69, 70]. While these side effects may dissipate over time, starting at a low dose, and titrating the dose slowly can help mitigate these side effects. Similarly, when lowering the dose, a slow taper is recommended to prevent discontinuation syndrome or withdrawal [71, 72]. In order to see the full effects of a medication, patients would need to be on a therapeutic dose of an antidepressant for about 4–6 weeks. Serotonin syndrome is a rare side effect of serotonergic medications such as SSRI's, however, should be closely monitored among frail cancer patients who are on other serotonergic agents such as fentanyl or tramadol. Serotonin syndrome is a potentially fatal drug-induced condition caused by too much serotonin in synapses in the brain. Patients present with a combination of neuromuscular, autonomic, and mental status symptoms. Most cases involve two drugs that increase serotonin in different ways or an overdose of one serotonin drug. Monoamine oxidase inhibitors, serotonin-norepinephrine reuptake inhibitors, and selective serotonin reuptake inhibitors are the most common culprits. The use of two high-dose serotonin drugs at the same time should be avoided. Prevention of serotonin toxicity is key. Education of prescribers and patients is important to avoid and detect serotonin toxicity [73].

Another consideration for pharmacological treatment of depression in cancer patients is the use of psychostimulants which can target symptoms such as depressed mood, fatigue, and cognitive slowing [74, 75]. Psychostimulants like methylphenidate and dextroamphetamines should be initiated at low dosages and titrated slowly as well. When considering psychostimulants in frail older adults with cancer, it is essential to monitor for potential side effects such impairments in sleep, worsening of anxiety, as well tics and paranoia [76]. The main benefit of using psychostimulants in cancer patients is the ability to see improvements in relatively short periods of time. Therefore, in palliative care settings, they may be preferred to antidepressants given the onset of action with antidepressants would be weeks as opposed to days with psychostimulants. Modafinil and armodafinil, known as wakefulness-promoting agents, can be considered in older cancer patients who primarily present with fatigue, amotivation, and depressive symptoms. Anecdotally, modafinil and armodafinil are well tolerated among older cancer patients.

Suicide

The rates of suicidal ideation are higher among older patients with cancer compared to the general population. Suicide completion rates are on average 50% higher in cancer patients than in the healthy population [77]. Characteristics associated with suicide in the cancer population, such as older age and male sex, are similar to those in the general population. Suicide risk among patients with cancer as a group is highest in the years immediately after diagnosis, but remains increased for more than 15 years as compared with the suicide rates in the general population. Suicide rates are also higher among patients with advanced disease at diagnosis.

While there are many different contributing factors to suicidal ideation such as poor physical function and lack of control, utilizing social supports to ensure monitoring and maintaining a safe environment is vital. A history of prior suicide attempts increases the risk for suicide. Personal or family history of mental illness and history of psychiatric hospitalization are additional risk factors. Delirium, cognitive impairment due to other etiologies, such as brain lesions also place patients at higher risk for suicide due to poor impulse control and increased risk of disinhibition. Desire for hastened death is an important construct to assess for in frail older adults with cancer. Patients who present with a desire for hastened death should be screened for common risk factors such as depression or history of psychiatric illness, hopelessness, physical distress (including pain and symptom burden), poor social support, fear of being a burden to others as well as existential concerns such as loss of meaning and loss of dignity. Studies have shown that when these factors are treated, patients show a decrease in desire for hastened death. Treating underlying conditions that compromise quality of life, such as pain, discomfort, fatigue, depression, and anxiety is essential as these conditions may exacerbate patients' negative views of the future and suicidal thoughts. The emphasis of intervention should be to aggressively attempt to prevent suicide that is driven by the desperation of uncontrolled physical and psychological symptoms such as uncontrolled pain, unrecognized delirium, and unrecognized and untreated depression. Prolonged suffering caused by poorly controlled symptoms may lead to such desperation, and it is the appropriate role of the clinician to provide effective management of physical and psychological symptoms as an alternative to desire for death, suicides, or requests for assisted suicide by their patient [78].

Suicidal ideation and behavior have traditionally been conceived as a unidimensional construct, with passive ideation, active intent, and behavior existing along a continuum screening tools such as Columbia Suicide Severity Rating Scale (C-SSRS) are helpful in stratifying suicide risk to identify patients who may require higher level of care and/or referral to psychiatry [78, 79]. The C-SSRS was designed to provide definitions of suicidal ideation and behavior and non-suicidal self-injurious behavior and corresponding probes; to quantify the full spectrum of suicidal ideation and suicidal behavior and gauge their severity over specified periods; to distinguish suicidal behavior and non-suicidal self-injurious behavior; and to employ a user-friendly format that allows integration of information from multiple sources (e.g., direct patient interview, family and other interviews, and medical records). In our institution, all cancer patients are screened for suicide by use of C-SSRS during all initial visits, and on a daily basis in the inpatient medical setting.

Sleep Disturbances

Sleep is often an issue for many patients with cancer but even more problematic with age. A history of cancer increases the likelihood of having sleep disturbance. Sleep disturbance is common, with a reported prevalence of between 30 and 72% in individuals with cancer [80]. In a sample of older cancer patients receiving treatment, the prevalence of sleep disturbance was reported to be 60%. In the general geriatric population, presence of sleep disturbance is associated with poor physical function, anxiety, depression and may predict cognitive decline [1, 81]. In cancer patients with sleep disturbance, there is higher rate of impairment in daytime functioning and cognitive functions such as concentration and memory [82, 83]. The National Comprehensive Cancer Network, Older Adult Oncology Guidelines recommend that older adults with cancer should be screened for sleep disturbances prior to the initiation of treatment and at regular intervals during the course of treatment [1]. The American Geriatric Society and the Pan-Canadian practice guidelines provide recommendations for the prevention, screening, assessment, and treatment of sleep disturbances in older adults, the latter guidelines focusing on older adults with cancer. In frail older adults with cancer, this holistic assessment is particularly important given impact of sleep disturbances on frailty and vice versa [84].

Regarding the assessment of sleep disturbance, patients whose sleep is disturbed by waking up in the middle of the night should be assessed further to rule out medical etiologies, such as frequent urination, pain, or gastrointestinal symptoms. However, if the patient has difficulty falling asleep and returning to sleep due to ruminative thoughts, or anxiety, then the sleep disruption may indicate a mood disorder. Sleep wake cycle disturbances may also be indicative of delirium or other cognitive syndromes. Moreover, some medications, such as corticosteroids which are widely used in cancer patients, can lead to insomnia. A sleep study may be considered to rule out sleep apnea especially for patients with head and neck cancers, comorbid obesity, or other medical comorbidities.

Once reversible causes have been ruled out, the primary focus should be on non-pharmacological interventions to improve sleep. Cognitive behavioral therapy for insomnia has proven effective among cancer patients and in older adults [85]. Sedative-hypnotics such benzodiazepines, should be avoided, if at all possible, given side effects associated with their use in frail older adults. Melatonin or melatonin agonists are safe alternative specifically for patients with sleep wake cycle changes. Mirtazapine, a sedating antidepressant, could be considered for older adults with comorbid insomnia, anorexia, and other depressive symptoms. Most patients with steroid-induced insomnia may require low dose antipsychotics for severe insomnia.

For further guidance, the American Geriatric Society has provided recommendations for the diagnosis, assessment, and management of insomnia in older adults [86]. The Pan-Canadian practice guidelines also provide recommendations for prevention, screening, assessment, and management of sleep disturbances in older patients with cancer [84].

Cancer-Related Fatigue

Cancer-Related Fatigue (CRF) is defined as "a distressing, persistent, subjective sense of physical, emotional, and cognitive tiredness or exhaustion related to cancer or cancer treatment that is not proportional to recent activity and interferes with usual functioning [87]." CRF is more severe and more distressing than the fatigue experienced by healthy individuals and is less likely to be relieved by rest. CRF is present at the time of diagnosis in approximately 50% of patients with cancer [88]. The reported prevalence of CRF is variable, with ranges depending on the specific cancer population studied and the methods of assessment [89]. Fatigue is highly prevalent in frail older adults with cancer [39, 90]. Studies have focused on understanding factors that contribute to fatigue, which include the cancer itself, cancer-related treatments, and a variety of physical and psychological comorbidities (e.g., anemia, pain, depression, anxiety, cachexia, sleep disturbances, and immobility) [91, 92].

All cancer patients should be screened for the presence and severity of fatigue at their initial visit, frequently during and following cancer treatment, and as clinically indicated [14]. One-dimensional scales, that are easy to use and brief to administer, are recommended in elderly patients. Some examples are the Functional Assessment of Cancer Therapy Fatigue subscale and the European Organization for Research and Treatment of Cancer Quality of Life Questionnaire Fatigue subscale (QLQ-C30) [93, 94]. The etiologies of fatigue are complex and varied but are generally related to cancer type and characteristics, patient factors (e.g., underlying comorbidities, psychological comorbidities), and treatment factors (e.g., medications, postoperative).

Potentially reversible causes of fatigue should be identified and treated, and non-essential centrally acting drugs (including prescription drugs, over-the-counter medications, and supplements) should be eliminated. Clinicians should ask and examine for alcohol, prescription, and illicit drug misuse. Non-pharmacological approaches have been recommended by guidelines for the treatment of CRF include physical activity and psychosocial interventions [87]. Pharmacological strategies include psychostimulants, which have been suggested to be effective for treating fatigue [95, 96], with close monitoring of patients with hypertension, underlying coronary artery disease, and tachyarrhythmias. A significant placebo response has been observed in randomized trials except for patients with severe levels of fatigue [97].

Substance-Use Disorders

Alcohol-use disorder, prescription drug misuse, and illicit drug use are growing health problems in later life yet may be overlooked by health care providers. Few studies examined substance use in cancer patients. In a systematic review, substance-use rates ranged from 2 to 35%, with a median opioid rate of 18 and 25.5% for alcohol in a mixed age patient population [98]. Although opioid abuse is growing among older adults, cannabis is currently the most frequently used illicit substance in this age group [99]. Alcohol-use disorder remains the most prevalent substance-use disorder in later life [100]. Since frail older adults are more likely to have multiple chronic health conditions and to be using prescription medications that can interact with alcohol and other substances, they are at increased risk for adverse consequences.

Unrecognized substance-use disorders can cause substantial harm to older adults in the form of an increased risk of falls, cognitive impairment, and medical morbidity, which can contribute to hospitalizations and health care costs, as well as loss of independence. All clinicians who care for older adults must be alert for possible signs and symptoms of substance-use disorders in their patients. Use of prescription drug monitoring programs help identify persons who obtain multiple prescriptions for medications with high misuse potential.

The management of opioid use disorder can be challenging in cancer patients because pain is a multidimensional experience encompassing physical and psychological domains. An interdisciplinary team approach is most effective, and management strategies may include harm reduction, including opioid switching, avoiding concurrent sedative use, and using adjuvant medications for their opioid-sparing potential, managing psychological distress with an interdisciplinary team and risk mitigation by pill counts, frequent clinic visits, and accessing statewide prescription drug monitoring plans [101]. Research is needed to develop targeted screening methods and to identify the best treatment models for substance-use disorders in frail older adults with cancer. Treatment plans must incorporate care for older patients with coexisting medical and psychiatric illnesses [102].

Social Support

Social frailty is a multidimensional concept where social resources (or restrictions), behaviors, and activities make people more vulnerable [103]. It is important to consider how the social determinants of health [104] (SDOH) may play a central role in preventing or predicting deterioration into a physically frail state. SDOH include education; health care; neighborhood and environment; social and community context; and economic stability, and have been shown to play a critical role in health [105] and aging [106, 107]. Woo et al. [108] identified that for older men, increasing frailty was observed for those from non-white collar occupations, with limited social support, and low socioeconomic status. For older women, little contact with relatives and absence of participation in religious and community activities were also risk factors. Therefore, social frailty also warrants close consideration by cancer clinicians.

The assessment of social frailty is conducted during the social history aspect of the clinical interview. Although there is no definitive tool to assess social frailty [109], validated tools for the assessment of social network [110, 111], social support [112], and SDOH [113] exist in the literature, and may serve as proxies for it in the older adult population. An increase of SDOH screening has shown to be cost-effective and has been associated with earlier diagnosis, treatment, and improved health outcomes with significant gains in quality-of-life-adjusted-years in Breast, Cervical, and Colorectal cancer patients [114].

Interventions aimed toward the improvement of outcomes associated with social frailty and SDOH include group interventions of provided volunteer, educational and physical activities, and have shown improvement in social participation, social isolation, and loneliness in elderly minority groups [115]. Consensus on the determination of social frailty, its assessment, and research on interventions aimed to improve it in the elderly cancer population are needed.

Conclusion

Oncology clinicians play an essential role in the identification, assessment, and management of psychosocial aspects of care. Close attention to the psychosocial dimension at all stages of cancer, from early cancer diagnosis to survivorship, from early conversations of palliative care till the terminal stages of cancer, improves care of older cancer patients, particularly those with frailty. The paucity of research in this highly vulnerable patient population, not just for those with active cancer but also for cancer survivors [116], is of concern and calls for urgent collaboration between oncologists, geriatricians, and psychosocial care providers to conduct studies and improve outcomes for older cancer patients with frailty.

References

1. National Comprehensive Cancer Network. Older adult oncology guidelines (Version 1.2020). 2020. https://www.nccn.org/professionals/physician_gls/pdf/senior.pdf. Accessed 23 Oct 2020.
2. Handforth C, Clegg A, Young C, Simpkins S, Seymour MT, Selby PJ, et al. The prevalence and outcomes of frailty in older cancer patients: a systematic review. Ann Oncol. 2015;26(6):1091–101. https://doi.org/10.1093/annonc/mdu540.
3. Extermann M, Hurria A. Comprehensive geriatric assessment for older patients with cancer. J Clin Oncol. 2007;25(14):1824–31. https://doi.org/10.1200/jco.2007.10.6559.

4. Miller KD, Nogueira L, Mariotto AB, Rowland JH, Yabroff KR, Alfano CM, et al. Cancer treatment and survivorship statistics, 2019. CA Cancer J Clin. 2019;69(5):363–85. https://doi.org/10.3322/caac.21565.
5. Valdivieso M, Kujawa AM, Jones T, Baker LH. Cancer survivors in the United States: a review of the literature and a call to action. Int J Med Sci. 2012;9(2):163–73. https://doi.org/10.7150/ijms.3827.
6. Hall J, Kellett S, Berrios R, Bains MK, Scott S. Efficacy of cognitive behavioral therapy for generalized anxiety disorder in older adults: systematic review, meta-analysis, and meta-regression. Am J Geriatr Psychiatry. 2016;24(11):1063–73. https://doi.org/10.1016/j.jagp.2016.06.006.
7. Warner DF, Schiltz NK, Stange KC, Given CW, Owusu C, Berger NA, et al. Complex multi-morbidity and health outcomes in older adult cancer survivors. Fam Med Community Health. 2017;5(2):129–38. https://doi.org/10.15212/fmch.2017.0127.
8. Riba MB, Donovan KA, Andersen B, Braun I, Breitbart WS, Brewer BW, et al. Distress management, version 3.2019, NCCN clinical practice guidelines in oncology. J Natl Compr Canc Netw. 2019;17(10):1229–49. https://doi.org/10.6004/jnccn.2019.0048.
9. Meier C, Taubenheim S, Lordick F, Mehnert-Theuerkauf A, Götze H. Depression and anxiety in older patients with hematological cancer (70+)—geriatric, social, cancer- and treatment-related associations. J Geriatr Oncol. 2020;11(5):828–35. https://doi.org/10.1016/j.jgo.2019.11.009.
10. Zhao W, Zhang Y, Liu X, Yue J, Hou L, Xia X, et al. Comorbid depressive and anxiety symptoms and frailty among older adults: findings from the West China health and aging trend study. J Affect Disord. 2020;277:970–6. https://doi.org/10.1016/j.jad.2020.08.070.
11. Bakkane Bendixen A, Engedal K, Selbæk G, Hartberg CB. Anxiety symptoms in older adults with depression are associated with suicidality. Dement Geriatr Cogn Disord. 2018;45(3-4):180–9. https://doi.org/10.1159/000488480.
12. Oncology ASoC: screening, assessment, and care of anxiety and depressive symptoms in adults with cancer. 2014. https://www.asco.org/sites/new-www.asco.org/files/content-files/practice-and-guidelines/documents/depression-anxiety-summary-of-recs-table.pdf. Accessed 17 Mar 2021.
13. Radue R, Walaszek A, Asthana S. Neuropsychiatric symptoms in dementia. Handb Clin Neurol. 2019;167:437–54. https://doi.org/10.1016/b978-0-12-804766-8.00024-8.
14. Network NCC: Cancer-Related Fatigue V.2. 2020. https://www.nccn.org/professionals/physician_gls/pdf/fatigue.pdf. Accessed 1 Oct 2020.
15. Cuijpers P, Karyotaki E, Pot AM, Park M, Reynolds CF 3rd. Managing depression in older age: psychological interventions. Maturitas. 2014;79(2):160–9. https://doi.org/10.1016/j.maturitas.2014.05.027.
16. Esser P, Hartung TJ, Friedrich M, Johansen C, Wittchen HU, Faller H, et al. The Generalized Anxiety Disorder Screener (GAD-7) and the anxiety module of the Hospital and Depression Scale (HADS-A) as screening tools for generalized anxiety disorder among cancer patients. Psychooncology. 2018;27(6):1509–16. https://doi.org/10.1002/pon.4681.
17. Annunziata MA, Muzzatti B, Bidoli E, Flaiban C, Bomben F, Piccinin M, et al. Hospital Anxiety and Depression Scale (HADS) accuracy in cancer patients. Support Care Cancer. 2020;28(8):3921–6. https://doi.org/10.1007/s00520-019-05244-8.
18. Zigmond AS, Snaith RP. The hospital anxiety and depression scale. Acta Psychiatr Scand. 1983;67(6):361–70. https://doi.org/10.1111/j.1600-0447.1983.tb09716.x.
19. Beck AT, Epstein N, Brown G, Steer RA. An inventory for measuring clinical anxiety: psychometric properties. J Consult Clin Psychol. 1988;56(6):893–7. https://doi.org/10.1037//0022-006x.56.6.893.
20. Pachana NA, Byrne GJ, Siddle H, Koloski N, Harley E, Arnold E. Development and validation of the Geriatric Anxiety Inventory. Int Psychogeriatr. 2007;19(1):103–14. https://doi.org/10.1017/s1041610206003504.

21. Muntingh AD, van der Feltz-Cornelis CM, van Marwijk HW, Spinhoven P, Penninx BW, van Balkom AJ. Is the Beck Anxiety Inventory a good tool to assess the severity of anxiety? A primary care study in the Netherlands Study of Depression and Anxiety (NESDA). BMC Fam Pract. 2011;12:66. https://doi.org/10.1186/1471-2296-12-66.
22. Krasucki C, Howard R, Mann A. The relationship between anxiety disorders and age. Int J Geriatr Psychiatry. 1998;13(2):79–99. https://doi.org/10.1002/(sici)1099-1166(199802)13:2<79::aid-gps739>3.0.co;2-g.
23. Spitzer RL, Kroenke K, Williams JB, Löwe B. A brief measure for assessing generalized anxiety disorder: the GAD-7. Arch Intern Med. 2006;166(10):1092–7. https://doi.org/10.1001/archinte.166.10.1092.
24. Andersen BL, DeRubeis RJ, Berman BS, Gruman J, Champion VL, Massie MJ, et al. Screening, assessment, and care of anxiety and depressive symptoms in adults with cancer: an American Society of Clinical Oncology guideline adaptation. J Clin Oncol. 2014;32(15):1605–19. https://doi.org/10.1200/jco.2013.52.4611.
25. Lambiase MJ, Kubzansky LD, Thurston RC. Prospective study of anxiety and incident stroke. Stroke. 2014;45(2):438–43. https://doi.org/10.1161/strokeaha.113.003741.
26. Tully PJ, Cosh SM, Baune BT. A review of the affects of worry and generalized anxiety disorder upon cardiovascular health and coronary heart disease. Psychol Health Med. 2013;18(6):627–44. https://doi.org/10.1080/13548506.2012.749355.
27. Rosenberg PB, Mielke MM, Appleby BS, Oh ES, Geda YE, Lyketsos CG. The association of neuropsychiatric symptoms in MCI with incident dementia and Alzheimer disease. Am J Geriatr Psychiatry. 2013;21(7):685–95. https://doi.org/10.1016/j.jagp.2013.01.006.
28. Mausbach BT, Decastro G, Schwab RB, Tiamson-Kassab M, Irwin SA. Healthcare use and costs in adult cancer patients with anxiety and depression. Depress Anxiety. 2020;37(9):908–15. https://doi.org/10.1002/da.23059.
29. Moorey S, Greer S. Cognitive behaviour therapy for people with cancer. New York: Oxford University Press; 2002.
30. Breitbart W, Pessin H, Rosenfeld B, Applebaum AJ, Lichtenthal WG, Li Y, et al. Individual meaning-centered psychotherapy for the treatment of psychological and existential distress: a randomized controlled trial in patients with advanced cancer. Cancer. 2018;124(15):3231–9. https://doi.org/10.1002/cncr.31539.
31. Gonçalves DC, Byrne GJ. Interventions for generalized anxiety disorder in older adults: systematic review and meta-analysis. J Anxiety Disord. 2012;26(1):1–11. https://doi.org/10.1016/j.janxdis.2011.08.010.
32. Pinquart M, Duberstein PR. Treatment of anxiety disorders in older adults: a meta-analytic comparison of behavioral and pharmacological interventions. Am J Geriatr Psychiatry. 2007;15(8):639–51. https://doi.org/10.1097/JGP.0b013e31806841c8.
33. Andreescu C, Lee S. Anxiety disorders in the elderly. Adv Exp Med Biol. 2020;1191:561–76. https://doi.org/10.1007/978-981-32-9705-0_28.
34. Alexopoulos GS, Borson S, Cuthbert BN, Devanand DP, Mulsant BH, Olin JT, et al. Assessment of late life depression. Biol Psychiatry. 2002;52(3):164–74. https://doi.org/10.1016/s0006-3223(02)01381-1.
35. Atag E, Mutlay F, Soysal P, Semiz HS, Kazaz SN, Keser M, et al. Prevalence of depressive symptoms in elderly cancer patients receiving chemotherapy and influencing factors. Psychogeriatrics. 2018;18(5):365–70. https://doi.org/10.1111/psyg.12329.
36. Parajuli J, Berish D, Valenti KG, Jao YL. Prevalence and predictors of depressive symptoms in older adults with cancer. J Geriatr Oncol. 2021;12(4):618–22. https://doi.org/10.1016/j.jgo.2020.12.009.
37. American Psychiatric Association. Diagnostic and statistical manual of mental disorders. Arlington, VA: American Psychiatric Association; 2013.
38. Canoui-Poitrine F, Reinald N, Laurent M, Guery E, Caillet P, David JP, et al. Geriatric assessment findings independently associated with clinical depression in 1092 older patients with cancer: the ELCAPA Cohort Study. Psychooncology. 2016;25(1):104–11. https://doi.org/10.1002/pon.3886.

39. Williams GR, Deal AM, Sanoff HK, Nyrop KA, Guerard EJ, Pergolotti M, et al. Frailty and health-related quality of life in older women with breast cancer. Support Care Cancer. 2019;27(7):2693–8. https://doi.org/10.1007/s00520-018-4558-6.
40. Godby RC, Dai C, Al-Obaidi M, Giri S, Young-Smith C, Kenzik K, et al. Depression among older adults with gastrointestinal malignancies. J Geriatr Oncol. 2021;12(4):599–604. https://doi.org/10.1016/j.jgo.2020.10.020.
41. Barboza MS, Cittadini J, de Hertelendy M, Farías MS, Loiacono N. Liaison psychiatry: playing "hide and seek" with delirium. In: Gargiulo P, Mesones-Arroyo H, editors. Psychiatry and neuroscience update. Cham: Springer; 2017.
42. Haigh EAP, Bogucki OE, Sigmon ST, Blazer DG. Depression among older adults: a 20-year update on five common myths and misconceptions. Am J Geriatr Psychiatry. 2018;26(1):107–22. https://doi.org/10.1016/j.jagp.2017.06.011.
43. Saracino RM, Rosenfeld B, Nelson CJ. Towards a new conceptualization of depression in older adult cancer patients: a review of the literature. Aging Ment Health. 2016;20(12):1230–42. https://doi.org/10.1080/13607863.2015.1078278.
44. American Psychiatric Association. Anxiety disorders. 5 ed. Diagnostic and statistical manual of mental disorders. Washington, DC: American Psychiatric Association; 2013.
45. Saracino RM, Weinberger MI, Roth AJ, Hurria A, Nelson CJ. Assessing depression in a geriatric cancer population. Psychooncology. 2017;26(10):1484–90. https://doi.org/10.1002/pon.4160.
46. Nelson CJ, Cho C, Berk AR, Holland J, Roth AJ. Are gold standard depression measures appropriate for use in geriatric cancer patients? A systematic evaluation of self-report depression instruments used with geriatric, cancer, and geriatric cancer samples. J Clin Oncol. 2010;28(2):348–56. https://doi.org/10.1200/jco.2009.23.0201.
47. Balentine CJ, Hermosillo-Rodriguez J, Robinson CN, Berger DH, Naik AD. Depression is associated with prolonged and complicated recovery following colorectal surgery. J Gastrointest Surg. 2011;15(10):1712–7. https://doi.org/10.1007/s11605-011-1640-5.
48. Horney DJ, Smith HE, McGurk M, Weinman J, Herold J, Altman K, et al. Associations between quality of life, coping styles, optimism, and anxiety and depression in pretreatment patients with head and neck cancer. Head Neck. 2011;33(1):65–71. https://doi.org/10.1002/hed.21407.
49. Brown LF, Kroenke K. Cancer-related fatigue and its associations with depression and anxiety: a systematic review. Psychosomatics. 2009;50(5):440–7. https://doi.org/10.1176/appi.psy.50.5.440.
50. Huo J, Hong Y, Xiao H, Wilkie DJ. The impact of post-diagnosis depression on survival and healthcare costs for patients diagnosed with late-stage cancer in the United States. Value Health. 2018;21:S25–S6. https://doi.org/10.1016/j.jval.2018.04.159.
51. Magnuson A, Sattar S, Nightingale G, Saracino R, Skonecki E, Trevino KM. A practical guide to geriatric syndromes in older adults with cancer: a focus on falls, cognition, polypharmacy, and depression. Am Soc Clin Oncol Educ Book. 2019;39:e96–e109. https://doi.org/10.1200/edbk_237641.
52. Miller M, Mogun H, Azrael D, Hempstead K, Solomon DH. Cancer and the risk of suicide in older Americans. J Clin Oncol. 2008;26(29):4720–4. https://doi.org/10.1200/jco.2007.14.3990.
53. Kiosses DN, Szanto K, Alexopoulos GS. Suicide in older adults: the role of emotions and cognition. Curr Psychiatry Rep. 2014;16(11):495. https://doi.org/10.1007/s11920-014-0495-3.
54. Zebrack B, Kayser K, Bybee D, Padgett L, Sundstrom L, Jobin C, et al. A practice-based evaluation of distress screening protocol adherence and medical service utilization. J Natl Compr Canc Netw. 2017;15(7):903–12. https://doi.org/10.6004/jnccn.2017.0120.
55. Kadan-Lottick NS, Vanderwerker LC, Block SD, Zhang B, Prigerson HG. Psychiatric disorders and mental health service use in patients with advanced cancer: a report from the coping with cancer study. Cancer. 2005;104(12):2872–81. https://doi.org/10.1002/cncr.21532.
56. Sharpe M, Strong V, Allen K, Rush R, Postma K, Tulloh A, et al. Major depression in outpatients attending a regional cancer centre: screening and unmet treatment needs. Br J Cancer. 2004;90(2):314–20. https://doi.org/10.1038/sj.bjc.6601578.

57. Tuinman MA, Gazendam-Donofrio SM, Hoekstra-Weebers JE. Screening and referral for psychosocial distress in oncologic practice: use of the Distress Thermometer. Cancer. 2008;113(4):870–8. https://doi.org/10.1002/cncr.23622.
58. Mausbach BT, Yeung P, Bos T, Irwin SA. Health care costs of depression in patients diagnosed with cancer. Psychooncology. 2018;27(7):1735–41. https://doi.org/10.1002/pon.4716.
59. Niazi S, Frank RD, Sharma M, Roy V, Ames S, Rummans T, et al. Impact of psychiatric comorbidities on health care utilization and cost of care in multiple myeloma. Blood Adv. 2018;2(10):1120–8. https://doi.org/10.1182/bloodadvances.2018016717.
60. Mausbach BT, Bos T, Irwin SA. Mental health treatment dose and annual healthcare costs in patients with cancer and major depressive disorder. Health Psychol. 2018;37(11):1035–40. https://doi.org/10.1037/hea0000670.
61. Fakoya OA, McCorry NK, Donnelly M. Loneliness and social isolation interventions for older adults: a scoping review of reviews. BMC Public Health. 2020;20(1):129. https://doi.org/10.1186/s12889-020-8251-6.
62. Trevino KM, Healy C, Martin P, Canin B, Pillemer K, Sirey JA, et al. Improving implementation of psychological interventions to older adult patients with cancer: convening older adults, caregivers, providers, researchers. J Geriatr Oncol. 2018;9(5):423–9. https://doi.org/10.1016/j.jgo.2018.04.007.
63. Bell AC, D'Zurilla TJ. Problem-solving therapy for depression: a meta-analysis. Clin Psychol Rev. 2009;29(4):348–53. https://doi.org/10.1016/j.cpr.2009.02.003.
64. Knight BG. Adapting older adults to cognitive behavior therapy and vice versa: the case of Geoffrey. Pragmatic Case Stud Psychother. 2008;4(module 3):40–3.
65. Nelson CJ, Saracino RM, Roth AJ, Harvey E, Martin A, Moore M, et al. Cancer and Aging: Reflections for Elders (CARE): a pilot randomized controlled trial of a psychotherapy intervention for older adults with cancer. Psychooncology. 2019;28(1):39–47. https://doi.org/10.1002/pon.4907.
66. Kim HF, Fisch MJ. Antidepressant use in ambulatory cancer patients. Curr Oncol Rep. 2006;8(4):275–81. https://doi.org/10.1007/s11912-006-0033-5.
67. Graves-Morris K, Stewart C, Soiza RL, Taylor-Rowan M, Quinn TJ, Loke YK, et al. The prognostic value of anticholinergic burden measures in relation to mortality in older individuals: a systematic review and meta-analysis. Front Pharmacol. 2020;11:570. https://doi.org/10.3389/fphar.2020.00570.
68. Cardwell K, Hughes CM, Ryan C. The association between anticholinergic medication burden and health related outcomes in the 'oldest old': a systematic review of the literature. Drugs Aging. 2015;32(10):835–48. https://doi.org/10.1007/s40266-015-0310-9.
69. Cipriani A, Furukawa TA, Salanti G, Chaimani A, Atkinson LZ, Ogawa Y, et al. Comparative efficacy and acceptability of 21 antidepressant drugs for the acute treatment of adults with major depressive disorder: a systematic review and network meta-analysis. Lancet. 2018;391(10128):1357–66. https://doi.org/10.1016/s0140-6736(17)32802-7.
70. Sobieraj DM, Martinez BK, Hernandez AV, Coleman CI, Ross JS, Berg KM, et al. Adverse effects of pharmacologic treatments of major depression in older adults. J Am Geriatr Soc. 2019;67(8):1571–81. https://doi.org/10.1111/jgs.15966.
71. Fava GA, Benasi G, Lucente M, Offidani E, Cosci F, Guidi J. Withdrawal symptoms after serotonin-noradrenaline reuptake inhibitor discontinuation: systematic review. Psychother Psychosom. 2018;87(4):195–203. https://doi.org/10.1159/000491524.
72. Maund E, Stuart B, Moore M, Dowrick C, Geraghty AWA, Dawson S, et al. Managing antidepressant discontinuation: a systematic review. Ann Fam Med. 2019;17(1):52–60. https://doi.org/10.1370/afm.2336.
73. Foong AL, Grindrod KA, Patel T, Kellar J. Demystifying serotonin syndrome (or serotonin toxicity). Can Fam Physician. 2018;64(10):720–7.
74. Masand PS, Tesar GE. Use of stimulants in the medically ill. Psychiatr Clin North Am. 1996;19(3):515–47. https://doi.org/10.1016/s0193-953x(05)70304-x.

75. Andrew BN, Guan NC, Jaafar NRN. The use of methylphenidate for physical and psychological symptoms in cancer patients: a review. Curr Drug Targets. 2018;19(8):877–87. https://doi.org/10.2174/1389450118666170317162603.
76. Breitbart W, Dickerman AL. Assessment and management of depression in palliative care. Emanuel EJ, Emanuel L, Roy-Byrne PR, section editors; Savarese DMF, Solomon D, deputy editors. 2017.
77. Misono S, Weiss NS, Fann JR, Redman M, Yueh B. Incidence of suicide in persons with cancer. J Clin Oncol. 2008;26(29):4731–8. https://doi.org/10.1200/jco.2007.13.8941.
78. McFarland DC, Walsh L, Napolitano S, Morita J, Jaiswal R. Suicide in patients with cancer: identifying the risk factors. Oncology (Williston Park). 2019;33(6):221–6.
79. Posner K, Brown GK, Stanley B, Brent DA, Yershova KV, Oquendo MA, et al. The Columbia-Suicide Severity Rating Scale: initial validity and internal consistency findings from three multisite studies with adolescents and adults. Am J Psychiatry. 2011;168(12):1266–77. https://doi.org/10.1176/appi.ajp.2011.10111704.
80. Savard J, Ivers H, Villa J, Caplette-Gingras A, Morin CM. Natural course of insomnia comorbid with cancer: an 18-month longitudinal study. J Clin Oncol. 2011;29(26):3580–6. https://doi.org/10.1200/jco.2010.33.2247.
81. Cricco M, Simonsick EM, Foley DJ. The impact of insomnia on cognitive functioning in older adults. J Am Geriatr Soc. 2001;49(9):1185–9. https://doi.org/10.1046/j.1532-5415.2001.49235.x.
82. Cheng KK, Lee DT. Effects of pain, fatigue, insomnia, and mood disturbance on functional status and quality of life of elderly patients with cancer. Crit Rev Oncol Hematol. 2011;78(2):127–37. https://doi.org/10.1016/j.critrevonc.2010.03.002.
83. Loh KP, Pandya C, Zittel J, Kadambi S, Flannery M, Reizine N, et al. Associations of sleep disturbance with physical function and cognition in older adults with cancer. Support Care Cancer. 2017;25(10):3161–9. https://doi.org/10.1007/s00520-017-3724-6.
84. Howell D, Oliver TK, Keller-Olaman S, Davidson J, Garland S, Samuels C, et al. A Pan-Canadian practice guideline: prevention, screening, assessment, and treatment of sleep disturbances in adults with cancer. Support Care Cancer. 2013;21(10):2695–706. https://doi.org/10.1007/s00520-013-1823-6.
85. Johnson JA, Rash JA, Campbell TS, Savard J, Gehrman PR, Perlis M, et al. A systematic review and meta-analysis of randomized controlled trials of cognitive behavior therapy for insomnia (CBT-I) in cancer survivors. Sleep Med Rev. 2016;27:20–8. https://doi.org/10.1016/j.smrv.2015.07.001.
86. Bloom HG, Ahmed I, Alessi CA, Ancoli-Israel S, Buysse DJ, Kryger MH, et al. Evidence-based recommendations for the assessment and management of sleep disorders in older persons. J Am Geriatr Soc. 2009;57(5):761–89. https://doi.org/10.1111/j.1532-5415.2009.02220.x.
87. Berger AM, Abernethy AP, Atkinson A, Barsevick AM, Breitbart WS, Cella D, et al. NCCN clinical practice guidelines cancer-related fatigue. J Natl Compr Canc Netw. 2010;8(8):904–31. https://doi.org/10.6004/jnccn.2010.0067.
88. Goedendorp MM, Gielissen MF, Verhagen CA, Peters ME, Bleijenberg G. Severe fatigue and related factors in cancer patients before the initiation of treatment. Br J Cancer. 2008;99(9):1408–14. https://doi.org/10.1038/sj.bjc.6604739.
89. Hofman M, Ryan JL, Figueroa-Moseley CD, Jean-Pierre P, Morrow GR. Cancer-related fatigue: the scale of the problem. Oncologist. 2007;12(Suppl 1):4–10. https://doi.org/10.1634/theoncologist.12-S1-4.
90. Giacalone A, Quitadamo D, Zanet E, Berretta M, Spina M, Tirelli U. Cancer-related fatigue in the elderly. Support Care Cancer. 2013;21(10):2899–911. https://doi.org/10.1007/s00520-013-1897-1.
91. Flechtner H, Bottomley A. Fatigue and quality of life: lessons from the real world. Oncologist. 2003;8(Suppl 1):5–9. https://doi.org/10.1634/theoncologist.8-suppl_1-5.

92. Henry DH, Viswanathan HN, Elkin EP, Traina S, Wade S, Cella D. Symptoms and treatment burden associated with cancer treatment: results from a cross-sectional national survey in the U.S. Support Care Cancer. 2008;16(7):791–801. https://doi.org/10.1007/s00520-007-0380-2.
93. Yellen SB, Cella DF, Webster K, Blendowski C, Kaplan E. Measuring fatigue and other anemia-related symptoms with the Functional Assessment of Cancer Therapy (FACT) measurement system. J Pain Symptom Manage. 1997;13(2):63–74. https://doi.org/10.1016/s0885-3924(96)00274-6.
94. Knobel H, Loge JH, Brenne E, Fayers P, Hjermstad MJ, Kaasa S. The validity of EORTC QLQ-C30 fatigue scale in advanced cancer patients and cancer survivors. Palliat Med. 2003;17(8):664–72. https://doi.org/10.1191/0269216303pm841oa.
95. Mücke M, Cuhls H, Peuckmann-Post V, Minton O, Stone P, Radbruch L. Pharmacological treatments for fatigue associated with palliative care. Cochrane Database Syst Rev. 2015;2015(5):Cd006788. https://doi.org/10.1002/14651858.CD006788.pub3.
96. Homsi J, Walsh D, Nelson KA. Psychostimulants in supportive care. Support Care Cancer. 2000;8(5):385–97. https://doi.org/10.1007/s005200050007.
97. de la Cruz M, Hui D, Parsons HA, Bruera E. Placebo and nocebo effects in randomized double-blind clinical trials of agents for the therapy for fatigue in patients with advanced cancer. Cancer. 2010;116(3):766–74. https://doi.org/10.1002/cncr.24751.
98. Yusufov M, Braun IM, Pirl WF. A systematic review of substance use and substance use disorders in patients with cancer. Gen Hosp Psychiatry. 2019;60:128–36. https://doi.org/10.1016/j.genhosppsych.2019.04.016.
99. Han BH, Sherman S, Mauro PM, Martins SS, Rotenberg J, Palamar JJ. Demographic trends among older cannabis users in the United States, 2006-13. Addiction. 2017;112(3):516–25. https://doi.org/10.1111/add.13670.
100. Moore AA, Karno MP, Grella CE, Lin JC, Warda U, Liao DH, et al. Alcohol, tobacco, and nonmedical drug use in older U.S. Adults: data from the 2001/02 national epidemiologic survey of alcohol and related conditions. J Am Geriatr Soc. 2009;57(12):2275–81. https://doi.org/10.1111/j.1532-5415.2009.02554.x.
101. Ulker E, Del Fabbro E. Best practices in the management of nonmedical opioid use in patients with cancer-related pain. Oncologist. 2020;25(3):189–96. https://doi.org/10.1634/theoncologist.2019-0540.
102. Lehmann SW, Fingerhood M. Substance-use disorders in later life. N Engl J Med. 2018;379(24):2351–60. https://doi.org/10.1056/NEJMra1805981.
103. Bunt S, Steverink N, Olthof J, van der Schans CP, Hobbelen JSM. Social frailty in older adults: a scoping review. Eur J Ageing. 2017;14(3):323–34. https://doi.org/10.1007/s10433-017-0414-7.
104. WHO. WHO Commission on Social Determinants of Health: closing the gap in a generation: health equity through action on the social determinants of health: Commission on Social Determinants of Health final report. World Health Organization; 2008.
105. Kirby MJ. The health of Canadians—The federal role: final report on the state of the health care system in Canada: recommendations for reform. Ottawa, Canada. 2002.
106. Northwood M, Ploeg J, Markle-Reid M, Sherifali D. Integrative review of the social determinants of health in older adults with multimorbidity. J Adv Nurs. 2018;74(1):45–60. https://doi.org/10.1111/jan.13408.
107. Marmot M, Wilkinson R. Social determinants of health in older age. Social determinants of health. Oxford University Press; 2006.
108. Woo J, Goggins W, Sham A, Ho SC. Social determinants of frailty. Gerontology. 2005;51(6):402–8. https://doi.org/10.1159/000088705.
109. Freer K, Wallington SL. Social frailty: the importance of social and environmental factors in predicting frailty in older adults. Br J Commun Nurs. 2019;24(10):486–92. https://doi.org/10.12968/bjcn.2019.24.10.486.
110. Cohen S, Doyle WJ, Skoner DP, Rabin BS, Gwaltney JM Jr. Social ties and susceptibility to the common cold. JAMA. 1997;277(24):1940–4.

111. Aung MN, Moolphate S, Aung TN, Katonyoo C, Khamchai S, Wannakrairot P. The social network index and its relation to later-life depression among the elderly aged ≥80 years in Northern Thailand. Clin Interv Aging. 2016;11:1067–74. https://doi.org/10.2147/cia.S108974.
112. Sherbourne CD, Stewart AL. The MOS social support survey. Soc Sci Med. 1991; 32(6):705–14. https://doi.org/10.1016/0277-9536(91)90150-b.
113. Barcelos WS. Social determinants of health assessment tool: implications for healthcare practice. Soc Work Public Health. 2019;34(5):395–408. https://doi.org/10.1080/19371918.2019.1614507.
114. Mohan G, Chattopadhyay S. Cost-effectiveness of leveraging social determinants of health to improve breast, cervical, and colorectal cancer screening: a systematic review. JAMA Oncol. 2020;6(9):1434–44. https://doi.org/10.1001/jamaoncol.2020.1460.
115. Pool MS, Agyemang CO, Smalbrugge M. Interventions to improve social determinants of health among elderly ethnic minority groups: a review. Eur J Public Health. 2017;27(6):1048–54. https://doi.org/10.1093/eurpub/ckx178.
116. Jacobsen PB, Rowland JH, Paskett ED, Van Leeuwen F, Moskowitz C, Katta S, et al. Identification of key gaps in cancer survivorship research: findings from the American Society of Clinical Oncology Survey. J Oncol Pract. 2016;12(3):190–3. https://doi.org/10.1200/jop.2015.009258.

Chapter 6
Comorbidity and Polypharmacy in Older Adults with Cancer and Frailty

Arielle S. Berger, Mark Pearce, Leonor Matos, and Shabbir M. H. Alibhai

Introduction

Comorbidity is one of the core elements contributing to frailty in older adults. Comorbidity refers to one or more co-existing medical conditions and it is the norm, rather than the exception, in older adults living in the community and becomes even more common among those in institutional settings. An increasing number of chronic illnesses can increase the risk of frailty and complicate the diagnosis, treatment, and prognosis of cancer in older adults. A higher number of comorbid medical conditions lead to greater medication use and therefore a greater risk of drug interactions, drug-related adverse events, and a higher risk of geriatric syndromes, such as falls. Polypharmacy refers to the total burden of medications or to specific types

A. S. Berger
Division of Geriatrics, Department of Medicine, University Health Network and Sinai Health Hospitals, Toronto, ON, Canada
e-mail: Arielle.Berger@uhn.ca

S. M. H. Alibhai (✉)
Department of Supportive Care, Princess Margaret Cancer Centre, University Health Network, Toronto, ON, Canada

Department of Medicine, Princess Margaret Cancer Centre, University Health Network, Toronto, ON, Canada

Department of Medicine, University of Toronto, Toronto, ON, Canada
e-mail: Shabbir.Alibhai@uhn.ca

M. Pearce
Pharmacy Department, The Christie NHS Foundation Trust, Manchester, UK
e-mail: Mark.Pearce5@nhs.net

L. Matos
Medical Oncology Department, Hospital São Francisco Xavier, Centro Hospitalar Lisboa Ocidental, Lisbon, Portugal

F. Gomes (ed.), *Frailty in Older Adults with Cancer*,
https://doi.org/10.1007/978-3-030-89162-6_6

of potentially inappropriate medications. This chapter will define comorbidity, establish its role within frailty, discuss common approaches to formally assessing it, and its impact on cancer treatment decision-making and its delivery. Similarly, it will define polypharmacy, review its role in frailty and its implications for cancer care and the approaches to its assessment. Another key aspect that will be covered is the role of de-prescribing and other aspects of medication optimization, alongside challenges in implementing such approaches within current models of care, considering its particular importance in older cancer patients with frailty.

Comorbidity

Definition and Its Role in Frailty

Comorbidity, defined as a medical condition that exists alongside an index disease, is highly prevalent in the older adult population, and a subject of growing importance in older cancer patients, who suffer from a higher burden of comorbidity compared with non-cancer patients [1–5]. The higher prevalence of comorbidity in older adults with cancer is possibly due to overlapping risk factors for both cancer and other diseases (e.g. smoking, obesity, alcohol use).

The term multimorbidity, commonly used interchangeably with comorbidity, can be defined as the coexistence of two or more conditions that may or may not have a cause-effect relationship, without any single one prevailing over others (Fig. 6.1). These two terms will be used in this chapter interchangeably.

The National Institute for Health and Care Excellence (NICE) guidelines on multimorbidity suggest that several areas of health must be considered to properly evaluate comorbidity, such as [7]:

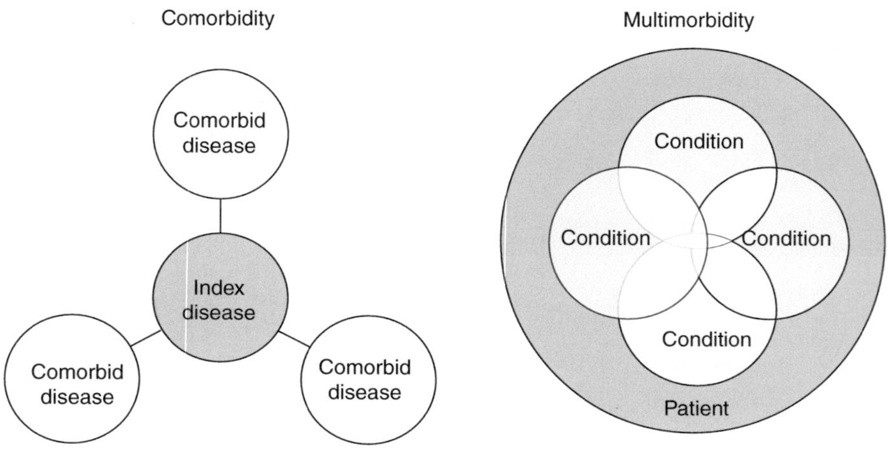

Fig. 6.1 Conceptual framework on comorbidity and multimorbidity (Adapted from [6])

- Defined physical and mental health conditions, such as diabetes or schizophrenia
- Active conditions, such as learning disabilities
- Sensory impairments, such as sight or hearing loss
- Alcohol and substance misuse
- Geriatric syndromes

Therefore, frailty should be integrated in the assessment of multimorbidity, as the latter is a major contributor to frailty, especially as accumulating diseases cause impairments in multiple organ systems, impact functional status, and contribute to psychological distress. The consensus is that although frailty and comorbidity are intimately related to one another, they are not the same. Though not all frailty definitions specifically include comorbidity, the Balducci criteria for frailty [8] clearly identifies the presence of three or more comorbidities as a criterion for frailty. Frailty and comorbidity can have a bidirectional causal relationship, with frailty both being caused by comorbidity and causing medical complications (i.e. comorbidity) (Table 6.1). Among these, depression and dementia are worth highlighting for a number of reasons: (a) they are extremely common in both the cancer population and the population with frailty; (b) they can cause significant impairments in global functioning; and (c) they are often missed by oncology teams [10–12].

Comorbidity Assessment

Comorbidity burden incorporates two unique concepts: (a) the number of independent comorbid conditions; and (b) the severity of each comorbidity. Standardized assessment tools approach these concepts in different ways. Many tools are described in the cancer literature but the most commonly used tools in clinical cancer care and cancer research are listed in Table 6.2.

Table 6.1 Diseases and conditions associated with frailty (Adapted from [9])

Diseases known to increase risk of frailty	Conditions caused by frailty
Congestive heart failure	Sarcopenia: loss of muscle mass
End-stage renal disease	Slowed motor processing, performance
Chronic obstructive pulmonary disease	Decreased strength, exercise tolerance
Diabetes	Slow gait speed, poor mobility
Dementia	Decreased balance
Depression	Low physical activity
Advanced cancer	Low mood
Tuberculosis, other chronic infections	Cognitive impairment
Pressure ulcers and chronic wounds	Cumulative illness
Hip fractures	
Chronic inflammatory diseases	

Table 6.2 Comorbidity scales used in oncology (Adapted from [5])

Index name	Items and rating	Advantages	Disadvantages
Not cancer-specific			
Charlson Comorbidity Index (CCI) [13]	19 conditions weighted 1–6	Easy to complete (<5 min) and can be applied retrospectively	Missing common comorbid diseases and severity of most conditions not considered
Cumulative Illness Rating Scale (CIRS) [14]	13 or 14 organ system categories, each rated 0–4	Comprehensive listing of conditions and organ systems	Weighted by physician's subjective judgement
Index of Coexistent Disease ICED) [15]	Disease severity sub-index: 14 diseases (rated 0–4) Functional severity sub-index: 12 conditions (rated 0–2) Total: 0–3	Incorporates a wide range of conditions and their severity	Limited validation in cancer setting
Cancer-specific			
Washington University Head and Neck Comorbidity (WUHNCI) [16, 17]	7 conditions, each rated 0–4	Predicts 5-year survival in patients with head and neck cancer	Limited scope to one oncology setting
Haematopoietic cell transplantation-comorbidity index (HCT-CI) [18]	17 conditions, each rated 0–3	Predicts 2-year non-relapse mortality in patients undergoing HCT	Limited scope to one oncology setting

It is important to note that when assessing comorbidity, it is also vital to incorporate a frailty assessment for several reasons. First, comorbidities often need to be optimized before any other approaches to reverse frailty (e.g. exercise, nutrition) are considered. Second, as the severity of frailty increases, comorbidity plays a smaller role in determining non-cancer prognosis. Third, goals to assess and optimize various comorbidities (e.g. hypertension, diabetes) must consider the patient's underlying frailty in order to minimize the risk of doing more harm than good.

There are few head-to-head studies in oncology comparing a formal comorbidity index to expert clinician evaluation in the clinical setting. Yet, one theoretical advantage of using a comorbidity index is the greater consistency in assessing different conditions, particularly for non-experts, although this has not been formally demonstrated in clinical practice [5].

Moreover, there is no clear evidence supporting the superiority of one comorbidity assessment tool over another. Each tool has its advantages and disadvantages, as summarized in Table 6.2. In the oncology setting, several studies, mostly retrospective, have examined a number of comorbidity indices and found generally a similar performance between them, in predicting survival in cancer populations, as well as surgical complications and chemotherapy outcomes [19].

Comorbidity Implications in Oncology

The diagnosis of cancer in an older person is often made in the context of multiple pre-existing health problems. Just as cancer and frailty are associated with aging, so too are diseases of the cardiovascular, cerebrovascular, and pulmonary systems, among others. What becomes apparent from clinical practice and is corroborated by available evidence is that comorbidity impacts cancer risk, treatment, and prognosis [3, 20, 21]. Comorbidity increases the risk of complications after surgery, radiation, and chemotherapy and frequently influences cancer treatment decisions. Moreover, cancer and cancer treatment can worsen comorbidities. These matters argue for the incorporation of systematic comorbidity assessment in routine evaluation of older adults with cancer throughout their cancer course [5, 22, 23].

Nonetheless, the impact of comorbid conditions in an older cancer patient can be extremely variable and may depend on multiple factors, such as the severity and degree of control of the comorbidities, the type of treatments targeted to the comorbidity, as well as the presence of frailty, the cancer and other patient-related factors, such as socioeconomic status and social support [24]. Thus, a patient with several comorbidities may be fit (i.e. not requiring oncologic treatment modifications), when all these underlying conditions are either mild or well controlled.

Comorbidity and Cancer-Specific Mortality

Observational studies demonstrate that cancer-specific mortality rates increase with increasing comorbidity. Piccirillo et al. [25] demonstrated a dose-dependent increase in cancer-specific mortality according to increasing comorbidity burden, with a hazard ratio of 1.21 for low comorbidity and of 2.56 for high comorbidity. Likewise, Satariano and Ragland [26] found that women with at least 3 comorbidities had a 20-fold higher rate of breast cancer mortality compared with patients with no comorbidity. Importantly, however, the prognostic importance of comorbidity is greatest in patients with early-stage cancer, when considering curative and adjuvant treatment. Once cancer has reached an advanced stage or is rapidly progressing, the cancer itself most commonly poses the highest risk to patient survival.

Comorbidity and Cancer Treatment Toxicity

In addition to mortality, increasing comorbidity is associated with poor cancer treatment tolerance, and comorbidity burden is a stronger predictor for toxicity than age [5]. For example, a systematic review by Lee et al. [19] showed an association between higher Charlson Comorbidity Index (CCI) and decreased rate of completion of chemotherapy, greater delays in chemotherapy, more dose reductions, greater grade 3–4 neutropenia, greater grade 3–4 constitutional symptoms, and incident grade 3–4 toxicity. Interestingly, although the most commonly used chemotherapy prediction tools, CARG and CRASH [5, 27], include some comorbidities, these tools do not include a metric for overall comorbidity burden. Moreover, not all clinical studies have shown a correlation between comorbidity burden and cancer treatment toxicity. Finally, although comorbidity is associated with higher cancer-specific mortality and treatment toxicity in most studies, some studies show that individuals with comorbidities who receive cancer treatment derive the same cancer-specific mortality benefit as those without comorbidity [28–31]. A limitation in these studies is that patients who were deemed fit enough to receive cancer treatment likely had lower levels of comorbidity than those who did not receive treatment, resulting in an upfront selection bias.

Cancer patients with significant comorbidity burden are routinely excluded from randomized controlled trials [32, 33]. Hernandez-Torres et al. [34] showed that "any significant comorbidity" excluded patients from 88.4% of the major randomized controlled trials of cancer treatment in Canada between 1990 and 2010. Additionally, comorbidity assessment is seldom reported or reported in non-standardized ways making it difficult for clinicians to apply trial results to individual patients [33]. Increasing the enrolment of patients with common comorbidities and systematically reporting on comorbidity burden and its interaction with treatment effects will provide needed evidence to direct cancer treatment for individuals with comorbidity.

Incorporating this seemingly conflicting data into clinical care is complex. Therefore, the authors suggest considering the following important points:

- The number of comorbidities may be less important compared to their severity and whether they are well-controlled.
- Other factors (for example, functional status or frailty) may be more important predictors than comorbidity alone, therefore assessments should incorporate functional and frailty measures.
- Specific comorbidities interact with cancer and cancer treatment in differing ways:
  - *Cytotoxic chemotherapy*: Comorbidity burden plays a role in the tolerability of chemotherapy. The chemotherapy toxicity prediction tools highlight a number of key comorbidities that confer a higher risk of toxicity. The CARG tool includes anaemia, moderate-severe renal impairment, and hearing loss as comorbid conditions that independently correlate with higher toxicity [5]. The CRASH tool includes diastolic hypertension as an independent predictor of haematologic toxicity [27]. Diabetes should be monitored closely during the course of chemotherapy: corticosteroids can destabilize well-controlled diabetes, and anorexia associated with chemotherapy can lead to hypoglycaemia, which can be life threatening. Additionally, the toxicities specific to each individual drug must be considered in the context of the individual patient and their comorbidities.

- *Targeted therapy and immune checkpoint inhibitors*: These novel cancer therapies are generally better tolerated than traditional cytotoxic chemotherapy. There are no standardized tools to predict toxicity, and clinical studies have not specifically evaluated the relationship between comorbidity and cancer-specific outcomes with these treatment categories. A few studies have shown that age alone is not predictive of toxicity [34]. As aging is a heterogeneous process, this is consistent with the literature showing that age is not a good surrogate marker for comorbidity. Hence, the individual drug profiles and known toxicity risks must be considered in the context of each individual patient and their comorbidities.
- *Radiotherapy*: Comorbidity burden is not consistently associated with poor tolerance of radiation therapy. It appears that nutritional status and functional status are more important predictors of radiation treatment tolerance [35]. An important exception is the underlying organ reserve of an organ undergoing radiation (e.g. pre-existing interstitial lung disease in a patient undergoing stereotactic body radiotherapy for lung cancer).
- *Surgery*: The comorbidities associated with cancer surgery risk are not unique to the cancer population. Like all surgical candidates, cardiac, pulmonary, and kidney diseases confer the greatest risk of perioperative complications including acute coronary syndromes, stroke, respiratory failure, and acute renal failure. In fact, comorbidity is often much more predictive of poor perioperative outcomes than age [36].

Polypharmacy

Definition and Its Role in Frailty

Polypharmacy is a common issue, particularly for older cancer patients with frailty. The prevalence of polypharmacy and potentially inappropriate medication use (PIMs) in cancer patients has been described as being up to 80% and 63%, respectively [37, 38].

Polypharmacy refers to both the number of medications a person is taking and medication appropriateness. Whilst there is no universally accepted definition, typically, polypharmacy is defined at 5 or more medications. Hyperpolypharmacy is commonly defined as 10 or more medications. Prescribing "cascades" may also occur, which is a scenario where medications are prescribed to manage the adverse effects from other prescribed medications; these in turn may cause further adverse effects requiring further medication to be prescribed. As patients are managed by multiple health care teams, there is increasing risk of breakdown in communication leading to therapeutic duplications, drug interactions, and continuation of inappropriate medications [39].

The use of multiple medications has a cumulative effect in terms of increasing the risk of medication-related adverse events, particularly in older cancer patients

Table 6.3 Examples of adverse events related to overlapping impairments from cancer, medications, and frailty

Adverse events	Cancer related	Medication related	Age and frailty related
Impaired cognition	– Central nervous system metastasis	– Opioid analgesia – Anticholinergic medications	– Short term memory loss
Falls	– Central nervous system metastasis affecting balance	– Platinum induced autonomic and peripheral neuropathy – Dehydration from nausea or diarrhoea	– Postural drop
Reduced drug excretion increasing drug toxicity	– Urinary obstruction by tumour	– Drug induced kidney injury	– Reduction in glomerular filtration rate
Reduced drug metabolism increasing drug toxicity	– Hepatic metastasis	– Enzyme inhibition by cancer therapy	– Reduced hepatic mass and blood flow

Table 6.4 Examples of pharmacokinetic considerations with ageing (Adapted from [41])

Stage	Change with ageing	Effect
Absorption	– Decreased gastrointestinal motility and blood flow	– Delay or reduction in drug absorption.
Distribution	– Reduced plasma protein binding as a result of malnutrition	– Increased free drug concentrations leading to toxicity
	– Increased body fat to muscle ratio	– Fat soluble drug accumulation (this shift is greater in women)
Metabolism	– Decreased hepatic blood flow and CYP450 function	– Reduced drug clearance
Excretion	– Decreased glomerular filtration rate via kidneys	

with frailty (Table 6.3) [40]. Pharmacodynamics, meaning the effect a medication has on the individual, can be less predictable in older adults and in those with multimorbidity and polypharmacy. Moreover, pharmacokinetic changes (the bodily absorption, distribution, metabolism, and excretion of drugs) due to ageing contribute towards adverse events for these patients (Table 6.4). These may require switching to alternate medications, reducing the dose or stopping the medication entirely.

Polypharmacy and drug interactions are closely associated. Some are avoidable but often a balance may need to be found between different treatments. Knowledge of pharmacokinetics and toxicity profiles is required in addition to checking databases to assess the risk/impact of interactions. Dedicated oncology drug interaction checkers [42], herbal medicine databases [43], and hepatic metabolic profiles of drugs are available [44]. It is important to also note that there is some uncertainty when assessing the effects of pharmacokinetics and pharmacodynamics in the older adult population with polypharmacy due to a lack of clinical studies [45]. Moreover, drug interactions do not occur exclusively with other drugs; they may also interact with diseases, food, and herbals.

Polypharmacy Assessment

Many tools have been developed and are available for the assessment of polypharmacy and PIMs (Table 6.5) [41, 46, 48]. These tools overlap in their scope and one is not recommended over another in oncology due to lack of comparative studies. Cancer patients are often taking several high-risk medications, in a context of particularly high levels of frailty and multimorbidity. This can limit the validity and applicability of these tools.

Nightingale and colleagues used a combination of the Screening Tool of Older Persons' Prescriptions (STOPP) and Beers criteria in order to identify an increased number of PIMs compared with either tool alone [52]. However clinical judgement is also required to implement the findings of any medication review [50, 53, 54].

One approach used Beers criteria followed by STOPP, before focusing on a more detailed tool like the Medicines Appropriateness Index (MAI); this approach has been shown to be effective at identifying PIMs [54]. Another strategy involved a pharmacist-led review with STOPP and the La Roche list in combination with an onco-geriatrician [55]. This was more effective at identifying PIMs than geriatrician review alone [55, 56]. While these approaches have increased the identification PIMs, impact on patient outcomes has yet to be demonstrated [51].

Time constraints and ease of use are significant limitations on the use of these tools in clinical practice, especially where a pharmacist is not included in the review

Table 6.5 Examples of PIM identification tools (Adapted from [47, 51])

Tool	Advantages	Disadvantages
Beers Criteria [46]	– Useful for identifying PIMs – Comprehensive list – Updated regularly	– Not always appropriate for oncology – No herbal medications
STOPP/START (Screening Tool of Older Persons' Prescriptions) [48]	– User friendly, systems-based approach – Covers duplications, omissions, drug interactions – Covers gaps in the Beers	– Not always appropriate for oncology – No herbal medications
MAI (Medicines Appropriateness Index) [47]	– Supports the role of clinical judgement – Complementary to other tools – Includes practical aspects of medication like administration	– Time consuming (10 min per medication)
OncPal De-prescribing guideline [49]	– Validated for the oncology population	– Only applicable if less than 6 months life expectancy

process. It is hoped that technological solutions will provide some automation and increase their use although as demonstrated in the SENATOR trial, this cannot yet serve as a replacement for clinician and pharmacist input [41, 57, 58].

Polypharmacy Implications in Oncology

Despite a high prevalence of polypharmacy in the oncology setting, problems are commonly missed by standard oncology care [5]. The older cancer patients, particularly with frailty, have an increased prevalence of comorbidity and are often started on several new medications as part of their cancer management [37, 40, 59]. These include not just the systemic anti-cancer treatment itself, but also an armamentarium of prophylactic and supportive medications, the latter particularly important for those with frailty. Many of these patients also use herbal medicines and supplements in addition to prescribed medications, which are often under-reported to the oncology team yet can cause toxicity and drug interactions [40]. As the number of medications increases, drug interactions become increasingly likely [37]. Falls risk, hospital admission, and outpatient visits related to adverse drug reactions also increase with polypharmacy [50, 60].

Polypharmacy and PIMs have been associated with physical function impairment, however causality has not been established, and further studies are required to establish if optimization can lead to an improvement in these outcomes [61]. Problems related to polypharmacy are compounded by a reduced physiological reserve in patients with frailty. This can be further exacerbated with complications arising from the cancer itself. For example, age-related cognitive decline may be exacerbated in patients with brain metastasis leading to increased susceptibility to a medication's anticholinergic effects (Table 6.3).

Overall, polypharmacy has been linked to multiple negative outcomes in the cancer population. It may hinder cancer treatment particularly through premature discontinuation or delays in chemotherapy due to increased toxicity [52]. Lu-Yao and colleagues recently demonstrated that increasing medication use prior to chemotherapy is linked to increased hospital admissions (OR 2.3), with evidence that it may be linked to frailty (OR 4.5), disability and depression (OR 1.6) [38]. A recent systematic review also demonstrated associations between polypharmacy and chemotherapy toxicity (including immunosuppression, nausea, vomiting, hair loss, renal toxicity, and hepatotoxicity) [62]. It has also been linked falls, poor medication adherence and caregiver burden (OR 2.2). Moreover, polypharmacy is independently associated with prolonged admission following surgery [63] and the risk of post-operative complications is almost doubled [64]. Patients with polypharmacy are also more likely to have non-surgical treatments such as radiotherapy over surgery, often reflecting their multimorbidity and/or frailty [64]. Consideration should also be given to medications that are potentially radiosensitizing (e.g. metronidazole) [65], as well as those that may lead to additive toxicity with the side effects from radiotherapy. However, there is currently less evidence about effects of polypharmacy on cancer survival with only two small studies showing an association between polypharmacy and mortality [64].

Pharmacogenomics testing is becoming more widely available and can involve assessing CYP450, metabolic enzymes, or HLA status. Over 90% of patients are thought to have a genetic variant that can contribute to drug response [66]. In oncology, some relevant examples include tamoxifen activation via CYP2D6, fluoropyrimidine metabolism (*DPYD*) and increased toxicity from drugs like allopurinol (HLA-B*5801) [67]. Pharmacogenomic assessment can identify patients at increased risk of hospital admissions over and above the effects of assessing polypharmacy alone [68, 69]. Current challenges include access, cost, and turnaround times for testing in routine practice.

Lastly, evidence linking PIMs in oncology and healthcare utilization are mixed with some, but not all, studies demonstrating an association [64]. A group in the United Kingdom were able to demonstrate a substantial saving in both healthcare utilization and medicine costs through medicines optimization by a pharmacist in a general population and quantifying resultant reduced admissions [70]. Newer oncology medications are now extremely costly, therefore it is prudent to try to maximize patient benefit through medicines optimization.

Medication Review and De-prescribing

Medications reviews may be conducted by appropriately trained pharmacists, doctors, or other healthcare professionals. Ideally medication review should be interdisciplinary [51] and be conducted in person [40]. The key elements of a medication review are summarized in Table 6.6.

The timing of medication reviews for oncology patients may in part be dictated by available resources in a healthcare system. A proactive approach has the advantage of preventing issues occurring but is more resource intensive. It is also unclear what the best screening method is, e.g. age, number of medications being taken or the identification of frailty. Reactive approaches focus resources on patients with active issues, but patients may suffer potentially avoidable morbidity or be missed entirely. Time can also present a barrier. Detailed medication reviews take on average 20–30 min per patient (but occasionally can exceed 2 h) [54, 56]. Additionally, prescribers can be reluctant to adjust or stop medications in the context of complex patients, such as an older cancer patient with frailty and multimorbidity. There is, however, evidence that patients are willing to consider changes [71]. Understanding a patient's priorities and the use of evidence-based resources can support discussions around de-prescribing [54]. In practice this can be incorporated into the comprehensive geriatric assessment of older cancer patients with frailty.

De-prescribing is the planned discontinuation of medication. This often comes about when a patient's medication is judged to be causing harm, likely to cause them harm in the future, or not providing a benefit. The risk of each of these is amplified in the older cancer patient with frailty. However, de-prescribing can cause

Table 6.6 Key elements of medication review

Patient goals – Establish priorities in the context of the potential cancer treatment and reduced prognosis – Educate on potential benefit of medication review
Identify essential drug therapy – Complete list of all medications (including those not prescribed) plus allergies and intolerances – Identify 'essential' drugs and ensure dose appropriate and titrated slowly – Identify underuse of medications – Consider consult with external teams before changing specialist medications
Identify unnecessary medication – Evaluate PIMs using one or more of the validated tools plus clinical judgement – Assess dose and durations of medications to ensure indication is still valid; consider time to benefit – Remove therapeutic duplication
Therapeutic goals – Prioritize control of disease related symptoms or treatment related side effects – Consider therapeutic switch to the most effective evidence-based therapies for an indication using number needed to treat and harm
Adverse drug reactions – Identify and address clinically significant drug interactions (use 2 or more databases) – Ensure medications are being monitored appropriately – Assess for signs, symptoms, or abnormal bloods results that could be medication related – Educate patient on 'sick-day rules' for relevant medications – Minimize prescribing cascade (scenario where medications are prescribed to manage the adverse effects from other prescribed medications)
Adherence – Assess if patient taking medication as prescribed (form, device, schedule, technique) and if there a role for compliance aides – Check they have appropriate support (relatives, carers)
Cost effectiveness – Check if treatment is within formulary and the most cost-effective option – Scrutinize if branded products, "specials" or non-standard formulations necessary for patient's adherence – Switch to equivalent, cheaper alternative if no concerns over safety or adherence
Agreement and implementation – Have patient and healthcare provider goals both been met? – Does the patient understand the outcomes of the review? – Consider resources (below) to assist in implementation of medicine changes – Communicate the outcome and any changes to medication and any actions to all relevant parties – Where possible, follow-up should be conducted to assess if the interventions were retained and effective and continue the process of optimization

harm if not done correctly. It is good practice to adjust one medication at a time to assess for benefit or harm; however this is not always practical and an 'all at once' approach can be used where follow-up may be difficult or if there is clinical urgency (e.g. during acute delirium) [54]. The following questions are helpful when prioritizing medications for de-prescribing: is a medication currently causing harm, does a medication have the potential to cause harm in the future, and patient preference regarding symptom or disease control [72].

In advanced cancer, drugs used as primary or secondary prevention, that are not providing symptom control and have longer 'time to benefit' can be stopped (e.g. anti-hypertensives, anti-lipidaemics). Stopping these drugs is unlikely to exacerbate underlying conditions or affect mortality [73]. Common scenarios include weight loss or decreased appetite, leading to withdrawal of antihypertensive medications and those that may suppress appetite [74]. Any changes should be communicated to the wider healthcare team promptly.

Some medications may require specific tapering schedules to avoid withdrawal symptoms such as antidepressants or benzodiazepines [75]. When switching medications, Hanlon et al. [76] outlined potential therapeutic switches for common PIMs. It is also important to consider non-pharmacological interventions (e.g. sleep hygiene for insomnia).

There may be instances where the addition of medications may be beneficial due to unmet therapeutic needs [47] e.g. bisphosphonates for management of cancer treatment related bone loss and risk of fracture in older patients (from aromatase inhibitors or androgen deprivation therapy). Certain groups are at particularly high risk for this, such as non-majority ethnic low socioeconomic groups and those in long-term care [77]. In these situations, consideration of frailty can be complex, as these patients have a higher risk of falling, yet limited life expectancy. Medication optimization in these patients is best done by a multidisciplinary team. Other common scenarios of unmet needs in older cancer patients include management of pain and constipation.

Adherence is another important consideration and is impacted by both the increasing numbers of medications and the frequency of administration [78]. Oncology medications frequently have stipulations on timing, in relation to food and other medications, adding further complexity. Reduced adherence can translate into a reduced therapeutic response. Some classes of medications (opioid analgesics, anxiolytics, antipsychotics and antidepressants) are particularly associated with reduced adherence [64]. Interventions include pill organizers, telephone reminders, educational materials, and adjustment of dosage forms, devices or packaging [39]. A systematic review of adherence interventions found that dose simplifications, patient education and electronic reminders were the most effective, however a Cochrane review found that behavioural or educational interventions may have some impact on adherence but overall the evidence was of low quality [79, 80]. Increasingly in oncology home delivery and administration of medications are utilized along with telemedicine and home monitoring. This places greater burden on patients and carers to manage medications and conditions as face-to-face interaction is reduced.

Resources for healthcare professionals and patients are available. These are generally not oncology-specific but provide guidance that can be applied to the older cancer patient with frailty.

– Canadian De-prescribing Network (www.deprescribingnetwork.ca)

- https://deprescribing.org
- NHS Scotland De-prescribing (https://polypharmacy.scot.nhs.uk)
- Rxisk (https://rxisk.org)
- Choosing Wisely (www.choosingwisely.org)

Models of Care for the Management of Polypharmacy

The National Comprehensive Cancer Network (NCCN) guidance for older adults includes medication review as part of the geriatric assessment [81]. Two key components are: (1) a thorough review of the medical history, including assessing for active or decompensated chronic diseases, and (2) a thorough medication review with a focus on adherence concerns, PIMs, and drug interactions. This may require substantial skill and input from a multidisciplinary team, and algorithmic approaches are not possible given the complexity and multitude of scenarios. A medication review is advised where there is any change in the patient's condition or treatment. There is a growing body of evidence that pharmacist-led review with use of medication review tools should form a key component of a geriatric assessment in the general population, however this has not yet been shown in oncology [56]. This complements the work of geriatricians and may help to alleviate physician workload. Different models of care have been attempted, which can be tailored to the available resources and skill set:

- *Review of all patients seen in an oncology clinic by a pharmacist*

  This has the advantage of capturing all patients. It does however result in a high demand of resources. Some patients may not require review making this potentially inefficient. Nightingale et al followed this approach, however in this case the medications reviews were conducted retrospectively rather than contemporaneously [52].
- *Triage model with polypharmacy tool applied to identify patients at high risk*

  High risk may be defined, for example, as 5 or more medications or problematic medications according to PIMs tools. This allows targeting those patients most likely to benefit from review. Identified patients then have a full medication review involving a pharmacist, doctor, or the wider multidisciplinary team as indicated [54, 62]. There are some resource implications for the process of triaging. But the key limitation is that currently there are no robustly validated methods for identifying these patients, so there is a risk of some patients being missed.
- *Referral based geriatric assessment by pharmacist in conjunction with multidisciplinary team*

  One study by Whitman and colleagues had referral by the primary oncologist; patients then had pharmacist review before interventions were confirmed with a geriatrician [54]. This method could be quite resource intensive depending on the level of geriatrician input required in addition to a detailed pharmacist review.

- *Referral based geriatric assessment by doctor/nurse (with pharmacist in exceptional cases)*

  Patients at high risk or who have had a medicines-related adverse event are referred. Many geriatric oncology teams do not include a pharmacist so including them within the review process may not be feasible. If there is a specific concern about a medication that cannot be addressed within the team, then a pharmacist may be consulted for guidance.

Impact of Interventions Addressing Comorbidity and Polypharmacy

Patients with comorbidities and polypharmacy are at risk of both under- and over-treatment [71]. Furthermore, studies evaluating the impact of geriatric assessment on cancer outcomes have highlighted the need to address comorbidity and polypharmacy. Alibhai et al. [82] found that comorbidity management was addressed in 95% of patients seen in a geriatric oncology clinic. Chapman et al. [83] showed that medication adjustments were made in 75% of patients seen in a multidisciplinary geriatric oncology program. A prospective study in oncology demonstrated improved chemotherapy tolerance by stopping PIMs [84]. However there are less data currently supporting its role in improving quality of life, health services utilization, or reducing major clinical events, particularly in older cancer patients with frailty [39]. In the non-cancer population there is evidence that medication reviews and de-prescribing have significant clinical effects including reduced adverse drug reactions, falls risk, and in one study, lower mortality [39, 85].

Considering the frequency of comorbidity and polypharmacy in the cancer population with frailty, the relative inattention paid to these domains by the primary cancer team and the frequency of geriatric assessment addressing these domains, it is therefore proposed that comorbidity management and medication optimization may be mechanisms through which cancer treatment is enhanced. This may be accomplished by reducing adverse effects of PIMs and optimizing symptoms related to poorly controlled comorbidities. Further evaluations of this impact are needed to elucidate the processes further. Moreover, prospective studies are needed following the current best practices to fully assess the benefits on clinical outcomes rather than on surrogate measures for these interventions.

Recently, three pivotal randomized trials of geriatric assessment and management in older cancer patients were presented at the 2020 American Society of Clinical Oncology annual scientific meeting. A core feature of each geriatric assessment was comorbidity assessment and management. Although details specific to the impact of comorbidity and polypharmacy management were not provided, all three trials demonstrated reductions in oncologic treatment toxicity and one study demonstrated improved quality of life [86–89]. Peer-reviewed publication of these trials and results of other ongoing trials are eagerly awaited.

Conclusion

Comorbidity and polypharmacy are common in older adults with cancer, particularly those who also have frailty. A careful approach to understanding the presence and severity of comorbid illnesses in cancer patients is paramount. This knowledge can highlight risks of treatment toxicity and can identify potential competing mortality risks which may alter the treatment trajectory. At present no one specific comorbidity index or measure can be recommended but several have shown utility in different settings. Polypharmacy is associated with multiple adverse outcomes in older cancer patients. Ideally a careful review of medications by a pharmacist or a multidisciplinary team should be performed to identify opportunities to optimize medications and de-prescribe particularly inappropriate medications, thereby improving symptom management and quality of life and reducing risks of cancer treatment toxicity. Although several tools exist to aid medication review and identifying PIMs, time and resources are major barriers to routine implementation. Further research into the optimal assessment and management of both comorbidity and polypharmacy in older cancer patients with frailty, as well as their subsequent benefit in the outcomes of these patients is needed.

References

1. Topaloğlu US, Özaslan E. Comorbidity and polypharmacy in patients with breast cancer. Breast Cancer. 2020;27:477–82.
2. Arinc S, Ece F, Ertugrul M, Erdal N, Oruc O, Hatabay N, Derince D, Arpag H, Taylan M, Hazar A. Analysis of young and elderly advanced stage nonsmall-cell lung carcinoma cases. South Med J. 2009;102:1019–22.
3. Koroukian SM, Murray P, Madigan E. Comorbidity, disability, and geriatric syndromes in elderly cancer patients receiving home health care. J Clin Oncol. 2006;24:2304–10.
4. Jorgensen TL, Hallas J, Friis S, Herrstedt J. Comorbidity in elderly cancer patients in relation to overall and cancer-specific mortality. Br J Cancer. 2012;106:1353–60.
5. Williams GR, Mackenzie A, Magnuson A, et al. Comorbidity in older adults with cancer. J Geriatr Oncol. 2016;7:249–57.
6. Boyd CM, Fortin M. Future of multimorbidity research: how should understanding of multimorbidity inform health system design? Public Health Rev. 2011;33:451–74.
7. Multimorbidity: clinical assessment and management. 2020.
8. Balducci L, Extermann M. Management of cancer in the older person: a practical approach. Oncologist. 2000;5:224–37.
9. Blaum C. The intersection between comorbidity, multimorbidity and frailty. In: U13 Gemsstar Conf. 2015.

10. Jia Y, Li F, Liu YF, Zhao JP, Leng MM, Chen L. Depression and cancer risk: a systematic review and meta-analysis. Public Health. 2017;149:138–48.
11. McWilliams L, Farrell C, Grande G, Keady J, Swarbrick C, Yorke J. A systematic review of the prevalence of comorbid cancer and dementia and its implications for cancer-related care. Aging Ment Health. 2018;22:1254–71.
12. Rosario CO, Puts M, Jang R, Bezjak A, Yokom D, Alibhai SMH. Exploring the geriatric needs of oncology inpatients at an academic cancer centre. J Geriatr Oncol. 2018; https://doi.org/10.1016/j.jgo.2018.12.001.
13. Charlson ME, Pompei P, Ales KL, MacKenzie CR. A new method of classifying prognostic comorbidity in longitudinal studies: development and validation. J Chronic Dis. 1987;40:373–83.
14. Miller MD, Paradis CF, Houck PR, Mazumdar S, Stack JA, Rifai AH, Mulsant B, Reynolds CF. Rating chronic medical illness burden in geropsychiatric practice and research: application of the Cumulative Illness Rating Scale. Psychiatry Res. 1992;41:237–48.
15. Miskulin DC, Athienites NV, Yan G, Martin AA, Ornt DB, Kusek JW, Meyer KB, Levey AS. Comorbidity assessment using the index of coexistent diseases in a multicenter clinical trial. Kidney Int. 2001;60:1498–510.
16. Piccirillo JF, Lacy PD, Basu A, Spitznagel EL. Development of a new head and neck cancer-specific comorbidity index. Arch Otolaryngol Head Neck Surg. 2002;128:1172–9.
17. Sanabria A, Carvalho AL, Vartanian JG, Magrin J, Ikeda MK, Kowalski LP. Validation of the Washington University Head and Neck Comorbidity Index in a cohort of older patients. Arch Otolaryngol Head Neck Surg. 2008;134:603–7.
18. Sorror ML, Maris MB, Storb R, Baron F, Sandmaier BM, Maloney DG, Storer B. Hematopoietic cell transplantation (HCT)-specific comorbidity index: a new tool for risk assessment before allogeneic HCT. Blood. 2005;106:2912–9.
19. Lee L, Cheung WY, Atkinson E, Krzyzanowska MK. Impact of comorbidity on chemotherapy use and outcomes in solid tumors: a systematic review. J Clin Oncol Off J Am Soc Clin Oncol. 2011;29:106–17.
20. Extermann M. Interaction between comorbidity and cancer. Cancer Control. 2007;14:13–22.
21. Søgaard M, Thomsen RW, Bossen KS, Sørensen HT, Nørgaard M. The impact of comorbidity on cancer survival: a review. Clin Epidemiol. 2013;5:3–29.
22. Guiding principles for the care of older adults with multimorbidity: an approach for clinicians: American Geriatrics Society Expert Panel on the Care of Older Adults with Multimorbidity. J Am Geriatr Soc. 2012;60:E1–25.
23. Boyd CM, Darer J, Boult C, Fried LP, Boult L, Wu AW. Clinical practice guidelines and quality of care for older patients with multiple comorbid diseases: implications for pay for performance. J Am Med Assoc. 2005;294:716–24.
24. Geraci J, Escalante C, Freeman J, Goodwin J. Comorbid disease and cancer: the need for more relevant conceptual models in health services research. J Clin Oncol. 2005;23:7399–404.
25. Piccirillo JF, Tierney RM, Costas I, Grove L, Spitznagel EL Jr. Prognostic importance of comorbidity in a hospital-based cancer registry. JAMA. 2004;291:2441–7.
26. Satariano WA, Ragland DR. The effect of comorbidity on 3-year survival of women with primary breast cancer. Ann Intern Med. 1994;120:104–10.
27. Hurria A, Mohile S, Gajra A, et al. Validation of a prediction tool for chemotherapy toxicity in older adults with cancer. J Clin Oncol. 2016;34:2366–71.
28. Extermann M, Boler I, Reich RR, et al. Predicting the risk of chemotherapy toxicity in older patients: the Chemotherapy Risk Assessment Scale for High-Age Patients (CRASH) score. Cancer. 2012;118:3377–86.
29. Chen H, Cantor A, Meyer J, et al. Can older cancer patients tolerate chemotherapy? A prospective pilot study. Cancer. 2003;97:1107–14.
30. Sargent DJ, Goldberg RM, Jacobson SD, Macdonald JS, Labianca R, Haller DG, Shepherd LE, Seitz JF, Francini G. A pooled analysis of adjuvant chemotherapy for resected colon cancer in elderly patients. N Engl J Med. 2001;345:1091–7.

31. Feliu J, Gómez LL, Madroñal C, Espinosa E, Espinosa J, Girón CG, Martinez B, Castro J, De La Gándara I, Barón MG. Gemcitabine plus vinorelbine in nonsmall cell lung carcinoma patients age 70 years or older or patients who cannot receive cisplatin. Cancer. 1999;86:1463–9.
32. Earle CC, Tsai JS, Gelber RD, Weinstein MC, Neumann PJ, Weeks JC. Effectiveness of chemotherapy for advanced lung cancer in the elderly: instrumental variable and propensity analysis. J Clin Oncol Off J Am Soc Clin Oncol. 2001;19:1064–70.
33. Rodrigues G, Sanatani M. Age and comorbidity considerations related to radiotherapy and chemotherapy administration. Semin Radiat Oncol. 2012;22:277–83.
34. Hernandez-Torres C, Cheung WY, Kong S, O'Callaghan CJ, Hsu T. Accrual of older adults to cancer clinical trials led by the Canadian Cancer Trials Group—is trial design a barrier? J Geriatr Oncol. 2019;4–11.
35. Elias R, Morales J, Rehman Y, Khurshid H. Immune checkpoint inhibitors in older adults. Curr Oncol Rep. 2016; https://doi.org/10.1007/s11912-016-0534-9.
36. Szumacher E, Sattar S, Neve M, Do K, Ayala AP, Gray M, Lee J, Alibhai S, Puts M. Use of comprehensive geriatric assessment and geriatric screening for older adults in the radiation oncology setting: a systematic review. Clin Oncol. 2018;30:578–88.
37. Alibhai SMH, Leach M, Tomlinson G, Krahn MD, Fleshner N, Holowaty E, Naglie G. 30-day mortality and major complications after radical prostatectomy: influence of age and comorbidity. J Natl Cancer Inst. 2005;97:1525–32.
38. Lu-Yao G, Nightingale G, Nikita N, Keith S, Gandhi K, Swartz K, Zinner R, Sharma S, Kelly WMK, Chapman A. Relationship between polypharmacy and inpatient hospitalization among older adults with cancer treated with intravenous chemotherapy. J Geriatr Oncol. 2020;11:579–85.
39. Rochon PA, Gurwitz JH. Optimising drug treatment for elderly people: the prescribing cascade. BMJ. 1997;315:1096–9.
40. Steinman MA, Hanlon JT. Managing medications in clinically complex elders: "There's got to be a happy medium". JAMA. 2010;304:1592–601.
41. Kumar S. Problem solving in older cancer patients. 1st ed. Oxford: Atlas Medical; 2016.
42. Balducci L, Goetz-Parten D, Steinman MA. Polypharmacy and the management of the older cancer patient. Ann Oncol. 2013;24:40–4.
43. University of Liverpool. Cancer drug interactions. 2020.
44. Memorial Sloane Kettering Cancer Centre. Integrative medicine. 2020.
45. Flockhart DA. Drug interactions: cytochrome P450 drug interaction table. Indiana University School of Medicine; 2007.
46. Curtin D, Gallagher PF, O'Mahony D. Explicit criteria as clinical tools to minimize inappropriate medication use and its consequences. Ther Adv Drug Saf. 2019;10:2042098619829431.
47. Whitman AM, DeGregory KA, Morris AL, Ramsdale EE. A comprehensive look at polypharmacy and medication screening tools for the older cancer patient. Oncologist. 2016;21:723–30.
48. American Geriatrics Society 2019 Updated AGS Beers Criteria® for potentially inappropriate medication use in older adults. J Am Geriatr Soc. 2019;67:674–94.
49. O'Mahony D, O'Sullivan D, Byrne S, O'Connor MN, Ryan C, Gallagher P. STOPP/START criteria for potentially inappropriate prescribing in older people: version 2. Age Ageing. 2014;44:213–8.
50. Samsa GP, Hanlon JT, Schmader KE, Weinberger M, Clipp EC, Uttech KM, Lewis IK, Landsman PB, Cohen HJ. A summated score for the medication appropriateness index: development and assessment of clinimetric properties including content validity. J Clin Epidemiol. 1994;47:891–6.
51. Miller MG, Kneuss TG, Patel JN, Parala-Metz AG, Haggstrom DE. Identifying potentially inappropriate medication (PIM) use in geriatric oncology. J Geriatr Oncol. 2020; https://doi.org/10.1016/j.jgo.2020.06.013.
52. Lindsay J, Dooley M, Martin J, Fay M, Kearney A, Khatun M, Barras M. The development and evaluation of an oncological palliative care deprescribing guideline: the 'OncPal deprescribing guideline'. Support Care Cancer. 2015;23:71–8.

53. Nightingale G, Hajjar E, Swartz K, Andrel-Sendecki J, Chapman A. Evaluation of a pharmacist-led medication assessment used to identify prevalence of and associations with polypharmacy and potentially inappropriate medication use among ambulatory senior adults with cancer. J Clin Oncol. 2015;33:1453–9.
54. Van Loveren FMAM, Van Berlo IRF, De Laar V, Imholz ALT, Van E, Taxis K, Jansman FGA. Journal of Geriatric Oncology Prevalence and follow-up of potentially inappropriate medication and potentially omitted medication in older patients with cancer—the PIM POM study. J Geriatr Oncol. 2020; https://doi.org/10.1016/j.jgo.2020.06.014.
55. Whitman A, DeGregory K, Morris A, Mohile S, Ramsdale E. Pharmacist-led medication assessment and deprescribing intervention for older adults with cancer and polypharmacy: a pilot study. Support Care Cancer. 2018;26:4105–13.
56. Choukroun C, Leguelinel-Blache G, Roux-Marson C, Jamet C, Martin-Allier A, Kinowski JM, Le Guillou C, Richard H, Antoine V. Impact of a pharmacist and geriatrician medication review on drug-related problems in older outpatients with cancer. J Geriatr Oncol. 2020; https://doi.org/10.1016/j.jgo.2020.07.010.
57. Laroche ML, Charmes JP, Merle L. Potentially inappropriate medications in the elderly: a French consensus panel list. Eur J Clin Pharmacol. 2007;63:725–31.
58. O'Mahony D, Gudmundsson A, Soiza RL, et al. Prevention of adverse drug reactions in hospitalized older patients with multi-morbidity and polypharmacy: the SENATOR* randomized controlled clinical trial. Age Ageing. 2020;49:605–14.
59. Dalton K, Curtin D, O'Mahony D, Byrne S. Computer-generated STOPP/START recommendations for hospitalised older adults: evaluation of the relationship between clinical relevance and rate of implementation in the SENATOR trial. Age Ageing. 2020;49:615–21.
60. Sharma M, Loh KP, Nightingale G, Mohile SG, Holmes HM. Polypharmacy and potentially inappropriate medication use in geriatric oncology. J Geriatr Oncol. 2016;7:346–53.
61. Damián J, Pastor-barriuso R, Valderrama-gama E, De Pedro-cuesta J. Factors associated with falls among older adults living in institutions. BMC Geriatr. 2013;13:6.
62. Mohamed MR, Ramsdale E, Loh KP, et al. Associations of polypharmacy and inappropriate medications with adverse outcomes in older adults with cancer: a systematic review and meta-analysis. Oncologist. 2020;25:94–108.
63. Shrestha S, Shrestha S, Khanal S. Polypharmacy in elderly cancer patients: challenges and the way clinical pharmacists can contribute in resource-limited settings. Aging Med. 2019;2:42–9.
64. Mohamed MR, Ramsdale E, Loh KP, et al. Association of polypharmacy and potentially inappropriate medications with physical functional impairments in older adults with cancer. J Natl Compr Canc Netw. 2021;19:1–8.
65. Badgwell B, Stanley J, Chang GJ, Katz MHG, Lin HY, Ning J, Klimberg SV, Cormier JN. Comprehensive geriatric assessment of risk factors associated with adverse outcomes and resource utilization in cancer patients undergoing abdominal surgery. J Surg Oncol. 2013;108:182–6.
66. Radiosensitizers, radioprotectors, and radiation mitigators. Indian J Dent Res. 2014;25:83–90.
67. Hocum BT, White JR, Heck JW, Thirumaran RK, Moyer N, Newman R, Ashcraft K. Cytochrome P-450 gene and drug interaction analysis in patients referred for pharmacogenetic testing. Am J Heal Pharm. 2016;73:61–7.
68. Whirl-Carrillo M, Huddart R, Gong L, Sangkuhl K, Thorn CF, Whaley R, Klein TE. Anevidence-based framework for evaluating pharmacogenomics knowledge for personalized medicine. Clin Pharmacol Ther. 2021. (online ahead of print).
69. Liu J, Friedman C, Finkelstein J. Pharmacogenomic approaches for automated medication risk assessment in people with polypharmacy. AMIA Jt Summits Transl Sci Proc. 2018;2017:142–51.
70. Brixner D, Biltaji E, Bress A, Unni S, Ye X, Mamiya T, Ashcraft K, Biskupiak J. The effect of pharmacogenetic profiling with a clinical decision support tool on healthcare resource utilization and estimated costs in the elderly exposed to polypharmacy. J Med Econ. 2016;19:213–28.

71. Turner JP, Kantilal K, Holmes HM, Koczwara B. Optimising medications for patients with cancer and multimorbidity: the case for deprescribing. Clin Oncol. 2020;32:609–17.
72. Qi K, Reeve E, Hilmer SN, et al. Older peoples' attitudes regarding polypharmacy, statin use and willingness to have statins deprescribed in Australia. Int J Clin Pharm. 2015;37:949–57. https://doi.org/10.1007/s11096-015-0147-7.
73. Reeve E, Wolff JL, Skehan M, Bayliss EA, Hilmer SN, Boyd CM. Assessment of attitudes toward deprescribing in older medicare beneficiaries in the United States. JAMA Intern Med. 2018;178:1673–80.
74. Garfinkel D, Ilhan B, Bahat G. Routine deprescribing of chronic medications to combat polypharmacy. Ther Adv drug Saf. 2015;6:212–33.
75. Alibhai SMH, Greenwood C, Payette H. An approach to the management of unintentional weight loss in elderly people. CMAJ. 2005;172:773–80.
76. Best Practice Advocacy Centre New Zealand. A practical guide to stopping medicines in older people. Best Practice Advocacy Centre New Zealand. 2010.
77. Hanlon JT, Semla TP, Schmader KE. Alternative medications for medications in the use of high-risk medications in the elderly and potentially harmful drug-disease interactions in the elderly quality measures. J Am Geriatr Soc. 2015;63:e8–e18.
78. Coleman R, Hadji P, Body J-J, et al. Bone health in cancer: esmo clinical practice guidelines. Ann Oncol. 2020;85:34–65.
79. Claxton AJ, Joyce Cramer CP. A systematic review of the associations between dose regimens and medication compliance. Clin Ther. 2001;23:1296–310.
80. Anderson LJ, Nuckols TK, Coles C, et al. A systematic overview of systematic reviews evaluating medication adherence interventions. Am J Heal Pharm. 2020;77:138–47.
81. Cross AJ, Elliott RA, Petrie K, Kuruvilla L, George J. Interventions for improving medication-taking ability and adherence in older adults prescribed multiple medications. Cochrane Database Syst Rev. 2020; https://doi.org/10.1002/14651858.CD012419.pub2.
82. NCCN Older Adult Oncology. NCCN Clinical Practice Guidelines in Oncology. Version 1.
83. Alibhai SMH, Jin R, Loucks A, Yokom DW, Watt S, Puts M, Timilshina N, Berger A. Beyond the black box of geriatric assessment: understanding enhancements to care by the geriatric oncology clinic. J Geriatr Oncol. 2018;9:679–82.
84. Chapman AE, Swartz K, Schoppe J, Arenson C. Development of a comprehensive multidisciplinary geriatric oncology center, the Thomas Jefferson University experience. J Geriatr Oncol. 2013;4:S96–7.
85. Kalsi T, Babic-Illman G, Ross PJ, Maisey NR, Hughes S, Fields P, Martin FC, Wang Y, Harari D. The impact of comprehensive geriatric assessment interventions on tolerance to chemotherapy in older people. Br J Cancer. 2015;112:1435–44.
86. Page AT, Clifford RM, Potter K, Schwartz D, Etherton-Beer CD. The feasibility and effect of deprescribing in older adults on mortality and health: a systematic review and meta-analysis. Br J Clin Pharmacol. 2016;82:583–623.
87. Soo W-K, King M, Pope A, Parente P, Darzins P, Davis ID. Integrated geriatric assessment and treatment (INTEGERATE) in older people with cancer planned for systemic anticancer therapy. J Clin Oncol. 2020;38:12011.
88. Li D, Sun C-L, Kim H, et al. Geriatric assessment-driven intervention (GAIN) on chemotherapy toxicity in older adults with cancer: a randomized controlled trial. J Clin Oncol. 2020;38:12010.
89. Mohile SG, Mohamed MR, Culakova E, et al. A geriatric assessment (GA) intervention to reduce treatment toxicity in older patients with advanced cancer: a University of Rochester Cancer Center NCI community oncology research program cluster randomized clinical trial (CRCT). J Clin Oncol. 2020;38:12009.

Chapter 7
Malnutrition, Cachexia, and Sarcopenia in Older Adults with Cancer and Frailty

Vérène Dougoud-Chauvin, Roman Dubianski, and Anne-Catherine Barras-Moret

Introduction

Older patients with cancer often have unintentional weight loss and this comprises three primary syndromes: malnutrition, cachexia, and sarcopenia. These different concepts have a complex degree of overlap but are not interchangeable concepts. However, over the years, an unsettling number of different definitions have caused confusion in this field.

Cancer and ageing are commonly associated with malnutrition, cachexia, and sarcopenia. Among these, malnutrition is the most widely assessed in cancer patients and it can affect about 40% of older patients [1]. Importantly, malnourished patients are also more likely to have frailty (OR = 3.82, 95% CI 1.35–10.84; $p = 0.01$) [1]. Cancer-related cachexia and sarcopenia also play an important role in these older cancer patients. This results in a complex interplay between cancer, ageing, frailty, and unintentional weight loss [2]. Therefore, understanding the leading cause of unintentional weight loss is challenging and often multifactorial. But this is important, as it may guide the subsequent management of weight loss and the cancer itself.

Assessing the nutritional status of an older patient with cancer, particularly with frailty, is key as it is associated with cancer-specific outcomes, such as treatment tolerability, quality of life, and mortality [3]. In fact, nutritional status is one of the

V. Dougoud-Chauvin (✉)
Division of Medical Oncology, HFR Fribourg Hospital, Fribourg, Switzerland

R. Dubianski
Department of Breast Cancer and Reconstructive Surgery, Maria Sklodowska-Curie National Research Institute of Oncology, Warsaw, Poland

A.-C. Barras-Moret
Division of Internal Medicine, HFR Fribourg Hospital, Fribourg, Switzerland
e-mail: anne-catherine.barras-moret@h-fr.ch

F. Gomes (ed.), *Frailty in Older Adults with Cancer*,
https://doi.org/10.1007/978-3-030-89162-6_7

core components of a comprehensive geriatric assessment (CGA), which supports the decision-making process regarding cancer treatment [4–6].

This chapter will discuss the topics of malnutrition, cachexia, and sarcopenia in older patients with cancer, covering their role in patients with frailty and the negative impact on cancer outcomes. Lastly, key assessment tools for these conditions will be presented with an emphasis on the importance of interventions, in order to improve outcomes for older adults with cancer and frailty.

Defining Malnutrition, Cachexia, Sarcopenia, and the Role of Frailty

An unintentional weight loss comprises three primary syndromes: malnutrition, cachexia, and sarcopenia, which have a complex degree of overlap but are not interchangeable concepts.

Malnutrition is defined by the Global Leadership Initiative in Malnutrition (GLIM) by three criteria [7]: a positive malnutrition screening test combined with at least one phenotypical and one etiological criterion (Table 7.1). Etiological criteria are used to differentiate starvation-type (with protein-sparing metabolism) from cachexia-type or disease-associated malnutrition, characterized by accelerated protein breakdown and the hallmark of muscle loss driven by metabolic changes, most notably systemic inflammation [8].

The prevalence of malnutrition in the general older population ranges between 30 and 80% with considerable differences depending on the setting (e.g., rehabilitation 50%; hospital 38%; nursing home 13%; community 5–8%) [9]. Predisposing factors for a poor nutritional status in older patients are multiple: ageing-associated decreased olfactive and gustative perception, poor dental status, cognitive impairment, reduced functional status affecting cooking or shopping and often social isolation [10].

Table 7.1 Criteria to define malnutrition by the Global Leadership Initiative in Malnutrition [7, 8]

Malnutrition is defined by the combination of 3 criteria	
1. A mandatory positive malnutrition screening	Malnutrition risk predicted by a validated screening test
2. One phenotypical criterion	Loss of or low body mass as defined by at least one of the following: A1: weight loss >5% in 6 months A2: body mass index below 20 kg/m^2 A3: low muscle mass
3. One etiological criterion	Reduced food availability (B1) and/or increased catabolism (B2) B1 (starvation type): reduction in food availability B1a: food intake <50% for > 1 week B1b: any reduction in food intake for >2 weeks B1c: chronic malabsorption B2 (cachexia type): increased acute or chronic systemic inflammation

Cachexia is a multifactorial syndrome defined by an ongoing loss of skeletal muscle mass (with or without loss of fat mass) that cannot be fully reversed by conventional nutritional support, leading to functional impairment. There is a negative protein and energy balance driven by a variable combination of reduced food intake and abnormal metabolism in the context of systemic inflammation which is disease-related, such as related with cancer (cancer cachexia) [11]. The defining criterion is a weight loss greater than 5% in the previous 6 months, or a weight loss greater than 2% with either a body mass index (BMI) <20 kg/m^2 or the evidence of muscle mass depletion [11]. This classification was then validated in cancer patients through a multicenter international follow-up study of more than 800 subjects [12].

The above-described GLIM definition of malnutrition is a helpful approach as it encompasses cachexia as a disease-related sub-type of malnutrition. By using the same criteria described in Table 7.1, cachexia is diagnosed in the presence of a positive malnutrition screening, at least one phenotypical criterion and the etiological criteria being systemic inflammation [7, 8]. In the setting of cancer, which particularly in more advanced stages results in significant systemic inflammation, this is entitled cancer cachexia. Another important consideration is that cachexia may evolve through several phases, from pre-cachexia to advanced cachexia, depending on its severity which often follows the progression of cancer [11].

Sarcopenia consists of low muscle strength combined with low muscle mass or quality [13]. This is another common problem observed in older adults and can be caused by a multitude of factors. Primary sarcopenia is related to normal aging with reduced physical activity and is commonly found in older adults. Conversely, secondary sarcopenia is caused by an underlying disease. Other subcategories of sarcopenia have been identified, with acute sarcopenia (lasting less than 6 months) being related with an acute illness or injury, and chronic sarcopenia (lasting more than 6 months) being related to a chronic condition, like cancer [13]. The histopathological changes of sarcopenia include both a reduction in muscle fiber length and in number of fibers, where the type 2 fiber is the most affected [14]. This is defined as a progressive and generalized skeletal muscle disorder that is associated with increased likelihood of adverse outcomes including falls, fractures, physical disability, and mortality [13]. Moreover, the diagnosis of sarcopenia is probable with low muscle strength but is confirmed with low muscle quantity, while severe sarcopenia is confirmed with reduced muscle strength and muscle quantity with reduced physical performance [13].

What Is the Relationship Between Malnutrition, Cachexia, and Sarcopenia?

While these different conditions may appear phenotypically similar, they are distinct yet partially overlapping. Cachectic patients suffer from malnutrition, but cachexia is not present in all malnourished patients. The weight loss in malnutrition results from the lack of nutrients and is therefore amenable to be improved with intervention [15]. But the weight loss in cachexia and sarcopenia is less amenable to being reversed by simple nutritional support [16].

Sarcopenia is often confused with cachexia since both conditions have muscle loss. But cachexia is often associated with both muscle and fat mass wasting and is associated with chronic illness, such as cancer, resulting in a state of systemic inflammation [16]. Sarcopenia is limited to muscle mass wasting and can occur with ageing [2]. Of note, sarcopenia is a disorder of muscle function and strength [17]. Moreover, whilst patients with cachexia are sarcopenic, most sarcopenic individuals do not have cachexia.

Lastly, the co-existence of malnutrition, cachexia, and sarcopenia may lead to substantial negative patient outcomes, such as decreased quality of life, functional ability, and increased morbidity and mortality, along with an increased hospital rates and costs.

What Is the Relationship Between These Conditions and Frailty?

These conditions can contribute to the development or deterioration of frailty. Fried et al. [18] defined the frailty phenotype based on the following physical criteria: weight loss, exhaustion, physical activity, walking time, and grip strength. People are classified as having frailty if they meet three or more of these features.

Regarding malnutrition, the importance of appropriate nutrition as a means of postponing the development of frailty in older adults is well established [19]. A systematic review looked for evidence pertaining to the association between nutritional status, nutrition measurements (e.g., micronutrients, macronutrients/protein intake, diet quality), and frailty syndrome [20]. It showed that low intake of specific micronutrients increased the risk of frailty and that higher protein intake was associated with a lower frailty risk. One important implication of the inverse association between micronutrients and frailty is that the intake of specific nutrients affects the health of older people and may lead to the development of frailty, among other important conditions. A multicenter study explored the association between protein or amino acid intake and frailty and showed that a higher intake of total protein was significantly associated with a lower prevalence of frailty among older Japanese women, regardless of the protein source or the amino acid that composed the protein [21]. In addition, the quality of the diet is inversely associated with the risk of frailty, thus providing evidence that a potentially modifiable factor such as dietary intake may play a significant role in frailty [22–24]. Cancer cachexia and sarcopenia are also associated with frailty as it is directly associated with functional impairment. One study showed a significantly different prevalence of cachexia between patients without any impairment in Instrumental Activities of Daily Living (IADL) compared to those with >1 impairment (48.5 vs. 72.5%) [25]. In fact, the loss of muscle mass is associated with physical frailty [26, 27] which is considered a pre-disability (with the definition of disability as the need of assistance with basic ADL).

Therefore, the management of malnutrition, cachexia, and sarcopenia is recommended as a key component of the comprehensive care plan for older patients with frailty [28]. In addition, older patients have a higher prevalence of cancer and other chronic illness, which all play an important role in this complex interplay.

Malnutrition, Cancer Cachexia, and Sarcopenia in Patients with Cancer

In the setting of oncology, malnutrition is one of the most common issues for older adults due to its high prevalence and its negative impact on prognosis and treatment tolerability [3, 29]. The incidence varies in studies between 30 and 65% [25, 30–32]. The prevalence of sarcopenia in this population also varies widely from 5 to 89% [33], similarly to cachexia with a prevalence between 40 and 87%, depending on several factors, such as tumor site and stage [34].

Overall, the risk of unintentional weight loss is higher in older cancer patients, particularly those with frailty. The reasons for this are multifactorial, some are related with aging and frailty, whilst others are related with the cancer itself and its treatments (Fig. 7.1).

This risk is particularly high in those patients with symptoms from head and neck or gastrointestinal cancers [30, 35, 36]. Depression, anxiety, and pain can preclude an adequate food intake [37]. Reduced food intake is a key aspect and it can have multiple causes, including poor oral health, medication side effects, depression, dysphagia, gastrointestinal complaints, anorexia, and inadequate nutrition support [7]. A limited food intake can be due to a structural and/or structurally or

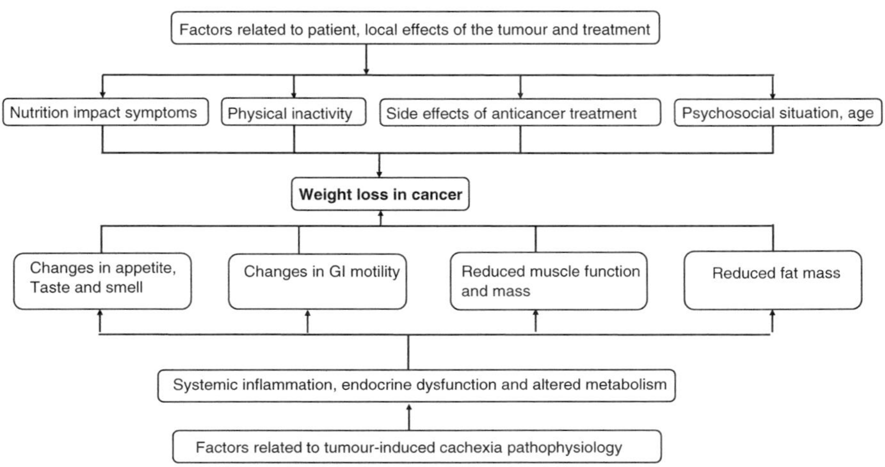

Fig. 7.1 Causes contributing to weight loss in patients with cancer (Adapted from [8])

functional impairment (i.e., mucositis, obstruction, altered intestinal transit, etc.) [38]. Moreover, cancer treatment side effects may cause or aggravate symptoms resulting in reduced food intake [1]. Anorexia is another key multifactorial aspect, which is associated with disturbances of the central physiological mechanisms controlling food intake [37]. Food intake is regulated by long- and short-term acting mediators, involving complex associations between neuropeptides and other neurotransmitters in the central nervous system (CNS). Altered CNS appetite signals can be related to cancer or its treatment and the disturbances of these neuroendocrine pathways lead to anorexia [37].

Malnutrition is a known poor prognostic factor in older patients with cancer and there is a significant correlation between malnutrition and mortality [39, 40]. It can lead to increased incidence of perioperative morbidity, poorer tolerance or more toxicities to treatments, poorer quality of life and higher mortality [41]. It is also associated with a higher rate of hospital admissions and length of stay, which can be improved with nutritional support [30]. Malnutrition has been identified as a risk factor to develop chemotherapy-related toxicity, where a low BMI or a low albumin level is associated with a higher risk of high-grade toxicity [42]. A systematic review and meta-analysis by Hamaker et al. confirmed the significant association between impaired nutritional status (based on validated malnutrition screening tools) and outcomes in older patients with cancer [3]. The presence of malnutrition (or high risk of) significantly increased the intermediate- and long-term mortality (hazard ration 1.87 (95% CI 1.62–2.17). Moreover, those with poorer nutritional status were less likely to complete anticancer treatment according to the plan and had higher use of health care resources. Similarly, in older patients with cancer, sarcopenia is strongly associated with a higher risk of adverse events, such as chemotherapy-related toxic effects, surgical complications, and generally poorer overall survival [33, 43–46].

Earlier identification and appropriate nutritional support may help to reverse or halt the malnutrition trajectory and the above-mentioned negative outcomes associated with poor nutritional status in older patients with cancer [47, 48]. In addition, poor performance status has been directly correlated with weight loss, suggesting that muscle loss may impact the level of activity [38, 48]. Therefore, it is recommended to evaluate the nutritional status of all cancer patients undergoing oncological treatment from the time of cancer diagnosis and repeated as clinically indicated.

Assessment Strategies

In the context of cancer, there are a myriad of causes that contribute to unintentional weight loss. The cancer may cause, for example, a gastrointestinal obstruction which may prohibit adequate nutritional intake; the cancer treatment may cause a severe oral mucositis; cancer-related symptoms such as nausea and anorexia may contribute to a reduced nutritional intake; or there may be cancer cachexia. Alternatively, the unintentional weight loss may not be primarily due to cancer or its treatment, but other conditions. Therefore, in terms of assessment it is key to attempt establishing not just the cause(s) but also a timeline for the nutritional status. The presence of frailty and other geriatric factors such as cognitive impairment or functional dependence is also relevant. This will help establish if cancer is the driving factor in the event of a more recent and rapid decline in the absence of other signs of frailty; instead of a slower process over the course of years associated with other signs of frailty. For these reasons implementing assessment strategies early on is paramount in the management of cancer, particularly for older patients with frailty [5].

There are no screening tools able to accurately distinguish between these three conditions: malnutrition, cachexia, and sarcopenia. Whilst for malnutrition, nutritional assessment alone may be sufficient, though other assessments may also be important. In the case of cachexia and sarcopenia, nutritional assessments alone are insufficient. Therefore, a stepwise assessment of nutritional status, oral intake, age, muscle mass, and function is key [16].

Assessment of Malnutrition

Nutrition is one of the core domains of a comprehensive geriatric assessment and it is also recommended as part of brief geriatric assessments. In fact, elements of nutritional assessment are present in geriatric screening tools, such as the Geriatric-8 (G8) and the CARG chemotherapy toxicity predictive tool. Moreover, nutritional assessment should be done upfront at diagnosis, but also repeated regularly, particularly at key events in the cancer pathway, such as hospital admissions and cancer progression. This will ultimately promote delivering a personalized treatment plan for these complex older adults with cancer and frailty (or at high risk of frailty).

There are several tools available to assess for malnutrition, such as the Nutritional Risk screening 2002 (NRS-2002), the Malnutrition Universal Screening Tool (MUST), short Nutritional Assessment Questionnaire (SNAQ), the Nutritional Risk Screening (NRS), and the Mini Nutritional Assessment (MNA). Regardless of which assessment tool is used, ultimately the nutritional assessment aim is to cover weight loss, body composition (anthropometry and/or imaging), food intake, energy and protein intake, nutritional deficiencies, and the factors contributing to the unintentional weight loss.

One of the most widely used assessments is the MNA, which is a tool validated in older cancer adults that can detect patients at risk of malnutrition before severe weight loss [49]. The MNA is composed of 18 brief questions that can be completed in less than 10 min. It is validated to provide a single and a rapid assessment of nutritional status for patients in outpatient clinics, inpatients, and nursing homes. It has been translated into several languages and validated around the world [49]. This tool is advantageous because diet, protein intake, as well as medications, mobility, the presence of depression and polypharmacy can be assessed, thus leading to potential dietary and other appropriate interventions. The high positive predictive value for detecting pre-frailty may also represent a clinical advantage and lead to early intervention in order to prevent frailty. Therefore two geriatric syndromes can be assessed with this test, malnutrition, and frailty [50]. This comprehensive assessment has been validated in the geriatric population and is commonly used in various studies of older adults with cancer [38]. A short version of this screening tool, entitled MNA-short, with only six questions has also been developed to screen only the malnutrition and can be completed in 5 min (Table 7.2). This can be delivered by any health care professional with a sensitivity of 89%, specificity of 82%, and a high inter-observer reliability of 0.89 [51]. A final score of 0–7 indicates malnutrition, 8–11 at risk of malnutrition, and 12–14 normal nutrition status. Dietary counseling is recommended for scores 11 and below for patients planned to be actively treated with anticancer therapies.

Alternatively, the other NRS-2002 [52] is another option often used which assesses the risk of malnutrition with a BMI < 20.5, weight loss over the last 3 months, low dietary intake during last week and disease severity.

Table 7.2 Mini Nutritional Assessment—short version [49]

(A) Has food intake declined over the past 3 months due to loss of appetite, digestive problems, chewing or swallowing difficulties?	0 = severe decrease in food intake 1 = moderate decrease in food intake 2 = no decrease in food intake
(B) Weight loss during the last 3 months	0 = weight loss greater than 3 kg (6.6 lb.) 1 = does not know 2 = weight loss between 1 and 3 kg (2.2 and 6.6 lb.) 3 = no weight loss
(C) Mobility	0 = bed or chair bound 1 = able to get out of bed/chair 2 = goes out
(D) Has suffered psychological stress or acute distress I the past 3 months?	0 = yes 2 = no
(E) Neuropsychological problems	0 = severe dementia or depression 1 = mild dementia 2 = no psychological problems
(F-1) Body mass Index (BMI) (weight in kg) / (height in m^2)	0 = BMI less than 19 1 = BMI 19 to less than 21 2 = BMI 21 to less than 23 3 = BMI 23 or greater
If BMI is not available, replace question F1 with question F2. Do not answer question F2 if question F1 is already completed	
(F-2) Calf circumference (CC) in cm	0 = CC < 31 1 = CC > 31

Assessment of Cancer Cachexia

Since cachexia is a sub-type of malnutrition with weight loss, systemic inflammation, and sarcopenia, its assessment is multimodal. As part of the assessment of cachexia, a nutritional assessment as above described, should be included, but additionally it is important to investigate the presence of systemic inflammation, using, for example, the Modified Glasgow Prognostic Score or estimate energy expenditure using indirect calorimetry. Moreover, due to its feature of muscle mass loss, understanding the functional status and physical performance of the patients is key, alongside markers of muscle mass and muscle strength as described in more detail bellow.

Assessment of Sarcopenia

The assessment of sarcopenia includes functional status and physical performance based on muscle strength and function which can be assessed via questionnaires and a wide range of tests. Additionally, muscle mass can be assessed with imaging tests.

Regarding questionnaire, the SARC-F is the most widely used and is a simple screening type questionnaire which comprised of five components: Strength, Assistance with walking, Rise from a chair, Climb stairs and Falls [53]. Another available questionnaire consisting of 14 questions is the SarcoPRO, where patients report on measures associated with limitations in IADLS [54]. This is particularly relevant in older adults with cancer and it can be very useful in situations when imaging is not easily obtained.

There is a range of physical performance assessments to assess sarcopenia, where the isokinetic muscle strength testing is the standard for muscle strength testing. The muscle strength can be assessed very easily and extremely cheaply by measuring grip strength using a calibrated handheld dynamometer. The handgrip is indeed often used as marker of sarcopenia [55] and it has been reported that low grip strength is a predictor of poor patient outcomes such as longer hospital stays, increased functional limitations, poor health-related quality of life, and death [56, 57]. Because of its ease of use, grip strength is advised for routine use in hospital practice, as well as another very easily performed test: the chair stand test (or Sit to Stand 5 test) that measures the amount of time needed for a patient to rise five times from a seated position without using the arms. Another variation of this test is the timed chair stand test that counts how many times a patient can sit and rise and in the chair over a 30-s period of time. The Short Physical Performance Battery (SPPB) is a composite test that includes assessment of gait speed, a chair stand test, and a balance test. The maximum score is 12 points, and a score of ≤8 points indicates poor physical performance [58]. Other examples of tests include a 6-min walk test or bioelectrical impedance analysis (BIA), the latter does not measure muscle mass directly but instead derives an estimate of muscle mass based on whole-body electrical conductivity.

Regarding the radiological assessment of sarcopenia, this can be assessed by various methods: computed tomography (CT), magnetic resonance imaging (MRI), or dual energy X-ray absorptiometry (DEXA). Radiological examination with CT or MRI is considered the gold standard to accurately assess muscle and fat mass and to detail individual muscle/muscle groups. Total skeletal muscle mass can be assessed in cross-sectional imaging by measuring muscle area on a single image slice (usually at the L3 vertebra) and, after accounting for stature, is reported as the skeletal muscle index. It has been proven that images of a specific lumbar vertebral landmark (L3) significantly correlate with whole-body muscle [11, 59] and it can also predict prognosis [46, 60]. Another radiological measurement used in some research studies is the mid-thigh imaging by CT and MRI, which is a good predictor of whole-body skeletal muscle mass and very sensitive to change [46, 59, 61, 62]. Opinions about the CT-based measurement of the psoas muscle as simple and predictive of morbidities in sarcopenia are divided [63–65]. Cross sectional radiological imaging can also assess the body composition which is crucial in the diagnostic process of cachexia. Moreover, radiological imaging can be used not only to measure muscle cross-sectional area, but also muscle quality by assessing muscle radiodensity. It has been proven that muscle density measured by Hounsfield units on CT is inversely related to muscle lipid content and is a surrogate for muscle quality [66]. However, the costs of CT/MRI and the requirement of specialized personnel to use the equipment limit the use of those measurement in the sarcopenia diagnosis.

Intervention Strategies

Intervention on Malnutrition

Malnutrition is reversible, therefore once malnutrition or a high risk of malnutrition has been identified, a dietary/nutritionist counseling is key to implement a personalized nutritional care and to evaluate the indications for further nutritional support. The goal of a specialized dietary counseling is to evaluate the nutritional status, to assess all the potential barriers for an adequate and sufficient food intake, to determine qualitatively and quantitatively the food intake, and to determine the adequate nutritional support according to the treatment plan and prognosis. Intensive individualized nutritional counseling requires a nutritional professional with specific experience in oncology. Evidence from other settings, particularly inpatient acute care and rehabilitation settings, has shown the importance of systematically identifying malnutrition and targeting it with protein-calorie supplementation, which can improve functional recovery, quality of life, and survival in specific settings [67, 68].

If the patient is not able to cover his caloric needs with regular food despite dietary counseling, nutritional supplements should be considered and prescribed. They can represent a useful support, when food intake is a problem, to cover about one third of the caloric and protein needs [67]. Nutritional supplementation should be enteral, with the oral route preferred. For patients who are unable to ingest adequate calories, tube feeding should be considered, either with a temporary nasojejunal tube or a more permanent access with a percutaneous gastric or jejunal tube [69]. Tube feeding may be indicated in the case of dysphagia due to obstruction, motility dysfunction, or mucosal inflammation and patients with head and neck or upper gastrointestinal cancers are at particular risk of developing it. Parenteral nutrition should be reserved for highly selected patients. Such nutritional assistance should be set up if the food intakes are significantly below the nutritional needs (at least 60% below), which may occur in the setting of some advanced gastrointestinal cancers [70]. Indications for prolonged parenteral nutrition in these patients is restricted to severe intestinal failure induced by cancer treatment (surgical resection, radiation enteritis) or impossibility to reach the gastrointestinal tract for an enteral nutrition [71]. A multidisciplinary discussion is mandatory before introducing a parenteral nutrition, and its associated risks must be considered, such as catheter-related infection and thrombosis, chronic hepatopathy and osteopathy, derangements of substrate and electrolyte levels and fluid overload.

One of the key problems in the success of nutritional supplements especially in older patients is the compliance. In older patients the taste is an important consideration, therefore the availability of supplements with different tastes is helpful. But patients need to be educated to understand that nutritional supplements play a complementary role to regular food, but they should not be replacing meals. Oral nutritional supplements are easy to implement and to organize as they can be delivered directly at home. Doses can be split over the day to the patients' convenience or even be given in small portions each time the patient has to take a medication. In the older population with frailty, oral nutritional supplements should be continued for a minimum of 1 month and compliance should be regularly assessed [15]. If the addition of oral nutritional supplements is not enough to cover the caloric needs, enteral nutrition should be considered, if indicated. The indication for a prolonged enteral nutrition is part of the general cancer care and must be discussed interdisciplinary depending on the cancer stage and the patient's condition. Prolonged enteral nutrition indications usually include dysphagia and intestinal failure, both induced by cancer treatment. The European Society for Clinical Nutrition and Metabolism (ESPEN) guidelines on enteral nutrition in the geriatric population state that for long-term nutritional support, gastrostomy tubes may be preferred to nasogastric tubes because they are associated with fewer treatment failures, better nutritional status, and are more convenient for the patient [72]. Long-term artificial nutrition should be performed at home or in an institution, not in the hospital. For older patients, the family member should also be trained for the home management. The poor compliances with the tubes and the frequent failure (obstruction, accidental withdrawal) can compromise the success of the artificial nutrition support.

For older cancer patients, factors to consider in tailoring interventions include disease status, cancer site, cancer treatment, comorbidity, physiological age, psychosocial factor, and frailty. In advanced cancer, patient quality of life is one of the highest priorities. Ultimately, the goal of nutritional counseling and artificial nutrition is this patient population is to diminish the impact of adverse effects from treatments and to improve outcomes, in particular quality of life [3, 73, 74]. In fact, a corrective intervention improves health outcomes, prevents the onset of disability, improves quality of life, and saves healthcare costs [75].

A systematic review on the association between nutritional status and outcomes in older patients with cancer and on the benefit of nutritional interventions in improving those outcomes found a strong association between nutritional status and intermediate- and long-term mortality [3]. In hospitalized medical patients, a strategy based on screening and individualized nutritional intervention improved clinical outcome and even mortality as shown in the EFFORT study [75]. Several other studies showed positive outcome for nutritional interventions [3]. Improvement of quality of life was found in three of six studies assessing this outcome [76–78]. One study showed a significantly higher chemotherapy completion rate in the intervention group compared to the standard of care group [79]. One other study suggested that dietary counseling reduced radiotherapy toxicity [80]. An association between treatment-related complications, i.e. wound infections in surgical patients was also shown [81, 82]. Parenteral nutrition as intervention has also demonstrated an improvement in quality of life for patients with incurable gastrointestinal disease [83].

Therefore, providing individualized dietary counseling to avoid a further deterioration of nutritional state is paramount [77]. Dietary counseling as a nutritional intervention has the potential to improve quality of life and to improve treatment completion rates. Nutritional support may also decrease post-operative complication rates. However, the effect on patients already malnourished is very limited and the interventions may not significantly improve prognosis [3]. In fact, neither interventions with specialized dietary counseling (versus usual care) nor oral nutritional support has shown an improvement in patient survival [3]. Lastly, it is key to identify the possible co-existence of cachexia and/or sarcopenia, which could affect patient outcomes in addition to malnourishment.

Intervention on Cancer Cachexia

The intervention on cancer cachexia must be personalized with a multitargeted and multimodal approach [84]. As cachexia is linked with systemic inflammation caused by the cancer, the anti-cancer treatment itself is a key aspect on the intervention plan. But other interventions should be included when anti-cancer treatment is offered to a cachectic patient. These include dietary counseling and nutritional support, physical exercise, anti-catabolic and anti-inflammatory treatments, as well as psychological and social support [85].

The previously described dietary counseling and nutritional support for those with malnutrition is part of the intervention plan. In summary, patients should receive guidance on choosing high-energy, high-protein and enriching foods and on the use of oral nutritional supplements [85]. The use of oral supplements can be effective in inducing weight gain and increasing dietary intake [86]. Specialized oral supplements enriched in protein and containing N-3 fatty acids have been studied in cancer cachexia and some trials suggest benefits of using them on weight, lean body mass and some aspects of quality of life when given to patients receiving chemotherapy, radiotherapy or chemoradiotherapy [87, 88]. In case this proves inadequate, interventions such as tube feeding or, in selected cases, parenteral nutrition should be offered [85]. Tube feeding is associated with a risk of serious mechanical (e.g., tube blockage), gastrointestinal (e.g., diarrhea), infectious (e.g., aspiration pneumonia), and metabolic (e.g., refeeding syndrome) complications [89]. In some patients with severely compromised gastrointestinal function adequate nutrition by the oral or enteral route may be not efficient and, in that case, parenteral nutrition may be considered.

Pharmacological interventions in the treatment of cancer cachexia include corticosteroids, progestins, cannabinoids, olanzapine, non-steroidal anti-inflammatory drugs (NSAIDs), and prokinetics. Corticosteroids such as prednisolone, methylprednisolone, and dexamethasone may be used to increase appetite but only for a short period of up to 2–3 weeks. They are also recommended for the control of cancer-related fatigue [90]. Medroxyprogesterone acetate and megestrol acetate are well known progestins frequently used to increase appetite and body weight. Unfortunately, no improvement in quality of life was observed while using them [91] and their potential risk of thromboembolic events should be always considered before prescribing these drugs. Cannabinoids are not recommended for the treatment of cancer related cachexia due to the insufficient evidence of their significant effect on the improvement of appetite or quality of life [92, 93]. Olanzapine is an atypical antipsychotic drug acting on dopamine and serotonin receptors which could be considered to treat appetite and nausea in patients with advanced cancer [94]. Due to the insufficient evidence recent recommendations [85] suggest no use of NSAIDs and prokinetics (such as metoclopramide) alone in the treatment of the cancer cachexia.

Intervention on Sarcopenia

The aim of those interventions is to improve muscle mass, strength, function, and overall physical performance. Multimodal interventions are required due to the pathogenesis of sarcopenia and the intervention should be focused on nutrition and exercise. Physical exercise prevents the loss of muscle mass and helps to improve the muscle strength and function therefore every older cancer patient should be encouraged and trained to perform physical exercises, which, as has been proven, can reduce the incidence of mobility disabilities [95]. Nutrition, particularly the intake of proteins, also plays a role in the maintenance of muscle mass. In this setting, it is currently recommended to increase the daily protein intake in older patients to 1–1.2 g/kg/day, and in patients with conditions characterized by enhanced catabolism, such as cancer, to increase this even to 1.2–1.5 g/kg/day [96, 97]. An adequate duration of the protein supplementation is also crucial. Unfortunately, no recommended pharmacological intervention exists to treat sarcopenia. The most frequently used agents such as testosterone or myostatin inhibitors show only partial improvement on some of the secondary outcome measures.

Conclusion

Malnutrition, cachexia, and sarcopenia are highly prevalent in older patients with cancer. There is a complex and multifactorial interplay between these, frailty and cancer. Moreover, these are of major concern in cancer patients, particularly for those also with frailty, because of their negative impact on outcomes, such as quality of life, treatment complications, and prognosis. Therefore, assessments and interventions regarding the nutritional status of an older patient are a key component of the geriatric assessments. The final goal is to recognize these conditions early on, tailor a personalized cancer treatment plan, and initiate the adequate support interventions to improve positively the global quality of life and prognosis of these older cancer patients.

References

1. Zhang X, Edwards BJ. Malnutrition in older adults with cancer. Curr Oncol Rep. 2019;21(9):80.
2. Gingrich A, Volkert D, Kiesswetter E, Thomanek M, Bach S, Sieber CC, et al. Prevalence and overlap of sarcopenia, frailty, cachexia and malnutrition in older medical inpatients. BMC Geriatr. 2019;19(1):120.
3. Hamaker ME, Oosterlaan F, van Huis LH, Thielen N, Vondeling A, van den Bos F. Nutritional status and interventions for patients with cancer—a systematic review. J Geriatr Oncol. 2021;12(1):6–21.
4. Wildiers H, Heeren P, Puts M, Topinkova E, Janssen-Heijnen MLG, Extermann M, et al. International Society of Geriatric Oncology consensus on geriatric assessment in older patients with cancer. J Clin Oncol Off J Am Soc Clin Oncol. 2014;32(24):2595–603.
5. Mohile SG, Dale W, Somerfield MR, Schonberg MA, Boyd CM, Burhenn PS, et al. Practical assessment and management of vulnerabilities in older patients receiving chemotherapy: ASCO guideline for geriatric oncology. J Clin Oncol Off J Am Soc Clin Oncol. 2018;36(22):2326–47.
6. Hamaker ME, Te Molder M, Thielen N, van Munster BC, Schiphorst AH, van Huis LH. The effect of a geriatric evaluation on treatment decisions and outcome for older cancer patients—a systematic review. J Geriatr Oncol. 2018;9(5):430–40.
7. Cederholm T, Jensen GL, Correia MITD, Gonzalez MC, Fukushima R, Higashiguchi T, et al. GLIM criteria for the diagnosis of malnutrition—a consensus report from the global clinical nutrition community. Clin Nutr. 2019;38(1):1–9.
8. Cancer cachexia in adult patients: ESMO Clinical Practice Guidelines☆—ESMO Open [Internet]. [cité 14 juill 2021]. Disponible sur: https://www.esmoopen.com/article/S2059-7029(21)00049-1/fulltext
9. Agarwal E, Miller M, Yaxley A, Isenring E. Malnutrition in the elderly: A narrative review. Maturitas. 2013;76(4):296–302.
10. Liposits G, Orrevall Y, Kaasa S, Österlund P, Cederholm T. Nutrition in cancer care: a brief, practical guide with a focus on clinical practice. JCO Oncol Pract. 2021. https://doi.org/10.1200/OP.20.00704

11. Fearon K, Strasser F, Anker SD, Bosaeus I, Bruera E, Fainsinger RL, et al. Definition and classification of cancer cachexia: an international consensus. Lancet Oncol. 2011;12(5):489–95.
12. Blum D, Stene GB, Solheim TS, Fayers P, Hjermstad MJ, Baracos VE, et al. Validation of the consensus-definition for cancer cachexia and evaluation of a classification model—a study based on data from an international multicentre project (EPCRC-CSA). Ann Oncol Off J Eur Soc Med Oncol. 2014;25(8):1635–42.
13. Cruz-Jentoft AJ, Bahat G, Bauer J, Boirie Y, Bruyère O, Cederholm T, et al. Sarcopenia: revised European consensus on definition and diagnosis. Age Ageing. 2019;48(1):16–31.
14. Dhillon RJS, Hasni S. Pathogenesis and Management of Sarcopenia. Clin Geriatr Med. 2017;33(1):17–26.
15. Volkert D, Beck AM, Cederholm T, Cruz-Jentoft A, Goisser S, Hooper L, et al. ESPEN guideline on clinical nutrition and hydration in geriatrics. Clin Nutr. 2019;38(1):10–47.
16. Miller J, Wells L, Nwulu U, Currow D, Johnson MJ, Skipworth RJE. Validated screening tools for the assessment of cachexia, sarcopenia, and malnutrition: a systematic review. Am J Clin Nutr. 2018;108(6):1196–208.
17. Rosenberg IH. Sarcopenia: origins and clinical relevance. J Nutr. 1997;127(5 Suppl):990S–1S.
18. Fried LP, Tangen CM, Walston J, Newman AB, Hirsch C, Gottdiener J, et al. Frailty in older adults: evidence for a phenotype. J Gerontol A Biol Sci Med Sci. 2001;56(3):M146–56.
19. Kelaiditi E, Guyonnet S, Cesari M. Is nutrition important to postpone frailty? Curr Opin Clin Nutr Metab Care. 2015;18(1):37–42.
20. Lorenzo-López L, Maseda A, de Labra C, Regueiro-Folgueira L, Rodríguez-Villamil JL, Millán-Calenti JC. Nutritional determinants of frailty in older adults: A systematic review. BMC Geriatr. 2017;17(1):108.
21. Kobayashi S, Asakura K, Suga H, Sasaki S. Three-generation study of women on diets and health study group. High protein intake is associated with low prevalence of frailty among old Japanese women: a multicenter cross-sectional study. Nutr J. 2013;12:164. Recherche Google [Internet] [cité 15 juill 2021].
22. Bollwein J, Diekmann R, Kaiser MJ, Bauer JM, Uter W, Sieber CC, et al. Dietary quality is related to frailty in community-dwelling older adults. J Gerontol A Biol Sci Med Sci. 2013;68(4):483–9.
23. Chan R, Leung J, Woo J. Dietary patterns and risk of frailty in Chinese community-dwelling older people in Hong Kong: a prospective cohort study. Nutrients. 2015;7(8):7070–84.
24. Shikany JM, Barrett-Connor E, Ensrud KE, Cawthon PM, Lewis CE, Dam T-TL, et al. Macronutrients, diet quality, and frailty in older men. J Gerontol A Biol Sci Med Sci. 2014;69(6):695–701.
25. Dunne RF, Roussel B, Culakova E, Pandya C, Fleming FJ, Hensley B, et al. Characterizing cancer cachexia in the geriatric oncology population. J Geriatr Oncol. 2019;10(3):415–9.
26. Masson E. Sarcopenia: A useful paradigm for physical frailty [Internet]. EM-Consulte. [cité 11 avr 2021]. Disponible sur: https://www.em-consulte.com/article/808170/article/sarcopenia-a-useful-paradigm-for-physical-frailty
27. Morley JE, von Haehling S, Anker SD, Vellas B. From sarcopenia to frailty: a road less traveled. J Cachexia Sarcopenia Muscle. 2014;5(1):5–8.
28. Dent E, Morley JE, Cruz-Jentoft AJ, Woodhouse L, Rodríguez-Mañas L, Fried LP, et al. Physical frailty: ICFSR international clinical practice guidelines for identification and management. J Nutr Health Aging. 2019;23(9):771–87.
29. Nutritional aspects of the cancer/aging interface. J Geriatr Oncol. [Internet]. [cité 29 juin 2020]. Disponible sur: https://www.geriatriconcology.net/article/S1879-4068(11)00026-9/fulltext
30. Pressoir M, Desné S, Berchery D, Rossignol G, Poiree B, Meslier M, et al. Prevalence, risk factors and clinical implications of malnutrition in French Comprehensive Cancer Centres. Br J Cancer. 2010;102(6):966–71.
31. Bozzetti F, Mariani L, Lo Vullo S, SCRINIO Working Group, Amerio ML, Biffi R, et al. The nutritional risk in oncology: a study of 1,453 cancer outpatients. Support Care Cancer Off J Multinatl Assoc Support Care Cancer. 2012;20(8):1919–28.

32. Paillaud E, Caillet P, Campillo B, Bories PN. Increased risk of alteration of nutritional status in hospitalized elderly patients with advanced cancer. J Nutr Health Aging. 2006;10(2):91–5.
33. Rier HN, Jager A, Sleijfer S, Maier AB, Levin M-D. The prevalence and prognostic value of low muscle mass in cancer patients: a review of the literature. The Oncologist. 2016;21(11):1396–409.
34. Ni J, Zhang L. Cancer cachexia: definition, staging, and emerging treatments. Cancer Manag Res. 2020;12:5597–605.
35. Palesty JA, Dudrick SJ. What we have learned about cachexia in gastrointestinal cancer. Dig Dis Basel Switz. 2003;21(3):198–213.
36. Stewart GD, Skipworth RJE, Fearon KCH. Cancer cachexia and fatigue. Clin Med Lond Engl. 2006;6(2):140–3.
37. Nicolini A, Ferrari P, Masoni MC, Fini M, Pagani S, Giampietro O, et al. Malnutrition, anorexia and cachexia in cancer patients: A mini-review on pathogenesis and treatment. Biomed Pharmacother. 2013;67(8):807–17.
38. Mislang AR, Di Donato S, Hubbard J, Krishna L, Mottino G, Bozzetti F, et al. Nutritional management of older adults with gastrointestinal cancers: An International Society of Geriatric Oncology (SIOG) review paper. J Geriatr Oncol. 2018;9(4):382–92.
39. Norman K, Pichard C, Lochs H, Pirlich M. Prognostic impact of disease-related malnutrition. Clin Nutr Edinb Scotl. 2008;27(1):5–15.
40. Gu W, Zhang G, Sun L, Ma Q, Cheng Y, Zhang H, et al. Nutritional screening is strongly associated with overall survival in patients treated with targeted agents for metastatic renal cell carcinoma. J Cachexia Sarcopenia Muscle. 2015;6(3):222–30.
41. French Speaking Society of Clinical Nutrition and Metabolism (SFNEP). Clinical nutrition guidelines of the French Speaking Society of Clinical Nutrition and Metabolism (SFNEP): summary of recommendations for adults undergoing non-surgical anticancer treatment. Dig Liver Dis Off J Ital Soc Gastroenterol Ital Assoc Study Liver. 2014;46(8):667–74.
42. Dotan E, Tew WP, Mohile SG, Ma H, Kim H, Sun C-L, et al. Associations between nutritional factors and chemotherapy toxicity in older adults with solid tumors. Cancer. 2020;126(8):1708–16.
43. Kazemi-Bajestani SMR, Mazurak VC, Baracos V. Computed tomography-defined muscle and fat wasting are associated with cancer clinical outcomes. Semin Cell Dev Biol. 2016;54:2–10.
44. Shachar SS, Deal AM, Weinberg M, Nyrop KA, Williams GR, Nishijima TF, et al. Skeletal muscle measures as predictors of toxicity, hospitalization, and survival in patients with metastatic breast cancer receiving taxane-based chemotherapy. Clin Cancer Res Off J Am Assoc Cancer Res. 2017;23(3):658–65.
45. Brown JC, Cespedes Feliciano EM, Caan BJ. The evolution of body composition in oncology-epidemiology, clinical trials, and the future of patient care: facts and numbers. J Cachexia Sarcopenia Muscle. 2018;9(7):1200–8.
46. Kim EY, Kim YS, Park I, Ahn HK, Cho EK, Jeong YM. Prognostic significance of CT-determined sarcopenia in patients with small-cell lung cancer. J Thorac Oncol Off Publ Int Assoc Study Lung Cancer. 2015;10(12):1795–9.
47. Zhang X, Sun M, McKoy JM, Bhulani NNA, Valero V, Barcenas CH, et al. Malnutrition in older patients with cancer: appraisal of the mini nutritional assessment, weight loss, and body mass index. J Geriatr Oncol. 2018;9(1):81–3.
48. Dewys WD, Begg C, Lavin PT, Band PR, Bennett JM, Bertino JR, et al. Prognostic effect of weight loss prior to chemotherapy in cancer patients. Am J Med. 1980;69(4):491–7.
49. Guigoz Y, Vellas BJ. [Malnutrition in the elderly: the mini nutritional assessment (MNA)]. Ther Umsch Rev Ther. 1997;54(6):345–50.
50. Soysal P, Isik AT, Arik F, Kalan U, Eyvaz A, Veronese N. Validity of the mini-nutritional assessment scale for evaluating frailty status in older adults. J Am Med Dir Assoc. 2019;20(2):183–7.
51. Kaiser MJ, Bauer JM, Ramsch C, Uter W, Guigoz Y, Cederholm T, et al. Validation of the Mini Nutritional Assessment short-form (MNA-SF): a practical tool for identification of nutritional status. J Nutr Health Aging. 2009;13(9):782–8.

52. Kondrup J, Rasmussen HH, Hamberg O, Stanga Z, Ad Hoc ESPEN Working Group. Nutritional risk screening (NRS 2002): a new method based on an analysis of controlled clinical trials. Clin Nutr Edinb Scotl. 2003;22(3):321–36.
53. Malmstrom TK, Miller DK, Simonsick EM, Ferrucci L, Morley JE. SARC-F: a symptom score to predict persons with sarcopenia at risk for poor functional outcomes. J Cachexia Sarcopenia Muscle. 2016;7(1):28–36.
54. Gewandter JS, Dale W, Magnuson A, Pandya C, Heckler CE, Lemelman T, et al. Associations between a patient-reported outcome (PRO) measure of sarcopenia and falls, functional status, and physical performance in older patients with cancer. J Geriatr Oncol. 2015;6(6):433–41.
55. Norman K, Stobäus N, Smoliner C, Zocher D, Scheufele R, Valentini L, et al. Determinants of hand grip strength, knee extension strength and functional status in cancer patients. Clin Nutr Edinb Scotl. 2010;29(5):586–91.
56. Ibrahim K, May C, Patel HP, Baxter M, Sayer AA, Roberts H. A feasibility study of implementing grip strength measurement into routine hospital practice (GRImP): study protocol. Pilot Feasibility Stud. 2016;2:27.
57. Leong DP, Teo KK, Rangarajan S, Lopez-Jaramillo P, Avezum A, Orlandini A, et al. Prognostic value of grip strength: findings from the Prospective Urban Rural Epidemiology (PURE) study. Lancet Lond Engl. 2015;386(9990):266–73.
58. Beaudart C, McCloskey E, Bruyère O, Cesari M, Rolland Y, Rizzoli R, et al. Sarcopenia in daily practice: assessment and management. BMC Geriatr. 2016;16(1):170.
59. Mourtzakis M, Prado CMM, Lieffers JR, Reiman T, McCargar LJ, Baracos VE. A practical and precise approach to quantification of body composition in cancer patients using computed tomography images acquired during routine care. Appl Physiol Nutr Metab Physiol Appl Nutr Metab. 2008;33(5):997–1006.
60. Baracos V, Kazemi-Bajestani SMR. Clinical outcomes related to muscle mass in humans with cancer and catabolic illnesses. Int J Biochem Cell Biol. 2013;45(10):2302–8.
61. Lee SJ, Janssen I, Heymsfield SB, Ross R. Relation between whole-body and regional measures of human skeletal muscle. Am J Clin Nutr. 2004;80(5):1215–21.
62. Baracos VE, Reiman T, Mourtzakis M, Gioulbasanis I, Antoun S. Body composition in patients with non-small cell lung cancer: a contemporary view of cancer cachexia with the use of computed tomography image analysis. Am J Clin Nutr. 2010;91(4):1133S–7S.
63. Hanaoka M, Yasuno M, Ishiguro M, Yamauchi S, Kikuchi A, Tokura M, et al. Morphologic change of the psoas muscle as a surrogate marker of sarcopenia and predictor of complications after colorectal cancer surgery. Int J Colorectal Dis. 2017;32(6):847–56.
64. Baracos VE. Psoas as a sentinel muscle for sarcopenia: a flawed premise. J Cachexia Sarcopenia Muscle. 2017;8(4):527–8.
65. Rutten IJG, Ubachs J, Kruitwagen RFPM, Beets-Tan RGH, Olde Damink SWM, Van Gorp T. Psoas muscle area is not representative of total skeletal muscle area in the assessment of sarcopenia in ovarian cancer. J Cachexia Sarcopenia Muscle. 2017;8(4):630–8.
66. Aubrey J, Esfandiari N, Baracos VE, Buteau FA, Frenette J, Putman CT, et al. Measurement of skeletal muscle radiation attenuation and basis of its biological variation. Acta Physiol Oxf Engl. 2014;210(3):489–97.
67. Milne AC, Potter J, Vivanti A, Avenell A. Protein and energy supplementation in elderly people at risk from malnutrition [Internet]. Vol. 2009, Cochrane Database Syst Rev. Wiley; 2009 [cited 2020 Oct 4]. Available from: https://pubmed.ncbi.nlm.nih.gov/19370584/
68. Kou K, Momosaki R, Miyazaki S, Wakabayashi H, Shamoto H. Impact of nutrition therapy and rehabilitation on acute and critical illness: A systematic review. J UOEH. 2019;41(3):303–15.
69. Bouras EP, Lange SM, Scolapio JS. Rational approach to patients with unintentional weight loss. Mayo Clin Proc. 2001;76(9):923–9.
70. Gerard S, Steinmeyer Z, Lozano S, et al. Digestive organ ageing and cancer. In: Extermann M, editor. Geriatric oncology. Cham: Springer; 2020.
71. Nutritional support of the elderly cancer patient: Long-term nutritional support—ClinicalKey [Internet]. [cité 12 août 2020]. Disponible sur: https://www.clinicalkey.fr/#!/content/journal/1-s2.0-S0899900714004985

72. Howard L, Malone M. Clinical outcome of geriatric patients in the United States receiving home parenteral and enteral nutrition. Am J Clin Nutr. 1997;66(6):1364–70.
73. Ravasco P, Monteiro-Grillo I, Marques Vidal P, Camilo ME. Impact of nutrition on outcome: a prospective randomized controlled trial in patients with head and neck cancer undergoing radiotherapy. Head Neck. 2005;27(8):659–68.
74. Presley CJ, Dotan E, Soto-Perez-de-Celis E, Jatoi A, Mohile SG, Won E, et al. Gaps in nutritional research among older adults with cancer [Internet]. J Geriatr Oncol. 2016;7:281–92. Elsevier Ltd [cited 2020 Oct 4].
75. Schuetz P, Fehr R, Baechli V, Geiser M, Deiss M, Gomes F, et al. Individualised nutritional support in medical inpatients at nutritional risk: a randomised clinical trial. Lancet. 2019;393(10188):2312–21.
76. Furness K, Silvers MA, Savva J, Huggins CE, Truby H, Haines T. Long-term follow-up of the potential benefits of early nutritional intervention in adults with upper gastrointestinal cancer: a pilot randomised trial. Support Care Cancer Off J Multinatl Assoc Support Care Cancer. 2017;25(11):3587–93.
77. Isenring EA, Capra S, Bauer JD. Nutrition intervention is beneficial in oncology outpatients receiving radiotherapy to the gastrointestinal or head and neck area. Br J Cancer. 2004;91(3):447–52.
78. Kabata P, Jastrzębski T, Kąkol M, Król K, Bobowicz M, Kosowska A, et al. Preoperative nutritional support in cancer patients with no clinical signs of malnutrition—prospective randomized controlled trial. Support Care Cancer Off J Multinatl Assoc Support Care Cancer. 2015;23(2):365–70.
79. Xie F-L, Wang Y-Q, Peng L-F, Lin F-Y, He Y-L, Jiang Z-Q. Beneficial effect of educational and nutritional intervention on the nutritional status and compliance of gastric cancer patients undergoing chemotherapy: a randomized trial. Nutr Cancer. 2017;69:1–10.
80. Ravasco P, Monteiro-Grillo I, Camilo M. Individualized nutrition intervention is of major benefit to colorectal cancer patients: long-term follow-up of a randomized controlled trial of nutritional therapy. Am J Clin Nutr. 2012;96(6):1346–53.
81. Burden ST, Gibson DJ, Lal S, Hill J, Pilling M, Soop M, et al. Pre-operative oral nutritional supplementation with dietary advice versus dietary advice alone in weight-losing patients with colorectal cancer: single-blind randomized controlled trial. J Cachexia Sarcopenia Muscle. 2017;8(3):437–46.
82. Burden ST, Hill J, Shaffer JL, Campbell M, Todd C. An unblinded randomised controlled trial of preoperative oral supplements in colorectal cancer patients. J Hum Nutr Diet Off J Br Diet Assoc. 2011;24(5):441–8.
83. Obling SR, Wilson BV, Pfeiffer P, Kjeldsen J. Home parenteral nutrition increases fat free mass in patients with incurable gastrointestinal cancer. Results of a randomized controlled trial. Clin Nutr Edinb Scotl. 2019;38(1):182–90.
84. Arends J. Struggling with nutrition in patients with advanced cancer: nutrition and nourishment-focusing on metabolism and supportive care. Ann Oncol. 2018;29(suppl_2):ii27–34.
85. Arends J, Strasser F, Gonella S, et al. Cancer cachexia in adult patients: ESMO Clinical Practice Guidelines. ESMO Open. 2021 Jun;6(3):100092. https://doi.org/10.1016/j.esmoop.2021.100092.
86. de van der Schueren MAE, Laviano A, Blanchard H, et al. Systematic review and meta-analysis of the evidence for oral nutritional intervention on nutritional and clinical outcomes during chemo(radio) therapy: current evidence and guidance for design of future trials. Ann Oncol. 2018;29(5):1141–53.
87. Blackwood HA, Hall CC, Balstad TR, et al. A systematic review examining nutrition support interventions in patients with incurable cancer. Support Care Cancer. 2020;28(4):1877–89.
88. de Aguiar Pastore Silva J, Emilia de Souza Fabre M, Waitzberg DL. Omega-3 supplements for patients in chemotherapy and/or radiotherapy: a systematic review. Clin Nutr. 2015;34(3):359–66.
89. Blumenstein I, Shastri YM, Stein J. Gastroenteric tube feeding: techniques, problems and solutions. World J Gastroenterol. 2014;20(26):8505–24.

90. Fabi A, Bhargava R, Fatigoni S, et al. Cancer-related fatigue: ESMO clinical practice guidelines for diagnosis and treatment. Ann Oncol. 2020;31(6):713–23.
91. Ruiz Garcia V, López-Briz E, Carbonell Sanchis R, et al. Megestrol acetate for treatment of anorexia-cachexia syndrome. Cochrane Database Syst Rev. 2013;2013(3):Cd004310.
92. Jatoi A, Windschitl HE, Loprinzi CL, et al. Dronabinol versus megestrol acetate versus combination therapy for cancer-associated anorexia: a North Central Cancer Treatment Group study. J Clin Oncol. 2002;20(2):567–73.
93. Strasser F, Luftner D, Possinger K, et al. Comparison of orally administered cannabis extract and delta-9-tetrahydrocannabinol in treating patients with cancer-related anorexia-cachexia syndrome: a multicenter, phase III, randomized, double-blind, placebo-controlled clinical trial from the Cannabis-In-Cachexia-Study-Group. J Clin Oncol. 2006;24(21):3394–400.
94. Navari RM, Pywell CM, Le-Rademacher JG, et al. Olanzapine for the treatment of advanced cancer-related chronic nausea and/or vomiting: a randomized pilot trial. JAMA Oncol. 2020;6(6):895–9.
95. Pahor M, Guralnik JM, Ambrosius WT, Blair S, Bonds DE, Church TS, et al. Effect of structured physical activity on prevention of major mobility disability in older adults: the LIFE study randomized clinical trial. JAMA. 2014;311(23):2387–96.
96. Bauer J, Biolo G, Cederholm T, Cesari M, Cruz-Jentoft AJ, Morley JE, et al. Evidence-based recommendations for optimal dietary protein intake in older people: a position paper from the PROT-AGE Study Group. J Am Med Dir Assoc. 2013;14(8):542–59.
97. Deutz NEP, Bauer JM, Barazzoni R, Biolo G, Boirie Y, Bosy-Westphal A, et al. Protein intake and exercise for optimal muscle function with aging: recommendations from the ESPEN Expert Group. Clin Nutr Edinb Scotl. 2014;33(6):929–36.

Chapter 8
Physical Performance and Functional Status in Older Adults with Cancer and Frailty

Jenny Welford, Jennifer Woods, Sofia Duque, and Fabio Gomes

Introduction

Maintenance of physical performance and function is crucial for older adults to remain autonomous and independent in managing their everyday activities and roles, which in turn is key in the promotion of quality of life and well-being. Whilst chronological age does not reflect physiological reserve or health status, physical performance and functional status can be considered surrogate markers of physiological reserve and biological age. Older adults with the same chronological age can have markedly different levels of physical performance and functionality, which highlights the need for holistic and objective assessments to be undertaken prior to considering cancer treatment, to ensure that health and wellbeing can be optimised and to inform shared decision-making. However, even though these markers can be predictive of patient outcomes in oncology, cancer treatment decisions for older

J. Welford (✉)
Occupational Therapy Department, Northern Centre for Cancer Care, Freeman Hospital, Newcastle, UK
e-mail: jenny.welford1@nhs.net

J. Woods
Christie NHS Foundation Trust, Manchester, UK
e-mail: Jennifer.woods8@nhs.net

S. Duque
Internal Medicine Department, Hospital Cuf Descobertas, Lisbon, Portugal

Preventive Medicine and Public Health Institute, Faculty of Medicine, Universidade de Lisboa, Lisbon, Portugal

F. Gomes
Medical Oncology Department, The Christie NHS Foundation Trust, Manchester, UK
e-mail: fabio.gomes2@nhs.net

F. Gomes (ed.), *Frailty in Older Adults with Cancer*,
https://doi.org/10.1007/978-3-030-89162-6_8

adults are often based on subjective assessments and clinical impressions, as well as some preconceptions primarily based on chronological age [1].

Many older adults may experience physical performance and functional deterioration at the first stage of their oncological disease, even prior to diagnosis, because of their cancer, chronic conditions, and geriatric syndromes such as frailty. This has the potential to impair the person's ability to tolerate oncological treatments, their quality of life and in some cases their survival. Moreover, it is important to recognise that changes to a person's physical performance and function can occur at any stage during the cancer care pathway and are key manifestations of frailty, which warrant specialist assessment and intervention to improve outcomes. Intervention can increase a person's ability to manage their symptoms, enable them to engage in both basic and meaningful activities and can support future planning based on what matters to them most.

This chapter will highlight the critical factors that influence physical performance and function within an oncological setting and their significance for older adults, particularly those with frailty. It will also provide an overview of key assessments and interventions to maintain or improve a person's physical performance and function.

Physical Performance and Functional Status

Physical performance is defined as an objective measure of whole-body function related to strength, mobility and transfers, which involves multiple systems (such as, muscle, bones, and the neurological and cardiovascular systems). These objective measures are also incorporated in the diagnostic criteria of frailty [2].

Functional status is defined as the ability to perform essential tasks of self-care and daily life. It includes basic activities of daily living (BADL), instrumental activities of daily living (IADL) and advanced activities of daily living (AADL). BADL are required for survival on a day-to-day basis such as bathing, dressing, toileting, feeding and transferring. IADL are activities required to live independently in the community such as shopping, managing finances, managing medication, cooking or using transport. IADL requires a higher level of cognitive capacity, whilst BADL relies more on physical performance. AADL is more complex activities, subdivided into physical, leisure, social and productive domains, requiring higher levels of cognitive, physical and social capacities, such as: skills to maintain working and planning trips, participation in community groups, driving or planning events.

The ability to perform ADL independently is vital; hence, the World Health Organisation (WHO) [3] defined the goal of healthy ageing as helping people in "*developing and maintaining the functional ability that enables well-being*". However, dependency in ADL can be a result of poor physical performance, cognitive impairment, physical symptoms or social disruption [4, 5].

Physical performance and functional status are key domains of a comprehensive geriatric assessment (CGA), which is the standard methodology for assessment and planning of care in geriatrics. Hence that the recommendations by the International Society of Geriatric Oncology (SIOG) include these parameters to also be assessed in oncology practice [6]. Moreover, some tools designed specifically for oncology, such as the frailty screening Geriatric-8 (G8) and the CARG chemotherapy toxicity prediction tool, incorporated some of these assessments, in particular mobility [7–10].

To implement effective strategies to maintain or improve physical performance and functional status, it is critical to recognise a variety of determinants (Table 8.1) and to intervene in every factor that is contributing to the impairment [11]. The multifactorial nature of functional status requires a holistic assessment and intervention, which can be facilitated using a CGA. In fact, the impairments in different domains of the CGA such as polypharmacy, multimorbidity, nutrition, mood, cognition, and social isolation, all have the potential to negatively impact on a person's physical performance, function and quality of life. Moreover, these often overlap and influence one another.

Cardiorespiratory capacity in older patients may be impaired due to deconditioning, lifestyle habits, high body mass index, cardiac diseases, lung diseases and premorbid anaemia [12]. This can then be aggravated due to cancer complications or treatment side-effects [13]. Furthermore, cardiorespiratory capacity declines between 5 and 26% during exposure to various systemic chemotherapy regimens and may not recover following treatment cessation [13].

Musculoskeletal and neurological conditions are more common in older people and can lead to variable disability in physical performance, mobility and ADL [14, 15]. These conditions can be exacerbated (or even triggered) by cancer or the side effects of its treatment, which can then impact physical performance and function. Chemotherapy-induced neuropathy and cancer cachexia are common examples [16, 17]. Moreover, many drugs frequently prescribed in older adults with cancer may affect musculoskeletal and neurological status such as corticosteroids, anticholinergics, sedative antidepressants, antipsychotics, barbiturates, benzodiazepines,

Table 8.1 Physical performance and functional status determinants in older adults

- Cardiorespiratory capacity
- Musculoskeletal and neurological status
- Cancer-related symptoms
- Multimorbidity
- Medication and polypharmacy
- Nutritional status
- Cognitive status
- Psychological status
- Social support/isolation
- Motivation
- Hearing and vision
- Environment barriers
- Urinary and faecal continence

metoclopramide, meperidine, muscle relaxants, etc. Although multifactorial, musculoskeletal and neurological status often leads to a risk of falls. People aged 65 and older are at greater risk of experiencing falls [18] and it is estimated that older adults with a cancer diagnosis are at a 15–20% greater risk of falling [19].

Cancer-related symptoms, either caused directly by cancer or indirectly by its treatments, can play an important role in the physical performance and functional status of older adults with cancer. Cheng et al. [20] identified a cluster of symptoms in an older cohort of patients with cancer that are relevant determinants of functional status including pain, fatigue, insomnia and mood disturbance. Moreover, other prevalent symptoms, such as gastrointestinal or respiratory, can be particularly impactful in patients with gastrointestinal or lung cancer respectively. For example, between 19 and 51% of patients with advanced cancer experience dyspnoea (shortness of breath) [21]. A major consequence of breathlessness is physical inactivity, which can precipitate a downward spiral of disease-causing muscle deconditioning, leading to reduced activity and increased disability [22].

Frailty, Disability and Cancer

Frailty is related to poor physical performance and functional status, but these concepts are not interchangeable. Frailty corresponds to a state of increased vulnerability to stressful events (e.g. infection, fall, new medication, hospitalisation or cancer diagnosis) due to the decline of physiological and functional reserve and an increased risk of developing dependency in ADL and poor health outcomes. Fried [23] described frailty in terms of phenotypes, which include weakness (low grip strength), slowness (reduced walking speed), shrinking (unintentional weight loss) and low physical activity. Most definitions of frailty emphasise its physical component; however, the concept of frailty also includes cognitive, psychological and social domains, which are often interlinked and can have just as great an impact on day-to-day life.

According to the clinical course of frailty (Fig. 8.1), physical performance and functional ability progressively decline, leading to disability that may end up in dependency. Therefore, frailty is often regarded as a pre-dependency condition; disability is an intermediate stage of functional impairment or limitation and usually precedes dependency in ADL as illustrated by the disablement process conceptualised by Verbrugge and Jette [24]. Conceptually, disability is a social process and is established when the impairment or limitation culminates in the loss or minimisation of the ability to play expected social roles [11]. Disability can be operationalised as the condition of having difficulty or experiencing dependency in carrying out ADL, which is required to maintain the person in their home environment and contribute to their quality of life [25].

Whilst assessing the patient, functional status provides useful information regarding disability and therefore prognosis, rehabilitation needs or additional support—the focus of these tools is on functional limitations and disability and are

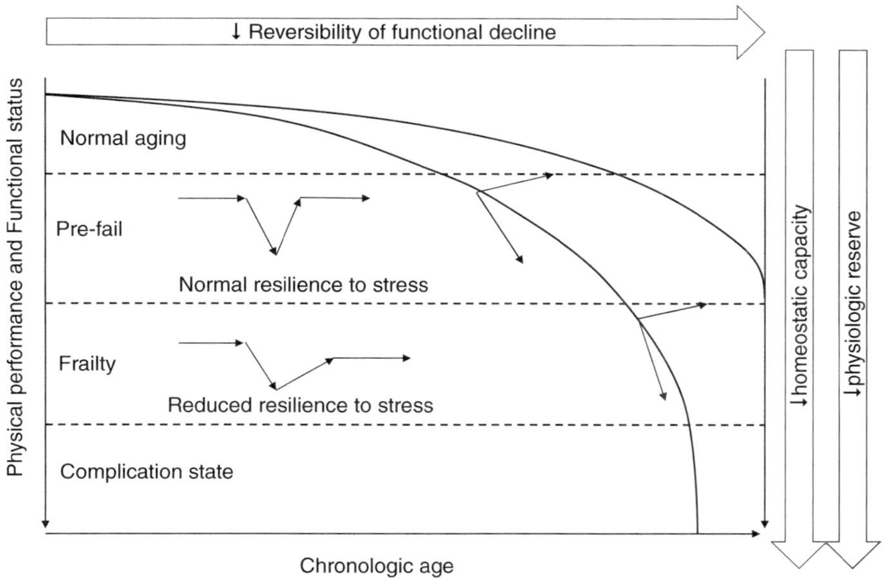

Fig. 8.1 Schematic graphic about the frailty clinical course (Adapted from [30])

unlikely to identify older adults who may be in the early phases of impairment [26]. Therefore, the use of physical performance assessments is crucial to identify patients, who may present as with pre-frailty or frailty, who may not yet be demonstrating functional decline or disability. In doing so, it enables clinicians to identify any potential issues earlier on within the pathway and mitigate potential adverse treatment outcomes by either improving physical performance through prehabilitation [27] or referring the person for geriatric assessment.

For older adults living with frailty, physical performance and functional status can be impacted as a result of a relatively minor stressor, such as a fall, urinary tract infection or changes in medication. Moreover, their recovery is more prolonged and often incomplete which can therefore result in a disability. A frequent example is the older adult who has experienced a fall. This can result in physical injury and pain, which if not appropriately addressed, may further impact their ability to mobilise and perform ADL, ultimately resulting in disability.

Importantly, cancer often presents not just as a major stressor for these patients with frailty, but also as a significant contributing factor [28]. Hence, that these patients represent a high-risk group where considerations about physical performance and function should be incorporated as part of their care, which helps to guide diagnostic and treatment decisions.

When thinking about decision-making, for some severely frail patients with advanced or end-stage chronic diseases, proceeding with diagnosis workup and cancer treatments may be of no benefit to their survival and quality of life near the end-of-life. In this case, morbidity and mortality are likely to rely more on other chronic conditions rather than cancer. Moreover, cancer diagnostics and treatment procedures can decompensate chronic conditions further [29], impacting quality of life and accelerating death.

The assessment of physical performance and functional status is often extrapolated as a physiological and functional reserve, but these often do not overlap (Fig. 8.1) [30]. In fact, patients with cancer often present with a recent deterioration due to, for example, cancer-related anaemia or breathlessness, which can be reversible (at least partially) and does not reflect their reserve. Therefore, when assessing these domains to aid decision-making, it is key to also explore the patients' baseline status prior to a recent deterioration (premorbid status). Premorbid status is more reliable to infer physiological and functional reserve and can therefore be more helpful at determining vulnerability or tolerance to cancer treatments. However, some older patients may remain independent in ADL for example but have poor reserves and be highly vulnerable to adverse events and at high risk of developing disability. In this case, the patient may not be a suitable candidate for certain more aggressive treatments, or they may benefit from prehabilitation interventions to improve physiological reserve and increase resilience [31, 32]. Frailty assessment is, therefore, a better marker of physiological reserve and resistance to cancer treatments, as it enables clinicians to categorise patients into fit, vulnerable/intermediate and frail [33], which can then determine the most appropriate cancer treatment and rehabilitation strategy.

Lastly, when deciding upon a specific cancer treatment and its intensity, decisions must be taken according to patient expectations, attitudes towards the burden of treatment and their goals of care regarding not only survival but also functionality [34]. It has been shown that about 75% of older adults with cancer and/or advanced chronic diseases would not accept a treatment, if severe functional impairment was expected, even though their survival could increase [34]. These findings were reinforced in a recent study, which highlighted that older adults with a cancer diagnosis prioritised autonomy, cognitive ability and functional independence over survival [35].

Physical Performance and Functional Status in Cancer Outcomes

In oncology, it is important to consider the physiological stress caused by anticancer treatments, such as chemotherapy drugs, radiotherapy and surgery. Such stressors can be particularly problematic for older patients who have frailty or a pre-frailty status, resulting in poor health outcomes.

An assessment of functional status, based on ADL scales, adds substantially to the functional information provided by the traditional oncological assessment using the Eastern Cooperative Oncology Group (ECOG) or the Karnofsky performance status and it has a predictive role for cancer outcomes. A landmark review by

Extermann et al. [36] highlighted the benefit particularly of IADL versus ECOG performance status as an independent predictor of cancer outcomes in multivariate analysis, such as chemotoxicity, post-operative morbidity, survival and early death. Cesari et al. [37] found that in older women with gynaecological cancer, IADL had a better prognostic value for survival than the ECOG or Karnofsky performance status. Furthermore, Tinquaut et al. [38] reported the results of a pooled analysis of three multicentric prospective phase II studies that evaluated the prognostic value of several geriatric variables for overall survival in older patients with advanced ovarian cancer, treated with carboplatin-based first-line chemotherapy. In the multivariate analysis, an impaired functional status measured by IADL (score <25) was confirmed to be associated with decreased survival. Similarly, Giannotti et al. [39] found that IADL was one the most significant predictors of 1-year mortality on multivariate analysis for older adults with cancer who underwent surgery for gastrointestinal cancer, alongside cancer stage. The prediction of functional recovery after cancer surgery specifically in older adults with cancer is being investigated in the international multicentric GOSAFE study, which included a significant proportion of patients with frailty and results are awaited [40]. Several other studies in the settings of lung cancer, haematological cancer and colorectal cancer have also highlighted the relationship between functional status and mortality [41–43]

A more recent systematic review by Couderc et al. [44] examining functional status in geriatric oncology, included 40 out of 4061 identified studies across multiple cancer types. This review showed that functional status is of prognostic value in a geriatric oncology setting despite heterogeneous methodology and inclusion criteria. It also suggested a need for a consensus in terms of the assessment and methodology used. Moreover, some evidence points towards the predictive value of BADL with regards to overall survival and outcomes of postoperative complications, whereas IADL seems to be predictive of treatment feasibility and chemotoxicity outcomes in older patients treated for cancer.

In terms of physical performance markers, gait speed and grip strength have been widely studied. In a recent large study by Hantel et al. [45], gait speed was shown to significantly predict survival in multivariable analysis for older adults with haematological cancers. Similarly, Liu et al. [46] found gait speed to be a predictor of unplanned hospitalisations and emergency department visits, as well as higher mortality in patients with haematological malignancies. In addition, for patients with good ECOG performance status (0 or 1), every 5kg decrease in grip strength was associated with worse survival, but not unplanned hospital or emergency department visits. Apart from a prognostic value in assessing survival outcomes, a review by Caillet et al. [47] highlighted that physical performance and functional status also had predictive value in terms of cancer treatment tolerability and toxicity. These impairments were correlated with the risk of post-surgical complications, disability after starting chemotherapy and a lower likelihood of chemotherapy completion.

Whilst one may argue a possible superiority of these physical and functional assessments for older adults with cancer regarding outcome prediction, in oncology, the most widely used measure is ECOG performance status [48]. However, ECOG performance status is also increasingly recognised as a limited assessment, particularly for older sub-groups, as it fails to consider multimorbidity, cognition or frailty [49]. It is therefore highly valuable and in line with what is used in the field of geriatrics to use a range of other physical and functional assessments [49]. The use of geriatric assessment is advocated by the ASCO [10] as traditional oncology performance measures such as the ECOG or Karnosfky do not accurately predict those older adults who are at greatest risk from adverse cancer treatment outcomes. Moreover, the use of the geriatric assessment within an oncology setting provides healthcare professionals the opportunity to explore what is important to the person, which thereby helps facilitate shared decision discussions around balancing cancer treatment and potential cancer treatment toxicity against the quality of life.

Assessment of Physical Performance and Functional Status

The use of physical performance and function assessments in addition to performance status measures has already been advocated in this chapter. Preserving functional decline is considered to be the goal of geriatric care and is a marker of well-being [50] and within an oncology setting maintaining and improving physical performance and function, has the potential to minimise adverse outcomes and enhance the quality of life [51]. It is advocated that older adults undergoing cancer treatment have regular functional and physical performance assessments undertaken, as they can often experience rapid deterioration in a short period of time [51].

Physical Performance Assessments

Hand Grip strength is a measure of muscle strength widely used in research and within clinical settings [2]. Grip strength is measured during muscular isotonic contraction using a dynamometer. When using handgrip, it is advocated that a standardised measurement protocol be used, such as the Southampton protocol [52]. Grip strength has been found to be a predictive tool for cognitive decline, functional status, and mortality for individuals with a cancer diagnosis [46, 53–56]. Low hand grip strength in cancer patients has also been associated with increased hospital admissions and length of stay in hospital [46] as well as impaired health-related quality of life [53].

The Short Physical Performance Battery (SPPB) consists of three measures, which include gait speed, timed chair stand and balance tests [2]. In a systematic review exploring the use of physical performance measures in predicting outcomes for cancer patients, the SPPB was shown to be a predictor for survival, treatment complications and functional decline [57]. Moreover, the SPPB can also be used as a diagnostic tool for sarcopenia [58], which can have a negative impact on the level of function.

The Gait Speed test is a key measure when undertaking a CGA as it enables clinicians to develop risk profiles and establish care plans [59]. Moreover, gait speed is an appropriate measurement in clinical settings as it is quick and inexpensive to administer. For older adults with a cancer diagnosis the gait speed test has been shown to be a predictive tool in relation to the quality of life, mortality, falls and physical and cognitive decline [45, 46, 60, 61]. The Gait Speed test may also be used as a screening tool to identify older adults undergoing colorectal surgery, who are at risk from preoperative complications and who would benefit from a comprehensive geriatric assessment [62].

The 10-metre walk test can be used across a wide range of patient populations. A 14m stretch of walkway is required to perform this test. Markers are set at 2 and 8m. The individual walks without assistance for 10m; however, a time is only recorded between the 2 and 8m mark to allow for an acceleration and deceleration phase. The patient is asked to walk the distance at a comfortable walking speed and at a fast-walking speed. The slower the person takes to mobilise the 6m, the higher the risk of falls and functional decline [63] which can lead to dependency in ADL.

Timed Up and Go (TUG) is a simple test to assess a person's mobility and balance and is reported to have high inter-rater reliability [2]. In older cancer patients the TUG has been demonstrated to be a predictive tool for identifying patients who are at an increased risk of post-operative complications [64] and is a predictor of falls in older breast cancer survivors [65]. This assessment is used to assess dynamic balance and requires the individual to rise from a chair and walk 3m, turn around and return to the starting point. Older adults who take longer than 15 seconds to complete the TUG are at greater risk of falling; however, it should be noted that evidence suggests that the TUG has limited ability to predict falls in community settings [66]. Therefore, it is recommended that this assessment is used in conjunction with other physical performance assessments [66]. For older adults with a cancer diagnosis, a TUG score of greater than 20 seconds has been associated with an increased risk of major post-operative complications and decreased survival rates [64, 67]. In a multicentre study undertaken by Hurria et al. [7], which explored chemotoxicity in older adults it was identified that individuals with a TUG score of greater than 10 seconds were at an increased risk of chemotoxicity.

Turn 180 degree test is commonly used in geriatric settings; however, its use in oncology settings appears to be limited. It aims to identify difficulty in turning, which can indicate reduced mobility and function and increased dependency in managing ADL in older adults [68]. Falls are of significant concern in older adults with cancer as they can lead to oncological treatment disruptions, morbidity and mortality [69]. Turning has been identified as one of the leading causes of older adults experiencing a fall [70]. Undertaking this test enables the assessment of dynamic posture stability [71], which can identify if tailored fall management intervention would be beneficial. The individual is asked to stand up and step around so that they are facing the opposite direction. If the person needs to take more than four steps to complete this, they are considered at risk of experiencing a fall [68].

The *Chair-Stand test* is quick and easy to administer in a clinic setting and it consists of counting the number of sit-to-stands that the person completes within

30 seconds. The individual is required to have their arms across their body, placing their hands on the opposite shoulders and completing as many sit-to-stands as they can in 20 seconds [51]. This assessment measures the person's lower body power, balance and endurance, which relate to the most physically demanding ADL [2]. This test has been demonstrated to be a predictor of falls; however, its use may be limited for individuals with moderate to severe mobility impairment [2].

Functional Status Assessments

Performance Status is commonly measured within the oncology setting using either the Karnosfky Performance Scale or the ECOG performance status. The Karnosfky Performance Scale [72] categorises patients in regard to their functional impairment and rates individuals on a linear scale of 0 (Dead) to 100 (normal activity). The ECOG performance status scale [48] is a widely used assessment in oncology to establish how the person's disease affects their ability to perform ADL as their disease progresses. Individuals are graded between 0 and 5 (0 = fully independent to 5 = dead). The ECOG primarily focuses on the person's level of function and how their symptoms may be impacting the ability to engage in everyday activities. The ECOG has been considered to be a valuable tool, which offers a quick and simplistic method of assessment, which has provided prognostic and predictive utility in regard to survival [49]. However, both the Karnosfky Performance Scale and ECOG are based on functional ability and due to their subjectivity and openness to bias [49], there is the potential for an overestimation of functional ability. It is therefore advocated that when assessing and managing older adults with cancer, the use of other physical and functional assessments should be used to support diagnostic and treatment decisions [10, 49].

The *Barthel Index (BI) of ADL* consists of ten items that measure daily functioning, in particular the ability to manage self-care ADL, such as washing, dressing, toileting, feeding and mobility [73]. In cancer, the BI can be administered by the patient self-reporting their level of independence; however, it is recommended that patients over the age of 75 should be assessed by rehabilitation specialists, due to the potential discrepancy between self-report scores and actual ADL performance scores [74]. Clinicians can complete the BI by direct observation, which can take up to 20 minutes. Scores are awarded based on the individual's level of independence, with a maximum score of 20 available. Lower scores indicate a higher level of disability. Within cancer patients, the BI is a useful tool to identify ADL domains that would benefit from rehabilitation [50, 75] to maintain the person's function and thereby increase the quality of life.

The *Katz Index of Independence in ADL* was originally designed for assessing functional status in older adults and has been used extensively throughout the research as an effective tool to identify the functional capabilities of older adults in clinical and community settings [76] and is used within oncology research to consider the level of disability amongst adults with a cancer diagnosis [50, 77, 78].

Lower scores in ADL independence are associated with poorer health-related quality of life [79–81]. The Katz Index of Independence in ADL focuses on performance in six functions: bathing, dressing, toileting, transferring, continence, and feeding. An important consideration in the utilisation of the Katz Index of Independence in ADL as a standardised measurement of physical function and performance in cancer care is that the tool is sensitive to changes in declining health and functional status; however, it is limited in its ability to demonstrate small changes made through the older person engaging in rehabilitation [76]. Therefore, it is important to utilise this assessment in conjunction with a physical performance assessment.

Lawton's IADL assesses the older person's ability to live independently in their community. There are eight areas of function included in this tool, which include the ability to use a telephone, shopping, food preparation, housekeeping, laundry, transport, responsibility for medications and ability to manage finances [82]. However, one of the limitations of this is that as it is a self-report measure, it has the potential to lead to an overestimation or underestimation of ability [82].

Interventions to Optimise Physical Performance and Function

As discussed throughout this chapter, physical performance and function in older adults can have a significant impact on treatment compliance, overall survival and quality of life. It is therefore crucial that older adults undergoing cancer treatment have timely access throughout the cancer pathway to rehabilitation professionals, such as occupational therapists, physiotherapists and dietitians, to address potentially modifiable functional deficits, which could potentially reduce mortality, morbidity and enhance quality of life [50, 51].

Intervention planning must be personalised, integrated and global, covering cancer and the CGA domains, in order to optimise physical performance and function and to improve clinical and patient outcomes, such as quality of life, treatment compliance and survival.

Physical Activity

It is advocated that physical activity can benefit patients at all stages of any cancer pathway [83]. Keeping active can improve survival rates [84–86], help maintain quality of life, improve sleep [87], can enhance psychological wellbeing [87] and reduce cancer-related fatigue [88]. Moreover, physical activity can help individuals with a cancer diagnosis to return to their pre-treatment health more quickly [83].

It is recommended that older cancer patients and survivors gradually increase their physical activity over time until they can achieve 150 minutes (moderate intensity) or 75 minutes (high intensity) aerobic exercise, in addition to 20–30 minutes muscle strengthening training 2–3 times per week; and regular stretching daily [89].

For older adults, physical activity interventions have the potential to prevent, delay or treat frailty through improving physical performance [90]. A recent study suggests that there are long-term benefits in older adults with cancer engaging in physical activity programmes during their treatment [91]. The preliminary data collated by Arrieta et al. [91] suggests the use of telephone physical activity advice during and after cancer treatment for older adults undergoing cancer treatment, may prevent long-term physical performance decline.

Older adults with a cancer diagnosis generally have a positive perception regarding physical activity [92]; however are often faced with multiple barriers to engaging in physical activity, such as fatigue, a lack of mental energy and social support or a fear of experiencing harm as a result of undertaking exercise [92]. This may prevent them from achieving the recommended exercise guidelines, which can lead to a deterioration in their physical performance, functional ability and lead to the person becoming frail. It is therefore important that any programme of physical activity is personalised to what is realistic for each person's needs. It should also be noted that these needs will change over time depending on treatment and disease progression. Support to identify realistic goals can be undertaken by different healthcare professionals including dietitians, occupational therapists, physiotherapists and nurses, who must also consider that older adults living with frailty and cancer may experience barriers to engagement such as poor transport links, financial constraints or as a result of their physical or cognitive function [93].

Modifying ADL

Occupational therapists specialising in oncology possess a range of skills in addition to in-depth knowledge about cancer and cancer treatments, and the impact that this has on an individual's function [94, 95]. When occupational therapists assess an older person with cancer, they do so using a holistic approach, focusing on physical, psychological, emotional, social and cognitive needs, which then form the basis of activity modification and goal setting [96]. Although evidence is lacking, it is thought that patients benefit from being referred to occupational therapy services as early as possible in the cancer pathway, either when there is a high suspicion of upcoming functional disruption or as soon as this disruption is evident [94, 95]. This enables potentially modifiable functional deficits to be addressed, through either education, rehabilitation or the use of compensatory techniques, such as using adaptive equipment [51, 94, 95, 97].

Cancer-Related Symptoms

Dyspnoea Underlying causes of breathlessness should be tackled prior to non-pharmacological interventions, which can include positioning, breathing techniques, equipment provision and muscle strengthening. Such interventions can prevent deconditioning and functional decline as a result of the person being able to remain physically active. Between five and seven out of every ten patients with lung cancer experience dyspnoea, rising to 90% in those with advanced disease [98]. Current literature also tells us that older adults with lung cancer are most likely to experience a decline in ADLs, specifically bathing, dressing, getting in and out of a chair and using the toilet due to symptoms such as dyspnoea and fatigue [99].

Cancer-Related Fatigue The provision of cancer-related fatigue education to all patients undergoing cancer treatment is recommended [100] and is sought by patients themselves. Data from several studies highlight the value of educational interventions, particularly the provision of anticipatory guidance and coping skills training, in assisting patient self-management of fatigue [101–104] and is particularly important for those individuals receiving systemic therapies [105]. Fatigue management education may include energy conservation techniques, such as planning activities that result in the individual balancing rest and activity, prioritising or delegating tasks, as well as prescribing adaptive equipment or modifying the person's environment. Sleep hygiene and nutritional advice are also key components to fatigue management. It may also be beneficial for the individual to have a medication review and the de-prescribing of some drugs that can contribute to cancer-related fatigue. In addition, there is strong evidence that supports the benefits of exercise in the management of cancer-related fatigue [88, 106–109]. A combination of aerobic walking and resistance band training, not only reduces cancer-related fatigue but can also improve muscular strength [110], which in turn can positively influence the person's physical performance, functional status and reduce their frailty status [111, 112].

Pain Management Older adults with cancer are more susceptible to pain than their younger counterparts as a result of having multiple comorbidities in addition to the ageing process [113]. Pain management in older adults with cancer is often complex and poorly managed [114]. This can lead to the person experiencing psychological distress and a withdrawal from everyday activities. This can consequently result in a deterioration in the person's level of function and performance status and a worsening level of frailty negatively impacting upon their quality of life [114]. It is advocated that when considering pain management for older adults, a multidisciplinary approach is the gold standard [115, 116].

Occupational therapists are able to provide pain management strategies for older adults with cancer, such as activity management and adaptation, lifestyle management and developing coping strategies to enable the individual to continue to engage or re-engage in everyday meaningful activities [117]. Coping strategies may include the use of mindfulness or other relaxation and visualisation techniques, which have been found to be beneficial in chronic and neuropathic pain [118]. The provision of adaptive equipment may also aid pain management as a result of activities being undertaken in a more ergonomically effective manner. Physiotherapists use a range of techniques to support pain relief. This may include working with individuals to improve balance and posture, enhancing muscle strength around the affected area and developing personalised exercise programmes to reduce muscle tightness and joint stiffness [119]. Non-pharmacological interventions can reduce the need for pain medication, which can induce many side effects that potentially impair physical performance and function like sedation and constipation.

Conclusion

Physical performance and functional status are two distinct concepts that are linked with frailty. Both have a strong predictive and prognostic value in respect to cancer treatment toxicity and mortality. These can and should be used to support treatment decisions and to facilitate shared decision-making, particularly in older adults with frailty. These assessments are part of CGA and there are multiple factors that influence physical performance and functional status, which strengthens the need to undertake a CGA prior to commencing cancer treatment. This not only helps to understand the benefits and risks to the individual by undergoing cancer treatment but also helps to identify potentially modifiable deficits. Even for oncology teams without access to geriatric services, there are several simple and brief physical performance and functional assessments that can be undertaken in the clinical setting, that can make a difference in developing treatment plans for those older patients who have frailty or pre-frailty. This, together with having access to the specialist skills of occupational therapists, physiotherapists and dietitians, can have a significant impact on optimising the person's health and wellbeing throughout the cancer treatment pathway, thereby contributing to improving patient and clinical outcomes.

References

1. Hamaker ME, van Rixtel B, Thunnissen P, Oberndorff AH, Smakman N, ten Bokkel HD. Multidisciplinary decision-making on chemotherapy for colorectal cancer: an age-based comparison. J Geriatr Oncol. 2015; https://doi.org/10.1016/j.jgo.2015.01.002.
2. Beaudart C, Rolland Y, Cruz-Jentoft AJ, et al. Assessment of muscle function and physical performance in daily clinical practice. Calcif Tissue Int. 2019; https://doi.org/10.1007/s00223-019-00545-w.
3. World Health Organisation. World report on ageing and health. 2015.
4. Ćwirlej-Sozańska A, Wiśniowska-Szurlej A, Wilmowska-Pietruszyńska A, et al. Determinants of ADL and IADL disability in older adults in southeastern Poland. BMC Geriatr. 2019; https://doi.org/10.1186/s12877-019-1319-4.
5. Wang D, Yao J, Zirek Y, Reijnierse EM, Maier AB. Muscle mass, strength, and physical performance predicting activities of daily living: a meta-analysis. J Cachexia Sarcopenia Muscle. 2020;11:3–25.
6. Wildiers H, Heeren P, Puts M, et al. International society of geriatric oncology consensus on geriatric assessment in older patients with cancer. J Clin Oncol. 2014; https://doi.org/10.1200/JCO.2013.54.8347.
7. Hurria A, Togawa K, Mohile SG, et al. Predicting chemotherapy toxicity in older adults with cancer: a prospective multicenter study. J Clin Oncol. 2011; https://doi.org/10.1200/JCO.2011.34.7625.

8. Soubeyran P, Bellera C, Goyard J, et al. Validation of the G8 screening tool in geriatric oncology: the ONCODAGE Project. J Clin Oncol. 2011; https://doi.org/10.1200/jco.2011.29.15_suppl.9001.
9. Burhenn PS, McCarthy AL, Begue A, Nightingale G, Cheng K, Kenis C. Geriatric assessment in daily oncology practice for nurses and allied health care professionals: opinion paper of the Nursing and Allied Health Interest Group of the International Society of Geriatric Oncology (SIOG). J Geriatr Oncol. 2016; https://doi.org/10.1016/j.jgo.2016.02.006.
10. Mohile SG, Dale W, Somerfield MR, Schonberg MA, Boyd CM, Burhenn PS, Canin B, Cohen HJ, Holmes HM, Hopkins JO, Janelsins MC, Khorana AA, Klepin HD, Lichtman SM, Mustian KM, Tew WP, Hurria A. Practical assessment and management of vulnerabilities in older patients receiving chemotherapy: ASCO guideline for geriatric oncology. J Clin Oncol. 2018;36:2326–47.
11. Manini T. Development of physical disability in older adults. Curr Aging Sci. 2012; https://doi.org/10.2174/1874609811104030184.
12. Zeiher J, Ombrellaro KJ, Perumal N, Keil T, Mensink GBM, Finger JD. Correlates and determinants of cardiorespiratory fitness in adults: a systematic review. Sports Med Open. 2019; https://doi.org/10.1186/s40798-019-0211-2.
13. Scott JM, Nilsen TS, Gupta D, Jones LW. Exercise therapy and cardiovascular toxicity in cancer. Circulation. 2018; https://doi.org/10.1161/CIRCULATIONAHA.117.024671.
14. Stanton BR. The neurology of old age. Clin Med J R Coll Phys Lond. 2011;1:54–6.
15. Minetto MA, Giannini A, McConnell R, Busso C, Torre GM. Common musculoskeletal disorders in the elderly: the star triad. J Clin Med. 2020;4:1216.
16. Cruz-Jentoft AJ, Baeyens JP, Bauer JM, et al. Sarcopenia: European consensus on definition and diagnosis. Age Ageing. 2010; https://doi.org/10.1093/ageing/afq034.
17. Hile ES, Fitzgerald GK, Studenski SA. Persistent mobility disability after neurotoxic chemotherapy. Phys Ther. 2010;90:1649–57.
18. NICE. NICE clinical guideline 161. Falls: assessment and prevention of falls in older people National Institute of Health and Care Excellence. 2013. https://doi.org/10.7748/nop.26.6.18.e586
19. Mohile SG, Lin F, Reeve E, Jean-Pierre P, Mustian K, Peppone L, Janelsins M, Morrow G, Hall W, Dale W. Association of cancer with geriatric syndromes in older Medicare beneficiaries. J Clin Oncol. 2011;29:1458–64.
20. Cheng KKF, Lee DTF. Effects of pain, fatigue, insomnia, and mood disturbance on functional status and quality of life of elderly patients with cancer. Crit Rev Oncol Hematol. 2011; https://doi.org/10.1016/j.critrevonc.2010.03.002.
21. Kathiresan G, Clement RF, Sankaranarayanan MT. Dyspnea in lung cancer patients: a systematic review. Lung Cancer Targets Ther. 2010;1:141.
22. John M, Jolley C. Breathlessness, fatigue and the respiratory muscles. Clin Med J. 2009;9:448.
23. Fried LP, Tangen CM, Walston J, et al. Frailty in older adults: evidence for a phenotype. J Gerontol Ser A Biol Sci Med Sci. 2001; https://doi.org/10.1093/gerona/56.3.m146.
24. Verbrugge LM, Jette AM. The disablement process. Soc Sci Med. 1994;38:1–14.
25. Tas Ü, Verhagen AP, Bierma-Zeinstra SMA, Odding E, Koes BW. Prognostic factors of disability in older people: a systematic review. Br J Gen Pract. 2007;57:319–23.
26. Reuben DB, Seeman TE, Keeler E, Hayes RP, Bowman L, Sewall A, Hirsch SH, Wallace RB, Guralnik JM. The effect of self-reported and performance-based functional impairment on future hospital costs of community-dwelling older persons. Gerontologist. 2004; https://doi.org/10.1093/geront/44.3.401.
27. Crevenna R, Palma S, Licht T. Cancer prehabilitation—a short review. Memo Mag Eur Med Oncol. 2021;14:39–43.
28. Ethun CG, Bilen MA, Jani AB, Maithel SK, Ogan K, Master VA. Frailty and cancer: implications for oncology surgery, medical oncology, and radiation oncology. CA Cancer J Clin. 2017;67:362–77.
29. Sarfati D, Koczwara B, Jackson C. The impact of comorbidity on cancer and its treatment. CA Cancer J Clin. 2016;337–50.

30. Lang PO, Michel JP, Zekry D. Frailty syndrome: a transitional state in a dynamic process. Gerontology. 2009; https://doi.org/10.1159/000211949.
31. Singh SJ, Danjoux G, Durrand J. Prehabilitation. Clin Med J R Coll of Phys Lond. 2019;19:458–64.
32. Santa Mina D, Alibhai SMH. Prehabilitation in geriatric oncology. J Geriatr Oncol. https://doi.org/10.1016/j.jgo.2019.05.017.
33. Ferrat E, Paillaud E, Caillet P, et al. Performance of four frailty classifications in older patients with cancer: prospective elderly cancer patients cohort study. J Clin Oncol. 2017; https://doi.org/10.1200/JCO.2016.69.3143.
34. Fried TR, Bradley EH, Towle VR, Allore H. Understanding the treatment preferences of seriously ill patients. N Engl J Med. 2002; https://doi.org/10.1056/NEJMsa012528.
35. Soto Perez De Celis E, Li D, Sun C-L, et al. Patient-defined goals and preferences among older adults with cancer starting chemotherapy (CT). J Clin Oncol. 2018; https://doi.org/10.1200/jco.2018.36.15_suppl.10009.
36. Extermann M, Hurria A. Comprehensive geriatric assessment for older patients with cancer. J Clin Oncol. 2007; https://doi.org/10.1200/JCO.2007.10.6559.
37. Cesari M, Cerullo F, Zamboni V, di Palma R, Scambia G, Balducci L, Antonelli Incalzi R, Vellas B, Gambassi G. Functional status and mortality in older women with gynecological cancer. J Gerontol Ser A Biol Sci Med Sci. 2013; https://doi.org/10.1093/gerona/glt073.
38. Tinquaut F, Freyer G, Gane N, Pujade-Lauraine E, Falandry C. Prognostic factors for overall survival in elderly patients with advanced ovarian cancer treated with chemotherapy: results of a pooled analysis of three GINECO phase II trials. Gynecol Oncol. 2016;143:22–6.
39. Giannotti C, Sambuceti S, Signori A, et al. Frailty assessment in elective gastrointestinal oncogeriatric surgery: predictors of one-year mortality and functional status. J Geriatr Oncol. 2019; https://doi.org/10.1016/j.jgo.2019.04.017.
40. Montroni I, Rostoft S, Spinelli A, et al. GOSAFE—Geriatric Oncology Surgical Assessment and Functional rEcovery after Surgery: early analysis on 977 patients. J Geriatr Oncol. 2020;11:244–55.
41. Maione P, Perrone F, Gallo C, et al. Pretreatment quality of life and functional status assessment significantly predict survival of elderly patients with advanced non-small-cell lung cancer receiving chemotherapy: a prognostic analysis of the multicenter Italian lung cancer in the elderly study. J Clin Oncol. 2005; https://doi.org/10.1200/JCO.2005.02.527.
42. DuMontier C, Liu MA, Murillo A, Hshieh T, Javedan H, Soiffer R, Stone RM, Driver JA, Abel GA. Function, survival, and care utilization among older adults with hematologic malignancies. J Am Geriatr Soc. 2019; https://doi.org/10.1111/jgs.15835.
43. Aparicio T, Jouve JL, Teillet L, et al. Geriatric factors predict chemotherapy feasibility: ancillary results of FFCD 2001-02 phase III study in first-line chemotherapy for metastatic colorectal cancer in elderly patients. J Clin Oncol. 2013; https://doi.org/10.1200/JCO.2012.42.9894.
44. Couderc AL, Boulahssass R, Nouguerède E, Gobin N, Guérin O, Villani P, Barlesi F, Paillaud E. Functional status in a geriatric oncology setting: a review. J Geriatr Oncol. 2019;10:884–94.
45. Hantel A, DuMontier C, Odejide OO, Luskin MR, Sperling AS, Hshieh T, Chen R, Soiffer R, Driver JA, Abel GA. Gait speed, survival, and recommended treatment intensity in older adults with blood cancer requiring treatment. Cancer. 2021;127:875–83.
46. Liu MA, DuMontier C, Murillo A, Hshieh TT, Bean JF, Soiffer RJ, Stone RM, Abel GA, Driver JA. Gait speed, grip strength, and clinical outcomes in older patients with hematologic malignancies. Blood. 2019;134:374–82.
47. Caillet P, Laurent M, Bastuji-Garin S, Liuu E, Culine S, Lagrange JL, Canoui-Poitrine F, Paillaud E. Optimal management of elderly cancer patients: usefulness of the comprehensive geriatric assessment. Clin Interv Aging. 2014; https://doi.org/10.2147/CIA.S57849.
48. Oken MM, Creech RH, Davis TE. Toxicology and response criteria of the Eastern Cooperative Oncology Group. Am J Clin Oncol Cancer Clin Trials. 1982; https://doi.org/10.1097/00000421-198212000-00014.
49. Simcock R, Wright J. Beyond performance status. Clin Oncol. 2020;32:553–61.

50. Nightingale G, Battisti NML, Loh KP, et al. Perspectives on functional status in older adults with cancer: an interprofessional report from the International Society of Geriatric Oncology (SIOG) nursing and allied health interest group and young SIOG. J Geriatr Oncol. 2020;12:658–65.
51. Pergolotti M, Sattar S. Measuring functional status of older adults with cancer with patient and performance-based measures, a how-to guide: a young society of geriatric oncology and nursing and allied health initiative. J Geriatr Oncol. 2021;12:473–8.
52. Roberts HC, Denison HJ, Martin HJ, Patel HP, Syddall H, Cooper C, Sayer AA. A review of the measurement of grip strength in clinical and epidemiological studies: towards a standardised approach. Age Ageing. 2011; https://doi.org/10.1093/ageing/afr051.
53. Paek J, Choi YJ. Association between hand grip strength and impaired health-related quality of life in Korean cancer survivors: a cross-sectional study. BMJ Open. 2019;9:30938.
54. Yang L, Koyanagi A, Smith L, et al. Hand grip strength and cognitive function among elderly cancer survivors. PLoS One. 2018; https://doi.org/10.1371/journal.pone.0197909.
55. Kilgour RD, Vigano A, Trutschnigg B, Lucar E, Borod M, Morais JA. Handgrip strength predicts survival and is associated with markers of clinical and functional outcomes in advanced cancer patients. Support Care Cancer. 2013;21:3261–70.
56. le Zhuang C, Zhang FM, Li W, Wang KH, Xu HX, Song CH, Guo ZQ, Shi HP. Associations of low handgrip strength with cancer mortality: a multicentre observational study. J Cachexia Sarcopenia Muscle. 2020;11:1476–86.
57. Verweij NM, Schiphorst AHW, Pronk A, van den Bos F, Hamaker ME. Physical performance measures for predicting outcome in cancer patients: a systematic review. Acta Oncol. 2016; https://doi.org/10.1080/0284186X.2016.1219047.
58. Phu S, Kirk B, Bani Hassan E, Vogrin S, Zanker J, Bernardo S, Duque G. The diagnostic value of the Short Physical Performance Battery for sarcopenia. BMC Geriatr. 2020;20:1–7.
59. Peel NM, Kuys SS, Klein K. Gait speed as a measure in geriatric assessment in clinical settings: a systematic review. J Gerontol Ser A Biol Sci Med Sci. 2013; https://doi.org/10.1093/gerona/gls174.
60. Studenski S, Perera S, Patel K, et al. Gait speed and survival in older adults. JAMA J Am Med Assoc. 2011;305:50–8.
61. Pamoukdjian F, Lévy V, Sebbane G, Boubaya M, Landre T, Bloch-Queyrat C, Paillaud E, Zelek L. Slow gait speed is an independent predictor of early death in older cancer outpatients: results from a prospective cohort study. J Nutr Health Aging. 2017;21:202–6.
62. Bessems SAM, Konsten JLM, Vogelaar JFJ, Csepán-Magyar R, Maas HAAM, van de Wouw YAJ, Janssen-Heijnen MLG. Frailty screening by Geriatric-8 and 4-meter gait speed test is feasible and predicts postoperative complications in elderly colorectal cancer patients. J Geriatr Oncol. 2020;12:592–8.
63. Karpman C, le Brasseur NK, de Pew ZS, Novotny PJ, Benzo RP. Measuring gait speed in the out-patient clinic: methodology and feasibility. Respir Care. 2014; https://doi.org/10.4187/respcare.02688.
64. Huisman MG, van Leeuwen BL, Ugolini G, Montroni I, Spiliotis J, Stabilini C, Carino NDL, Farinella E, de Bock GH, Audisio RA. "Timed Up & Go": a screening tool for predicting 30-day morbidity in onco-geriatric surgical patients? A multicenter cohort study. PLoS One. 2014; https://doi.org/10.1371/journal.pone.0086863.
65. Blackwood J, Rybicki K. Assessment of Gait Speed and Timed Up and Go measures as predictors of falls in older breast cancer survivors. Integr Cancer Ther. 2021; https://doi.org/10.1177/15347354211006462.
66. Barry E, Galvin R, Keogh C, Horgan F, Fahey T. Is the Timed Up and Go test a useful predictor of risk of falls in community dwelling older adults: a systematic review and meta-analysis. BMC Geriatr. 2014; https://doi.org/10.1186/1471-2318-14-14.
67. Soubeyran P, Fonck M, Blanc-Bisson C, et al. Predictors of early death risk in older patients treated with first-line chemotherapy for cancer. J Clin Oncol. 2012;30:1829–34.
68. Simpson JM, Worsfold C, Reilly E, Nye N. A standard procedure for using TURN180. Physiotherapy. 2002; https://doi.org/10.1016/s0031-9406(05)60747-x.

69. Sattar S, Haase K, Kuster S, Puts M, Spoelstra S, Bradley C, Wildes TM, Alibhai S. Falls in older adults with cancer: an updated systematic review of prevalence, injurious falls, and impact on cancer treatment. Support Care Cancer. 2021;29:21–33.
70. Chua-Tuan JL. Video capture of the circumstances of falls in elderly people residing in long-term care: an observational study: Robinovitch SN, Feldman F, Yang Y, Schonnop R, et al. Lancet 2013;381:47–54. J Emerg Med. 2013; https://doi.org/10.1016/j.jemermed.2013.03.011.
71. Simpson JM, Worsfold C, Reilly E, Nye N. A standard procedure for using TURN180: testing dynamic postural stability among elderly people. Physiotherapy. 2002; https://doi.org/10.1016/S0031-9406(05)60747-X.
72. Karnosfky DA, Burchenal JH. The clinical evaluation of chemotherapeutic agents in cancer. In: MacLeod CM, editor. Evaluation of chemotherapeutic agents. New York: Columbia University Press; 1948.
73. Mahoney FI, Barthel DW. Functional evaluation: the Barthel Index. Md State Med J. 1965;14:61–5.
74. Sinoff G, Ore L. The Barthel activities of daily living index: self-reporting versus actual performance in the old-old (≤ 75 years). J Am Geriatr Soc. 1997; https://doi.org/10.1111/j.1532-5415.1997.tb01510.x.
75. Shimoda K, Imai H, Tsuji T, Tsuchiya K, Tajima H, Kanemaki H, Tozato F. Factors affecting the performance of activities of daily living in patients with advanced cancer undergoing inpatient rehabilitation: results from a retrospective observational study. J Phys Ther Sci. 2019;31:795–801.
76. Wallace M, Shelke M. Katz Index of independence in activities of daily living (ADL). Urol Nurs. 2007;1:93–4.
77. Blackwood J, Karczewski H, Huang MH, Pfalzer L. Katz activities of daily living disability in older cancer survivors by age, stage, and cancer type. J Cancer Surviv. 2020;14:769–78.
78. Neo J, Fettes L, Gao W, Higginson IJ, Maddocks M. Disability in activities of daily living among adults with cancer: a systematic review and meta-analysis. Cancer Treat Rev. 2017;61:94–106.
79. Aminisani N, Nikbakht H, Jafarabadi MA, et al. Functional deficits and quality of life among cancer survivors: implications for occupational therapy in cancer survivorship care. Oncologist. 2017;109:266–70.
80. Brekke MF, la Cour K, Brandt Å, Peoples H, Wæhrens EE. The association between ADL ability and quality of life among people with advanced cancer. Occup Ther Int. 2019;2019:2629673.
81. Pergolotti M, Deal AM, Williams GR, Bryant AL, Bensen JT, Muss HB, Reeve BB. Activities, function, and health-related quality of life (HRQOL) of older adults with cancer. J Geriatr Oncol. 2017;8:249–54.
82. Lawton MP, Brody EM. Assessment of older people: self-maintaining and instrumental activities of daily living. Gerontologist. 1969; https://doi.org/10.1093/geront/9.3_Part_1.179.
83. Macmillan Cancer Support. Prehabilitation for people with cancer. Principles and guidance for prehabilitation within the management and support of people with cancer. 2019.
84. Meyerhardt JA, Giovannucci EL, Holmes MD, Chan AT, Chan JA, Colditz GA, Fuchs CS. Physical activity and survival after colorectal cancer diagnosis. J Clin Oncol. 2006;24:3527–34.
85. Eickmeyer SM, Gamble GL, Shahpar S, Do KD. The role and efficacy of exercise in persons with cancer. PM R. 2012;4:874–81.
86. Ibrahim EM, Al-Homaidh A. Physical activity and survival after breast cancer diagnosis: meta-analysis of published studies. Med Oncol. 2010; https://doi.org/10.1007/s12032-010-9536-x.
87. Buffart LM, Kalter J, Sweegers MG, et al. Effects and moderators of exercise on quality of life and physical function in patients with cancer: an individual patient data meta-analysis of 34 RCTs. Cancer Treat Rev. 2017;52:91–104.
88. Tomlinson D, Diorio C, Beyene J, Sung L. Effect of exercise on cancer-related fatigue. Am J Phys Med Rehabil. 2014;93:675–86.

89. Mustian K, Lin PJ, Cole C, Loh KP, Magnuson A. Exercise and the older cancer survivor. In: Extermann M, editor. Geriatric oncology. Cham: Springer; 2020. p. 917–38.
90. Angulo J, el Assar M, Álvarez-Bustos A, Rodríguez-Mañas L. Physical activity and exercise: strategies to manage frailty. Redox Biol. 2020; https://doi.org/10.1016/j.redox.2020.101513.
91. Arrieta H, Astrugue C, Regueme S, et al. Effects of a physical activity programme to prevent physical performance decline in onco-geriatric patients: a randomized multicentre trial. J Cachexia Sarcopenia Muscle. 2019;10:287–97.
92. Mikkelsen MK, Nielsen DL, Vinther A, Lund CM, Jarden M. Attitudes towards physical activity and exercise in older patients with advanced cancer during oncological treatment—a qualitative interview study. Eur J Oncol Nurs. 2019;41:16–23.
93. Moschny A, Platen P, Klaaßen-Mielke R, Trampisch U, Hinrichs T. Barriers to physical activity in older adults in Germany: a cross-sectional study. Int J Behav Nutr Phys Act. 2011; https://doi.org/10.1186/1479-5868-8-121.
94. Pergolotti M, Williams GR, Campbell C, Munoz LA, Muss HB. Occupational therapy for adults with cancer: why it matters. Oncologist. 2016;21:314–9.
95. Pergolotti M, Williams GR, Campbell C, Munoz LA, Muss HB. Geriatric oncology occupational therapy for adults with cancer: why it matters. Oncologist. 2016;21:314–9.
96. Taylor K, Currow D. A prospective study of patient identified unmet activity of daily living needs among cancer patients at a comprehensive cancer care centre. Aust Occup Ther J. 2003;50:79–85.
97. Pergolotti M, Deal AM, Lavery J, Reeve BB, Muss HB. The prevalence of potentially modifiable functional deficits and the subsequent use of occupational and physical therapy by older adults with cancer. J Geriatr Oncol. 2015; https://doi.org/10.1016/j.jgo.2015.01.004.
98. About shortness of breath | Cancer Research UK | Coping physically. https://www.cancerresearchuk.org/about-cancer/coping/physically/breathing-problems/shortness-of-breath. Accessed 23 May 2021
99. Pergolotti M, Cutchin MP, Weinberger M, Meyer AM. Occupational therapy use by older adults with cancer. Am J Occup Ther. 2014;68:597–607.
100. National Cancer Comprehensive Network. NCCN clinical practice guidelines in oncology (NCCN guidelines) cancer-related fatigue. 2018.
101. Kuiper AJ, Wolvers MDJ, Vonk D, Hagenbeek A. Untire: an all-embracing self-management eHealth program to cope with cancer-related fatigue. ecancermedicalscience. 2018; https://doi.org/10.3332/ecancer.2018.ed81.
102. Bruggeman-Everts FZ, Wolvers MDJ, van de Schoot R, Vollenbroek-Hutten MMR, van der Lee ML. Effectiveness of two web-based interventions for chronic cancer-related fatigue compared to an active control condition: results of the "Fitter na kanker" randomized controlled trial. J Med Internet Res. 2017; https://doi.org/10.2196/jmir.7180.
103. Goedendorp MM, Knoop H, Gielissen MFM, Verhagen CAHHVM, Bleijenberg G. The effects of cognitive behavioral therapy for postcancer fatigue on perceived cognitive disabilities and neuropsychological test performance. J Pain Symptom Manage. 2014; https://doi.org/10.1016/j.jpainsymman.2013.02.014.
104. Kangas M, Bovbjerg DH, Montgomery GH. "Cancer-related fatigue: a systematic and meta-analytic review of non-pharmacological therapies for cancer patients": correction to Kangas, Bovbjerg, and Montgomery (2008). Psychol Bull. 2009; https://doi.org/10.1037/a0014650.
105. Bower JE. Cancer-related fatigue—mechanisms, risk factors, and treatments. Nat Rev Clin Oncol. 2014;11:597–609.
106. Larkin D, Lopez V, Aromataris E. Managing cancer-related fatigue in men with prostate cancer: a systematic review of non-pharmacological interventions. Int J Nurs Pract. 2014; https://doi.org/10.1111/ijn.12211.
107. Gerritsen JKW, Vincent AJPE. Exercise improves quality of life in patients with cancer: a systematic review and meta-analysis of randomised controlled trials. Br J Sports Med. 2016;50:796–803.
108. Meneses-Echávez JF, González-Jiménez E, Ramírez-Vélez R. Effects of supervised exercise on cancer-related fatigue in breast cancer survivors: a systematic review and meta-analysis. BMC Cancer. 2015; https://doi.org/10.1186/s12885-015-1069-4.

109. Kessels E, Husson O, van der Feltz-Cornelis CM. The effect of exercise on cancer-related fatigue in cancer survivors: a systematic review and meta-analysis. Neuropsychiatr Dis Treat. 2018;14:479–94.
110. Lin P-J, Loh KP, Inglis JE, et al. Effects of exercise on cancer-related fatigue and muscular strength in patients with breast cancer. J Clin Oncol. 2019;37:11507.
111. Haider S, Grabovac I, Dorner TE. Effects of physical activity interventions in frail and pre-frail community-dwelling people on frailty status, muscle strength, physical performance and muscle mass—a narrative review. Wien Klin Wochenschr. 2019;131:244.
112. Giacalone A, Quitadamo D, Zanet E, Berretta M, Spina M, Tirelli U. Cancer-related fatigue in the elderly. Support Care Cancer. 2013; https://doi.org/10.1007/s00520-013-1897-1.
113. Kumar A, Allcock N. Pain in older people. 2008.
114. el Hachem G, Rocha FO, Pepersack T, Jounblat Y, Drowart A, Dal Lago L. Advances in pain management for older patients with cancer. ecancermedicalscience. 2019; https://doi.org/10.3332/ecancer.2019.980.
115. Taylor LEV, Stotts NA, Humphreys J, Treadwell MJ, Miaskowski C. A Biopsychosocial-spiritual model of chronic pain in adults with sickle cell disease. Pain Manag Nurs. 2013; https://doi.org/10.1016/j.pmn.2011.06.003.
116. Keefe FJ, Porter L, Somers T, Shelby R, Wren A. Psychosocial interventions for managing pain in older adults: outcomes and clinical implications. Br J Anaesth. 2013; https://doi.org/10.1093/bja/aet129.
117. Hill W. The role of occupational therapy in pain management. Anaesth Intensive Care Med. 2016; https://doi.org/10.1016/j.mpaic.2016.06.008.
118. Dunford E, Thompson M. Relaxation and mindfulness in pain: a review. Rev Pain. 2010; https://doi.org/10.1177/204946371000400105.
119. Semmons J. The role of physiotherapy in the management of chronic pain. Anaesth Intensive Care Med. 2016; https://doi.org/10.1016/j.mpaic.2016.06.006.

Part II
Frailty Implications, Challenges and the Multidisciplinary Approach

Chapter 9
Prehabilitation and Rehabilitation in Older Adults with Cancer and Frailty

Zoe Merchant, Linda Denehy, Daniel Santa Mina, Shabbir Alibhai, and John Moore

Z. Merchant (✉)
Prehab4Cancer and Recovery Programme, Greater Manchester Cancer alliance Hosted by The Christie NHS Foundation Trust, Greater Manchester, UK
e-mail: zoe.merchant@nhs.net

L. Denehy
Department of Physiotherapy, Melbourne School of Health Sciences, Faculty of Medicine, Dentistry & Health Sciences, The University of Melbourne, Parkville, VIC, Australia

Allied Health Research Team, Peter McCallum Cancer Centre, Melbourne, VIC, Australia
e-mail: l.denehy@unimelb.edu.au

D. Santa Mina
Faculty of Kinesiology and Physical Education, University of Toronto, Toronto, ON, Canada

Department of Anesthesia and Pain Management, University Health Network, Toronto, ON, Canada
e-mail: daniel.santamina@utoronto.ca

S. Alibhai
Geriatric Medicine/Geriatric Oncology, Princess Margaret Cancer Centre, UHN (University Health Network), Toronto, ON, Canada

Department of Medicine, University of Toronto, Toronto, ON, Canada
e-mail: shabbir.alibhai@uhn.ca

J. Moore
Prehab4Cancer and Recovery Programme, Greater Manchester Cancer alliance, Greater Manchester, UK

Division for Anaesthesia, Peri-Operative Medicine and Critical Care Services, Manchester Royal Infirmary, Manchester University NHS Foundation Trust, Manchester, UK
e-mail: john.moore@mft.nhs.uk

F. Gomes (ed.), *Frailty in Older Adults with Cancer*,
https://doi.org/10.1007/978-3-030-89162-6_9

Introduction

It is well-accepted that the adverse effects of cancer and associated treatment(s) are essentially ubiquitous across disease types and can be highly deleterious to quality of life (QoL). For many people with cancer, the significant physical and psychosocial morbidity associated with the cancer compromise functional ability across these domains. Functional impairments are highly prevalent and can be due to the disease or treatment, such as the new onset or exacerbation of fatigue, pain, neuropathy, lymphoedema, urinary or bowel dysfunction, difficulty with speech or eating, aerobic and musculoskeletal deconditioning, sexual dysfunction, distress, anxiety, depression and cognitive deficits [1, 2]. Screening, assessment, and intervention approaches that aim to identify and prevent dysfunction, as well as maintain or recover pre-diagnosis levels of function, are recommended. Such services and practices are classified as prehabilitation (prior to treatment) or rehabilitation (during or after treatment). The goals of prehabilitation (prehab) and rehabilitation (rehab) are to manage functional changes associated with cancer and optimise health across the cancer continuum.

Recommendations for referral to prehab and rehab, as well as evidence-based clinical practice guidelines that direct such care, have grown rapidly in recent years [3, 4]. However, only a few have specifically focused on the needs of older adults with cancer [5, 6]. This subset of cancer survivors has been historically unaccounted for in research and in tailored clinical programmes, despite their growing prevalence and their complex needs, from age-related changes to physiology, function, cognition and concomitant comorbidities [4, 7–10]. For example, Pergolotti and colleagues found that approximately two-thirds of older adults with cancer report functional limitations [11], and in a systematic review of 20 studies and nearly 3000 older patients by Handforth et al, over 40% were identified as frail or prefrail [12]. Moreover, when combined with disease and treatment-related adverse effects, frail older adults with cancer and functional limitations are more likely to have surgical complications, treatment intolerance, chronic disability and hastened mortality [12–14]. In light of the prevalence of dysfunction and frailty in older adults with cancer, combined with their associated increased risk for poor health outcomes, there is a compelling need for prehab and rehab to optimise health and prevent, mitigate or ameliorate loss of function throughout the cancer continuum. Older adults with functional impairments are historically not referred to rehab [15], although it is understood that referral behaviour varies internationally.

This chapter aims to provide considerations for the integration of prehab and rehab delivery for frail older adults with cancer into clinical care plans citing examples from the scientific literature. The Dietz's phases of rehabilitation [16] are used to structure chapter sections given their nuanced considerations across the cancer continuum. The chapter concludes with recommendations highlighting priorities in advancing prehab and rehab care and research for older cancer patients with frailty.

Prehabilitation, Rehabilitation and Frailty

A commonly used definition for cancer rehabilitation is '[a care strategy] that aims to allow the patient to achieve optimal physical, social, physiological and vocational functioning within the limits imposed by the disease and its treatment [17]'. The essence of this definition was subsequently applied to distinct contexts related to patients' circumstances and needs [16] (Box 9.1). Importantly, early cancer rehabilitation conceptualisations acknowledged the importance of preventing or minimising the adverse effects of cancer treatment with interventions implemented prior to treatment—a strategy now referred to as 'prehab'.

Box 9.1. Dietz Phases of Cancer Rehabilitation

- *Preventative phase*: Limiting the impact of potential complications and morbidity which could be acquired as the result of treatment.
- *Restorative phase*: A person being facilitated to resume their pre-morbid level of functional ability.
- *Supportive phase*: Where continued treatment is needed, the aim is to maximise independence and functional ability whilst also ensuring the necessary support is in place.
- *Palliative phase*: Symptom management as a person is expected to deteriorate in response to the disease progression, maximising quality of life where possible.

Cancer prehab is defined as a 'process on the cancer continuum of care that occurs between the time of cancer diagnosis and the beginning of acute treatment and includes physical and psychological assessments that establish a baseline functional level, identify impairments, and provide interventions that promote physical and psychological health to reduce the incidence and/or severity of future impairments [1]'. Contemporary approaches to prehab and rehab for people with cancer emphasise individualisation of programming for person-centred, goal-directed care, whilst discouraging a 'one-size-fits-all' approach [2]. Accordingly, prehab and rehab are often 'multimodal' and incorporate two or more intervention components specifically selected for their potential cumulative or synergistic effects on health outcomes for a given patient. Multimodal care is inherently inter-professional, requiring the coordinated efforts of a variety of professions (Fig. 9.1).

Following a cancer diagnosis, resilience to the inherent stressors of treatment and lifestyle changes is needed to preserve health and QoL. For patients who are older and frail, prehab and rehab can target resiliency to support adaptive capacity as depicted in the schematic of frailty and its relationship with stress and treatment outcomes (Fig. 9.2). Whilst adaptive capacity may be commonly interpreted as resilience to physiological stressors, the importance of psychosocial and cognitive resilience may be particularly relevant to the older adult with cancer given the

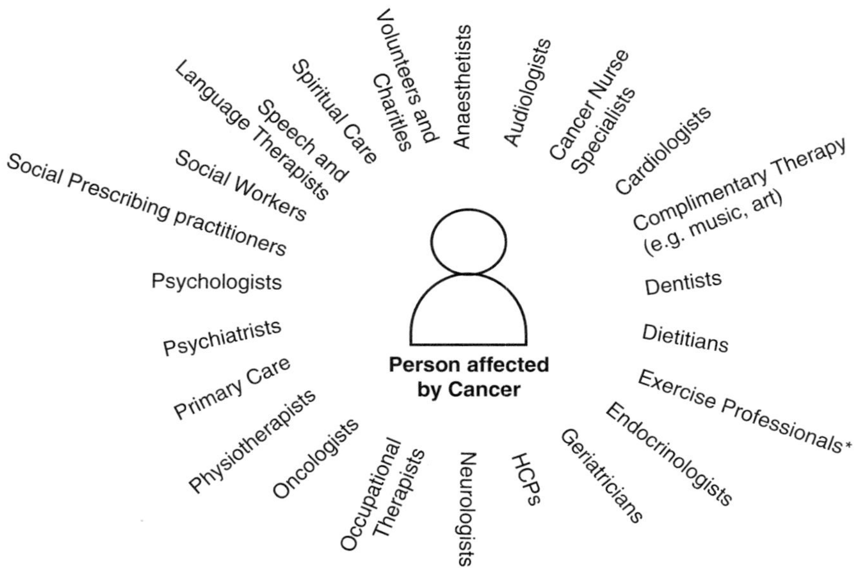

Fig. 9.1 The interdisciplinary team. *Exercise Professionals: Including but not limited to exercise physiologists, kinesiologists, fitness instructors and sport rehabilitators

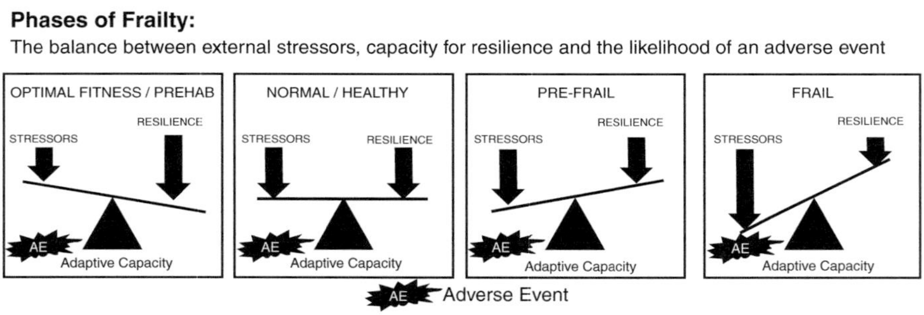

Fig. 9.2 Phases of frailty and the correlation with an older persons' adaptive capacity to be resilient to adverse events (Adapted from [24])

likelihood for social isolation and age/co-morbid or treatment-related cognitive decline [18–21]. Accordingly, assessments must be multidimensional to capture the breadth of health, psychosocial and functional factors, to appropriately design prehab and rehab interventions in this population. The National Comprehensive Cancer Network (NCCN) and the American Society of Clinical Oncology (ASCO) specifically recommend geriatric screening and assessment tools to appraise functional status across physical, cognitive, medical and social domains [5, 6]. Frailty screening, as a minimum, is recommended when older adults are diagnosed with cancer and also when a referral to prehab/rehab is being considered. These evaluations, including determining the support a patient needs, aids to avoid over- or under-treatment of cancer, a well-known problem in geriatric oncology [22]. In particular, the Comprehensive Geriatric Assessment (CGA) is recommended as standard of care in this population to identify vulnerabilities beyond usual oncological assessments [5]; however, due to potential time requirements of the CGA and the balance of overall data, clinicians are recommended to prioritise the assessment of function, comorbidity, falls, mood, cognition and nutrition [5]. CGA is a key component in the identification of patients for referral to prehab and rehab and an important assessment tool within prehab and rehab programmes. Therefore, it is unsurprising that referrals to physiotherapy, occupational therapy, nutrition or dietetics and speech-language pathology or speech and language therapy (grouped as 'Allied Health Professionals—AHPs') are commonly advised for patients with functional deficits identified during geriatric assessments [23].

Ultimately, when managing cancer patients, particularly if older and with frailty, both the patient and the family/carers should be involved in discussions around treatment planning, adopting the mantra of 'no decision without me, about me' as suggested by Cancer Research UK [25]. The findings from the CGA better identify the risks and the unmet needs for patients, such as additional support required in order to undergo specific treatments, which aids treatment-related decisions. Overall, important considerations for frail or pre-frail older adults with cancer include: (a) their capacity for decision-making [26]; (b) the need for a patient-centred approach assessing the person holistically (not just their needs, but also their wishes and goals) and (c) the focus on functional independence and QoL which are often more important than length of survival for this group of patients [27].

Preventative Phase of Cancer Rehabilitation (Prehab)

The aim of prehab is to improve and or prevent physical, mental wellbeing and nutritional dysfunction, increase the likelihood of a return to functional baseline and optimise the patient's ability to undergo additional oncology treatments [20, 21, 27].

Prehab should be multimodal and incorporate aerobic and resistance exercise, nutritional support and mental wellbeing interventions (to support anxiety and mood disturbance), as well as behaviour change strategies to promote adherence and longer-term lifestyle changes [10]. For healthy lifestyle modification smoking cessation and alcohol intake management [28] where applicable should be included, and medical optimisation of other health conditions. Prehab for older cancer patients with frailty should be guided by the CGA, with programmes starting as early as possible in the cancer pathway to ameliorate the often quick decline between the onset of symptoms, diagnosis and eventual treatment [29]. Prehab interventions should be routinely assessed and adapted based upon the findings of additional dynamic risk assessments, re-considered at the start of each patient contact using pre-agreed risk criteria such as changes in symptoms, medication etc., to ensure optimal programme effects and to prevent harm [29].

Exercise interventions and advice within the context of prehab require several considerations and adaptations for the frail older adult with cancer. Traditionally, there has been a dominance for cardiovascular-based aerobic exercise (walking, cycling) interventions. However, with the increasingly recognised prevalence of sarcopenia in older patients with cancer, an equal focus on resistance training combined with nutritional protein supplements is recommended to improve muscle function and potentially reverse frailty [29, 30]. Prehab programmes may be outpatient, community or home-based, and safety guidelines are important so as to ascertain potential cautions or contraindications [29]. For those prescribing or delivering the exercise programme, relevant physiological parameters (blood pressure, heart rate, oxygen saturation (SaO2)) should be specified as part of local standard operating procedures with attention to potential changes in the patients' condition and screening for agreed 'red flags' which might escalate the patient back to the clinical team and temporarily suspend them from the programme. Where a prehab programme does not currently exist, 'home based exercises' for older people with a focus on achievable goals based on their CGA is still valuable. These may range from a simple exercise prescription inclusive of ascending stairs at home a set number of times daily, to asking a patient to increase their completion of physically challenging Instrumental Activities of Daily Living (IADLs), which may enhance their level of independence in the community, such as walking to the local shops. Similarly, comprehensive prehab services may incorporate such occupation-based 'physical activities' as a method to effectively engage and achieve programme aims for older adults experiencing frailty. Other obstacles to prehab may be identified in the holistic needs assessment within a CGA such as financial burden, reliance on family members and reduced volition, all of which could present as potential blocks to engagement for this vulnerable group [12, 31].

Sequencing difficulties are a common deficit component experienced by patients with cognitive impairment and new activities such as prehab may be difficult to 'initiate' if they are unfamiliar to the patient. Thus, it may be necessary to 'activate' the patient to engage in interventions, through verbal and physical prompting and demonstration from another person. A trial of a digital solution 'Fit4Surgery TV' has been successful in actively prompting older colorectal cancer patients with frailty to complete prehab tasks [30]. Similarly, wearable activity tracker trials have been shown to be a motivating factor for increased physical activity [32]. These studies are small but show an emerging technology-driven methodology to support prehab and rehab in older patients [33].

Nutrition is an important consideration in older adults with cancer undergoing either prehab or rehab, and there are several important considerations regarding this topic. First, malnutrition is common in older adults with cancer [34, 35], and is a major risk factor for frailty [36]. Second, malnutrition is associated with multiple adverse outcomes, including post-operative outcomes, reduced tolerance to and greater adverse events from chemotherapy, functional decline and worse QoL [34]. Third, malnutrition is more common in advanced cancer, and is sometimes difficult to separate from the cancer anorexia and cachexia syndrome [35]. Finally, there are major gaps in knowledge of how to optimise nutrition in older adults with cancer, but dietary counselling and nutritional supplementation have shown to be valuable [34]. Moreover, evidence in other settings, particularly inpatient acute care and rehabilitation settings, has shown the importance of systematically identifying undernutrition and targeting it with protein-calorie supplementation, which can improve functional recovery, QoL and survival in specific settings [37, 38].

'Social frailty', the concept of losing one's resources required for social requirements such as engagement in social activities [39], needs to be addressed as it may indeed precede and be implicated in the development of physical and/or cognitive frailty. Depression and social isolation lead to apathy, reduced self-management and self-neglect with compromised adherence to medication and other advice. Additional considerations important for older adults include health literacy and education, digital exclusion, management of social communication, nutritional and swallowing difficulties and adapting assessments and interventions to account for hearing and vision loss [25]. By addressing these potential 'barriers to engagement' for this cohort, there will be greater likelihood of goal achievement and subsequent improved clinical outcomes and QoL.

In Europe, in-patient and community programmes for both prehab and rehab exist, whereas in Australia these are predominately out-patient. Some examples of prehabilitation programmes can be found in Table 9.1. Unfortunately, there are too few programmes to meet the increasing demand in oncology [40]. The environmental setting is an important consideration for the successful delivery of prehab (and rehab) for older cancer patients, with and without frailty, as clinicians and administrators aim to support high adherence whilst still delivering the most effective programme. This is traditionally felt to be optimal within face-to-face programmes, where group activities, often based in community settings, bring a number of additional benefits including better social interaction, peer support and the promotion of self-management skills. If travel is a barrier to attendance at community-based prehab or patient preference, which can often be the case for this population, then a home-based programme with phone and digital options can be considered. Achieving intervention and adherence targets is more challenging in home-based (unsupervised) programmes, however, home-based rehab has been shown to achieve improved outcomes in patients with lung cancer [41]. There is minimal research that compares efficacy between out-patient, community and home-based prehab or rehab [42]. For patients who are frail, it would seem that, given their higher risk already discussed, that outpatient or community-based programmes may be preferred to rapidly identify and manage risk [43] and to maximise their engagement and exercise dose safely. Reports from research in non-frail patients demonstrate prehab is generally safe, with adverse events mostly relating to musculoskeletal injury, with a smaller number of serious adverse events such as falls [44]. In frail patients, caution is warranted since the few studies completed have not discussed the rate of adverse events [45].

Table 9.1 Examples of prehabilitation programmes

Country and leads(s)	UK; Moore, J and Merchant, Z	Australia; Crowe, J and Denehy, L
Programme name and patient cohorts	Prehab4Cancer and recovery service Colorectal, Lung and Oesophago-Gastric surgery with curative intent; Lung alternative curative intent treatment incl. SABR, radical radiotherapy and concurrent chemo/radiotherapy. Age 17 years and above. Registered with a Greater Manchester GP	Fit4surgery and Fit4transplant Adults having pelvic exenteration, Oesophago-Gastric surgery, hepatectomy, colorectal, retroperitoneal sarcoma, Autologous stem cell transplants (lymphoma, multiple myeloma)
Workforce	Exercise Specialist Instructors (Level 4 Cancer Rehabilitation qualified) Co-designed and supported by Anaesthetist, EP, OT, PT, GP, Dietitians, Oncology Psychologist, Surgeons, Respiratory Physician, CNSs, ERAS nurses, and other members of cancer MDTs	The interdisciplinary team includes Anaesthetists, Oncologists, Surgeons, pain specialists, Haematologists, PT, EP, Oncology Dietitians, and clinical Psychologists, ERAS nurses, nurse/coordinators and nurse consultants
Referral source	Single Point of Access via https://prehab4cancer.co.uk/how-to-refer/ Clinical MDTs from 10 different acute hospitals in Greater Manchester Named referrer normally patients' keyworker (CNS or equivalent)	Surgical to allied health through Fit4surgery email: More broadly Anaesthetists, surgical liaison nurses, Preoperative and tumour stream nurse coordinators and consultants including CPET and PAC clinic, Fit4transplant referrals from Haematologists and AuSCT nurse consultant All from the tertiary hospital
Setting, frequency and stratified patient pathways	Delivered in local leisure facility close to participants' residential postcode. Available in 87+ leisure facilities in Greater Manchester conurbation. Free gym membership for prehab phase (from referral to break for treatment) and rehab phase (12 weeks) Recommended 2–3 sessions/week for all participants Targeted pathway—supervised, 3× sessions/week F2F Universal pathway—self-managed, independent exercise sessions with regular (at least weekly) contact with an exercise specialist, which can include F2F	Tertiary hospital OP, and/or group programme; 60 min; 2–3 sessions/week OR telehealth service; Patients reviewed weekly if high risk unless attending F2F supervised sessions If a surgical patient, they also attend 'Surgery School' which involves group sessions by webinar or face to face where individual members of the MDT provide education about the upcoming surgery and perioperative care process by video or face to face
Objective physiological outcome measures	CPET ISWT or 6MWT (ISWT preferential but can be contraindicated for patients with musculoskeletal injury/weakness, reduced baseline fitness levels and other co-morbidities). 60 s STS. Handgrip strength Rockwood Clinical Frailty Scale, PG-SGA	CPET (surgical—VO_2 peak, AT), 30 s STS, 6MWT, handgrip strength, post-operative complications, weight, height, clinical frailty scale, DASI, PG-SGA

(continued)

Table 9.1 (continued)

Patient-reported outcomes	EQ5D-5L, IPAQ, Self-Efficacy Scale for Exercise, WHODAS 2.0, EORTCQLQ-C30, PG-SGA	EORTC-QLQ-C30, IPAQ, meeting activity guidelines (Y:N), PG-SGA GAD-7, PHQ-9
Aerobic exercise	Prehab: Either re-HIIT interval training using exercise bike (or alternative ergometer if required) or Progressive/Continuous steady-state cardiovascular exercise, dependent upon fitness baseline Rehab: Personalised exercise prescription using a range of equipment/group sessions/PA based on patient preference, for prolonged behavioural change post-discharge	Supervised: Treadmill walking or cycling at moderate/high intensity prescribed at Borg 3–5/10 and/or 60–80% max heart rate for a total of 20 min (Continuous exercise or HIIT dependent upon fitness baseline)
Resistance exercise	Muscle groups targeted in the upper body and lower body, mainly related to functional tasks including bed, chair and toilet transfers, mobility, stairs. Resistance bands were issued and range of weights and other resistance equipment were utilised in local leisure facilities. Swimming and other PA recommended which addresses muscle strengthening	Muscle groups targeted based on individual deficits assessed using objective outcomes (see below) at first assessment session by the allied health team. In general, functional exercises in the upper and lower limb including: sit to stand, heel-raises, squats, step-ups, bench push ups, bicep curls, overhead press, shoulder abduction. Dumb-bells and resistance bands were provided for patients to take home as indicated. Commenced at 80% of the 10-repetition maximum 8–12 repetitions, 2–3 sets. 2–3 × week
Home-based instructions	Personalised Home Exercise Pack (https://prehab4cancer.co.uk/coronavirus-covid-19/) issued to each patient and adapted for participants changing exercise ability through their engagement in the service All advised to engage in daily PA walking in around exercise prescription and as medical treatment regime, i.e. radiotherapy allows	Home based: progressive increase to 150 min of continuous moderate intensity BORG 3–4/10 per week. Walking, exercise bike, swimming, jogging based on patient equipment and preference. Start level based upon assessment Individual resistance programme prescribed as above: in general functional exercises of the UL and LL. Commenced at 80% of the 10-repetition maximum. 8–12 repetitions, 2–3 sets. 2–3 × week

(continued)

Table 9.1 (continued)

Nutrition	PG-SGA and 'traffic light system': Green—Provide low-risk nutritional advice sheet as per https://prehab4cancer.co.uk/nutrition-2/, continue to monitor weight regularly and PG-SGA at regular time points Amber—Provide 'Eating Help Yourself' diet booklet, contact named referrer to escalate concern Red—As above, request a dietetic referral or make this directly All patients all receive 1:1 advice verbally re. diet and exercise	1:1 advice from a registered oncology dietician for 1–4 sessions based on need Dietetics OP clinic or telehealth; 20 min sessions then follow up as needed
Psychosocial and mental well-being	All exercise specialists completed level 1 psychological communication training, able to notice distress, listen, be empathetic, signpost to appropriate service or escalate back to named referrer based on unmet need identified. Utilise exercise, group support and relaxation PA to address mental well-being Staff receives reflective sessions with psychologist and OT bimonthly for CPD and their emotional well-being includes case study discussion	1:1 advice and strategies if PHQ4 score > 2 at screening from a registered clinical Psychologist. Initial 60 min session then follow up as needed. All patients preparing for a Pelvic exenteration automatically qualify for initial clinical psychology assessment. 1–5 sessions based on needs

BMT, bone marrow transplant; PT, physiotherapist; EP, exercise physiologist; PA, physical activity; PHQ4, Patient Health Questionnaire (4-item) measure anxiety and depression; CPET, cardiopulmonary exercise test; VO_2 peak, peak oxygen uptake; AT, anaerobic threshold; 6MWT, six-minute walk test; PG-SGA, patient-generated subjective global assessment (nutrition assessment); EORTC, European Organization for Research and Treatment of Cancer quality of life questionnaire; IPAQ, international physical activity questionnaire; SABR, stereotactic ablative radiotherapy; CNS, cancer nurse specialists; ERAS nurse, enhanced recovery after surgery nurse; ISWT, Incremental Shuttle Walk Test; STS, Sit to Stand test; EQ-5D-5L, EuroQoL outcome measure; IPAQ, International Physical Activity Questionnaires; WHODAS 2.0, World Health Organisation Disability Assessment Schedule version 2

Prehab Considerations Regarding Surgical Cancer Treatments

Cancer surgery for older patients benefits from integrating assessment and care [46]. A meta-analysis found that perioperative pathways in older patients (>60 years), specifically those with elements of prehab and enhanced recovery programmes in multicomponent interventions, reduced hospital stay for elective surgery by an average of 1.5 days amongst people having colorectal surgery and an average of 5 days in those having upper abdominal surgery [47].

The evidence base for the benefits of prehab is growing [48], particularly for colorectal, lung and oesophageal surgical patients but also in haematologic and prostate cancers. Preoperative frailty is associated with 2.5 times the risk of postoperative complications and increased length of hospital stay after abdominal surgery [49]. In a recent systematic review examining prehab prior to abdominal surgery, the authors suggest that high-risk patients should be targeted for prehab as those are most likely to benefit [50]. The complex presentation and often inherent co-morbidities present in older people experiencing frailty place them in a high-risk group leading to a greater likelihood of complications or side effects of aggressive cancer treatment (including major surgery, radical radiotherapy and other systemic cancer therapies).

There are currently limited research studies that include older patients with frailty in prehabilitation for cancer surgery, and even less feature in trials for patients receiving prehab as part of chemo-, radio- or immunotherapy. A recent randomised controlled trial by Carli et al examined prehabilitation in a frailty cohort undergoing predominantly minimally invasive colorectal resection surgery. Patients identified as frail (using Fried Frailty Index) were randomised to receive a multimodal prehabilitation intervention delivered pre-op versus no-prehab. The no-prehab group was offered the same intervention delivered post-op as a rehabilitation package. Although there was a physical improvement in 6MWT in the prehab group, in this study this did not translate into a reduction in post-operative complications or length of stay (4 days in both groups), which were used as primary outcome measures. The authors considered that the use of minimally invasive surgery within enhanced recovery pathways mitigated the effect of the prehabilitation programme on the primary endpoints in this group [45]. There was a tendency to a reduction in hospital readmissions within the prehab group and it is important to consider what the endpoints of rehabilitation should be with a focus on longer patient impact. Despite the limitations to the current body of evidence, clinicians are increasingly supportive of prehab for older patients. This is exemplified in a Delphi survey, 80% of colorectal surgeons recommended exercise prehabilitation be included for patients from 40 years of age to > 80 years and should include aerobic training [51].

Furthermore, all patients should be offered Enhanced Recovery programmes when undergoing major cancer resection [52], which should dovetail with prehab to optimise surgical preparation [53]. They offer in-hospital, stepped recovery for patients with a focus on daily goal setting around early mobilisation, early nutrition and chest recovery in an attempt to reduce perioperative complications and support early discharge [54]. Enhanced recovery programmes have been shown to be safe when applied to older frail patients and demonstrated to reduce post-operative complications and shorten the length of hospital stay [55].

Detecting higher risk older surgical patients, using previously described methods such as cardiopulmonary exercise testing, clinical frailty tools and performance scores [56], will determine which patients will benefit most from the involvement of a geriatrician within their perioperative care alongside a more standard Enhanced Recovery programme. Various models incorporating geriatrician involvement exist, including additional ward level care, daily board round, weekly interdisciplinary meeting, targeted geriatrician-led ward rounds and a geriatric surgery checklist. These models have been associated with reduced post-operative complications and hospital length of inpatient stay [57].

Post-operative delirium is an extremely common complication in older patients following all types of cancer and non-cancer anaesthesia and surgery, with an incidence as high as 65% in patients aged 65 years and older [58]. Delirium in the post-op periods increases hospital length of stay, induces functional decline [58] and can increase the incidence of long-term cognitive impairment and dementia [59]. Perioperative interventions to reduce delirium encompass support for cognitive and sensory domains (e.g. orientation and hearing aids), enhanced recovery after surgery principles including patient and family information, reducing medication load, improving pain management, sleep and circadian rhythm maintenance. Further, in older patients (70 years or greater) prehab has been shown to improve post-operative delirium [45].

Prehab Considerations Regarding Non-surgical Cancer Treatments

It is acknowledged within cancer clinical practice that older adults experiencing frailty and diagnosed with cancer are less likely to be able to be offered curative surgical options due to their presenting performance status and high risk of post-operative complications. Thus this cohort is more likely to be treated using oncological treatment such as chemotherapy, immunotherapy and radiotherapy. The aims of prehab prior to such treatment modalities include improving tolerance and adherence to oncological treatments with subsequent longer-term survival, maintaining optimised QoL through treatment due to the reduction in the experience of side effects and ultimately reducing the risk of toxicity and other harmful treatment complications. Whilst the aims of prehab for people undergoing non-surgical cancer treatments might be different to the surgical cohort the interventions are similar, maintained where possible during the same time period as whilst the cancer patient is undergoing chemotherapy and radiotherapy treatment. However, evidence from prehab programmes is still very limited in the non-surgical setting.

The cohort of patients in this non-surgical pathway is often older and more frail, which may limit some of the more standard prehab approaches. Therefore, often there will need to be some adjustment within the patient's programme particularly in the physical training aspects of prehab and rehab. Moreover, treatments such as chemotherapy are delivered over prolonged periods of time, which is different from surgery for example. Therefore, components of both prehab and rehab are often merged in this setting and they should be further tailored according to the patient's response to treatment and the ability for the participant to remain engaged dependent on emerging treatment-related side-effects (Fig. 9.3) [29]. For patients entering non-surgical cancer treatment including radiotherapy and chemotherapy, one should aim for interventions to be maintained for as long as possible, with close monitoring during this period. It may also become less feasible and acceptable for patients to maintain engaging in community-based interventions whilst also having to travel for daily radiation doses for several weeks or more.

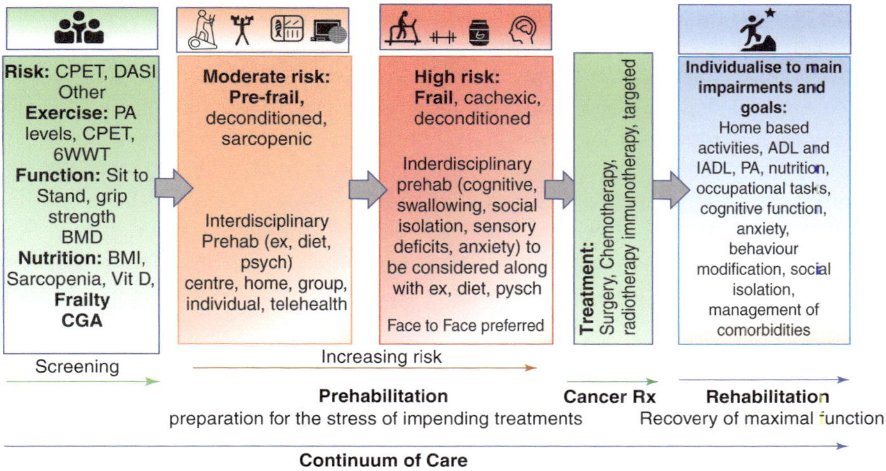

Fig. 9.3 Suggested model for prehab and rehab assessments and interventions. CPET, cardiopulmonary exercise testing; DASI, Dike activity status index; PA, physical activity; 6MWT, six minutes' walk test; BMD, bone mineral density; CGA, comprehensive geriatric assessment; ex, exercise; psych, psychology; ADL, activities of daily living; IADL, instrumental activities of daily living; Rx, treatment

Personalisation of prehab and rehab for the older patients with frailty particularly will support their ongoing participation. Where possible this should be led by an interdisciplinary team approach as described above in close liaison with the patient, cancer care delivery team and the patient's care network to support realistic goal setting. Continued prehab may further promote a greater sense of wellbeing, self-control, with reduced experience of anxiety and mood disturbance, and better tolerance of common cancer treatment symptoms including cancer-related fatigue, nausea, peripheral neuropathy, pain and in general a patient's tolerance to treatment [35]. Another potential benefit is the patient being able to complete a chemo or radiotherapy treatment sequence if they are fitter and less fatigued although this remains to be robustly established in trials.

Ongoing dynamic risk assessment continues to be essential to ensure that if prehab interventions are maintained by an individual, that they are done so safely, taking into consideration risk of cardiac toxicity and other potential significant complications of cancer treatment [29].

Restorative Phase of Cancer Rehabilitation

Rehab is widely evidenced to be positive for people with cardiac, pulmonary, heart failure, and neurological conditions [50, 60]. Geriatric patients mobilising as soon as possible in hospitals is supported from studies examining 'pyjama paralysis' where patients are dressed in 'street' clothes and sat out of bed rather than staying in bed in their pyjamas [61]. Promoting the achievement of generic older adult physical activity recommendations coupled with targeted additions such as reducing sedentary behaviour improving cognition and improving strength and balance to prevent falls is a reasonable approach [62] utilised in many rehab programmes.

Once the patient has completed their medical treatment they should be re-assessed including reviewing pre-treatment function and QoL goals to clarify whether these are still relevant, or whether goal-adjustment is required [63]. For older patients with a more complicated recovery from surgery, in-patient rehabilitation led by AHPs will be necessary, supported ideally by a geriatrician as part of a co-ordinated pathway. This team will then support patient recovery and the transition to home or residential/nursing care facility. The subsequent 'seamless transfer of care' with a community-based prehab–rehab team will benefit from a close handover from hospital-based services as the patient aims to step back into facilitated community-based rehab. Restorative and adaptive principles may be needed to enable a patient to resume basic ADLs. It should be expected that a patient's lowest functional ability will be immediately post-treatment [64]. Short- and longer-term agreed goals can set expectations for the patient [63] and motivate them as they make progress in a graded fashion. They will also help dictate which member(s) of the interdisciplinary team should be involved at this stage and the interventions required.

Restorative rehabilitation may focus on the impact on function of the common cancer-specific side effects already listed. As such, healthcare and exercise professionals should have a heightened awareness of cancer-related fatigue, peripheral neuropathy and pain, especially given the greater probability of these being experienced by a frail, older adult post-treatment [31]. There needs to be understanding that such symptoms may signal disease progression, and may delay patients' safely resuming activities such as exercise. Fatigue and anxiety management are likely additional interventions required during this phase [10].

Supportive Phase of Cancer Rehabilitation

Behavioural change is a psychological feature of prehab/rehab (probably even more so for rehab as the expectation is long-term adherence, well beyond the acute phase) programmes, with the engagement in healthy lifestyle activities enabling the added wider goal of secondary prevention of other long-term health conditions or comorbidities [10] and even the aspiration to reduce the reoccurrence of cancers. The patient may prefer to adapt how they exercise so this fits within their daily and weekly routine. Indeed within the Prehab4Cancer and recovery programme, although patients resume exercise in a leisure facility for 12 weeks prior to discharge during their rehab phase, they are then encouraged to engage in physical activities which suits their preferences both habitually and volitionally [53] (e.g. joining a local walking group). Through change in a patient's behaviour they are encouraged to be independent exercisers, with as little support as is required for this cohort, and less involvement, if any, from healthcare services.

As the patient achieves their newly adjusted rehabilitation goals and is on the verge of discharge then it will be important to re-assess their holistic unmet needs and agree on an 'exit' strategy, identifying what further support the patient may require and how they will receive this. This is where social prescribing, support from voluntary and charitable organisations, from existing family and friends' networks and potentially even ongoing digital support could be what is required for maintenance purposes and to address any outstanding needs for the patient. In the UK there is a focus on improved self-management for patients, through the personalised care agenda [10]. In some situations, where a patient is experiencing pronounced frailty, a carer or family member may be involved in rehabilitation sessions as the patient learns to adapt their completion of ADLs, either with dependence on someone else's assistance or adaptive equipment for optimised self-management.

Importantly at this stage in a patient's care, they may no longer have oncological treatment options, likely in part due to their frailty and reduced fitness, but this does not mean that they do not have rehabilitation potential. A patient may still be able to engage in some interventions such as the rehab elements of exercise, nutrition and psychological support, which will achieve their functional goals and maximise their QoL, in advance of the palliative phase. Anecdotally, it has been observed that patients are often not referred for rehabilitation in this phase, when they should be.

Palliative Phase of Cancer Rehabilitation

In most cases, older people experiencing non-curative cancer and combined frailty, approaching the end of their life, will significantly deteriorate in their functional ability as they transition into palliative care. At this stage specialist rehabilitation may be beneficial to ameliorate the symptoms of cancer progression and the cumulative side effects of treatment (if being offered) [23], with the overarching short-term goal of optimal QoL. Complex management is required including applying orthopaedic, respiratory, neurological and lymphoedema expertise as indicated by the patient's prognosis, adverse effect profile and tolerance [23].

Family members may require additional support at this time also and once again it is important to understand their and the patient's wishes including end-of-life planning and the role of hospice care. In the United Kingdom, hospices can offer patients the opportunity to attend during the day and many have rehabilitation teams with a mixture of nursing staff and AHPs available to address needs that become present during this cancer stage, as well as complimentary therapeutic provision such as music therapy. Additional referrals may be needed for dietetic or speech and language therapy input if a patient becomes unable to swallow or if their communication deteriorates. Social work professionals are often pivotal at this point, whether to facilitate practical assistance or in some countries provide emotional and spiritual support. The rehabilitation offered to patients at this stage should still be goal based, although it is likely these will be focused on immediate needs such as reducing pain, managing anxiety and maximising time spent with family members. In-depth interviews with patients with advanced cancer concluded that symptom control and palliation should be viewed as mechanisms to optimise active participation in essential and valued activities. Participants in this qualitative study were adamant they did not want to languish and wanted to be able to do '… the everyday things….' [65]. Low-level physical activity or exercise can still be a method to achieve these short-term ADL goals, such as chair-based exercise [58]. Risk assessment is paramount, with consideration being paid to potential metastatic spinal cord compression and other bone fractures, which could exacerbate pain and other associated symptoms during this phase.

Research Needs

More evidence needs to be accrued detailing which intervention or combination of interventions is most feasible, efficacious and cost effective, and crucially, which are most important to older patients [66]. Beyond specific interventions, the measurement of important outcomes (i.e. what to measure and how to measure it) is controversial. Indeed, for all prehab populations the development of a patient facing common core outcome dataset is long overdue. Similarly, in frail populations, agreement in screening instruments and longer-term outcomes that have high clinical utility are needed. Further, longitudinal research in frailty is important, since patients may dynamically transition between frailty and pre-frail states [66] and prehab and rehab strategies should be intuitive and personalised across the continuum of frailty and cancer.

Whilst recent systematic reviews and meta-analyses support the role of interdisciplinary prehab and rehab in several tumour sites, there are many aspects of this care that require further research. In particular; the impact of prehab and rehab for older and /or frail patient subgroups, the fidelity of individual components of the treatments, the most patient-centred and effective implementation strategies, the growing role of technology in delivering such services, and their effectiveness across the range of tumour sites and treatments. Improvements in outcomes need to be sustained across different stages of cancer survivorship and aligned with patient goals. Figure 9.4 summarises a list of research unmet needs that will help close the evidence–practice gap across prehab, particularly in the setting of frailty.

Multiple prehab randomised clinical trials for patients with frailty are currently recruiting including McIsaac et al. [67] using a single centre, parallel-arm randomised clinical trial to test the efficacy of home-based exercise prehab for older people undergoing intra-abdominal or intrathoracic cancer at The Ottawa Hospital [67] and Wang et al investigating the impact of nutritional optimisation and exercise training on the early and long-term outcomes on older patients undergoing 'digestive' surgery [68]. The majority of existing trials are limited to cancer surgery and whilst we await their findings with interest it is further recommended for

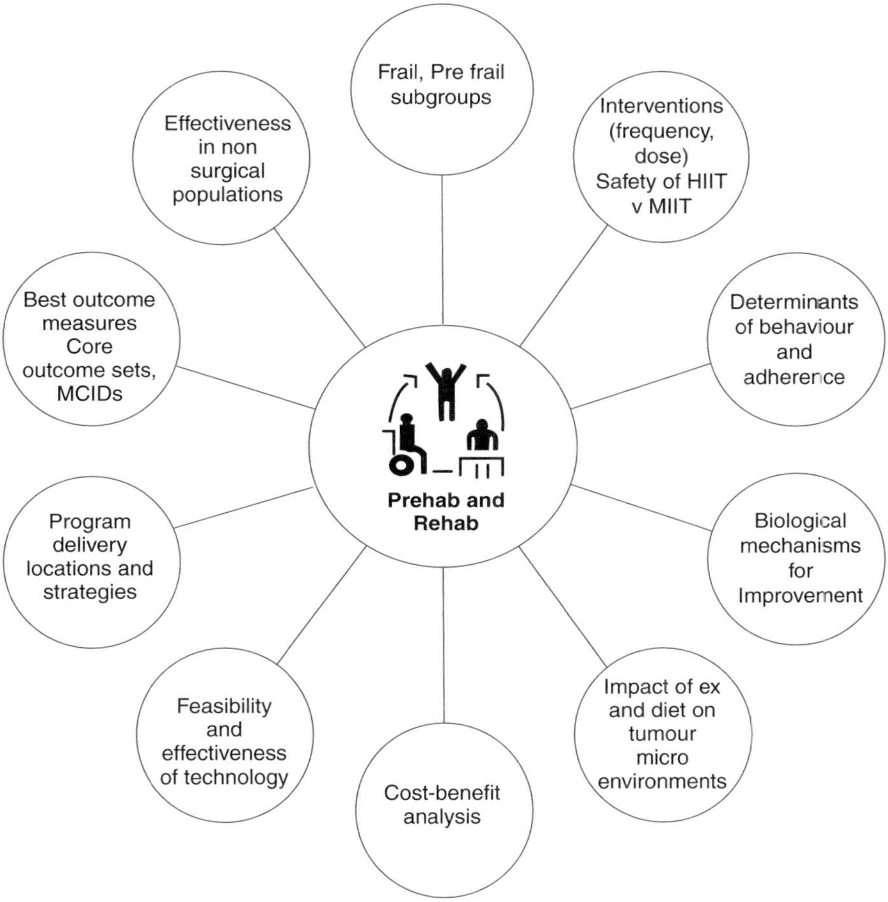

Fig. 9.4 Suggested research areas for prehab and rehab

frailty-focused prehab (and rehab) randomised clinical trials to be completed within other cancer treatment modalities.

Conclusion

Older adults with cancer are commonly frail with reduced resilience and adaptive capacity to stressors and seem to be an ideal group to benefit from prehab and rehab. Identifying and optimising the management of comorbidities and their associated medications, promoting the achievement of generic older adult physical activity recommendations coupled with targeted additions are important in the management of this cohort of cancer patients [62].

Use of CGA and frailty screening is recommended in the prescription of prehab and rehab, prioritising the assessment of function, comorbidity, falls, depression, cognition and nutrition [5], in addition to other more standard risk assessment tools.

Personalised therapy is perhaps the most important aspect of maximising functional outcomes for people in any programme, but especially in frail patients, to target the main impairments aligned with the individual's goals. As above-described, frailty is multidimensional including physical, social, environmental, and psychological factors. Some risks for frailty may be preventable, treatable and/or reversible. However, the current provision of rehab often does not specifically address frailty factors, instead of being delivered by a large team often not able to provide frailty-focused individualised care. Growing evidence recommends to improve effectiveness, prehab or rehab programmes for older people should identify and target specific factors for frailty [69].

It is acknowledged that the above-described models of prehab and rehab may not be available globally, despite this being an aim of worldwide initiatives, such as the World Health Organisation rehab recommendations [70]. In the absence of established 'prehab' and 'rehab' services available locally there can still be an aspiration for good care for cancer patients, particularly those older with (or at high risk) of frailty. This can include successful secondary care initiatives such as 'Making Every Contact Count' which obligate healthcare professionals working within hospital settings to focus on improved independence and the adoption of healthy behaviours. Furthermore, there are digital resources available which patients and family members/carers can be signposted to (Prehab4Cancer website [71]), as well as websites designed to upskill and give confidence to healthcare providers to empower them to give basic exercise advice applicable to the patients they are treating, such as the Moving Medicine website [72].

References

1. Silver JK, Baima J, Mayer RS. Impairment-driven cancer rehabilitation: an essential component of quality care and survivorship. CA Cancer J Clin. 2013;63(5):295–317.
2. Alfano CM, Pergolotti M. Next-generation cancer rehabilitation: a giant step forward for patient care. Rehabil Nurs. 2018;43(4):186–94.
3. Stout NL, Santa Mina D, Lyons KD, Robb KA, Silver JK. A systematic review of rehabilitation and exercise recommendations in oncology guidelines. CA J Cancer Clin. 2020. https://doi.org/10.3322/caac.21639
4. Introduction—delivering high-quality cancer care—NCBI Bookshelf [Internet]. [cited 30 Sept 2020]. Available from: https://www.ncbi.nlm.nih.gov/books/NBK202150/
5. Mohile SG, Dale W, Somerfield MR, Schonberg MA, Boyd CM, Burhenn PS, et al. Practical assessment and management of vulnerabilities in older patients receiving chemotherapy: ASCO guideline for geriatric oncology. J Clin Oncol. [Internet] 2018;36(22):2326–47 [cited 30 Sept 2020]. Available from: https://pubmed.ncbi.nlm.nih.gov/29782209/
6. NCCN clinical practice guidelines in oncology [Internet] [cited 4 Oct 2020]. Available from: https://www.nccn.org/professionals/physician_gls/default.aspx
7. Talarico L, Chen G, Pazdur R. Enrollment of elderly patients in clinical trials for cancer drug registration: a 7-year experience by the US Food and Drug Administration. J Clin Oncol.

[Internet] 2004;22(22):4626–31 [cited 30 Sept 2020]. Available from: https://pubmed.ncbi.nlm.nih.gov/15542812/
8. Quaglia A, Tavilla A, Shack L, Brenner H, Janssen-Heijnen M, Allemani C, et al. The cancer survival gap between elderly and middle-aged patients in Europe is widening. Eur J Cancer. [Internet] 2009;45(6):1006–16 [cited 30 Sept 2020]. Available from: https://pubmed.ncbi.nlm.nih.gov/19121578/
9. Hutchins LF, Unger JM, Crowley JJ, Coltman CA, Albain KS. Underrepresentation of patients 65 years of age or older in cancer-treatment trials. N Engl J Med. [Internet] 1999;341(27):2061–7 [cited 30 Sept 2020]. Available from: http://www.nejm.org/doi/abs/10.1056/NEJM199912303412706
10. Internet [cited 30 Sept 2020]. Available from: https://www.macmillan.org.uk/documents/get-involved/campaigns/ageoldexcuse/ageoldexcusereport-macmillancancersupport.pdf
11. Pergolotti M, Deal AM, Lavery J, Reeve BB, Muss HB. The prevalence of potentially modifiable functional deficits and the subsequent use of occupational and physical therapy by older adults with cancer. J Geriatr Oncol. [Internet] 2015;6(3):194–201 [cited 30 Sept 2020]. Available from: https://pubmed.ncbi.nlm.nih.gov/25614296/
12. Handforth C, Clegg A, Young C, Simpkins S, Seymour MT, Selby PJ, et al. The prevalence and outcomes of frailty in older cancer patients: a systematic review. Ann Oncol. [Internet] 2015;26(6):1091–101 [cited 30 Sept 2020]. Available from: https://pubmed.ncbi.nlm.nih.gov/25403592/
13. Clough-Gorr KM, Stuck AE, Thwin SS, Silliman RA. Older breast cancer survivors: geriatric assessment domains are associated with poor tolerance of treatment adverse effects and predict mortality over 7 years of follow-up. J Clin Oncol. [Internet] 2010;28(3):380–6 [cited 30 Sept 2020]. Available from: https://www.ncbi.nlm.nih.gov/pmc/articles/PMC2815700/?report=abstract
14. Kenis C, Milisen K, Flamaing J, Wildiers H, Decoster L, Van Puyvelde K, et al. Performance of two geriatric screening tools in older patients with cancer. J Clin Oncol. [Internet] 2014;32(1):19–26 [cited 30 Sept 2020]. Available from: https://pubmed.ncbi.nlm.nih.gov/24276775/
15. Mariano C, Williams G, Deal A, Alston S, Bryant AL, Jolly T, et al. Geriatric assessment of older adults with cancer during unplanned hospitalizations: an opportunity in disguise. Oncologist. [Internet] 2015;20(7):767–72 [cited 4 Oct 2020]. Available from: https://pubmed.ncbi.nlm.nih.gov/26032136/
16. Dietz JH. Rehabilitation oncology. Wiley; 1981 (Wiley medical publication).
17. Cromes GFJ. Implementation of interdisciplinary cancer rehabilitation. Rehabil Couns Bull. 1978;21(3):230–7.
18. Hshieh TT, Jung WF, Grande LJ, Chen J, Stone RM, Soiffer RJ, et al. Prevalence of cognitive impairment and association with survival among older patients with hematologic cancers. JAMA Oncol. [Internet] 2018;4(5):686–93 [cited 30 Sept 2020]. Available from: https://jamanetwork.com/
19. Magnuson A, Mohile S, Janelsins M. Cognition and cognitive impairment in older adults with cancer. Curr Geriatr Rep. [Internet] 2016;5:213–9 [cited 30 Sept 2020]. New York: Springer. Available from: https://link.springer.com/article/10.1007/s13670-016-0182-9
20. Kumar Pal S, Katheria V, Hurria A. Evaluating the older patient with cancer: understanding frailty and the geriatric assessment. CA Cancer J Clin. [Internet] 2010;60(2):120–32 [cited 30 Sept 2020]. Available from: http://doi.wiley.com/10.3322/caac.20059
21. Nicholson NR. A review of social isolation: an important but underassessed condition in older adults. J Prim Prev. [Internet] 2012;33:137–52 [cited 30 Sept 2020]. Springer. Available from: https://link.springer.com/article/10.1007/s10935-012-0271-2
22. DuMontier C, Poh Loh K, Bain PA, Silliman RA, Hshieh T, Abel GA, et al. Defining undertreatment and overtreatment in older adults with cancer: a scoping literature review. J Clin Oncol. [Internet] 2020;38:2558–69 [cited 4 Oct 2020]. American Society of Clinical Oncology. Available from: https://pubmed.ncbi.nlm.nih.gov/32250717/

23. Rankin J, Gracey J. Rehabilitation in oncology and palliative care. In: Rankin J, Robb K, Murtagh N, Cooper J, Lewis S, editors. Rehabilitation in cancer care. 1st ed. Oxford: Blackwell; 2008. p. 24–43.
24. Ethun CG, Bilen MA, Jani AB, Maithel SK, Ogan K, Master VA. Frailty and cancer: implications for oncology surgery, medical oncology, and radiation oncology. CA Cancer J Clin. [Internet] 2017;67(5):362–77 [cited 4 Oct 2020]. Available from: https://pubmed.ncbi.nlm.nih.gov/28731537/
25. Cancer Research UK. Advancing care, advancing years: improving cancer treatment and care for and ageing population. 2018;(1089464):19. Available from: https://www.cancerresearchuk.org/sites/default/files/advancing_care_advancing_years_briefing.pdf
26. Mental Capacity Act 2005 [Internet] [cited 30 Sept 2020]. Available from: https://www.legislation.gov.uk/ukpga/2005/9/contents
27. Rønning B, Wyller TB, Nesbakken A, Skovlund E, Jordhøy MS, Bakka A, et al. Quality of life in older and frail patients after surgery for colorectal cancer-A follow-up study. J Geriatr Oncol. [Internet] 2016;7(3):195–200. Available from: https://doi.org/10.1016/j.jgo.2016.03.002
28. Hayes SC, Newton RU, Spence RR, Galvão DA. The Exercise and Sports Science Australia position statement: exercise medicine in cancer management. J Sci Med Sport. 2019;22:1175–99. Elsevier
29. Santa Mina D, Alibhai SMH. Prehabilitation in geriatric oncology. J Geriatr Oncol. 2020;11(4):731–4.
30. Bruns ERJ, Argillander TE, Schuijt HJ, Van Duijvendijk P, Van Der Zaag ES, Wassenaar EB, et al. Fit4SurgeryTV at-home prehabilitation for frail older patients planned for colorectal cancer surgery: a pilot study. Am J Phys Med Rehabil. 2019;98(5):399–406.
31. Overcash J, Cope DG, Van Cleave JH. Frailty in older adults. Clin J Oncol Nurs. 2018;22(6):8–17.
32. Richards S, Jerram P, Brett C, Falloon M, Frizelle F. The association between low pre-operative step count and adverse post-operative outcomes in older patients undergoing colorectal cancer surgery. Perioper Med. 2020;9(1):1–10.
33. Steffens D, Delbaere K, Young J, Solomon M, Denehy L. Evidence on technology-driven preoperative exercise interventions: are we there yet? Br J Anaesth. 2020;125(5):646–9. Elsevier.
34. Hamaker ME, Oosterlaan F, van Huis LH, Thielen N, Vondeling A, van den Bos F. Nutritional status and interventions for patients with cancer—a systematic review. J Geriatr Oncol. [Internet] 2020 [cited 4 Oct 2020]. Elsevier. Available from: https://pubmed.ncbi.nlm.nih.gov/32616384/
35. Presley CJ, Dotan E, Soto-Perez-de-Celis E, Jatoi A, Mohile SG, Won E, et al. Gaps in nutritional research among older adults with cancer. J Geriatr Oncol. [Internet] 2016;7:281–92 [cited 4 Oct 2020]. Elsevier. Available from: https://pubmed.ncbi.nlm.nih.gov/27197919/
36. Lorenzo-López L, Maseda A, De Labra C, Regueiro-Folgueira L, Rodríguez-Villamil JL, Millán-Calenti JC. Nutritional determinants of frailty in older adults: a systematic review. BMC Geriatr. [Internet] 2017;17(1) [cited 4 Oct 2020]. Available from: https://pubmed.ncbi.nlm.nih.gov/28506216/
37. Milne AC, Potter J, Vivanti A, Avenell A. Protein and energy supplementation in elderly people at risk from malnutrition. Cochrane Database Syst Rev. [Internet] 2009 [cited 4 Oct 2020]. Wiley. Available from: https://pubmed.ncbi.nlm.nih.gov/19370584/
38. Kou K, Momosaki R, Miyazaki S, Wakabayashi H, Shamoto H. Impact of nutrition therapy and rehabilitation on acute and critical illness: a systematic review. J UOEH. [Internet] 2019;41:303–15 [cited 4 Oct 2020]. University of Occupational and Environmental Health. Available from: https://pubmed.ncbi.nlm.nih.gov/31548485/
39. Bunt S, Steverink N, Olthof J, van der Schans CP, Hobbelen JSM. Social frailty in older adults: a scoping review. Eur J Ageing. [Internet] 2017;14:323–34 [cited 6 Apr 2021]. Springer. Available from: https://pubmed.ncbi.nlm.nih.gov/28936141/
40. Dennett AM, Peiris CL, Shields N, Morgan D, Taylor NF. Exercise therapy in oncology rehabilitation in Australia: a mixed-methods study. Asia Pac J Clin Oncol. 2017;13(5):e515–27.

41. Edbrooke L, Aranda S, Granger CL, Mcdonald CF, Krishnasamy M, Mileshkin L, et al. Multidisciplinary home-based rehabilitation in inoperable lung cancer: a randomised controlled trial. Thorax. 2019;74(8).
42. Alibhai SMH, Santa Mina D, Ritvo P, Tomlinson G, Sabiston C, Krahn M, et al. A phase II randomized controlled trial of three exercise delivery methods in men with prostate cancer on androgen deprivation therapy. BMC Cancer. 2019;19(1):2.
43. Lopez C, Jones J, Alibhai SMH, Mina DS. What is the "home" in home-based exercise? The need to define independent exercise for survivors of cancer. J Clin Oncol. 2018;36:928–9. American Society of Clinical Oncology.
44. Santa Mina D, Au D, Auger LE, Alibhai SMH, Matthew AG, Sabiston CM, et al. Development, implementation, and effects of a cancer center's exercise-oncology program. Cancer. 2019;125(19):3437–47.
45. Carli F, Bousquet-Dion G, Awasthi R, Elsherbini N, Liberman S, Boutros M, et al. Effect of multimodal prehabilitation vs postoperative rehabilitation on 30-day postoperative complications for frail patients undergoing resection of colorectal cancer: a randomized clinical trial. JAMA Surg. 2020;155(3):233–42.
46. Harari D, Hopper A, Dhesi J, Babic-Illman G, Lockwood L, Martin F. Proactive care of older people undergoing surgery ('POPS'): designing, embedding, evaluating and funding a comprehensive geriatric assessment service for older elective surgical patients. Age Ageing. [Internet] 2007;36(2):190–6 [cited 30 Sept 2020]. Available from: https://pubmed.ncbi.nlm.nih.gov/17259638/
47. Nunns M, Shaw L, Briscoe S, Thompson Coon J, Hemsley A, McGrath JS, et al. Multicomponent hospital-led interventions to reduce hospital stay for older adults following elective surgery: a systematic review. Heal Serv Deliv Res. 2019;7(40):1–178.
48. Waterland JL, McCourt O, Edbrooke L, Granger CL, Ismail H, Riedel B, et al. Efficacy of prehabilitation including exercise on postoperative outcomes following abdominal cancer surgery: a systematic review and meta-analysis. Front Surg. [Internet] 2021;8:628848 [cited 2 Apr 2021]. Available from: https://www.frontiersin.org/articles/10.3389/fsurg.2021.628848/full
49. Makary MA, Segev DL, Pronovost PJ, Syin D, Bandeen-Roche K, Patel P, et al. Frailty as a predictor of surgical outcomes in older patients. J Am Coll Surg. 2010;210(6):901–8.
50. Thomas G, Tahir MR, Bongers BC, Kallen VL, Slooter GD, van Meeteren NL. Prehabilitation before major intra-abdominal cancer surgery. Eur J Anaesthesiol. 2019;36(12):933–45.
51. Boereboom CL, Williams JP, Leighton P, Lund JN. Forming a consensus opinion on exercise prehabilitation in elderly colorectal cancer patients: a Delphi study. Tech Coloproctol. 2015;19(6):347–54.
52. Overview | Perioperative care in adults | Guidance | NICE [Internet] [cited 4 Oct 2020]. Available from: https://www.nice.org.uk/guidance/ng180
53. Moore J, Merchant Z, Rowlinson K, McEwan K, Evison M, Faulkner G, et al. Implementing a system-wide cancer prehabilitation programme: the journey of Greater Manchester's 'Prehab4cancer'. Eur J Surg Oncol. 2021;47(3):524–32.
54. Moore JA, Conway DH, Thomas N, Cummings D, Atkinson D. Impact of a peri-operative quality improvement programme on postoperative pulmonary complications. Anaesthesia. [Internet] 2017;72(3):317–27 [cited 30 Sept 2020]. Available from: http://doi.wiley.com/10.1111/anae.13763
55. Bagnall NM, Malietzis G, Kennedy RH, Athanasiou T, Faiz O, Darzi A. A systematic review of enhanced recovery care after colorectal surgery in elderly patients. Colorectal Dis. [Internet] 2014;16:947–56 [cited 30 Sept 2020]. Blackwell. Available from: https://pubmed.ncbi.nlm.nih.gov/25039965/
56. Kalsi T, Harari D. Assessment methods and services for older people with cancer in the United Kingdom. World J Clin Oncol. [Internet] 2020;11(3):152–61 [cited 4 Oct 2020]. Available from: https://www.ncbi.nlm.nih.gov/pmc/articles/PMC7103526/?report=abstract
57. Braude P, Goodman A, Elias T, Babic-Illman G, Challacombe B, Harari D, et al. Evaluation and establishment of a ward-based geriatric liaison service for older urological surgical

patients: Proactive care of Older People undergoing Surgery (POPS)-urology. BJU Int. [Internet] 2017;120(1):123–9 [cited 30 Sept 2020]. Available from: https://pubmed.ncbi.nlm.nih.gov/27167854/
58. Rudolph JL, Marcantonio ER. Postoperative delirium: acute change with long-term implications. Anesth Analg. [Internet] 2011;112:1202–11 [cited 30 Sept 2020]. Lippincott Williams and Wilkins. Available from: https://www.ncbi.nlm.nih.gov/pmc/articles/PMC3090222/?report=abstract
59. Saczynski JS, Marcantonio ER, Quach L, Fong TG, Gross A, Inouye SK, et al. Cognitive trajectories after postoperative delirium. N Engl J Med. [Internet] 2012;367(1):30–9 [cited 30 Sept 2020]. Available from: http://www.nejm.org/doi/abs/10.1056/NEJMoa1112923
60. Luther A, Gabriel J, Watson RP, Francis NK. The impact of total body prehabilitation on post-operative outcomes after major abdominal surgery: a systematic review. World J Surg. [Internet] 2018;42:2781–91 [cited 4 Oct 2020]. New York: Springer. Available from: https://pubmed.ncbi.nlm.nih.gov/29546448/
61. Buchanan C, Kane C. Developing therapy services to support frail patients through an acute hospital admission. Physiotherapy. 2019;105:e131–2.
62. Dent E, Martin FC, Bergman H, Woo J, Romero-Ortuno R, Walston JD. Management of frailty: opportunities, challenges, and future directions. Lancet. [Internet] 2019;394:1376–86 [cited 30 Sept 2020]. Lancet Publishing. Available from: https://pubmed.ncbi.nlm.nih.gov/31609229/
63. Lyons KD, Newman RM, Kaufman PA, Bruce ML, Stearns DM, Lansigan F, et al. Goal attainment and goal adjustment of older adults during person-directed cancer rehabilitation. Am J Occup Ther. 2018;72(2).
64. Hunter EG, Gibson RW, Arbesman M, D'Amico M. Systematic review of occupational therapy and adult cancer rehabilitation: Part 2. Impact of multidisciplinary rehabilitation and psychosocial, sexuality, and return-to-work interventions. Am J Occup Ther. 2017;71(2).
65. Morgan DD, Currow DC, Denehy L, Aranda SA. Living actively in the face of impending death: constantly adjusting to bodily decline at the end-of-life. BMJ Support Palliat Care. [Internet] 2017;7(2):179–88 [cited 30 Sept 2020]. Available from: https://pubmed.ncbi.nlm.nih.gov/26182946/
66. Hoogendijk EO, Afilalo J, Ensrud KE, Kowal P, Onder G, Fried LP. Frailty: implications for clinical practice and public health. Lancet. 2019;394:1365–75. Lancet Publishing.
67. McIsaac DI, Saunders C, Hladkowicz E, Bryson GL, Forster AJ, Gagne S, et al. PREHAB study: a protocol for a prospective randomised clinical trial of exercise therapy for people living with frailty having cancer surgery. BMJ Open. 2018;8(6):1–8.
68. Multicomponent prehabilitation and outcomes in elderly patients with frailty—Full text view—ClinicalTrials.gov [Internet] [cited 6 Apr 2021]. Available from: https://clinicaltrials.gov/ct2/show/NCT04715581
69. Janssen TL, Mosk CA, Van Hoof-De Lepper CCHA, Wielders D, Seerden TCJ, Steyerberg EW, et al. A multicomponent prehabilitation pathway to reduce the incidence of delirium in elderly patients in need of major abdominal surgery: study protocol for a before-and-after study. BMC Geriatr. 2019;19(1):1–10.
70. WHO | World Health Organization [Internet] [cited 30 Sept 2020]. Available from: https://www.who.int/rehabilitation/rehab-2030/en/
71. Prehab4Cancer [Internet] [cited 30 Sept 2020]. Available from: https://prehab4cancer.co.uk/
72. Homepage—Moving Medicine [Internet] [cited 18 Aug 2020]. Available from: https://movingmedicine.ac.uk/

Chapter 10
Holistic Needs Assessment and Advance Care Planning in Older Adults with Cancer and Frailty

Jane Gibson, Sarah Wells, and Cassandra Ng

Introduction

Cancer and its treatment in older adults often result in physical deconditioning and increased dependency requiring longer periods to maintain medical stability and rehabilitation [1]. The focus of care in older adults living with frailty is more often that of health optimisation, maintaining independence and prioritising quality of life, as opposed to curative medicine in most cases via the provision of the gold standard Comprehensive Geriatric Assessment (CGA). A CGA is a multi-dimensional assessment and intervention, encompassing medical, functional capacity, social, environmental and psychological aspects [2, 3].

Cancer services are seeing more older adults with the rising incidence of cancers in an ageing population. With advancements in cancer treatment options, older adults with cancer are more likely to be considered for cancer treatments. International guidelines for the assessment and management of older adults with cancer advocate that all adults aged 65 years or older with cancer will benefit from geriatric assessment using validated assessment tools [4, 5]. For example, a recently published randomised clinical trial, the INTEGRATE trial has shown that older cancer patients undergoing CGA were less likely to be hospitalised and were able to continue cancer treatments for longer [6].

J. Gibson · S. Wells
Haemato-Oncology Department, The Christie NHS Foundation Trust, Manchester, UK
e-mail: jane.gibson2@nhs.net; s.wells7@nhs.net

C. Ng (✉)
Geriatric Department, Wythenshawe Hospital, Manchester NHS Foundation Trust, Manchester, UK
e-mail: Cassandra.Ng@mft.nhs.uk

F. Gomes (ed.), *Frailty in Older Adults with Cancer*,
https://doi.org/10.1007/978-3-030-89162-6_10

While it is feasible to deliver CGA in an oncology clinic [7], the extent to which oncology teams undertake CGA can be limited by factors such as time constraints within an already busy clinical workload, lack of training of healthcare professionals and financial constraints on services impacting on referral pathways.

However, it is likely that geriatric services alone will quickly be inundated and unlikely to match the needs of all older patients with cancer. Arguably, it is more sustainable to make identification of frailty 'everyone's business'. Developing new roles and dedicated geriatric teams take time and incur significant financial costs. The basic skills required for holistic care are already present in the existing workforce and can be expanded. Undeniably, up-skilling of pre-existing cancer services to identify frailty and assess for simple reversible causes through collaborative working within a multi-disciplinary team (MDT) is key.

Furthermore, training and empowering cancer specialist nurses who are already proficient with assessing holistic needs, and therapists as 'frailty champions' could be another way forward. The Nursing and Allied Health (NAH) Interest Group of the International Society of Geriatric Oncology (SIOG) recommends the integration of the assessment of geriatric domains into routine oncology assessments, and challenges nurses and allied health professionals to play a pertinent role in this field [8].

This chapter will review the similarities and differences between a CGA and the holistic needs assessment (HNA) in cancer care which is currently in use, for example, in the United Kingdom (UK). It will explore how HNA may provide a mechanism of identifying those older adults with cancer living with (or at high-risk of) frailty, who would benefit from a CGA. Finally, this chapter will also cover the Advance Care Planning, since the presence of frailty and cancer are key triggers to begin discussions about future medical care.

Holistic Needs Assessment (HNA)

HNA is a concept which has been developed as a direct result of a requirement for more person-centred care. It emerged as part of the UK government's commitment to invest and reform cancer services, and to therefore improve cancer survival and outcomes. This resulted from the UK Cancer Reform Strategy published in 2007 [9] and the Improving Outcomes Strategy for cancer in 2011 [10]. Moreover, the National Cancer Survivorship Initiative (NCSI) [11] aimed to develop services to address the unmet needs of patients living with and beyond cancer [12].

Being diagnosed with a cancer can be overwhelming for a patient and their family [13]. Patients are provided with a wealth of information that can often lead to information overload. Healthcare professionals (HCPs) inform patients of their diagnosis, investigations required, the increasingly more complex treatment options, as well as their efficacy and potential side effects. This information is important to keep patients safe and to ensure they consent to a treatment plan as informed as possible. However, HCPs can easily fail to understand what is most important to the patient. It may not be the side effects of treatment, but more often than not, their main concerns will be psychosocial. For example, who will feed their cat, how will this impact their loved ones, financial concerns or the concept of smoking cessation. Patients may have a long list of potential concerns and failure to acknowledge individual patient's concerns can result in a lack of concordance with a treatment plan, increased levels of anxiety and unmet needs [14].

The HNA is a process of gathering and discussing information with a patient to develop an understanding of what that person living with and beyond cancer knows, understands, and needs. This assessment is focused on the whole person, where their entire well-being is assessed and addressed including their physical, psychological, spiritual, mental, social, and environmental needs and concerns. Ultimately, this process's strength is that it is a patient-led assessment, and not driven by the medical team and what HCPs believe to be the patient's priorities. The results of the assessment are used to inform a written care plan shared with the patient and HCPs involved in their care throughout their cancer care pathway [11]. Assessments are ideally completed with the patient at set time points in their cancer care: at diagnosis, at treatment changes and on completion of treatment.

The HNA assessment does not need to be a prescriptive document, but rather a method that can guide the conversation between key worker and patient, to help identify their needs and develop a care plan. This assessment process is therefore patient-centred and addresses the principles outlined above, but it is more based on an open holistic discussion, rather than using specific assessment tools. However, some checklists and simple tools have been developed to better guide HCPs. These include the Concerns checklist [15], a Distress thermometer [16], the Sheffield Profile for Assessment and Referral to care (SPARC) [17] and the MacMillan HNA [18]. Overall, there is not an overarching HNA tool in use across the UK nor a standard set of tools, and each hospital may choose how best to deliver the principles of HNA.

Following completion of this assessment, a care plan is devised with the patients to address their concerns. Ultimately, this individualised care place focuses on what is important to the patient, optimising patient-centred care and it often involves referrals to other allied health professionals or support centres. The care plan is also shared with the patient and, with the patient's consent, their General Practitioner (or primary care physician). Reassessment is an important part of this process [18], to allow for changes in patient concerns at different time points in their care pathway. As described above, after an initial assessment, this should be repeated, in a flexible manner, at treatment changes and on completion of treatments.

The HNA is usually performed by the patient's key worker, which is defined as the patient's main point of contact with specialist knowledge in the disease group, its treatments and potential side effects. This is most commonly a clinical nurse specialist [19], however any member of the MDT involved in the patient's care can undertake the assessment and complete the care plan. But, completing an effective assessment requires the use of several advanced skills, which may result in some members of the MDT having reservations about being involved in this process. These include effective advanced communication skills, motivational interviewing skills, good clinical knowledge of the cancer type and knowledge around how to signpost to other services.

Whilst the HNA process can be seen as time consuming for HCPs, the time taken to carefully listen, identify and address patient concerns at the outset can significantly reduce patient anxiety and reduce preventable complications, saving time and resources in the longer term. Not only are the concerns of a patient explored and referrals initiated to other appropriate services, but patients also report feeling 'heard' with their concerns acknowledged and this can provide a therapeutic benefit [20].

With the refinement of anticancer therapies and supportive medications, there is a growing number of treatment options that may be offered to older cancer patients. Although age in itself should not be a barrier to treatment, treating older adults, particularly those with frailty, can be more challenging [21]. A well-timed HNA can be a helpful method to help exploring the older patient's goals of care, concerns around the treatment and unmet needs that could be relevant for their cancer management. Fear of cancer treatment in older patients may originate from many other concerns. Older patients often live independently or are isolated from support networks. The commitment, expense, travel, or inconvenience of treatment may often feel overwhelming for older adults. It is imperative to elicit these concerns and attempt to alleviate them by implementing an effective care plan. The side effects of cancer treatments may also bring additional worries, particularly for those patients more vulnerable or frail. Therefore, particularly for those complex older cancer patients with frailty, HCPs need to find the right balance between ensuring the safety of this potentially vulnerable group of people, without encroaching on their independence. Also, it is important to ensure this patient group maintain dignity and independence throughout their cancer pathway. However, the HNA has some limitations particularly in this group, since it is not targeting specifically older patients, it is relatively generic and it does not address specific frailty issues, which this patient group may experience. It is however a flexible assessment, where the key workers may potentially be upskilled to implement frailty assessments for older patients in order to flag those at high-risk.

Holistic Needs Assessment Versus Comprehensive Geriatric Assessment

The HNA and CGA have several key similarities and differences (Table 10.1). Both the HNA and CGA aim to provide a multi-dimensional person-centred approach to the assessment and management of adults with a cancer diagnosis, with the goal to optimise clinical outcomes, such as the quality of life of individuals. Both involve the development of an individualised plan of care in collaboration with the patient and their families and/or carers. The gathering and sharing of information should

Table 10.1 Similarities and differences between HNA and CGA

Holistic Needs Assessment (HNA)	Comprehensive Geriatric Assessment (CGA)
Similarities	
Multi-dimensional person-centred approach to the assessment and management of adults with a cancer diagnosis	
Goal to optimise patient outcomes, including enhanced quality of life	
Individualised plan of care in collaboration with the patient, their families and/or carers	
Information gathered and shared from diagnosis, through cancer treatment and beyond	
Should identify patients' own concerns and needs, not the perceptions of the professionals undertaking the assessment [22]	
Differences	
Not age specific	Focusses on older adults
Assessment encompasses the physical, psychological and social concerns and needs of the patient	Assessment focuses not just on the patient needs and concerns, but also on common issues and conditions, such as geriatric syndrome/frailty. Therefore, it also covers areas such as medical history, medications and cognition
Primary focus on assessment	Similar focus on assessment and subsequent interventions
Assessment often more generic	Specialised assessments with validated tools, questionnaires and tests
Assessment typically performed by a cancer clinical nurse specialist	Assessment by multi-disciplinary team with expertise in geriatric care
Performed at specific time points along the cancer patient's journey	Involves continuous assessments, delivery of interventions with regular reassessments

extend beyond the person's cancer diagnosis itself and include identifying what can help patients cope with their cancer treatment and beyond. The assessment should identify patients' own concerns and needs, not the perceptions of the professionals undertaking the assessment [22].

The HNA encompass the physical, psychological and social concerns and needs of the patient, not specifically focused on the particular needs of older adults. However, the CGA focuses not just on the concerns and needs, but also on identifying issues and conditions more specific to older cancer patients, such as frailty/geriatric syndromes. Moreover, CGA more often uses specialised validated tools, questionnaires and tests, and it also covers areas such as medical history, medications and cognition. Subsequently, the CGA has a more substantial interventional component, which is also more specialised. The HNA is typically performed by a single designated oncology specialist HCPs, usually a clinical nurse specialist, within a cancer disease team (who may then send some referrals to other teams, such as, for psychological support). The CGA, on the other hand, encompasses all the assessments and interventions, and it often requires an MDT to deliver these, particularly the targeted specialised interventions. This MDT often includes medical, nursing, physiotherapy, occupational therapy, pharmacy, dietetic and social work expertise within the speciality of geriatric care. The timing of the assessments is also potentially different, since HNA is often performed at baseline (before starting a treatment) and whenever the treatment changes or is completed. However, the CGA often includes more regular reassessments, particularly if problems have been identified previously that require intervention and monitoring.

As the principles of HNA and CGA are similar in terms of assessing the multidimensional needs of older adults with cancer to optimise clinical outcomes, the assessments should be used in a complementary way, to avoid duplication of the assessment process that may negatively impact on the patient and healthcare professional's time. Undertaking a HNA for older adults could be used to inform referrals to geriatric services for CGA, by the facilitation of initial assessment and prioritisation of referrals. This would be particularly relevant where oncology services do not have readily available access to geriatric assessment services and delays may ensue before an initial geriatric assessment is made. Moreover, HNAs performed at future time points in the patients' cancer journey could also inform the geriatric services of any changes relevant to individual patient care that may prompt further geriatric assessments that might not have otherwise been planned. This enhanced communication and collaboration between oncology and geriatric services would aim to streamline the older patient pathway from diagnosis, through treatment, remission or end of life care. It would also allow sharing of expertise, educational development and joint research opportunities between HCPs from both the geriatric and oncology specialities.

Advance Care Planning

Advance Care Planning (ACP) is universally accepted as 'enabling individuals to define goals and preferences for future medical treatment and care, to discuss these goals and preferences with family and healthcare providers, and to record and review these preferences if appropriate' [23]. ACP, like a will, can be discussed at any stage of life but major health crises such as cancer, hospitalisation or the presence of frailty are triggers to start these conversations. Healthcare organisations globally promote the proactive use of ACP with guidance on how best to do so including tools such as *The Conversation Project* (United States of America), *National Gold Standards Framework* (UK), and *My Voice Planning Ahead* (Canada) [24]. An ACP prepares patients (and their families) on their expectations in the event of deterioration in health, respects patient autonomy and promotes a good end of life care. This can be revised regularly while one has the capacity to do so.

However, the use of ACP is suboptimal [25, 26] due to multiple reasons including fear of causing distress, lack of time, lack of clinician's confidence and training, and the presence of prognostic uncertainties [27, 28]. An ACP is sometimes incorrectly perceived as exclusively for the context of limiting care, futility of treatment or withholding interventions; posing as a barrier to having these conversations early, especially when the cancer is treatable. The absence of ACP often leads to inappropriate and distressing life prolonging interventions, impeding on preferred place of care and patient-centred decisions [25].

Nonetheless, ACP is especially pertinent at the outset of the management of older cancer patients with frailty due to numerous factors. Older adults living with severe frailty are five times more likely to die within 1 year than their less frail counterparts [29]. Frailty is also associated with cognitive decline, and the lack of cognitive reserves places an older frail person at risk of lacking capacity to decide during an acute illness. The presence of frailty poses further complexity and clinical uncertainties, and treatment options do not only have impact on life expectancies but more importantly on quality of life. In fact, very often older patients and their families would have had thoughts about their future and welcome open conversations about their future medical care [30].

An effective ACP requires older adults to be adequately informed about their illness trajectory, acknowledging clinical uncertainties, and understanding the transition points between curative and palliative treatments. Additionally, one will require thorough information about the benefits and burdens of their treatment options, including the impact on quality of life, to be able to make an informed decision. Frailty plays a very significant role in all these considerations. In the UK, while ACP predominantly occurs in primary care through initiatives such as the above-mentioned *National Gold Standards Framework*, older cancer patients, particularly those more complex with frailty, benefit from personalised information coming from the specialists in their care, such as the treating oncology or geriatric teams.

Thus, ACP is deeply rooted within a CGA. The identification of frailty and recognition of an individual who is likely to be in the last year of life regularly leads on to honest conversations about the future. The MDT approach to a CGA, incorporating members from the Oncology and Geriatric teams, ensures the patient is well informed, and supported during and after the ACP process.

Similarly, the HNA provides a forum for the initiation of conversations around ACP. HNA addresses one's concerns, expectations and wishes, building the setting for further discussions with the oncology team in the following visits. At the very least, one can be signposted and supported to discuss one's ACP with the Oncologist or General Practitioner.

Conclusion

This chapter demonstrated that while HNA and CGA are two separate holistic assessments designed for different purposes, their underlying principles are not entirely dissimilar. In fact, these can and should be complementary, whenever available. The needs and priorities of older patients however vary hugely, particularly for those with frailty, and can only be met via personalised MDT assessments, ideally via CGA. There are benefits to be gained from integrating both assessments to provide a holistic and time efficient assessment for older adults with cancer who make up a major proportion of cancer service users. As many centres may not have the resources or an easy access to CGA, a HNA is a simpler and less resource-intense approach that may help identify some patients who may benefit from CGA. Moreover, the oncology key workers who perform HNA may be upskilled to deliver frailty screening assessments and work collaboratively with geriatric services to deliver the best care for these complex patients. Lastly, the presence of frailty and cancer should trigger ACP early on, which can be performed by these teams and not just at the level of primary care, in order to allow for realistic expectations and a good end of life care.

Case Study

Mrs G, 69 years old was admitted to hospital after presenting with a left middle cerebral artery infarct and a solitary left cerebellar peduncle lesion which prompted further investigations. This revealed a lung cancer with bilateral lung and liver metastases and a biopsy confirmed adenocarcinoma with positive epidermal growth factor receptor (EGFR) mutation. She was discharged home with follow-up with the oncology team.

Whilst she was living in her son's house independently with Clinical Frailty Score of 4, on discharge, Mrs G was walking with the aid of a stick with mild residual right-sided weakness, facial numbness and was now dysarthric.

Mrs G was offered treatment with an EFGR inhibitor called Gefitinib. Her cancer responded well to the treatment, but Mrs G was low in mood. Four months later, she developed a left eye neurotrophic ulcer requiring multiple hospital admissions. Her eye condition worsened despite topical antibiotics and steroids requiring a surgical procedure in which her left eyelids were partially sutured together to protect her cornea (tarsorrhaphy). This intervention led to cosmetic distress and vision impairment which had a further negative impact on her mood and also on her quality of life.

Sadly, 11 months after starting treatment, her cancer progressed, and Mrs G was offered another treatment. The goals of care were discussed, and Mrs G opted for best supportive care and died peacefully at home with her family present.

HNA Undertaken by Mrs G's Lung Cancer Team

Initial HNA

Mrs G completed a written HNA assessment form prior to her first visit to the oncology clinic. This was reviewed by her lung cancer clinical nurse specialist (key worker), who was present during the oncology consultation and spent time with Mrs G afterwards undertaking an assessment and formulated an action plan based on the priority concerns identified.

Priority concerns identified with agreed action plan included:

1. Anxiety and low mood.

   Mrs G's CNS assessed her mood and offered the opportunity to explore her feelings and worries. Mrs G's anxieties were related not only to her cancer diagnosis and treatment but were predominantly related to her stroke and the impact on her quality of life. It was at this point the HNA identified the requirement for geriatric specialist referral. Mrs G also agreed with a referral to psychological support services, but she preferred to access services local to her rather than additional hospital visits and a referral was therefore made to her local hospice counselling service. It was also agreed that she would have regular contacts with her key worker by telephone and when she attended the hospital.

2. Poor oral intake and weight loss

   Her usual dietary intake was reviewed, and the key worker provided some top-level suggestions on how to improve this, such as a high protein and high carbohydrate diet. A community dietician referral was also made at this time.

3. Constipation

   The key worker, who was also a non-medical prescriber, reviewed some of her medication, and agreed that before introducing laxatives, the initial goal would be to improve her diet and fluid intake.

Subsequent HNA

The key worker maintained regular contact with Mrs G where her needs were continuously assessed and evaluated. A formal HNA was undertaken when Mrs G attended for results of her CT scan which sadly showed progressive disease. The agreed priorities at that point were about receiving best supportive care and her preferred place was to be cared for at home. Community palliative care service referrals were made. The key worker remained in contact with the Mrs G, and with her son when she was to unwell to communicate, until her peaceful death at home.

CGA Undertaken by Geriatrician Within Lung Cancer Team

Mrs G was seen by the Geriatrician embedded within the lung cancer services.

Visit 1

A CGA was commenced by a Geriatrician with aid of the physiotherapy assessments during Mrs G's recent admission on the stroke rehabilitation unit. From the HNA, it was identified that Mrs G's main concern was around her stroke and recurrence, and she found it reassuring to be able to discuss her stroke management in detail. She was also referred to the community Speech and Language team for speech therapy. A medication review was also undertaken, and her Statin was stopped due to multiple liver metastases.

It was identified that Mrs G's was living in her son's house and did not require any social support. There were also no concerns around Mrs G's cognition, and she had the capacity to make decisions on her own health. She was feeling mildly anxious but was enjoying spending time with her family and new grandchild. She was aware of the cancer prognosis.

An ACP was commenced with Mrs G and she agreed that she would like to have all active treatments but not at the expense of her quality of life and did not want Cardiopulmonary Resuscitation in the event of a cardiac arrest. This was shared with her General Practitioner.

Visit 2

Mrs G's speech had improved, and she tolerated the treatment with Gefitinib well with no overt side effects. She reported constipation and lack of appetite resulting in weight loss. Therefore, she was given advice on increasing fibre in her diet, commenced on laxatives and provided with oral nutritional supplements and encouraged to have a high calorie, high protein diet.

Visit 3

Mrs G had an admission to the eye hospital with left eye neurotrophic ulcer and keratopathy which did not improve with topical eye drops. Due to involvements of multiple specialities including Ophthalmology, Oncology and Stroke services across different hospital sites, the role of the Geriatrician was central in coordinating care and piecing together the different clinical managements.

This situation aggravated Mrs G low mood, further affecting her diet and resulting in fatigue and more weight loss. She felt her quality of life had been significantly affected with her loss of vision, surgical eye intervention and multiple appointments at the eye clinic. Moreover, Mrs G was unable to administer her eye drops herself, hence that district nurses provided support with her eye care so that she could stay in her own home as she preferred.

Functionally, Mrs G had become weaker and more fatigue. Her Clinical Frailty Score was now 6. The lung cancer nursing team linked in with the community palliative care team for an environmental assessment and provided her with equipment to maintain her independence. She also contacted a Psychologist at her local hospice for support with her mood.

Visit 4

Mrs G's lung cancer progressed and became frailer and was depressed. Her ACP was revisited, and she expressed that she would not like further treatment or hospitalisations. She prioritised her quality of life and time at home with her family stating her preferred place of care and death as her home. She was commenced on mirtazapine 15 mg once at night to help with her mood and appetite.

In conclusion, the collaboration with pre-existing community and cancer services was key to provision of holistic care for Mrs G who benefitted from input from both the HNA and CGA at various stages of her cancer journey. In fact, several of the key issues were highlighted via the HNA. The role of the geriatric oncology service was crucial in leading and coordinating care across multiple medical specialties at the more complex timepoints. There was clearly a value in the integration of both assessments to allow for an effective holistic assessment.

References

1. van Abbema D, van Vuuren A, van den Berkmortel F, van den Akker M, Deckx L, Buntinx F, van Kampen R, Lambooij E, de Boer M, de Vos-Geelen J, Tjan-Heijnen VC. Functional status decline in older patients with breast and colorectal cancer after cancer treatment: a prospective cohort study. J Geriatr Oncol. 2017;8(3):176–84.
2. Decoster L, Van Puyvelde K, Mohile S, Wedding U, Basso U, Colloca G, Rostoft S, Overcash J, Wildiers H, Steer C, Kimmick G. Screening tools for multidimensional health problems warranting a geriatric assessment in older cancer patients: an update on SIOG recommendations. Ann Oncol. 2015;26(2):288–300.
3. International Society of Geriatric Oncology. Comprehensive Geriatric Assessment (CGA) of the older patient with cancer. 2006. http://siog.org/content/comprehensive-geriatric-assessment-cga-older-patient-cancer. Accessed 25 Aug 2020.
4. Mohile SG, Dale W, Somerfield MR, Schonberg MA, Boyd CM, Burhenn PS, Canin B, Cohen HJ, Holmes HM, Hopkins JO, Janelsins MC. Practical assessment and management of vulnerabilities in older patients receiving chemotherapy: ASCO guideline for geriatric oncology. J Clin Oncol. 2018;36(22):2326.
5. Wildiers H, Heeren P, Puts M, Topinkova E, Janssen-Heijnen ML, Extermann M, Falandry C, Artz A, Brain E, Colloca G, Flamaing J. International Society of Geriatric Oncology consensus on geriatric assessment in older patients with cancer. J Clin Oncol. 2014;32(24):2595.
6. Soo WK, King M, Pope A, Parente P, Darzins P, Davis ID. Integrated geriatric assessment and treatment (INTEGERATE) in older people with cancer planned for systemic anticancer therapy. J Clin Oncol. 2020;38(15):12011.
7. Torres CH, Hsu T. Comprehensive geriatric assessment in the older adult with cancer: a review. Eur Urol Focus. 2017;3(4-5):330–9.
8. Burhenn PS, McCarthy AL, Begue A, Nightingale G, Cheng K, Kenis C. Geriatric assessment in daily oncology practice for nurses and allied health care professionals: opinion paper of the Nursing and Allied Health Interest Group of the International Society of Geriatric Oncology (SIOG). J Geriatr Oncol. 2016;7(5):315–24.
9. UK Cancer Reform Strategy. Available at: https://www.nhs.uk/NHSEngland/NSF/Documents/Cancer%20Reform%20Strategy.pdf. Accessed 25 Aug 2020.
10. Improving Outcomes Strategy. Available at: https://www.gov.uk/government/publications/the-national-cancer-strategy. Accessed 25 Aug 2020.
11. National Cancer Survivorship Initiative. Assessment and care planning definitions. 2013. Available at: https://assets.publishing.service.gov.uk/government/uploads/system/uploads/attachment_data/file/181054/9333-TSO-2900664-NCSI_Report_FINAL.pdf. Accessed 25 Aug 2020.
12. Richards M, Corner J, Maher J. The National Cancer Survivorship Initiative: new and emerging evidence on the ongoing needs of cancer survivors. Br J Cancer. 2011;105(Suppl 1):S1–4. Published online 2011 Nov 3. https://doi.org/10.1038/bjc.2011.416.
13. Biddle L, Paramasivan S, Harris S, Campbell R, Brennan B, Hollingworth W. Patients' and clinicians' experiences of holistic needs assessment using a cancer distress thermometer and problem list: a qualitative study. Eur J Oncol Nurs. 2016;23:59–65.
14. Puts MTE, Papoutsis A, Springall E, Tourangeau AE. A systematic review of unmet needs of newly diagnosed older cancer patients undergoing active cancer treatment. Support Care Cancer. 2012;20(7):1377–94. https://doi.org/10.1007/s00520-012-1450-7.

15. Harrison J, Maguire P, Ibbotson T, MacLeod R, Hopwood P. Concerns, confiding and psychiatric disorder in newly diagnosed cancer patients: a descriptive study. Psychooncology. 1994;3:173–9.
16. NCCN Distress Thermometer. Available at: https://www.nccn.org/patients/resources/life_with_cancer/pdf/nccn_distress_thermometer.pdf
17. Ahmedzai SH, Payne SA, Bestall JC, Ahmed N, Clark D, Noble B. Improving access to specialist palliative care. Developing a screening measure to assess the distress caused by advance illness that may require referral to specialist palliative care. Sheffield: University of Sheffield; 2004.
18. Macmillan Cancer Support. Holistic needs assessment and care planning—introduction. 2012. Available at: https://www.macmillan.org.uk/documents/aboutus/health_professionals/macvoice/sharinggoodpractice-electronicholisticneedsassessmentandcareplanning.pdf. Accessed 25 Aug 2020.
19. Young J, Cund A, Renshaw M, Quigley A, Snowden A. Improving the care of cancer patients: holistic needs assessment. Br J Nurs. 2015;24(4):17–20.
20. Taylor C, Cummings R, McGilly C. Holistic needs assessment following colorectal cancer treatment. Gastrointest Nurs. 2012;10(9):42–9.
21. Goldbery J, Burhenn P, Ginex P. Nursing education, review of assessment, clinical care, and implications for practice regarding older adult patients with cancer. Clin J Oncol Nurs. 2018;22(6):19–25.
22. Doyle N, Henry R. Holistic needs assessment: rationale and practical implementation. Cancer Nurs Pract. 2014;13:16–21.
23. Sudore RL, Lum HD, You JJ, Hanson LC, Meier DE, Pantilat SZ, Matlock DD, Rietjens JA, Korfage IJ, Ritchie CS, Kutner JS. Defining advance care planning for adults: a consensus definition from a multidisciplinary Delphi panel. J Pain Symptom Manage. 2017;53(5):821–32.
24. Blackford J, Street AF. Advance care planning. In: Wittenberg E, editor. Textbook of palliative care communication. Oxford: OUP; 2015.
25. Narang AK, Wright AA, Nicholas LH. Trends in advance care planning in patients with cancer: results from a national longitudinal survey. JAMA Oncol. 2015;1(5):601–8.
26. Heyland DK, Barwich D, Pichora D, Dodek P, Lamontagne F, You JJ, Tayler C, Porterfield P, Sinuff T, Simon J, ACCEPT (Advance Care Planning Evaluation in Elderly Patients) Study Team. Failure to engage hospitalized elderly patients and their families in advance care planning. JAMA Intern Med. 2013;173(9):778–87.
27. De Vleminck A, Pardon K, Beernaert K, Deschepper R, Houttekier D, Van Audenhove C, Deliens L, Vander SR. Barriers to advance care planning in cancer, heart failure and dementia patients: a focus group study on general practitioners' views and experiences. PLoS One. 2014;9(1):e84905.
28. Lund S, Richardson A, May C. Barriers to advance care planning at the end of life: an explanatory systematic review of implementation studies. PLoS One. 2015;10(2):e0116629.
29. Clegg A, Bates C, Young J, Ryan R, Nichols L, Ann Teale E, Mohammed MA, Parry J, Marshall T. Development and validation of an electronic frailty index using routine primary care electronic health record data. Age Ageing. 2016;45(3):353–60.
30. Simon J, Porterfield P, Bouchal SR, Heyland D. 'Not yet' and 'Just ask': barriers and facilitators to advance care planning—a qualitative descriptive study of the perspectives of seriously ill, older patients and their families. BMJ Support Palliat Care. 2015;5(1):54–62.

Chapter 11
Multidisciplinary Onco-Geriatric Care Models

Carolina Gómez-Moreno, Raúl Córdoba, Javier Martínez-Peromingo, José Alberto Avila-Funes, and Enrique Soto-Perez-de-Celis

Introduction

The presence of frailty is associated with a higher risk of adverse health-related outcomes, however, a significant proportion of individuals with frailty, even those with a cancer diagnosis, have a reasonable probability of dying *with cancer* rather than dying *of cancer* itself [1].

Frailty in patients with cancer makes them more likely to experience severe cancer-related symptoms, which is associated with functional decline and a poor quality of life, and it has been identified as a predictor of chemotherapy intolerance, post-operative complications, and disease progression [2]. Unfortunately, despite the clear benefit of identifying frailty early in patients with cancer, there is a lack of awareness and consensus among oncology clinical care providers about the best ways in which to assess frailty and treat older adults with frailty. This might be partly because of the absence of a universal definition to identify it, making it confusing to review and cumbersome to implement in clinical practice, particularly for

---

C. Gómez-Moreno
Department of Emergency Medicine, Instituto Nacional de Ciencias Médicas y Nutrición Salvador Zubirán, Mexico City, Mexico

R. Córdoba
University Hospital Fundacion Jimenez Diaz, Madrid, Spain
e-mail: raul.cordoba@fjd.es

J. Martínez-Peromingo
Consejería de Sanidad, Comunidad de Madrid, Madrid, Spain
e-mail: fmperomingo@salud.madrid.org

J. A. Avila-Funes · E. Soto-Perez-de-Celis (✉)
Department of Geriatrics, Instituto Nacional de Ciencias Médicas y Nutrición Salvador Zubirán, Mexico City, Mexico
e-mail: alberto.avilaf@incmnsz.mx; enrique.sotop@incmnsz.mx

F. Gomes (ed.), *Frailty in Older Adults with Cancer*,
https://doi.org/10.1007/978-3-030-89162-6_11

non-geriatricians [2]. Furthermore, most centres lack the infrastructure necessary to appropriately coordinate the various healthcare workers and material resources needed to provide complex care to individuals with frailty, and many specialists lack training in geriatric skills and/or have ageist attitudes. Unfortunately, while most oncologists are aware of the relevance of frailty and its implications, they may be significantly less aware of how to identify it and what to do when it is detected in an older adult with cancer.

This chapter will provide an overview of the relevance of creating multidisciplinary teams for the management of older patients with cancer and frailty, and different models of care in geriatric oncology.

Evidence of the Effect of Multidisciplinary Teams on Frailty (Non-oncology)

Broadly speaking, the three core components of a geriatric interdisciplinary team are usually the physician, who obtains and interprets diagnostic information in order to implement treatments; the nurse (or nurse practitioner), who is in charge of maximizing the patient's functional status, obtaining essential assessments, and providing educational and therapeutic interventions; and the social worker, who serves as a facilitator, patient advocate, and case manager [3]. In addition to these core components, an extended multidisciplinary team should also include many other related disciplines depending on the type of patients and on the available resources at each centre. Lastly, when dealing with specific diseases, geriatric interdisciplinary teams must also coordinate care with other specialists, who often come from disciplines where geriatric expertise is not widely available.

Although the field of geriatric oncology is recent, other clinical areas of medicine have already taken some of the necessary steps to create fully integrated geriatric teams, which should serve as examples. The leading discipline in which collaborative multidisciplinary geriatric services were implemented successfully was orthogeriatrics, with the creation of integrated geriatric care for patients with hip fractures going back to the 1960s [4]. This integrated model started primarily targeting patients admitted with hip fractures. These patients are among the frailest and sickest patients in hospital wards and represent an excellent example of complex clinical care in geriatrics. Currently, international guidelines for the management of older patients with a hip fracture stress the need for the inclusion of a geriatrician into the team from the time of admission, and early geriatric interventions have been shown to reduce morbimortality in patients with hip fractures [5]. Multidisciplinary teams involved in providing clinical care for patients with hip fractures are extensive, and include admission for a joint assessment agreed upon by geriatrics, orthopaedics, and anaesthesia, as well as postoperative co-management by geriatricians, and an in-depth assessment of bone health, future fall risk, and reintegration in the community [6].

In the outpatient setting, integrated models of care have been created for other specialties, including, among others, geriatric cardiology, geriatric nephrology, and the care of older adults with dementia. Interdisciplinary teams for the management of dementia, for instance, have been created to provide support not only to the patient, but also to caregivers. The integration of geriatric care with nursing, social work, nutrition, psychology, rehabilitation, and even with legal support, has led to improved outcomes and to better care not only in hospital settings, but also in the community [7].

Another useful example of an area of medicine which has moved towards the creation of geriatric interdisciplinary teams is cardiology. The American Heart Association and the American College of Cardiology recognized the relevance of creating specific clinical practice guidelines for patients with cardiovascular disease who also have frailty [8]. The inclusion of geriatricians in cardiology teams can lead to a better assessment of patients with complex diseases and can lead to improved communication and to high-quality care that can better meet the specific needs of older patients [9]. Moreover, geriatric assessment helps to identify older patients who are only candidates for best supportive care.

The Importance of Multidisciplinary Care Teams for Older Adults with Cancer

Multidisciplinary care teams (MDT) can be defined as an integrated team approach to healthcare in which medical and allied healthcare professionals consider all relevant treatment options and develop an individual treatment plan for each patient collaboratively. Multidisciplinary care has been identified as a key enabler in the provision of high-quality treatment and care for patients with cancer, and its main aim is improving communication, coordination, and decision-making between healthcare professionals [10]. The use of MDT in cancer care is endorsed internationally, although uptake varies. It has been adopted in several countries in North American and Western Europe but is a less common model of care in other areas of the world, such as the Middle East. Research has shown that MDT decisions lead to revisions of cancer diagnoses and treatment plans in new cancer cases, and to better and individualized adherence to evidence-based guidelines. Importantly, patient satisfaction with the operation of MDT is shown to be excellent [11].

Multidisciplinary cancer care can be delivered using various models of care. These include multidisciplinary clinics staffed by a mix of different health professionals (Fig. 11.1), and MDT that hold regular meetings to discuss patient care plans prospectively. Overall, these MDT and clinics tend to be tumour or organ specific. In large metropolitan hospitals, MDT meetings are usually held weekly; while in smaller community hospitals, meetings may be held fortnightly or monthly. Rural hospitals may be linked to metropolitan cancer centres for regular meetings through teleconference or videoconferencing [12].

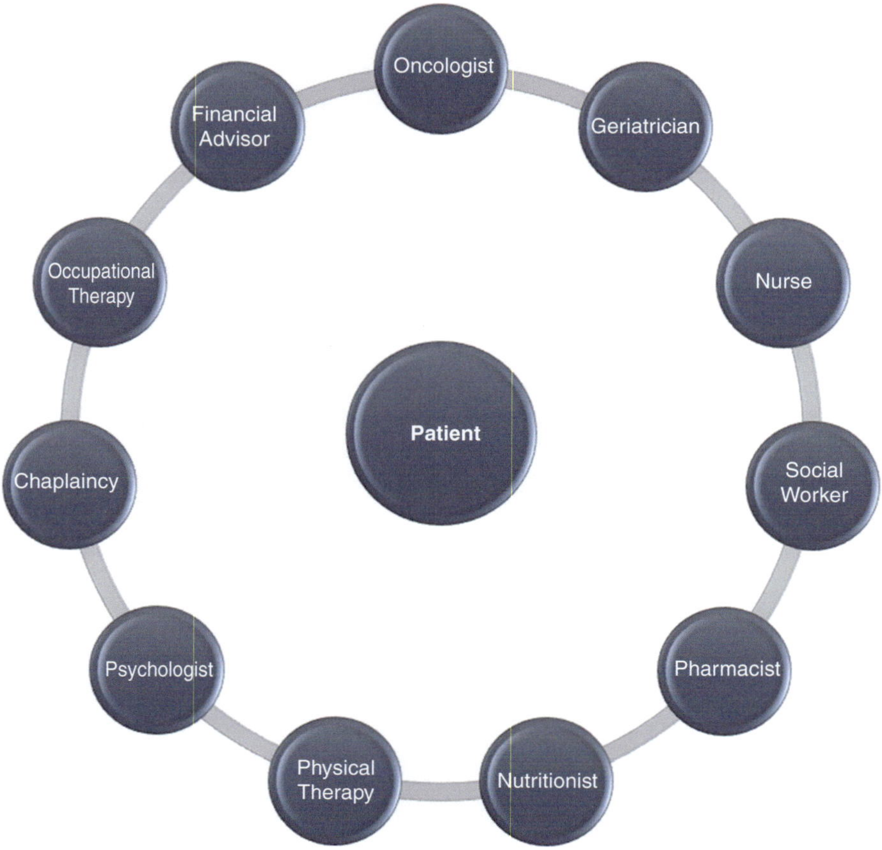

Fig. 11.1 Members of the geriatric oncology multidisciplinary team

Discussions of individual cases at the MDT meetings provide an excellent opportunity for training physicians and nurses. Also, team meetings assist in communication and information sharing between members, particularly between hospital-based specialists and primary care providers, which enhance referral and continuing care pathways.

Core members of the multidisciplinary cancer team should include an oncologist (medical, surgical, radiation), pathologist, radiologist, nurse, social worker, and geriatrician. The make-up of the team varies depending on the tumour type and on the healthcare services provided. Nurse coordinators are often the team members who bring patient information and concerns to the meeting. Communication with the patient's primary care provider is also important. In most western countries, the MDT recommendations are also discussed with each patient by an appropriate member of the care team after the meeting is concluded.

Outpatient Models of Care in Geriatric Oncology

Incorporating geriatric assessment into the care of older adults with cancer has been shown to be feasible and predictive of outcomes, with many domains of the traditional comprehensive geriatric assessment showing value as best predictors of adverse health-related outcomes in this population [13]. Caring for an older individual with cancer requires knowledge and expertise in both oncologic and geriatric issues. However, the goals of these two disciplines may vary significantly. Oncologists mostly focus on the assessment of cancer-related variables, such as tumour biology and staging, and develop cancer-specific treatment plans. On the other hand, geriatricians assess physiologic age, functional and cognitive status, and focus on optimising an individual's autonomy. Integration of these two skill-sets into one individualized care plan is key and can improve outcomes of the older patient with cancer, particularly those who have frailty [14].

The integration of geriatrics in oncology can have different aims depending on each centre's needs and on the available resources. It could be primarily targeted at patients who are about to start treatment in order to support treatment decision-making. In other cases, it can be targeted at older patients who develop geriatric syndromes or functional decline during treatment, as a part of supportive care.

The feasibility and impact of the geriatric assessment in oncology have been studied and proven as a valuable model to predict all-cause mortality and treatment tolerance in different studies evaluating older patients with cancer, as well as to identify important changes in treatment following geriatric recommendations. While many of these studies did not include frailty-specific measures or frailty phenotypes, all utilized geriatric assessments including the items needed to identify the phenotype of an older cancer patient with frailty, therefore providing important evidence about its usefulness in this population [15].

The clinical capacity of identifying frailty in a homogeneous cohort of older adults with cancer has been studied in patients undergoing surgery for oncological treatment. In a prospective study conducted by Kristjansson et al, patients aged 70 years or older who were scheduled for surgery for suspected or confirmed colorectal cancer underwent a pre-operative geriatric assessment [16]. Patients were categorized into three groups as "fit", "intermediate", or "frail" using a modification of criteria proposed by Balducci and Extermann [1, 17]. After data analysis and adjusting for the cancer stage and age, frailty status (defined using the accumulation of deficits in the geriatric assessment) remained an independent predictor of mortality [16]. However, there is no consensus regarding modifications in the type of treatment in vulnerable and frail patients once they are identified, and further research on how to use this information to improve oncological outcomes and prognosis is required [18]. The combination of the disease-oriented approach of oncologists and the patient-oriented approach of the geriatricians provides the adequate balance to deliver the optimal care for this specific group of patients and its various needs.

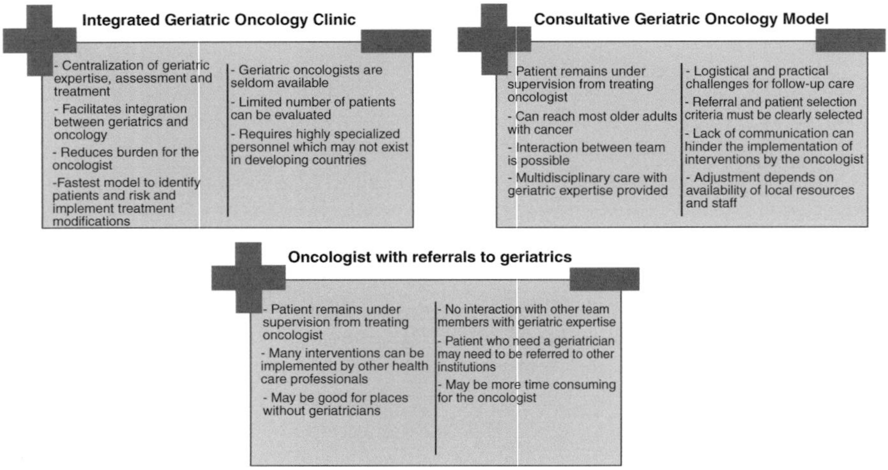

Fig. 11.2 Advantages and disadvantages of the various models of care in geriatric oncology [35]

There are several existing models for incorporating geriatrics skills into oncology care, including integrated geriatric oncology clinics, consultative geriatric oncology models, and the assessment and management of older adults with cancer by an oncologist with referrals to geriatricians when needed (Fig. 11.2) [19].

Integrated Geriatric Oncology Clinic

Several cancer centres have integrated a geriatrician into their oncology clinics, and this can be done in two different ways: (1) geriatricians are embedded and function as a member of the multidisciplinary oncology clinic and therefore patients may be seen by both the oncologist and the geriatrician as required and (2) geriatric oncologists, i.e. dual-trained physicians, perform both the oncological and geriatric assessments and plans, following the patient throughout their course of treatment. An example of this type of clinic is the Geriatrics Service at Memorial Sloan Kettering Cancer Center in New York [20].

The possibility of having a dual-trained geriatric oncologist facilitates integration between both specialities. However, this approach is limited due to the scarce number of dual-trained geriatric oncologists to perform this role, particularly in developing countries. While on one hand, this reduces the need to recruit multiple physicians with these complementing skill sets, on the other hand this also reduces the number of patients that can be seen by each geriatric oncologist due to this more comprehensive role. Therefore, when dual-trained physicians are not available, having a geriatrician integrated into the oncology clinic may reduce the time required by the oncologist to manage complex older patients with frailty, multimorbidity, geriatric syndromes, complex social situations, physical impairments, and cognitive issues. In addition, the geriatrician can easily interact with other team members with geriatric expertise, or work alongside a nurse with geriatrics training, thus providing a more comprehensive multidisciplinary approach to care.

Either way, having a geriatrician integrated into the oncology clinic simplifies communication and makes geriatrics an integral part of the decision-making process. This is the easiest and fastest model to identify patients at increased risk of treatment toxicity using geriatric assessment-based predictive models, and to utilize these models for tailoring cancer treatments. Moreover, it allows for the provision of better patient-centred care, since geriatric assessment provides a comprehensive health evaluation, and the geriatrician actively supports patients throughout their treatment journey.

Consultative Geriatric Oncology Model

In this extended model, the care of older adults with cancer is fundamentally multidisciplinary, with a key feature for effective care being communication and collaboration between geriatricians and oncologists. In consultative clinics, the treating oncologists refer patients to the geriatrics team to undergo a multidisciplinary geriatric assessment. Reasons for referral may vary, with some centres referring all patients over a certain age and others using screening tools before sending patients for a complete assessment [21]. Therefore, in this model, a separate geriatrics team conducts that assessment, and the recommendations for care are delivered back to the primary oncologist, who may take these onboard or not [22]. An example of this model is the Cancer Care in Elderly Clinic, in Mexico City [21].

The upside of this model is that collaboration between multidisciplinary geriatrics teams and the oncology team may allow for the assessment and support of large numbers of patients. The shortcomings of the consultative model include that, as mentioned above, the treatment plan will be determined by the oncologist, and it may not always reflect the recommendations made by the geriatrician [19]. However, some studies have shown positive results for this model, with over 60% agreement between the geriatrician's recommendations and final therapeutic decisions by treating oncologists [21, 23].

It is also important to highlight that for a consultative model to work, collaboration and communication between the geriatrics team and the oncology team is essential, and that this can be at times challenging. In addition, continuing education and training of both oncologists and geriatricians are also necessary to better understand treatment options and interventions. Knowledge of geriatric principles will provide oncologists with high awareness about the specific needs of the frail person. At the same time, possessing knowledge about oncology will provide the geriatrician with the tools to interpret cancer prognosis and implement interventions in busy oncology settings [18].

Another potential limitation is that the members of the geriatric team who performed the initial evaluation, may not be the same as the one(s) who provide(s) follow-up care. This may be a problem since changes in functional status through time are as or more important than basal functional performance, so it is very important to standardize healthcare workers in order to have homogeneous measures and practices [24].

Lastly, lack of resources is another barrier for the adoption of the geriatric assessment by a multidisciplinary geriatric team as standard of care. In some institutions, the geriatrician may be substituted by a specialized geriatrics-trained nurse or a physician with skills in gerontology, who helps oncologists obtain a geriatric assessment and implement some educational and therapeutic interventions. This variation in the model might be particularly useful in resource-limited settings, since geriatricians are scarce and often unavailable in oncology clinics [25].

Oncologist with Referrals to Geriatrics/Supportive Care

This model relies on validated screening tools to identify age-related problems, such as frailty, that may be beyond the clinical and therapeutic capabilities of oncologists [26]. When identified, the patient is referred to a geriatrician (or geriatrics team), who performs a geriatric assessment. In this type of model, the geriatrician is not embedded in the oncology clinic and thus less specialized geriatric resources are available. In some cases, referrals may need to be made to other institutions with geriatrics services. The main characteristic of this model is that not all older patients undergo a geriatric assessment performed by a multidisciplinary team. Instead, the oncologist utilizes screening tools to evaluate various geriatric-specific domains and refers patients to geriatricians or to a geriatrics team only when a problem is identified. In this model, the oncologist receives less feedback from geriatricians and oversees the initial assessment of patients, which means that some level of training and geriatric knowledge is needed to implement it.

Screening tools do not replace a full geriatric assessment but are recommended in a busy practice to identify those patients at high risk of having geriatric syndromes and other deficits upon the implementation of a full geriatric assessment. The most commonly used geriatric screening tools in oncology are the *Geriatric-8 (G8)*, the *Vulnerable Elder Survey-13* (VES-13), and the *Flemish version of the Triage Risk Screening Tool* (fTRST) [27, 28].

The G8 was developed for patients with cancer, it takes approximately 5 minutes to apply, and has been compared with the geriatric assessment in several studies, proving a sensitivity ranging from 65% to 92% and a specificity of over 60% to identify deficits in geriatric assessment domains. G8 scores ($\leq$14 is considered abnormal) predict several health-related outcomes such as functional decline and chemotherapy-related toxicity [27, 29, 30].

The VES-13 is a 13 item self-administered tool, developed for identifying people at an increased risk of health deterioration among community-dwelling older adults [31]. It has been compared to the geriatric assessment in patients with cancer, showing a sensitivity between 39% and 88% and a specificity of 62% to 100% for identifying functional decline [27]. However, it has not proven to predict morbidity or mortality in patients with cancer scheduled for surgical treatment [32].

The fTRST is a tool composed of five yes/no questions. A score of two or more points is considered abnormal. Just like the G8 and the VES-13, it shows an adequate performance in identifying vulnerable patients (i.e. those who require a more extensive geriatric assessment) but it has not shown to predict other important outcomes (such as mortality or functional decline) in older adults with cancer [27, 33].

The benefit of this model is that it allows the primary oncologist to perform a basic screening to identify those patients with increased vulnerability, without having to include a multidisciplinary team to perform more specialized assessments, which may be resource-consuming [27]. Although some tools might have some advantages for predicting specific outcomes, we believe that the most practical approach is to choose whichever tool makes more sense for the specific setting, the available personnel, and the existing capability to provide training to the staff who will implement the screening tool. The downside is that, while most of these tools are quite easy to implement, it makes the oncology consultation more time consuming, which may discourage the primary oncologist from performing geriatric screening. This limitation, however, might be overcome by adequate continuous training of oncologists on the relevance of performing the screening, and on the ease with which it can be performed even in the busiest clinical settings. On top of that, this type of model requires a strong network and reliable bidirectional communication between the primary oncologist and the geriatrics team to ensure a proper and timely referral and recommendations to impact the patient's treatment. If communication is not effective, relevant information may be lost in the process and the purpose of the referral may not be accomplished [34].

Implementation Across Different Healthcare Settings

One of the most significant barriers to the implementation of multidisciplinary geriatric oncology teams for the care of frail patients in everyday clinical practice is the limited availability of resources in most healthcare settings. Clinicians attempting to implement a geriatric oncology team, or a geriatric oncology clinic, must be aware of the many barriers and challenges they might face, and be prepared to tackle them (Table 11.1) [20]. As mentioned before, there are several models of geriatric oncology care, and the International Society of Geriatric Oncology (SIOG) has issued specific recommendations regarding how to design and coordinate each of these models across various settings [35].

Although there is now enough evidence to move these principles into everyday care, there is no universal solution, and resources (personnel, space, time, and money) are different everywhere. However, no matter what resources are available, an effort must be made for the implementation of geriatric oncology care due to its potential benefits for the patient, particularly the frail older person. A potentially useful solution is the adoption of a resource stratification framework in order to

Table 11.1 Challenges faced when implementing a geriatric oncology clinic and potential solutions [20]

Challenge	Potential solution
Lack of recognition from other physicians	• Provide data to back geriatric assessments and interventions • Engage in constant communication with colleagues • Improve the visibility of geriatric oncology by participating in tumour boards, multidisciplinary meetings, and educational sessions
Lack of trained personnel	• Educate all the staff in basic geriatric oncology principles • Teach oncologists or nurses how to undertake geriatric screening • Aim for the training and recruitment of additional personnel
Lack of clear referral criteria	• Develop clear written guidelines underlining who should be referred to the geriatric oncology clinic • Educate providers on the identification of vulnerable/frail patients • Set realistic aims regarding the number of patients that your clinic an assess/treat
Lack of adaptation to the oncologists' needs	• Establish clear limits regarding the responsibilities of the geriatric oncology clinic • Create mechanisms of subsequent referrals (such as to palliative care or other geriatric clinics)
Lack of space	• Optimise existing space within regular clinic hours (hallways, office space etc.) • Utilize telemedicine and digital tools to assess patients and perform interventions

select which interventions are the most appropriate depending on the availability of resources, and to adequate local recommendations and guidelines according to these principles. Resource stratification in cancer care was spearheaded by the Breast Health Global Initiative (BHGI) with the publication of their breast cancer resource-stratified guidelines in 2006 [36]. BHGI created a four-tier resource-stratification framework which divided settings into those with basic (essential services needed to provide the minimum standard of care); limited (additional services which produce major improvements in outcomes with little financial means); enhanced (optional services which can further improve outcomes); and maximal (services which provide gains in secondary outcomes) resources [36–38].

A resource-stratified approach to the management of older patients with cancer and frailty could potentially help implement multidisciplinary care even in settings where geriatric-specific teams are unavailable. The Young SIOG interest group has made some recommendations regarding how to resource-stratify geriatric assessments which are summarized in Fig. 11.3 [39]. According to this proposal, while resource-rich centres (mostly in developed nations) may be able to conduct a full geriatric assessment in all older adults with cancer, centres with resource constraints may need to use geriatric screening tools, and then refer patients to multidisciplinary team members that may not be specifically trained in geriatrics [39].

Data presented at the American Society of Clinical Oncology (ASCO) 2020 annual meeting provided further evidence demonstrating that multidisciplinary geriatric oncology care may provide benefits for patients regardless of the type of care model implemented. At least three randomized clinical trials (GAP-70,

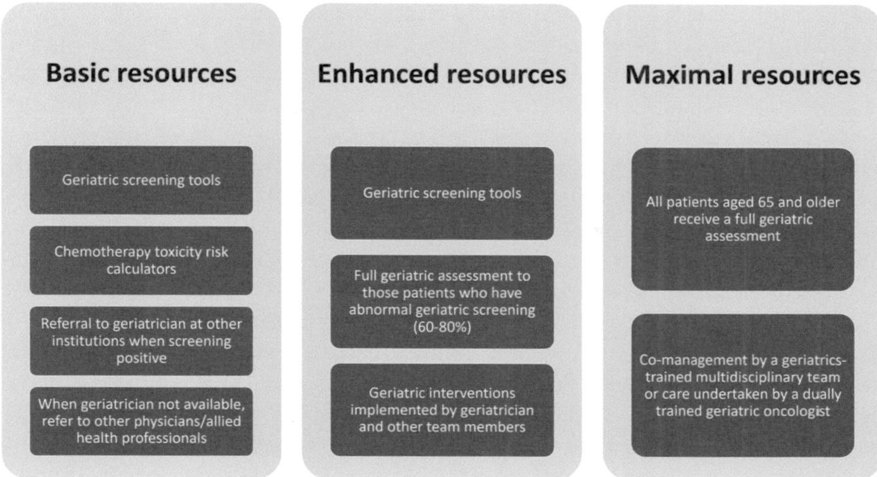

Fig. 11.3 Young International Society of Geriatric Oncology interest group proposal for the resource stratification of geriatric assessments and interventions [39]

INTEGERATE, and GAIN) demonstrated that multidisciplinary interventions led to significant reductions in severe chemotherapy-related toxicity, decreased healthcare utilization, and improved health-related quality of life among older adults receiving cancer treatment [40–42]. Importantly, although these trials utilized different types of interventions, all had positive outcomes. In GAP-70, for example a consultative model which involved a collaboration between community cancer clinics and a centralized geriatric oncology hub showed an improvement in toxicity among older adults who could be considered as vulnerable or frail according to their geriatric assessment [40]. In the Australian INTEGRATE trial, co-management by geriatricians and oncologists also showed an improvement in quality of life, with an important reduction in emergency room visits and hospitalizations [42]. Finally, GAIN showed that providing patients with a highly specialized and coordinated geriatric oncology team can lead to decreased toxicity [41]. Taken together, these trials show that, regardless of the type of resources available, providing some form of multidisciplinary geriatric oncology care may help frail older adults during treatment [43].

Conclusions

An increasing amount of evidence shows that implementing multidisciplinary geriatric oncology care for older adults with cancer may lead to a series of improvements in both cancer- and non-cancer-specific outcomes. These benefits are particularly relevant in older patients with cancer and frailty, for whom modifications in treatment plans, as well as the implementation of geriatric interventions, may lead to better health-related quality of life and decreased toxicity. It is important to highlight that one size does not fit all when deciding to implement a multidisciplinary geriatric oncology clinic, and that each centre may need to tailor the aforementioned models of care to existing resources and staff. That being said, current evidence and available recommendations strongly support the creation of some form of geriatric oncology team, which can go from a highly integrated model in which an oncologist with training in geriatrics implements interventions and treatment modifications, to a simpler model in which an oncologist conducts some basic geriatric assessments and leans on geriatricians or a geriatrics team to further evaluate those patients at higher risk of vulnerability.

Although many barriers still exist, international organizations have increasingly highlighted the relevance of multidisciplinary geriatric oncology care, and guidelines and toolkits have been developed in order to help clinicians implement these models in their everyday clinical practice taking advantage of the experience already demonstrated in geriatrics. In summary, teamwork is essential in geriatric oncology and, regardless of the existing resources, something can always be done to improve the quality of care and outcomes of frail older patients with cancer.

References

1. Balducci L, Extermann M. Management of the frail person with advanced cancer. Crit Rev Oncol Hematol. 2000;33(2):143–8.
2. Ethun CG, Bilen MA, Jani AB, Maithel SK, Ogan K, Master VA. Frailty and cancer: implications for oncology surgery, medical oncology, and radiation oncology. CA Cancer J Clin. 2017;67(5):362–77.
3. Dyer CB, Hyer K, Feldt KS, Lindemann DA, Busby-Whitehead J, Greenberg S, et al. Frail older patient care by interdisciplinary teams: a primer for generalists. Gerontol Geriatr Educ. 2003;24(2):51–62.
4. Sabharwal S, Wilson H. Orthogeriatrics in the management of frail older patients with a fragility fracture. Osteoporos Int. 2015;26(10):2387–99.
5. Riemen AH, Hutchison JD. The multidisciplinary management of hip fractures in older patients. Orthop Trauma. 2016;30(2):117–22.
6. Aw D, Sahota O. Orthogeriatrics moving forward. Age Ageing. 2014;43(3):301–5.
7. Crooks EA, Geldmacher DS. Interdisciplinary approaches to Alzheimer's disease management. Clin Geriatr Med. 2004;20(1):121–39.
8. Arnett DK, Goodman RA, Halperin JL, Anderson JL, Parekh AK, Zoghbi WA. AHA/ACC/HHS strategies to enhance application of clinical practice guidelines in patients with cardiovascular disease and comorbid conditions: from the American Heart Association, American College of Cardiology, and U.S. Department of Health and Human Services. J Am Coll Cardiol. 2014;64(17):1851–6.
9. Forman DE, Rich MW, Alexander KP, Zieman S, Maurer MS, Najjar SS, et al. Cardiac care for older adults. Time for a new paradigm. J Am Coll Cardiol. 2011;57(18):1801–10.
10. Jung SM, Hong YS, Kim TW, Park JH, Kim JH, Park SH, et al. Impact of a multidisciplinary team approach for managing advanced and recurrent colorectal cancer. World J Surg. 2018;42(7):2227–33.
11. Snelgrove RC, Subendran J, Jhaveri K, Thipphavong S, Cummings B, Brierley J, et al. Effect of multidisciplinary cancer conference on treatment plan for patients with primary rectal cancer. Dis Colon Rectum. 2015;58(7):653–8.

12. Gomes FM, Santos KTDO, Silva SME, Pinho CPS, Silva A. Fragilidad en ancianos oncológicos en tratamiento con quimioterapia. Rev Chil Nutr. 2019;46:384–91.
13. Bruijnen CP, van Harten-Krouwel DG, Koldenhof JJ, Emmelot-Vonk MH, Witteveen PO. Predictive value of each geriatric assessment domain for older patients with cancer: a systematic review. J Geriatr Oncol. 2019 Nov;10(6):859–73.
14. Caillet P, Canoui-Poitrine F, Vouriot J, Berle M, Reinald N, Krypciak S, et al. Comprehensive geriatric assessment in the decision-making process in elderly patients with cancer: ELCAPA study. J Clin Oncol. 2011;29(27):3636–42.
15. Hamaker ME, Vos AG, Smorenburg CH, de Rooij SE, van Munster BC. The value of geriatric assessments in predicting treatment tolerance and all-cause mortality in older patients with cancer. Oncologist. 2012;17(11):1439–49.
16. Kristjansson SR, Rønning B, Hurria A, Skovlund E, Jordhøy MS, Nesbakken A, et al. A comparison of two pre-operative frailty measures in older surgical cancer patients. J Geriatr Oncol. 2012;3(1):1–7.
17. Balducci L, Extermann M. Management of cancer in the older person: a practical approach. Oncologist. 2000;5(3):224–37.
18. Ruiz M, Reske T, Cefalu C, Estrada J. Management of elderly and frail elderly cancer patients: the importance of comprehensive geriatrics assessment and the need for guidelines. Am J Med Sci. 2013;346(1):66–9.
19. Magnuson A, Dale W, Mohile S. Models of care in geriatric oncology. Curr Geriatr Rep. 2014;3(3):182–9.
20. Korc-Grodzicki B, Tew W, Hurria A, et al. Development of a Geriatric Service in a Cancer Center: lessons learned. J Oncol Pract. 2017;13(2):107–12.
21. Verduzco-Aguirre HC, Navarrete-Reyes AP, Chavarri-Guerra Y, Ávila-Funes JA, Soto-Perez-de-Celis E. The effect of a geriatric oncology clinic on treatment decisions in Mexican older adults with cancer. J Am Geriatr Soc. 2019;67(5):992–7.
22. Terret C, Zulian GB, Naiem A, Albrand G. Multidisciplinary approach to the geriatric oncology patient. J Clin Oncol. 2007;25(14):1876–81.
23. Kenis C, Heeren P, Decoster L, Van Puyvelde K, Conings G, Cornelis F, et al. A Belgian survey on geriatric assessment in oncology focusing on large-scale implementation and related barriers and facilitators. J Nutr Health Aging. 2016;20(1):60–70.
24. Monfardini S, Balducci L. A comprehensive geriatric assessment (CGA) is necessary for the study and the management of cancer in the elderly. Eur J Cancer. 1999;35(13):1771–2.
25. Soto-Perez-de-Celis E, de Glas NA, Hsu T, Kanesvaran R, Steer C, Navarrete-Reyes AP, et al. Global geriatric oncology: achievements and challenges. J Geriatr Oncol. 2017;8(5):374–86.
26. Williams GR, Deal AM, Jolly TA, Alston SM, Gordon BB, Dixon SA, et al. Feasibility of geriatric assessment in community oncology clinics. J Geriatr Oncol. 2014;5(3):245–51.
27. Decoster L, Van Puyvelde K, Mohile S, Wedding U, Basso U, Colloca G, et al. Screening tools for multidimensional health problems warranting a geriatric assessment in older cancer patients: an update on SIOG recommendations†. Ann Oncol. 2015;26(2):288–300.
28. Kenis C, Decoster L, Van Puyvelde K, De Grève J, Conings G, Milisen K, et al. Performance of two geriatric screening tools in older patients with cancer. J Clin Oncol. 2014;32(1):19–26.
29. Bellera CA, Rainfray M, Mathoulin-Pélissier S, Mertens C, Delva F, Fonck M, et al. Screening older cancer patients: first evaluation of the G-8 geriatric screening tool. Ann Oncol. 2012;23(8):2166–72.
30. Soubeyran P, Bellera C, Goyard J, Heitz D, Curé H, Rousselot H, et al. Screening for vulnerability in older cancer patients: the ONCODAGE Prospective Multicenter Cohort Study. PLoS One. 2014;9(12):e115060.
31. Min LC, Elliott MN, Wenger NS, Saliba D. Higher vulnerable elders survey scores predict death and functional decline in vulnerable older people. J Am Geriatr Soc. 2006;54(3):507–11.
32. Mohile SG, Bylow K, Dale W, Dignam J, Martin K, Petrylak DP, et al. A pilot study of the vulnerable elders survey-13 compared with the comprehensive geriatric assessment for identifying disability in older patients with prostate cancer who receive androgen ablation. Cancer. 2007;109(4):802–10.

33. Meldon SW, Mion LC, Palmer RM, Drew BL, Connor JT, Lewicki LJ, et al. A brief risk-stratification tool to predict repeat emergency department visits and hospitalizations in older patients discharged from the emergency department. Acad Emerg Med. 2003;10(3):224–32.
34. Rodin MB, Mohile SG. A practical approach to geriatric assessment in oncology. J Clin Oncol. 2007;25(14):1936–44.
35. Wildiers H, Heeren P, Puts M, Topinkova E, Janssen-Heijnen ML, Extermann M, et al. International Society of Geriatric Oncology consensus on geriatric assessment in older patients with cancer. J Clin Oncol. 2014;32(24):2595–603.
36. Anderson BO, Shyyan R, Eniu A, Smith RA, Yip CH, Bese NS, et al. Breast cancer in limited-resource countries: an overview of the breast health global initiative 2005 guidelines. Breast J. 2006;12(Suppl 1):S3–15.
37. Anderson BO, Yip CH, Smith RA, Shyyan R, Sener SF, Eniu A, et al. Guideline implementation for breast healthcare in low-income and middle-income countries: overview of the Breast Health Global Initiative Global Summit 2007. Cancer. 2008;113(8 Suppl):2221–43.
38. Anderson BO, Cazap E, El Saghir NS, Yip CH, Khaled HM, Otero IV, et al. Optimisation of breast cancer management in low-resource and middle-resource countries: executive summary of the breast health global initiative consensus, 2010. Lancet Oncol. 2011;12(4):387–98.
39. Loh KP, Soto-Perez-de-Celis E, Hsu T, de Glas NA, Battisti NML, Baldini C, et al. What every oncologist should know about geriatric assessment for older patients with cancer: Young International Society of Geriatric Oncology Position Paper. J Oncol Pract. 2018;14(2):85–94.
40. Mohile SG, Mohamed MR, Culakova E, Xu H, Loh KP, Magnuson A, et al. A geriatric assessment (GA) intervention to reduce treatment toxicity in older patients with advanced cancer: a University of Rochester Cancer Center NCI community oncology research program cluster randomized clinical trial (CRCT). J Clin Oncol. 2020;38(15 suppl):12009.
41. Li D, Sun C-L, Kim H, Chung V, Koczywas M, Fakih M, et al. Geriatric assessment-driven intervention (GAIN) on chemotherapy toxicity in older adults with cancer: a randomized controlled trial. J Clin Oncol. 2020;38(15 suppl):12010.
42. Soo W-K, King M, Pope A, Parente P, Darzins P, Davis ID. Integrated geriatric assessment and treatment (INTEGERATE) in older people with cancer planned for systemic anticancer therapy. J Clin Oncol. 2020;38(15 suppl):12011.
43. Soto-Perez-de-Celis E, Aapro M, Muss H. ASCO 2020: the geriatric assessment comes of age. Oncologist. 2020;25(11):909–12.

Chapter 12
Decision-Making Process in Older Adults with Cancer and Frailty

Marije E. Hamaker, Grant Punnett, Janelle Yorke, and Fabio Gomes

Introduction

Cancer management has been revolutionised in recent decades with patients living longer and with a better quality of life particularly due to early diagnosis and advances in treatment, supportive and palliative care. However, having multiple options is both an opportunity and a challenge. Whilst cancer patients are facing the emotional stress of a cancer diagnosis, they must also make complex decisions about which treatment option is best for them.

In previous decades, the clinician typically made this decision unilaterally, due to a more paternalistic model of care [1]. Whilst the process of clinical decision-making is complex, multi-layered and part of the everyday clinical practice,

M. E. Hamaker (✉)
Department of Geriatric Medicine, Diakonessenhuis Utrecht/Zeist, Utrecht, the Netherlands
e-mail: mhamaker@diakhuis.nl

G. Punnett
Christie Patient-Centred Research Team, The Christie NHS Foundation Trust, Manchester, UK
e-mail: grant.punnett@nhs.net

J. Yorke
Christie Patient-Centred Research Team, The Christie NHS Foundation Trust, Manchester, UK

School of Health Sciences, University of Manchester, Manchester, UK
e-mail: Janelle.Yorke@nhs.net

F. Gomes
Christie Patient-Centred Research Team, The Christie NHS Foundation Trust, Manchester, UK

Medical Oncology Department, The Christie NHS Foundation Trust, Manchester, UK
e-mail: fabio.gomes2@nhs.net

F. Gomes (ed.), *Frailty in Older Adults with Cancer*,
https://doi.org/10.1007/978-3-030-89162-6_12

decisions must not be unilateral and should involve the patient. Physicians may hold the medical evidence, training and experience; but patients know what matters the most for themselves [1]. Since neither clinician nor patient holds all the information, sharing this knowledge in both directions is crucial. Reassuringly, patients' involvement in the decision-making has been improving over time, as reported in a survey in the United States based on patient perception [2].

Shared-decision making (SDM) is the process of incorporating the patient's preferences, values and circumstances into medical decisions putting the patients at the centre of care [1]. A recent systematic review identified that poor communication by physicians was a key barrier to SDM [3]. Without adequate communication to promote well-informed deliberations, patients are unable to construct informed preferences considering their values and circumstances. Information regarding diagnosis, treatment options and prognosis must be offered, and patients must be faced with choices. In oncology, the wide variety of treatment options, high risk of significant side effects and high costs present a challenge. In addition, the option of focussing on best supportive care instead should be considered and discussed.

The SDM process is particularly relevant in older cancer patients with frailty where medical decisions are more challenging. The complexity of these patients is aggravated by the limited level of scientific evidence for this sub-group as they are often excluded from clinical trials [4–8]. Therefore, patients' perceptions about the non-technical aspects of care are key to informing such decisions.

This chapter will review the different aspects (disease-, treatment-, physician- and patient-related) contributing to the challenge of SDM regarding cancer treatment decisions for older cancer patients with frailty. It will also highlight key questions that oncology teams can incorporate in their SDM process and discussions for this complex patient group.

Disease-Related Factors

Cancer type and tumour stage are usually the first elements taken into consideration by oncologists during the clinical decision process, often even before meeting the patient (Table 12.1). These two pieces of information immediately define a range of possible treatment options.

The type of cancer, determined by its organ of origin and its histological subtype, is a key determinant of access to treatments, since the clinical trials that led to the development of scientific knowledge during the last decades used this information as key eligibility. Molecular biomarkers beyond the above-mentioned morphological characteristics are also part of oncology daily practice for several types of cancer and define further sub-groups of cancer types, determining new treatment pathways. An example of this is the epidermal growth factor receptor (EGFR) in non-small cell lung cancer, which may acquire mutations that sensitise the cancer cells to treatment with EGFR-inhibitors [9]. The identification of genomic

Table 12.1 Factors contributing to the challenge of shared decision-making in frail older patients with cancer

Disease related	– Type of cancer – Molecular markers – Stage of disease – Pace of disease progression – Cancer burden and cancer-related symptoms
Treatment related	– Available treatment modalities – Potential benefit – Risk of toxicity – Risk of complications – Lack of evidence specific to older/frail patients – Treatment logistics
Physician related	– Reliance on evidence-based medicine – Personal preferences and priorities – Estimation of patient's level of fitness – Fear of undertreating patients – Time constraints and workload – Perception of patient's preferred decision-making role
Patient related	– Personal preferences and priorities – Beliefs and expectations – Decisional conflict – Preferred decision-making role – Frailty – Decision making capacity – Informal care givers and proxies

abnormalities with targeted treatments offers new treatment options and has led to the development of personalized cancer medicine. Using the example of non-small cell lung cancer, it means that this type of cancer is no longer treated as a single entity but as a complex disease with several histological and molecular sub-types with different treatment options and prognoses.

The cancer stage (i.e. localized versus locally advanced versus metastatic) also determines the treatment options upfront, mainly because the prognosis differs, and it therefore impacts the treatment intent (curative or palliative intent). There are some other elements related to the stage which are frequently included in the decision-making: (1) the pace of disease progression (this reflects how fast the cancer is growing, such as, the cancer doubling time); (2) the cancer burden (this reflects the number, volume and distribution of cancer lesions) and (3) cancer-related symptoms (this is often related with the cancer burden, but sometimes despite a low cancer burden, the cancer location may cause significant symptoms). As an example, a metastatic fast-growing cancer potentially involving multiple organs that may compromise their function and cause significant symptoms, will result in different treatment considerations compared to a metastatic cancer that has a slow and indolent behaviour and no imminent risk of causing symptoms to the patient.

Treatment-Related Factors

During a treatment decision, the toxicity and tolerability of potential treatment options are crucial considerations in the decision-making process when the oncology team is filtering the range of options available upfront based on the above-described disease-related factors (Table 12.1). This is often a key decision-making element for the patients, since treatments with a higher likelihood of controlling the cancer are often more intensive, associated with more toxicity and longer recovery times. This, in turn, will have a significant impact on determining the patients' quality of life.

The tolerability and risk of toxicity should be balanced with the possible benefits of the treatments. However, evidence on benefits and toxicity specific to older cancer patients with frailty is lacking. Older cancer patients are under-represented in clinical trials, which is not usually a matter of having an age limit in the eligibility but instead a selection of fit and less comorbid patients, more often younger [4–8]. Therefore, not just the trial populations are younger than the real-world cancer populations, but also fitter, hence the challenge in extrapolating such data for older cancer patients with frailty. For example, the multiple pivotal clinical trials that led to the worldwide implementation of immunotherapy with checkpoint inhibitors for the treatment of patients with non-small cell lung cancer, enrolled a population 10 years younger than the median age of lung cancer [10].

This is often a deliberate choice because inclusion of these older patients with frailty would raise more safety concerns and potentially hinder a prospective benefit of the treatment under investigation. Frailty and comorbidity limit the patient's ability to tolerate possible treatment toxicities and are also a competing cause of death, which could overall diminish the treatment benefits compared to younger, healthier patients [11]. Whilst some patients may benefit, others will die of causes other than cancer, regardless of cancer treatment, and some patients will not be able to complete the treatment because of unacceptable toxicity and some may die due to treatment-related complications.

This under-representation was confirmed by studies comparing real-life outcomes with those observed in clinical trial patients. In a study on metastatic colorectal cancer, trial data on the effect of various types of chemotherapy were compared to patients receiving the same treatment outside of the trial [12]. In this comparative study, patients who fulfilled the trial inclusion criteria but who did not participate, achieved similar results as the trial patients (median survival of 16 months compared to 17 months in trial participants). However, non-eligible non-participants—for example based on age or performance status yet considered by the oncology team as a fit for treatment—had significantly poorer results, with a median survival of only 9 months ($p < 0.01$) [12]. A similar result was seen in a Norwegian study in patients with metastatic colorectal cancer: trial patients had a 40% longer survival than non-trial patients receiving the same treatment [13]. Similarly, multiple studies have demonstrated incremental increases in complication rates with increasing age and increasing comorbidity burden [14–17]; further demonstrating that trial data may not be applicable to patients who are older and/or frail.

Lastly, another important treatment-related consideration is the treatment logistics which is often underestimated by oncology teams. This includes the number of visits to hospital, length of stay, frequency of treatment administration etc. These considerations are often of particular relevance for older cancer patients with frailty when they rely on the support of family and friends.

Physician-Related Factors

When learning to practice medicine, physicians are taught to base this on evidence (Table 12.1). However, as described above, evidence specific to older cancer patients with frailty is generally lacking. As a result, physicians may fall back on the evidence available, despite all its limitations. Critically evaluating the extent to which the study populations in clinical trials are similar to the individual patient for whom a treatment decision needs to be made is essential to avoid overestimating treatment benefit or underestimating its toxicity. This begins with estimating a patient's level of fitness and ability to tolerate treatment, which becomes increasingly complex as patients age and accumulate health issues. Here frailty becomes a key aspect to consider, as described in a subsequent section.

Patients and physicians may have different priorities when it comes to treatment outcomes. One study demonstrated that cancer patients prioritised outcomes such as symptom improvement and quality of life, instead of survival outcomes [18]. Moreover, other studies have shown that whilst physicians focus more on the physical effects of treatment, patients prioritise their mental health, emotional well-being, quality of life and vitality [19, 20]. This is particularly evident in older cancer patients with frailty.

However, data on these outcomes are often lacking: the majority of oncology studies still focus primarily on clinical outcomes such as survival and progression-free survival, and secondarily on toxicity [21, 22]. In an overview of 463 recent or ongoing breast cancer trials, only 20% included any patient-related endpoints, such as quality of life. Functional status or cognitive functioning were included in less than 5% of studies [23]. In addition, results with regards to quality of life often remain unpublished: in an analysis of 201 phase III trials in poor prognosis malignancies, less than half of studies that assessed the quality of life incorporated these results in trial publications [24], further highlighting the gap between evidence from research and patient priorities. When limited or even no evidence regarding patient-centred outcomes of oncologic treatment options is available, physicians may unconsciously prioritise the outcomes they do have evidence on.

Additionally, there may be concerns of undertreating patients, that is of precipitating an avoidable tragedy by withholding a treatment option that could be of benefit [25]. As a result, both physicians and even families are more prone to favour more intensive treatments than patients would [26, 27]. Being honest with oneself and the patient about what is known and tangible given the patient's health status and oncological situation is essential to provide the highest likelihood of achieving what the patient wants within the spectrum of what is possible in their situation.

Whilst the above factors may significantly influence physician's recommendations for patients, other underlying attitudes and beliefs held by physicians may preclude the sharing of decision-making with patients. Many of the beliefs physicians possess relate to the process of SDM and its practicalities; primarily that engaging in SDM with patients will significantly increase the length of consultations [28]. This is an undesirable outcome with increasing workload for physicians, however, there is little evidence that consultation times were significantly increased by interventions designed to facilitate SDM [29]. Furthermore, opposition to SDM may be a result of physicians believing limited resources are available to support the process [30]. Although interventions such as decision aids are not imperative for SDM to occur, readily available, evidence-based resources exist to facilitate the SDM process (as described in the subsequent section).

A prominent barrier of particular relevance to decision-making involving older adult patients is the physician's perceptions as to whether a patient is willing or able to be involved in decisions relating to their treatment [28]. An incorrect perception may result in discordance between patient's desire to be involved and actual involvement in the decision-making process. Discussions with patients about their preferred involvement in decision-making are therefore advised within the early stages of consultation.

Patient-Related Factors

Ageing is associated with an increased heterogeneity in health status and an increased prevalence of frailty. In addition, preferences and priorities may change as a person progresses through life. These patient-related factors are highly relevant to the shared decision-making process (Table 12.1).

Patient Preferences, Beliefs and Expectations

At the centre of SDM are the patient's own and preferences and beliefs. Asking a patient what matters most in his/her life, and subsequently linking this to treatment options and possible outcomes, is more appropriate than simply asking if he/she wants a specific treatment. Older patients are as willing to receive life-prolonging chemotherapy as younger patients [31], but less accepting of toxicity [32], particularly when this could affect their quality of life, independence, cognitive functioning or social situation [33–35].

Adequately assessing the patient's goals requires finding out what he/she understands about the choices available, and which personal priorities and motivations are driving these choices. Exploring below the surface of a patient's wishes will often uncover underlying concerns and assumptions that need to be addressed before a decision can be made. In some cases, the patient may have misconceptions about anti-cancer treatment toxicity based on past experiences with family or friends [36]. Preferences may also be influenced by misconceptions fueled by negative mindsets or depression. For example, patients may believe themselves to be a burden or "I'm too old so what's the point?" [36]. In other cases, patients may have goals and expectations which are not realistic particularly in the context of frailty. Balancing both hope and reality is an important component of the SDM process.

In addition, patient preferences may change over time, making it essential to re-evaluate treatment decisions periodically. Some patients may feel that having said "yes" to a certain treatment, they cannot change their mind or say "no" at a later point in the treatment trajectory or even change their minds once started. On the other hand, people have a remarkable capacity of adapting to their circumstances and finding ways to experience quality of life even in a situation that a priori would have seemed unacceptable to them; for example becoming care-dependent or bed-ridden. This reiterates the relevance of having an ongoing dialogue about what is important to the patient and what they want now and for their future.

As with physicians, patients may possess, and in some cases share, beliefs and attitudes towards sharing decisions regarding their treatment [30]. For example the desire to be perceived as a good or less difficult patient may result in patients deferring decisions to physicians, therefore, promoting a more paternalistic approach to decision-making [37]. Patients, like physicians, may also consider time restraints and adopt a more passive approach so as not to delay the consultations further. Furthermore, patients may feel ill-equipped and unqualified to be involved in decisions about cancer treatment, potentially feeling that the physician's medical training represents the only knowledge relevant for such a decision [30]. Whilst conveying the importance of the patients' knowledge and expertise about their own lives for the purposes of SDM, further steps may need to be taken in order to address the patients' self-efficacy to be involved in decisions.

Although little evidence exists confirming that older patients are more likely to regret treatment decisions, a lack of involvement in decisions, dissatisfaction with information provided, poor preparation for decision-making and higher decision conflict are associated with increased decision regret [38]. These attributes can be addressed by a collaborative approach to consultations which is championed by SDM models. For older cancer patient with frailty, the information provided about the risks and benefits of treatment options may be complex as a result of multiple morbidities. It is therefore essential that information is tailored to the individual's needs and understanding. Although higher decision regret is also associated with treatment complications [38], of which older patients with frailty have a higher risk of experiencing, appropriately informing patients to the risks and facilitating their involvement in decisions may diminish regret.

Patient Frailty

Ageing is associated with an increased heterogeneity in health status and an increased prevalence of frailty. Chronological age and performance status do not suffice as stratification tools when considering treatment options in older adults with cancer [17]. Frailty affects one's organ functional reserve and therefore such patients are at a higher risk in the event of complications with cancer treatments. Hence that frailty is a key consideration when assessing patients' fitness and suitability for cancer treatments.

Geriatric assessment assists in objectively determining the degree of frailty in an individual patient, which assists in estimating the risk of mortality and toxicity of cancer treatments, and therefore optimises treatment selection [39–41]. Geriatric assessment evaluates the individual patient's general health status through assessing the patient's functional status, mobility, comorbidities, polypharmacy, cognition, nutritional status, emotional status and social network in a structured way, and serves many purposes [42]. This helps to achieve upfront tailoring of treatment to the patient's vulnerability rather than modifying treatment only after complications demonstrate that the patient is unable to tolerate standard treatment [43]. Tools such as the CARG and CRASH scores, used for predicting chemotherapy toxicity, and tools for predicting remaining life expectancy in various clinical settings, make use of geriatric assessment data, demonstrating the importance of this information for establishing a patient's health status and optimising treatment selection [44–46].

Prior studies have shown that based on the results of a geriatric assessment, initial oncological treatment plans were altered in 8–54% of patients, more often resulting in a less intensive treatment option [47]. A study by Corre et al. which focussed explicitly on treatment allocation based on the outcome of the geriatric assessment, without further non-oncologic interventions, found that geriatric assessment-based allocation resulted in improved tailoring of care, with less over- and undertreatment [48]. Patients undergoing geriatric assessment had a higher rate of treatment completion and less overall toxicity with similar oncologic outcomes to the control arm [48]. More recently, Mohile et al. examined the impact of providing oncologists with a geriatric assessment and management recommendations on treatment-related toxicities among patients aged 70 years or older with cancer. They found that integrating GA findings in clinical decision-making resulted in less toxicity due to more upfront dose reductions in the geriatric assessment arm, without impacting survival [49]. Similar effects have been reported in two other studies, which also showed that increased rates of tailored treatment after GA resulted in significantly better treatment tolerance and a trend towards less toxicity, without affecting disease control at 6 months [50, 51].

In other studies, the geriatric assessment was used primarily to implement non-oncologic interventions in hopes of improving the patient's ability to tolerate and recover from treatment. Ability to tolerate treatment does appear to improve, with significant effect on treatment completion and a trend towards less treatment-related complications and toxicity [47]. This is interesting because the geriatric assessment generally yields a myriad of recommendations for non-oncologic interventions and previous studies outside oncology have demonstrated that the comprehensive GA as used in geriatric medicine is consistently beneficial for various health outcomes [52].

Decision-Making Capacity and the Role of Proxies

The defining criteria of most definitions or models of SDM involve at least a dyadic discussion, usually between the patient or caregiver and the physician, to discuss the risks and benefits of treatment options in light of the patient's priorities and values. Prominent models of SDM demonstrate several stages of information sharing between parties, which can occur multiple times across the patient's treatment pathway, until a preference-based decision is reached [30, 53, 54]. Cognitive impairment, even of mild severity, may reduce a person's ability to be actively involved in decisions about treatment to the extent these models promote. For example, a patient's comprehension of discussions about treatment options may be limited by impairments to executive functions such as memory, information processing and communication skills [55]. Impairments may be a result of the patient's oncological condition, such as tumours of the brain, medication-related (e.g. opioids or steroids), metabolic complications such as hypercalcemia, or from comorbid conditions such as dementia or other neuropsychiatric disorders.

Depending on the patient's cognitive impairment, usual verbal or written methods of presenting information may be inappropriate as a result of their inability to assimilate or retain the information. As discussed earlier in this chapter, this is particularly relevant to the older cancer patient with frailty where multiple morbidities may make discussions of treatment plans increasingly complicated or confused with other treatment plans. It is therefore essential to determine, where possible, a patient's preferred way of receiving information and what assistance may be required for them to interpret this.

Informal caregivers may adopt a number of roles in decision-making. This can include acting as an advocate for the patient in obtaining and relaying information between involved parties but may also assist patients in making a decision through discussions [56]. Patients and caregivers may prefer that the caregiver also adopts the role of proxy decision maker on behalf of the patient; for example where a patient is experiencing severe cognitive impairment [57, 58]. It could be assumed that informal caregivers, particularly family, are a reliable source of information regarding the patient's priorities and their quality of life thus ensuring patient preferences inform the eventual decisions. This is not always the case, with some patients and caregivers giving incongruent responses relating to the patient's preferences [59]. It is expected that caregivers will also have their own assumptions and concerns surrounding treatment options based on their own or others' experiences, which may need to be addressed as part of the consultation process [36]. Caregivers involved in the care of frail patients are likely to deal with increased adverse effects of any treatment plan devised as a result of the patient's impaired resilience whilst potentially addressing other pre-existing co-morbidities; this may factor in the decision making process to ensure relevant support is given.

Caregivers can play a valuable role in decision-making, however, caution is advised that this does not lead to the complete exclusion of the patient's involvement in decisions about their care. An altruistic motive of not wishing to burden the patient with decision responsibilities may be a premature reason not to involve them in decisions where they may still retain capacity and desire for some involvement in the process [58]. The basis of involvement will be dependent on the individual patient's desire for involvement in decision-making and their situation. This is indicative of a sliding scale analogy for involvement in decision-making, which has been suggested for patients with cognitive impairment [60] rather than a binary "yes or no" approach to involvement or capacity to decide. These states are fluid and can differ with different decision types and situations. Discussing a patient's individual information needs, values and preferred role in decision-making is therefore still important to older frail patients with cognitive impairment as it would be to those who have no impairments.

Preparatory Steps in the Shared Decision-Making Process

Decision-making regarding possible cancer treatments for older patients with frailty actually starts before a cancer diagnosis has been made. Depending on the patient's physical signs and symptoms, a physician may suspect the presence of a malignancy. Before a further diagnostic trajectory is initiated, it is important to take a moment to consider the burden of this trajectory and the benefit of making a diagnosis [61]. In some cases, if the burden is greater than the benefit or if it is clear at the onset that no primary oncologic treatment will be started irrespective of the diagnosis, the result of SDM might be not to investigate further but to focus instead on providing best supportive care. The same question can be relevant all through the diagnostic trajectory, especially in case of burdensome or invasive diagnostic procedures: if it is likely that the outcome of a routine, guideline-recommended test or procedure will not alter the care that may be provided, then it is worth questioning the reason for doing this test in this particular patient.

Discussions within multidisciplinary teams (MDT) focus primarily on therapeutic strategies informed by the characteristics of their disease rather than geriatric assessments or the patients' priorities. Prior to MDT meetings and a SDM conversation with the patient, it may be useful to contact the primary care physician, to double-check information provided by the patient and caregivers against the background knowledge the primary care physician has regarding the patient's history, past treatment decisions, and advance care directives. In addition, it is important to have an understanding of the patient's health status across somatic, psychosocial, cognitive and functional domains—for example by performing a geriatric assessment—in addition to the data regarding the (suspected) malignancy. Where possible, eliciting the patient's priorities prior to MDT discussions would be beneficial to ensure they are represented. Combined, these data can be used to make the best possible estimate regarding the potential benefit and risks of various diagnostic and treatment options [17].

In addition, the patient's decision-making capacity needs to be established and in case this is diminished, assessing who is the legal proxy in accordance with national guidelines. Irrespective of cognitive status, asking a patient to bring along a family member or caregiver may be quite helpful. They can facilitate this process by being a sparring partner to the patient and helping to verbalise which questions are relevant to them and what information is needed to be able to reach a decision [62].

The following questions should be considered by the treating physician and, preferably, the entire multidisciplinary oncology team, in order to determine which treatment options might be considered for a particular older cancer patient with frailty and a particular type and stage of cancer [63]:

- What is the patient's life expectancy without cancer?
- What is the patient's life expectancy if the cancer is left untreated?
- What is contributing to the patient's frailty, its severity and is there room to optimise this patient?
- What will be the burden of illness and quality of life if the cancer is left untreated (now and in the future)?
- What will the treatment contribute to the patient's life expectancy?
- What will the treatment contribute to alleviating the burden of illness (now and in the future) and maintaining quality of life for this specific patient?
- What is the burden of treatment in terms of hospitalisation, complications and side-effects, out-patient clinic visits, longer-term functional or cognitive decline, care needs and institutionalisation, for this specific patient?
- What is the likelihood that the patient will be able to complete the treatment as planned?
- What other treatment options are available (including palliative or best supportive care)?
- What are the patient's treatment goals, expectations and preferences?
- What are the patients' fears and concerns?

Tools to Support the Shared Decision-Making

Multiple interventions exist which aim to facilitate aspects of SDM between patients and health care professionals within consultations. Cancer decision interventions directed towards patients, such as decision aids, may convey information about treatment options and the associated risks and benefits to patients which are appropriate to their current clinical situation and the treatment intent. Although this information is available using clinical algorithms and risk prediction models, decision aids will present information relating to each option available to patients in an accessible way that allows for comparison. Decision aids are also likely to contain values clarification methods to ensure that treatment decisions are concordant with the patient's preferences.

Studies have shown that decision aids produce a benefit to patients in domains such as increased knowledge and a reduction in decision conflict [29]; however, most are adapted for use within all age ranges with no specific engagement with or consideration towards older adults noted in articles detailing their development [64]. Many may not take into account the needs of older patients with frailty, such as the addition of multiple co-morbidities as a factor in treatment decisions. Furthermore, there is also a scarcity of decision aids aimed for use with patients who have cognitive impairment [55]. Despite this, a recent systematic review and meta-analysis acknowledged that decision aids designed for the general population were predominantly effective in generating positive outcomes in study populations with a mean age of 65+ or a subsample of participants in the same age category [64]. Care must also be taken to ensure decision aids are accessible to those with lower health literacy [65].

In the context of cancer care, very few decision aids exist for older patients and of those that do exist they are predominantly focused on decisions relating to cancer screening choices rather than decisions for anti-cancer treatment [66–68].

Alternative interventions to decision aids for use with patients include various methods to enhance their ability for involvement in SDM by, for example, educating patients about SDM or developing patient abilities such as consultation preparation which might encourage an SDM process. Furthermore, interventions to facilitate SDM are not solely directed towards patients. Many educational courses or materials have been developed for physicians to promote the use of SDM in consultations with patients [69]. A recent Cochrane review did however indicate a high degree of uncertainty regarding the efficacy of these intervention types in encouraging the use of SDM by healthcare professionals [69].

Whilst few interventions exist which are specific to the older frail patient, a model of SDM for older patients with multiple morbidities has been developed by Van de Pol et al [70] where they demonstrate a framework that physicians can use within their consultations. Whilst the framework is not specific to cancer treatment, it provides a prompt for the conversations which are relevant to generic SDM conversations for older patients with multiple morbidities. Below are some examples of questions that may be useful in starting these conversations:

- Tell me about what matters most to you in your life right now?
- What aspects of your life are you concerned may be affected by your cancer and/or cancer treatment?
- What are you hoping that treatment/discontinuing treatment will achieve?

Using SDM frameworks in conjunction with patient-focused interventions such as decision aids may be beneficial and assist in conveying information to patients and their caregivers. At the time of printing a list of currently available decision aids is available from the Ottawa Hospital website [71].

Conclusion

Older adult patients with frailty present additional factors to be considered when making decisions about cancer treatment which can increase the complexity and uncertainty about the best course of action to take. Whilst patient co-morbidities and living situations may predict the tolerability and complications of available treatment options, discussions surrounding the risks and benefits of available treatment options may not be as comprehensive as desired due to the limited evidence available for this subgroup of patients. SDM allows treatment options to be considered in concordance with the patient's preferences, beliefs and priorities.

Although barriers may be encountered when incorporating SDM into consultations with frail older adults, many of these are modifiable. For example, the patient's self-efficacy to be involved in decision-making may be increased through communication tailored to the individual's level of understanding and by addressing beliefs about their role in decision-making. Decision support tools can also be used to assist this process and increase patient knowledge about their choices. Where unmodifiable barriers exist, such as cognitive impairment which limits the capacity for decision-making, an SDM approach is still appropriate to ensure that patient priorities are represented albeit tailored to the patient's situation or through proxy decision makers where necessary.

References

1. Barry MJ, Edgman-Levitan S. Shared decision making – pinnacle of patient-centered care. N Engl J Med. 2012;366:780–1.
2. Levine DM, Landon BE, Linder JA. Trends in patient-perceived shared decision making among adults in the United States, 2002-2014. Ann Fam Med. 2017;15:552–6.
3. Covvey JR, Kamal KM, Gorse EE, et al. Barriers and facilitators to shared decision-making in oncology: a systematic review of the literature. Support Care Cancer. 2019;27:1613–37.
4. Rothwell PM. External validity of randomised controlled trials: "to whom do the results of this trial apply?". Lancet. 2005;365:82–93.
5. Zulman DM, Sussman JB, Chen X, Cigolle CT, Blaum CS, Hayward RA. Examining the evidence: a systematic review of the inclusion and analysis of older adults in randomized controlled trials. J Gen Intern Med. 2011;26:783–90.
6. Schiphorst AH, Pronk A, Borel Rinkes IHM, Hamaker ME. Representation of the elderly in trials on laparoscopic surgery for colorectal cancer. Colorectal Dis. 2014;16:976–83.
7. Hamaker ME, Stauder R, van Munster BC. Exclusion of older patients from ongoing clinical trials for hematological malignancies: an evaluation of the National Institutes of Health Clinical Trial Registry. Oncologist. 2014;19:1069–75.
8. Schulkes KJ, Nguyen C, van den Bos F, van Elden LJ, Hamaker ME. Selection of patients in ongoing clinical trials on lung cancer. Lung. 2016;194:967–74.
9. Zhao Y, Liu J, Cai X, et al. Efficacy and safety of first line treatments for patients with advanced epidermal growth factor receptor mutated, non-small cell lung cancer: systematic review and network meta-analysis. BMJ. 2019;367:l5460.
10. https://www.nature.com/articles/s41416-020-0986-4. 2021. Ref Type: Online Source.

11. Lewis JH, Kilgore ML, Goldman DP, et al. Participation of patients 65 years of age or older in cancer clinical trials. J Clin Oncol. 2003;21:1383–9.
12. Mol L, Koopman M, van Gils CW, Ottevanger PB, Punt CJ. Comparison of treatment outcome in metastatic colorectal cancer patients included in a clinical trial versus daily practice in The Netherlands. Acta Oncol. 2013;52:950–5.
13. Sorbye H, Pfeiffer P, Cavalli-Bjorkman N, et al. Clinical trial enrollment, patient characteristics, and survival differences in prospectively registered metastatic colorectal cancer patients. Cancer. 2009;115:4679–87.
14. Hamaker ME, Schiphorst AH, Verweij NM, Pronk A. Improved survival for older patients undergoing surgery for colorectal cancer between 2008 and 2011. Int J Color Dis. 2014;29:1231–6.
15. Burhenn P, Sun CL, Scher KS, et al. Predictors of hospital readmission among older adults with cancer. J Geriatr Oncol. 2020;11(7):1108–14.
16. Sun V, Burhenn PS, Lai L, Hurria A. The impact of comorbidity on surgical outcomes in older adults with cancer. Semin Oncol Nurs. 2017;33:80–6.
17. Mohile SG, Dale W, Somerfield MR, et al. Practical assessment and management of vulnerabilities in older patients receiving chemotherapy: ASCO guideline for geriatric oncology. J Clin Oncol. 2018;36:2326–47.
18. Kool M, van der Sijp JR, Kroep JR, et al. Importance of patient reported outcome measures versus clinical outcomes for breast cancer patients evaluation on quality of care. Breast. 2016;27:62–8.
19. Rothwell PM, McDowell Z, Wong CK, Dorman PJ. Doctors and patients don't agree: cross sectional study of patients' and doctors' perceptions and assessments of disability in multiple sclerosis. BMJ. 1997;314:1580–3.
20. Akishita M, Ishii S, Kojima T, et al. Priorities of health care outcomes for the elderly. J Am Med Dir Assoc. 2013;14:479–84.
21. van Bekkum ML, van Munster BC, Thunnissen PL, Smorenburg CH, Hamaker ME. Current palliative chemotherapy trials in the elderly neglect patient-centred outcome measures. J Geriatr Oncol. 2015;6:15–22.
22. Hamaker ME, Stauder R, van Munster BC. On-going clinical trials for elderly patients with a hematological malignancy: are we addressing the right end points? Ann Oncol. 2014;25:675–81.
23. de Glas NA, Hamaker ME, Kiderlen M, et al. Choosing relevant endpoints for older breast cancer patients in clinical trials: an overview of all current clinical trials on breast cancer treatment. Breast Cancer Res Treat. 2014;146:591–7.
24. Hamaker ME, Schulkes KJ, ten Bokkel HD, van Munster BC, van Huis LH, van den Bos F. Evaluation and reporting of quality of life outcomes in phase III chemotherapy trials for poor prognosis malignancies. Qual Life Res. 2017;26:65–71.
25. Heath I. Role of fear in overdiagnosis and overtreatment--an essay by Iona Heath. BMJ. 2014;349:g6123.
26. Earle CC, Neville BA, Landrum MB, Ayanian JZ, Block SD, Weeks JC. Trends in the aggressiveness of cancer care near the end of life. J Clin Oncol. 2004;22:315–21.
27. Scherr KA, Fagerlin A, Hofer T, et al. Physician recommendations trump patient preferences in prostate cancer treatment decisions. Med Decis Mak. 2017;37:56–69.
28. Legare F, Ratte S, Gravel K, Graham ID. Barriers and facilitators to implementing shared decision-making in clinical practice: update of a systematic review of health professionals' perceptions. Patient Educ Couns. 2008;73:526–35.
29. Stacey D, Legare F, Lewis K, et al. Decision aids for people facing health treatment or screening decisions. Cochrane Database Syst Rev. 2017;4:CD001431.
30. Joseph-Williams N, Elwyn G, Edwards A. Knowledge is not power for patients: a systematic review and thematic synthesis of patient-reported barriers and facilitators to shared decision making. Patient Educ Couns. 2014;94:291–309.
31. Extermann M, Albrand G, Chen H, et al. Are older French patients as willing as older American patients to undertake chemotherapy? J Clin Oncol. 2003;21:3214–9.

32. Yellen SB, Cella DF, Leslie WT. Age and clinical decision making in oncology patients. J Natl Cancer Inst. 1994;86:1766–70.
33. Wildiers H, Mauer M, Pallis A, et al. End points and trial Design in Geriatric Oncology Research: a joint European Organisation for Research and Treatment of Cancer-Alliance for Clinical Trials in Oncology-International Society of Geriatric Oncology Position Article. J Clin Oncol. 2013;31:3711–8.
34. Chouliara Z, Miller M, Stott D, Molassiotis A, Twelves C, Kearney N. Older people with cancer: perceptions and feelings about information, decision-making and treatment: a pilot study. Eur J Oncol Nurs. 2004;8:257–61.
35. Fried TR, Bradley EH, Towle VR, Allore H. Understanding the treatment preferences of seriously ill patients. N Engl J Med. 2002;346:1061–6.
36. Rostoft S, van den Bos F, Pedersen R, Hamaker ME. Shared decision-making in older patients with cancer - what does the patient want? J Geriatr Oncol. 2021;12:339–42.
37. Frosch DL, May SG, Rendle KA, Tietbohl C, Elwyn G. Authoritarian physicians and patients' fear of being labeled 'difficult' among key obstacles to shared decision making. Health Aff (Millwood). 2012;31:1030–8.
38. Becerra Perez MM, Menear M, Brehaut JC, Legare F. Extent and predictors of decision regret about health care decisions: a systematic review. Med Decis Mak. 2016;36:777–90.
39. Hamaker ME, Jonker JM, de Rooij SE, Vos AG, Smorenburg CH, van Munster BC. Frailty screening methods for predicting outcome of a comprehensive geriatric assessment in elderly patients with cancer: a systematic review. Lancet Oncol. 2012;13:e437–44.
40. Hamaker ME, Buurman BM, van Munster BC, Kuper IM, Smorenburg CH, de Rooij SE. The value of a comprehensive geriatric assessment for patient care in acutely hospitalized older patients with cancer. Oncologist. 2011;16(10):1403–12.
41. Hamaker ME, Seynaeve C, Wymenga ANM, et al. Baseline comprehensive geriatric assessment to predict for toxicity of single-agent chemotherapy in elderly metastatic breast cancer patients: results from the OMEGA study of the Dutch Breast Cancer Trialists' Group. J Clin Oncol. 2012;30:15.
42. Wildiers H, Heeren P, Puts M, et al. International Society of Geriatric Oncology consensus on geriatric assessment in older patients with cancer. J Clin Oncol. 2014;32:2595–603.
43. Hoeben KW, van Steenbergen LN, van de Wouw AJ, Rutten HJ, Van Spronsen DJ, Janssen-Heijnen ML. Treatment and complications in elderly stage III colon cancer patients in the Netherlands. Ann Oncol. 2012;24(4):974–9.
44. Hurria A, Togawa K, Mohile SG, et al. Predicting chemotherapy toxicity in older adults with cancer: a prospective multicenter study. J Clin Oncol. 2011;29(25):3457–65.
45. Eprognosis. eprognosis.ucsf.edu. 2018. Ref Type: Online Source.
46. Extermann M, Boler I, Reich RR, et al. Predicting the risk of chemotherapy toxicity in older patients: the chemotherapy risk assessment scale for high-age patients (CRASH) score. Cancer. 2011;118(13):3377–86.
47. Hamaker ME, Te MM, Thielen N, van Munster BC, Schiphorst AH, van Huis LH. The effect of a geriatric evaluation on treatment decisions and outcome for older cancer patients - a systematic review. J Geriatr Oncol. 2018;9:430–40.
48. Corre R, Greillier L, Le CH, et al. Use of a comprehensive geriatric assessment for the management of elderly patients with advanced non-small-cell lung cancer: the phase III randomized ESOGIA-GFPC-GECP 08-02 study. J Clin Oncol. 2016;34:1476–83.
49. Giri S, Chakiba C, Shih YY, et al. Integration of geriatric assessment into routine oncologic care and advances in geriatric oncology: a young International Society of Geriatric Oncology Report of the 2020 American Society of Clinical Oncology (ASCO) annual meeting. J Geriatr Oncol. 2020;11(8):1324–8.
50. Kalsi T, Babic-Illman G, Ross PJ, et al. The impact of comprehensive geriatric assessment interventions on tolerance to chemotherapy in older people. Br J Cancer. 2015;112:1435–44.
51. Puts MTE, Sattar S, Kulik M, et al. A randomized phase II trial of geriatric assessment and management for older cancer patients. Support Care Cancer. 2018;26:109–17.

52. Pilotto A, Cella A, Pilotto A, et al. Three decades of comprehensive geriatric assessment: evidence coming from different healthcare settings and specific clinical conditions. J Am Med Dir Assoc. 2017;18:192.
53. Makoul G, Clayman ML. An integrative model of shared decision making in medical encounters. Patient Educ Couns. 2006;60:301–12.
54. Elwyn G, Durand MA, Song J, et al. A three-talk model for shared decision making: multistage consultation process. BMJ. 2017;359:j4891.
55. Mejia AM, Smith GE, Wicklund M, Armstrong MJ. Shared decision making in mild cognitive impairment. Neurol Clin Pract. 2019;9:160–4.
56. Hubbard G, Illingworth N, Rowa-Dewar N, Forbat L, Kearney N. Treatment decision-making in cancer care: the role of the carer. J Clin Nurs. 2010;19:2023–31.
57. Shin DW, Cho J, Roter DL, et al. Preferences for and experiences of family involvement in cancer treatment decision-making: patient-caregiver dyads study. Psychooncology. 2013;22:2624–31.
58. Miller LM, Whitlatch CJ, Lyons KS. Shared decision-making in dementia: a review of patient and family carer involvement. Dementia (London). 2016;15:1141–57.
59. Shin DW, Cho J, Kim SY, et al. Discordance among patient preferences, caregiver preferences, and caregiver predictions of patient preferences regarding disclosure of terminal status and end-of-life choices. Psychooncology. 2015;24:212–9.
60. Lahey T, Elwyn G. Sliding-scale shared decision making for patients with reduced capacity. AMA J Ethics. 2020;22:E358–64.
61. Hamaker ME, van Huis LH. Diagnostics in very old patients; when to apply it or not in cases of suspected malignancy? Ned Tijdschr Geneeskd. 2019;163:D3708.
62. Kane HL, Halpern MT, Squiers LB, Treiman KA, McCormack LA. Implementing and evaluating shared decision making in oncology practice. CA Cancer J Clin. 2014;64:377–88.
63. Festen S, Kok M, Hopstaken JS, van der Wal-Huisman H, van der Leest A, Reyners AKL, de Bock GH, de Graeff P, van Leeuwen BL. How to incorporate geriatric assessment in clinical decision-making for older patients with cancer. An implementation study. J Geriatr Oncol. 2019;10(6):951–9.
64. Kane HL, Halpern MT, Squiers LB, Treiman KA, McCormack LA. Implementing and evaluating shared decision making in oncology practice. CA Cancer J Clin. 2014;64:377–88.
65. McCaffery KJ, Holmes-Rovner M, Smith SK, et al. Addressing health literacy in patient decision aids. BMC Med Inform Decis Mak. 2013;13(Suppl 2):S10.
66. Lewis CL, Golin CE, DeLeon C, et al. A targeted decision aid for the elderly to decide whether to undergo colorectal cancer screening: development and results of an uncontrolled trial. BMC Med Inform Decis Mak. 2010;10:54.
67. Lewis CL, Kistler CE, Dalton AF, et al. A decision aid to promote appropriate colorectal cancer screening among older adults: a randomized controlled trial. Med Decis Mak. 2018;38:614–24.
68. Schonberg MA, Hamel MB, Davis RB, et al. Development and evaluation of a decision aid on mammography screening for women 75 years and older. JAMA Intern Med. 2014;174:417–24.
69. Legare F, Adekpedjou R, Stacey D, et al. Interventions for increasing the use of shared decision making by healthcare professionals. Cochrane Database Syst Rev. 2018;7:CD006732.
70. van de Pol MH, Fluit CR, Lagro J, Slaats YH, Olde Rikkert MG, Lagro-Janssen AL. Expert and patient consensus on a dynamic model for shared decision-making in frail older patients. Patient Educ Couns. 2016;99:1069–77.
71. https://decisionaid.ohri.ca/AZlist.html. 2020.

Chapter 13
Perioperative Care in Older Adults with Cancer and Frailty

Sherena Nair and Simon J. Howell

Introduction

Rapid global demographic transitions have witnessed an increased proportion of people above the age of 65 years, with a projected tripling of those aged 80 years and over by 2050 [1]. This significant increase of an ageing population will mean that hospitals and healthcare systems will be under pressure to meet the needs of older people often with frailty, dementia and multiple comorbidities complicating their acute illness. It is projected that by 2030, one-fifth of people aged above the age of 75 years and older will undergo surgery in England each year, at an approximate cost of €3·2 billion [2]. Moreover, it is estimated that up to 26% of the general population aged 85 years and over have frailty [3]. The identification and management of older people with frailty undergoing surgery have gained wider recognition since the National Confidential Enquiry into Patient Outcome and Death report was published in 2010 highlighting that older surgical patients experienced sub-standard care [3, 4].

Frailty is defined by a state of disruption to homeostasis and increased state of vulnerability due to stressor events that can significantly alter the physiology and function resulting in adverse outcomes including a reduction in mobility, cognitive decline (such as delirium) and an increased level of dependency (Fig. 13.1) [3, 5]. The two most widely known models of frailty are the 'phenotypic model' which includes the presence of three or more features (unintentional weight loss,

S. Nair (✉)
Elderly Medicine Department, Leeds Teaching Hospitals NHS Trust, Leeds, UK
e-mail: sherenanair@nhs.net

S. J. Howell
Leeds Institute of Medical Research, University of Leeds, Leeds, UK

Anaesthesiology Department, Leeds Teaching Hospitals NHS Trust, Leeds, UK
e-mail: s.howell@leeds.ac.uk

F. Gomes (ed.), *Frailty in Older Adults with Cancer*,
https://doi.org/10.1007/978-3-030-89162-6_13

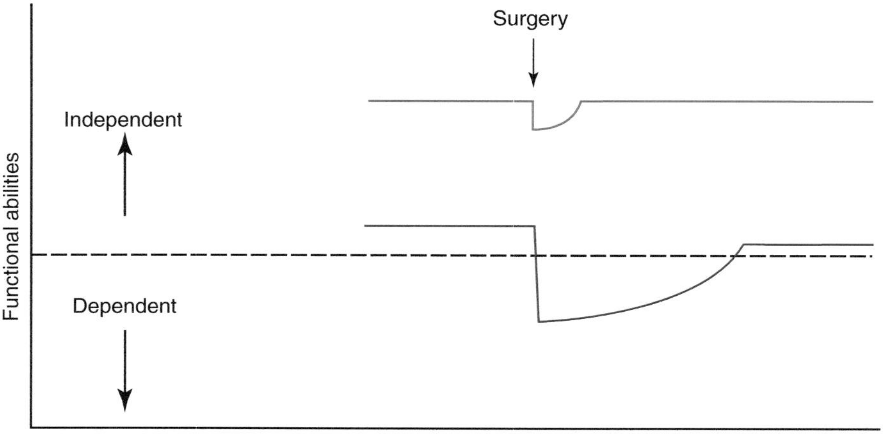

Fig. 13.1 A stressor event (such as surgery) can result in a poorer functional outcome in an older patient with frailty (in red) (Adapted from [3])

exhaustion, weakness, slow walking speed and low physical activity) and the 'cumulative deficit model' where frailty is defined by indices reflecting the accumulation of a broad range of functional and pathological deficits [6, 7]. As it is widely accepted that frailty is associated with worse outcomes for surgical patients [8], there is increasing recognition of the need for a holistic multidisciplinary approach to assessing and planning intervention in older patients with frailty undergoing cancer surgery. Risk stratification and pre- and post-surgery optimisation are key to addressing this challenge and multidisciplinary involvement is crucial in achieving a fully informed shared decision-making process [9–11]. Therefore, this chapter will discuss the implications of frailty, risk stratification, relevant investigations, as well as the multidisciplinary perioperative care required to manage the older adult with frailty undergoing cancer surgery.

Perioperative Physiology and Frailty

Frailty is a strong predictor of mortality, care home admission and hospitalisation although these outcomes may be improved and potentially reversed by appropriate interventions [5]. A meta-analysis of 16 studies found that frailty was associated with higher complication and all-cause mortality rates across multiple surgical specialties [8]. It is postulated that the reduction of physical reserve coupled with multiple comorbidities in a patient with frailty renders them more susceptible to post-op complications such as poor wound healing, myocardial infarction, pulmonary embolism and a higher rate of return to theatre.

The combination of anaesthesia and major surgery represents a significant physiological insult, and it is sometimes asked if a patient is 'fit for anaesthesia'. This is a spurious question as anaesthesia is always administered to allow a surgical or other therapeutic intervention and the effects of anaesthesia and surgery should be considered together. Anaesthetic drugs produce multiple changes across all organ systems [12]. Surgery causes direct tissue damage and triggers a systemic inflammatory response which may cause organ injury [13].

The cardiorespiratory effects of anaesthetic drugs are exaggerated in older patients. Almost all anaesthetic drugs cause vasodilatation and many produce a significant degree of myocardial depression; these changes can cause a reduction in cardiac output and blood pressure [12, 13]. Induction of anaesthesia produces significant changes in respiratory mechanics. The induction of general anaesthesia causes a reduction in functional residual capacity which may decrease below closing capacity, so producing significant airway closure and atelectasis which is more marked in the older patient [13]. Anaesthesia and surgery produce changes to autoregulation and organ blood flow. For example, splanchnic perfusion has been shown to be blood pressure dependence during colorectal surgery and major abdominal surgery is associated with reductions in renal blood flow [14]. Many older patients are exquisitely sensitive to both hypovolaemia and overload. Large-scale observational studies have repeatedly shown a robust association between perioperative hypotension and markers of renal and cardiac injury [14, 15]. Management can be challenging. The older surgical patient is also less able to regulate their body temperature and active warming may be needed not only during but after surgery [16].

Older patients display altered pharmacokinetics and pharmacodynamics. The binding of acidic drugs is reduced because of decreased albumin concentration with age; binding of basic drugs increases due to increased levels of α-1 acid glycoprotein [17]. The decrease in total body water with age, together with the increase in body fat and changes in hepatic and renal function produce pharmacokinetic changes [18]. Older patients are more sensitive to the effects of most anaesthetic drugs and display slow onset and offset times for drug action and fluid management can be challenging [15, 17, 18].

Major surgery precipitates a systemic inflammatory response (SIRS) that may cause organ injury. The perioperative oxidative stress and inflammatory responses can dampen the immune system and lead to endocrine dysregulation, and malnutrition and a reduction in mobility can all lead to acute sarcopenia [13, 19] The SIRS response to surgery has been implicated in perioperative myocardial injury and neuroinflammation may have a role in the aetiology of postoperative delirium [20, 21]. There is no specific anaesthetic technique that mitigates these effects. It is often held that local or regional anaesthesia is safer than general anaesthesia in high-risk patients. The evidence for outcome benefits from the use of regional anaesthesia is mixed. A case has been made that the use of regional anaesthesia reduces the incidence of cancer recurrence following surgery, but to date, this has not been demonstrated in randomised controlled trials [15, 22]. The judicious use of regional techniques to mitigate the use of opiates in the postoperative period in the older patient can certainly be of value and should be considered where possible. Epidural and spinal anaesthesia has a place but can be associated with intraoperative and postoperative hypotension that requires active management.

In summary, understanding the changes of ageing physiology is crucial for optimising and managing the older patient with frailty (or at high-risk) undergoing surgery. There is no specific anaesthetic technique that is appropriate for the management of older surgical patients, particularly those with frailty. What is important is close attention to detail and proactive management of deviations from physiological norms.

Preoperative Assessment

A clear distinction needs to be made between risk adjustment and risk stratification. Risk adjustment is used to 'determine the expected rate of an outcome for a provider or a population' while risk stratification 'predicts future adverse events that could be costly, undesirable and potentially preventable' [23, 24]. The key to translating risk adjustment and risk stratification into useful clinical tools is to apply these constructs into risk-stratification healthcare management tools which influence decision-making and support a tailored care plan for each patient [25]. This often involves a multidisciplinary team and approach to arrive at the final outcomes, but in the long term, it is resource and cost-effective. There are numerous risk prediction tools that are widely available to calculate surgical risk. These include the National Surgical Quality Improvement Program (NSQIP) surgical risk calculator, the American Society of Anaesthesiologists (ASA) classification and the Surgical Outcome Risk Tool (SORT) [26, 27]. However, only the NSQIP tool takes frailty into account using proxy markers such as level of dependence, mobility status, history of falls as well as any concomitant diagnosis of dementia or cognitive impairment. The evidence around the use of these tools to aid risk stratification unfortunately has not been consistently demonstrated across different surgical specialties in an older surgical population [28]. A collaborative approach is needed to achieve a general consensus around the use of such tools in clinical practice.

The role of preoperative assessment is to assess the fitness of high-risk patients undergoing surgery with the view to optimise any underlying medical comorbidities prior to surgery [29]. During such consultations, issues such as postoperative complications, suitability of anaesthesia and discussions around the risk of surgery are integral to the conversations with patients which enables a shared decision-making process. Routinely, basic investigations such as blood tests, and an electrocardiogram (ECG) are undertaken to measure the baseline physiological function of the patient [30]. More detailed investigations such as a quantified exercise tolerance test are also often conducted to predict outcomes and postoperative complications.

The multicentre international prospective cohort study entitled Measurement of Exercise Tolerance before Surgery (METS) published in 2018 was undertaken to assess preoperative functional capacity using cardiopulmonary testing (CPET), the Duke Activity Status Index (DASI) questionnaire and N-terminal pro-B-type natriuretic peptide (NT-pro-BNP) [31]. CPET was assessed using a bicycle or treadmill over 8–12 min on an incremental exercise with the two main indices of peak oxygen consumption (VO2 max) and anaerobic threshold measured by continuous spirometry monitoring. The DASI questionnaire is a 12-item questionnaire that uses activities of daily living to produce an estimate of functional capacity. NT pro-BNP is used as a marker for cardiac dysfunction. It was found that all three components of the METS study accurately identified patients with poor cardiopulmonary fitness and predicted 30-day mortality and myocardial injury and death; peak oxygen consumption during CPET was found to be a good predictor of moderate or severe postoperative complications [32]. These comprehensive tests are used to aid prehabilitation decisions where patients are given specific interventions, using a multimodal approach such as exercise and nutrition advice to optimise their cardiopulmonary fitness in order to ensure positive surgical outcomes [33].

However, general preoperative assessments may not always assess frailty and the related syndromes which contribute to poorer outcomes [29]. Therefore, comprehensive geriatric assessment, a gold standard of evaluating and optimising management of the surgical patient with frailty (or at high-risk), carried out alongside traditional preoperative assessments can reduce postoperative morbidity and mortality significantly [34].

Perioperative Care

Surgical Patient with Frailty

Data from the United States indicate that more than half of people in their last year of life undergo surgery when they are physically frail and on a downward health trajectory [35]. Surgical risk prediction tools that incorporate geriatric-specific variables tend to improve their predictive accuracy of adverse outcomes and may play a part in patient selection for surgery, but there is no 'one size fits all' and the scope of instruments is extensive [27]. A meta-analysis of 15 studies demonstrated different frailty scales showed a different prevalence of frailty within the same population although frailty phenotype and single-item scales (such as grip strength or gait tests) were associated with greater predictive risk of postoperative complications [36].

Some examples of frailty tools used in the surgical setting include the Rockwood Clinical Frailty Scale, the Edmonton Frail Scale and the more recently developed electronic frailty index (eFI) [6, 37, 38]. The choice of tool is dependent on several factors, which include predictive accuracy, time effectiveness, ease of use and local practice [39]. In the United Kingdom, there is growing use of the Edmonton Frail Scale because it encompasses elements that are modifiable preoperatively such as nutrition, medication optimisation, and gait velocity (a strong predictor of postoperative outcomes) [40]. In the United States, the Clinical Frailty Scale is a popular choice because it is easy to use, feasible and takes no more than 2 min to complete and is more straightforward in an emergency situation [41, 42]. The electronic frailty index (eFI) designed originally for use in primary care is available for primary care practitioners to use on the two main primary care electronic health records in England [38]. However, the programme has to be executed by primary care through the electronic health management system that derives the score through coding of medical conditions on the patient record and may not be updated regularly. Its use for preoperative assessment in secondary care is dependent on paper or electronic transmission of the index to the perioperative team. Unfortunately, the uptake of the eFI within England's primary care is variable; therefore, relying on it for secondary care use is not practical. Clinicians will continue to use frailty assessment tools that are suited to their experience, context and local practice but the large variability in these frailty measurements calls for more robust research towards a standardisation of such tools that is transferable across different surgical settings [43].

Increasing age is associated with a higher perioperative risk and is often used as a surrogate marker for a state of reduced physiological reserve. However, chronological age does not necessarily reflect biological age, frailty and the need for preoperative optimisation. Perioperative medical optimisation consists of four facets: assessment and optimisation of physiological reserve, assessment and optimisation of comorbidities, assessment and optimisation of geriatric syndromes and finally postoperative optimisation [44, 45]. The optimisation of physiological reserve requires the assessment of cardiorespiratory function either through cardiopulmonary exercise testing or measuring the gait speed. Many perioperative departments have established prehabilitation programmes that may involve supervised or unsupervised exercise. It is now well established that the fitness of patients can be improved before surgery but robust evidence of the cost-effectiveness of such programmes requires further clinical trials [46]. Individual chronic conditions such as heart failure, anaemia, hypertension and diabetes can affect perioperative outcomes, and collectively can significantly affect patient outcomes. Anaemia may need to be corrected preoperatively with iron infusions and heart failure medications titrated to optimise cardiac function prior to surgery [45, 47].

The assessment and optimisation of geriatric syndromes may be less straightforward as these are not defined as discrete entities and include cognitive impairment, nutrition, falls, and incontinence; these syndromes often require a multifaceted approach to manage them throughout the perioperative period [45, 48]. While not strictly under the umbrella of medical optimisation, psychological function and social support assessments also form a central component of the perioperative medicine care pathway. Postoperatively, a key element is continuity of care from a geriatrician to address any postoperative complications in the immediate post-surgical phase this is to support the surgical team with recovery, rehabilitation and discharge decisions [45].

Sarcopenia Considerations

Acute sarcopenia is defined by loss of muscle mass and muscle function within 28 days of a stressor event. This is an emerging disorder that is increasingly being considered in acutely unwell patients who are hospitalised and risk factors include surgery, medications (such as steroids), chronic diseases, malnutrition, and acute illness that exacerbate the rate of muscle mass loss [49] This can be particularly problematic for an older cancer patient with (or at high risk) of frailty. In general, sarcopenia is associated with adverse perioperative outcomes such as increased morbidity and mortality and in cancer and cancer surgery has a significant impact on postoperative outcomes; it is caused by mitochondrial dysfunction, protein synthesis alteration and lack of exercise [50].

Elective surgical patients with colorectal cancer and sarcopenia were found to have poorer 30-day mortality and survival at 1 year [51]. Besides postoperative outcomes, sarcopenia was also found to increase the risk of death from other causes following gastric cancer surgery, emphasising the correlation between sarcopenia and comorbidity [52].

The European Working Group on Sarcopenia in Older People (EWGSOP) updated its original definition of sarcopenia in early 2018 to reflect the scientific and clinical evidence synthesis over the last decade; this includes a focus on low muscle strength as a key characteristic of sarcopenia, and low muscle quantity to confirm the diagnosis through the uptake of available clinical tools that will support the diagnosis of sarcopenia [53]. The SARC-F questionnaire is a simple validated tool that can be used to screen for sarcopenia and severity graded by several performance measures which include the timed get up and go test, gait speed, and the 400-metre walk test [53–55]. The only current clinical tool that is recommended by the EWSOP to diagnose sarcopenia is the use of a dual-energy X-ray absorptiometry (DEXA) scan although this is not widely used.

Sarcopenia requires a multimodal approach of management but nutrition especially in the form of protein coupled with physical activity can stimulate anabolic muscle protein synthesis [56]. A review of patients undergoing hip fracture surgery demonstrated that nutritional supplementations and a higher protein intake improved postoperative complications both in the short term and positively impacted morbidity after discharge [57]. However, one of the main issues in any nutritional intervention in cancer surgery is a lack of standardisation of such protocols, particularly for older patients with frailty [58, 59]. Unfortunately the evidence for parenteral and enteral nutrition in older people with frailty is limited. However, enteral nutrition is preferred rather than parenteral nutrition due to better outcomes such as increased survival and reduced incidence of sepsis [60]. The European Society for Clinical Nutrition and Metabolism (ESPEN) guidelines suggest that while enteral and parental nutrition in older patients should be reserved for those who are completely unable to meet their nutritional needs, there are ethical and clinical considerations that need to be taken into account due to the risks and complications involved; and randomised controlled trials would be considered unethical in these instances and therefore consensus-based guidelines are urgently required to address this area of unmet need [61]. The potential risks and benefits of artificial nutrition need to be closely weighed in individual circumstances and assessed regularly when the patient's clinical condition changes.

Delirium and Postoperative Cognitive Deficits

Postoperative delirium occurs in 20–50% of patients aged 60 years and above who have undergone major surgery [62]. This can also be particularly problematic for older cancer patients with (or at high risk) of frailty. The pathophysiological processes underlying postoperative delirium remain unclear. Delirium can be hypoactive, hyperactive or of a mixed pattern. Preoperative factors associated with delirium include age, underlying cognitive impairment, frailty, electrolyte imbalances, cardiovascular dysfunction and anticholinergic drugs; intraoperative factors include the site of surgery (abdominal and cardiothoracic surgery) bleeding and cancer; and postoperative causes include poor management of pain and postoperative complications such as infection or electrolyte disturbances [63–65]. While the causal relationship between postoperative delirium and postoperative cognitive dysfunction cannot be established, the first remains a risk factor for the development of the later [63]. The incidence of postoperative cognitive dysfunction in older people undergoing non-cardiac surgery remains around 12 to 20% at 3 months although there are limited data about the longer-term effects of postoperative delirium on cognitive impairment of the development of dementia [66]. A more recent hypothesis for postoperative cognitive dysfunction has been investigated through the NeuroVISION study, which concluded that 1 in 14 patients who undergo non-cardiac surgery aged 65 years and overdeveloped a perioperative covert stroke, and this was associated with an increased risk of postoperative delirium and cognitive decline at 1 year postoperatively [67]. Further research is warranted to establish management and preventative strategies to avoid the incidence of covert strokes in frail older people.

Discharge Planning

Transitional care and discharge planning of older people with frailty is a particularly important consideration for patients when they are ready to leave hospital post-surgery. These services are implemented through the multidisciplinary involvement of allied health professionals including physiotherapists, occupational therapists, social workers and community teams. The aims are to ensure that patients leave the hospital sooner, reduce the rate of readmission and to improve their short- and medium-term outcomes. The most common models of care in the United Kingdom include: early supported discharge and home-based intermediate care, community-based rehabilitation and discharge to assess [68]. Early supported discharge enables patients to return home with therapy services that support them within their own home and provide support around activities of daily living. Community-based rehabilitation provides patients who have extended stays in the hospital or require a period of convalescence with the means to regain their physical function prior to returning to their home. A discharge-to-assess model of care has several pathways and has recently been championed to include providing a period of rehabilitation and assessment within bed-based settings of care homes for a period of time in order for long-terms discharge plans to be completed by a multidisciplinary team [69]. All of these models are delivered by a multidisciplinary team of professionals, are based on comprehensive assessment, and include a shared decision-making process with patients and families which may not always be possible and feasible in an acute setting.

Perioperative Programmes in the United Kingdom

In recognition of the need to address the growing complexity of older people undergoing surgery, surgical liaison is a developing field in the United Kingdom and was first developed in 2003 at Guys and St Thomas' hospital in London [70]. The main pillar of the perioperative care of older people undergoing surgery (POPS) model of care is a comprehensive geriatric assessment; through this process, the older surgical patient is assessed and optimised in preparation for surgery, while taking into consideration underlying chronic comorbidities, frailty and other geriatric syndromes [71]. This has been shown to reduce the length of stay, improve postoperative outcomes, and reduce intensive care utilisation through shared decision-making with a multidisciplinary team [71, 72].

POPS pre-assessment clinics are most effective when run through a multidisciplinary model with the involvement of anaesthetists, surgeons, geriatricians and allied healthcare professionals with the aim of optimising frail older patients who require specialist input due to underlying cancer or complex surgical needs [73]. Often, patients are seen by clinicians in the first instance, and subsequently referred to other services such as a dietician or therapist to meet any specific goals prior to surgery. There are various configurations of such services in the United Kingdom although the most common scenario is of joint assessment between geriatricians and anaesthetists. The main aims of such clinics are to provide a comprehensive assessment of the patient, assess the risks of surgery, identify optimisation opportunities using recognised evidence-based guidelines, and produce an individualised care plan tailored for the patient prior to surgery [74]. In some patients, these shared care plans may include a prehabilitation programme; which includes smoking and alcohol cessation advice, correction of preoperative malnutrition, cardiac and pulmonary rehabilitation, a tiered physical exercise programme as well as psychological support in preparation for surgery [75].

These shared care plans cover preoperative, intraoperative and postoperative management, are discussed with the patient, and inform all aspects of perioperative care. The different skills and experience that the anaesthetist and geriatrician bring to the table underpin clear plans about the mode of anaesthesia, pain management, delirium recognition, the management of postoperative complications and escalation of care. This advanced planning minimises any crisis situations throughout the perioperative pathway [47, 74, 76]. While the goal of the POPS clinic is to assess and develop a plan for preoperative optimisation, there is increasing recognition that there may be some patients who have severe frailty and are unfit for surgery; and although this is a complex and often difficult discussion, there is a moral obligation as clinicians to inform patients about these perspectives and to strive for shared decisions about the appropriateness of surgery, alternative treatments or move towards of palliation rather than cure [21]. The ideal POPS service should also include attendance and participation at surgical and anaesthetic governance meetings to ensure holistic care is delivered and to collaborate across specialities through research and quality improvement; this will promote better decision-making, guideline development, and enable more innovative pathways of care to improve postoperative outcomes in older patients with frailty [77, 78].

Traditional practices of perioperative care such as prolonged fasting, slow return to eating and mechanical bowel preparation are associated with increased pathophysiological stress on the body in the perioperative period surgery resulting in increased mortality and morbidity [15, 79]. This has led to the development of Enhanced Recovery After Surgery (ERAS) programmes. ERAS is a complex multimodal intervention with over 20 interventions spread across the surgical journey; key components include medical optimisation, the reduction or cessation of alcohol and tobacco consumption, active intraoperative warming, and opioid-sparing techniques with goal-directed perioperative fluid management, early ambulation, nutrition, multimodal management of pain and nausea, and early discharge [80]. ERAS was first developed in Denmark in the late 1990s by a colorectal surgeon, Henrik Kehlet, and subsequently introduced to the United Kingdom in the early 2000s with variable uptake of the programme; however, in 2011, 14 sites across the National Health Service with the support of the Department of Health signed up to the Enhanced Recovery Partnership Programme and has since become embedded in routine perioperative care across the United Kingdom [81, 82].

Although the development of ERAS predated that of POPS, the two have evolved and emerged as two separate entities of perioperative care for patients. ERAS is a paradigm shift in surgical practice for all surgical patients and POPS focusing on improving surgical outcomes of older people undergoing surgery, particularly those more vulnerable and potentially with frailty. While the principles of POPS and ERAS are similar considering their holistic approach and focus on improving surgical outcomes, the ERAS pathway is more generic and can be delivered by trained nurses and allied healthcare professionals across the pathway of care for all surgical patients undergoing surgery. On the other hand, POPS requires additional input from specialist geriatricians to identify and optimise the heterogenous and more complex group of older patients (often with a significant degree of vulnerability or frailty) undergoing surgery [83]. The nuanced approach of POPS enables early identification of complications in older patients with frailty, such as postoperative delirium. It also provides continuity of care that enables more clear clinical decision-making. Ultimately, elements of ERAS programmes can be combined with POPS to provide a comprehensive high-quality care for older people undergoing surgery.

Conclusion

The quality of perioperative care in older cancer patients with frailty has significant implications on surgical outcomes and the delivery of such care has developed over the last few decades to provide a more holistic, multidisciplinary and patient-centred approach. However, there are several challenges that need to be overcome, such as workforce planning, improved training, and the involvement of primary care. All these need to be addressed to streamline and standardise pathways to optimise the perioperative process for cancer surgery. Culture change and organisational investment will be crucial to expand these services to ensure that older cancer patients with frailty will have a more equitable and equal access to the care that they need. It is clear that a paradigm shift is taking place in how cancer surgery in older patients is managed. This radical transformation brings innovative models of care to address the unmet needs of these patients, and it provides equitable care through the seamless integration of services for those more complex older patients.

References

1. ONU. World population prospects 2019 [Internet]. Department of Economic and Social Affairs. World Population Prospects 2019. Available from http://www.ncbi.nlm.nih.gov/pubmed/12283219
2. Fowler AJ, Abbott TE, Prowle RPR. Age of patients undergoing surgery. Br J Surg. 2019;106(8):1012–8.
3. Clegg A, Young J, Iliffe S, Olde Rikkert MGM, Rockwood K. Frailty in older people summary. Lancet. 2013;381(9868):752–62.
4. Hewitt J, Long S, Carter B, Bach S, McCarthy K, Clegg A. The prevalence of frailty and its association with clinical outcomes in general surgery: a systematic review and meta-analysis. Age Ageing. 2018;47(6):793–800.
5. Hale M, Shah S, Clegg A. Frailty, inequality and resilience. Clin Med (Lond). 2019;19(3):219–23.
6. Rockwood K, Minitski A. Limits to deficint accumulation in elderly people. Mech Ageing Dev. 2006;127(5):494–6.
7. Hollinghurst J, Fry R, Akbari A, Clegg A, Lyons RA, Watkins A, et al. External validation of the electronic frailty index using the population of Wales within the secure anonymised information linkage databank. Age Ageing. 2019;48(6):922–6.
8. Panayi AC, Orkaby AR, Sakthivel D, Endo Y, Varon D, Roh D, et al. Impact of frailty on outcomes in surgical patients: a systematic review and meta-analysis. Am J Surg. 2019;218(2):393–400.
9. Shahrokni A, Tin A, Korc-Grodzicki B. Development and evaluation of a new frailty index for older surgical patients with cancer. JAMA Netw Open. 2019;2(5):e193545.
10. Kow AW. Prehabilitation and its role in geriatric surgery. Ann Acad Med Singap. 2019;48(11):386–92.
11. Ethun CG, Bilen MA, Jani AB, Maithel SK, Ogan K, Master VA. Frailty and cancer: implications for oncology surgery, medical oncology, and radiation oncology. CA Cancer J Clin. 2017;67(5):362–77.
12. Strøm C, Rasmussen LSSJ. Practical management of anaesthesia in the elderly. Drugs Aging. 2016;33(11):765–77.

13. Pilka R, Marek R, Adam T, Kudela M, Ondrová D, Neubert D, et al. Systemic inflammatory response after open, laparoscopic and robotic surgery in endometrial cancer patients. Anticancer Res. 2016;36(6):2909–22.
14. Gould TH, Grace K, Thorne GTM. Effect of thoracic epidural anaesthesia on colonic blood flow. Br J Anaesth. 2002;89(3):446–51.
15. McEvoy M, Gupta R, Koepke E, Feldheiser A, Michard F, et al. Perioperative Quality Initiative (POQI)-3 consensus statement on postoperative blood pressure: risk and outcomes for elective surgery. Br J Anaesth. 2019;122(5):563–74.
16. Sessler DI, Pei L, Huang Y, Fleischmann E, Marhofer P, Kurz A, et al. Recurrence of breast cancer after regional or general anaesthesia: a randomised controlled trial. Lancet. 2019;394(10211):1807–15.
17. Hughes SG. Prescribing for the elderly patient: why do we need to exercise caution? Br J Clin Pharmacol. 1998;46(6):531–3.
18. Mangoni AA, Jackson SHD. Age-related changes in pharmacokinetics and pharmacodynamics: basic principles and practical applications. Br J Clin Pharmacol. 2004;57(1):6–14.
19. Strøm C, Rasmussen LS, Steinmetz J. Practical management of anaesthesia in the elderly. Drugs Aging. 2016;33(11):765–77.
20. May SM, Abbott TEF, Del Arroyo AG, Reyes A, Martir G, Stephens RCM, et al. MicroRNA signatures of perioperative myocardial injury after elective noncardiac surgery: prospective observational mechanistic cohort study. Br J Anaesth. 2020;125(5):661–71.
21. Alam A, Hana Z, Jin Z, Suen KCMD. Surgery, neuroinflammation and cognitive impairment. EBioMedicine. 2018;37:547–56.
22. Buggy DJWT. Can anaesthetic-analgesic technique during cancer surgery of curative intent influence recurrence or metastasis? An update. Br J Anaesth. 2019;126(6):e525–6.
23. Lane-Fall M. Outcomes measures and risk adjustment. Int Anesthesiol Clin. 2013;51(4):10. https://doi.org/10.1097/AIA.0b013e3182a70a52.
24. NHS. New care models risk stratification: learning and impact study, 2017.
25. Dera D. Risk stratification: a two-step process for identifying your sickest patients. Am Acad Fam Phys. 2019.
26. Protopapa KL, Simpson JC, Smith NCE, Moonesinghe SR. Development and validation of the surgical outcome risk tool (SORT). Br J Surg. 2014;101(13):1774–83.
27. Hornor MA, Ma M, Zhou L, Cohen ME, Rosenthal RA, Russell MM, et al. Enhancing the American College of Surgeons NSQIP surgical risk calculator to predict geriatric outcomes. J Am Coll Surg. 2020;230(1):88–100.e1. https://doi.org/10.1016/j.jamcollsurg.2019.09.017.
28. Eamer G, Al-Amoodi MJH, Holroyd-Leduc J, Rolfson DB, Warkentin LM, Khadaroo RG. Review of risk assessment tools to predict morbidity and mortality in elderly surgical patients. Am J Surg. 2018;216(3):585–94. https://doi.org/10.1016/j.amjsurg.2018.04.006.
29. Kim S, Brooks AK, LG. Preoperative assessment of the older surgical patient: honing in on geriatric syndromes. Clin Interv Aging. 2015;10:13–27.
30. Kumar A, Srinivastava U. Role of routine laboratory investigations in preoperative evaluation. J Anaesthesiol Clin Pharmacol. 2011;27(2):174–9.
31. Wijeysundera DN, Pearse RM, Shulman MA, Abbott TEF, Torres E, Croal BL, et al. Measurement of exercise tolerance before surgery (METS) study: a protocol for an international multicentre prospective cohort study of cardiopulmonary exercise testing prior to major non-cardiac surgery. BMJ Open. 2016;6(3):e010359.
32. Wijeysundera DN, Pearse RM, Shulman MA, Abbott TEF, Torres E, Ambosta A, et al. Assessment of functional capacity before major non-cardiac surgery: an international, prospective cohort study. Lancet. 2018;391(10140):2631–40.
33. Carli F, Baldini GFL. Redesigning the preoperative clinic. JAMA Surg. 2021;156(2):191–2.
34. Partridge JSL, Harari D, Martin FC, Peacock JL, Bell R, Mohammed A, et al. Randomized clinical trial of comprehensive geriatric assessment and optimization in vascular surgery. Br J Surg. 2017;104(6):679–87.
35. Deshpande R, Asch WS, Malinis M. Frailty and perioperative outcomes. Curr Anesthesiol Rep. 2018;8(2):225–31.

36. Rocha V, Marmelo F, Leite-Moreira A, Moreira-Gonçalves D. Clinical utility of frailty scales for the prediction of postoperative complications: systematic review and meta-analysis. Rev Port Cir Cardiotorac Vasc. 2017;24(3–4):132.
37. Rolfson DB, Majumdar SR, Tsuyuki RT, Adeel Tahir KR. Validity and reliability of the Edmonton frail scale. Age Ageing. 2006;35(5):526–9.
38. Clegg A, Young J, Iliffe S. Marcel Olde Rikkert and KR. Frailty in elderly people. Lancet. 2013;381(9868):752–62.
39. Mcisaac DI, Harris EP, Hladkowicz E, Moloo H, Lalu MM, Bryson GL, et al. Prospective comparison of preoperative predictive performance between 3 leading frailty instruments. Anesth Analg. 2020;131(1):263–72.
40. The British Geriatrics Society. Fit for frailty: consensus best practice guidance for the care of older people living with frailty in community and outpatient settings. 2014;26 p.
41. Rockwood K, Song X, MacKnight C, Bergman H, Hogan DB, McDowell I, et al. A global clinical measure of fitness and frailty in elderly people. CMAJ. 2005;173(5):489–95.
42. McIsaac DI, Macdonald DB, Aucoin SD. Frailty for perioperative clinicians: a narrative review. Anesth Analg. 2020;130(6):1450–60.
43. Faller JW, do Nascimento Pereira D, de Souza S, Nampo FK, de Souza Orlandi F, Matumoto S. Instruments for the detection of frailty syndrome in older adults: a systematic review. PLoS One. 2019;14(4):1–23.
44. Levy N, Grocott MPW, Carli F. Patient optimisation before surgery: a clear and present challenge in peri-operative care. Anaesthesia. 2019;74:3–6.
45. Gordon AL, Evans BJ, Dhesi J. The physician's role in perioperative management of older patients undergoing surgery. Clin Med (Lond). 2017;17(4):357–9.
46. Milder DA, Pillinger NL, Kam PCA. The role of prehabilitation in frail surgical patients: a systematic review. Acta Anaesthesiol Scand. 2018;62(10):1356–66.
47. Chan SP, Ip KY, Irwin MG. Peri-operative optimisation of elderly and frail patients: a narrative review. Anaesthesia. 2019;74(1):80–9.
48. Cheung JTK, Yu R, Wu Z, Wong SYS, Woo J. Geriatric syndromes, multimorbidity, and disability overlap and increase healthcare use among older Chinese. BMC Geriatr. 2018;18(1):1–8.
49. Welch C, Hassan-Smith ZK, Greig CA, Lord JM, Jackson TA. Acute sarcopenia secondary to hospitalisation - an emerging condition affecting older adults. Aging Dis. 2018;9(1):151–64.
50. Mohd Nawi SN, Khow KS, Lim WS, Yu SC. Screening tools for sarcopenia in community-dwellers: a scoping review. Ann Acad Med Singap. 2019;48(7):201–16.
51. Dolan DR, Knight KA, Maguire S, Moug SJ. The relationship between sarcopenia and survival at 1 year in patients having elective colorectal cancer surgery. Tech Coloproctol. 2019;23(9):877–85. https://doi.org/10.1007/s10151-019-02072-0.
52. Kuwada K, Kuroda S, Kikuchi S, Yoshida R, Nishizaki M, Kagawa S, et al. Sarcopenia and comorbidity in gastric cancer surgery as a useful combined factor to predict eventual death from other causes. Ann Surg Oncol. 2018;25(5):1160–6. https://doi.org/10.1245/s10434-018-6354-4.
53. Cruz-Jentoft AJ, Bahat G, Bauer J, Boirie Y, Bruyère O, Cederholm T, et al. Sarcopenia: revised European consensus on definition and diagnosis. Age Ageing. 2019;48(1):16–31.
54. Martone AM, Marzetti E, Calvani R, Picca A, Tosato M, Bernabei R, et al. Assessment of sarcopenia: from clinical practice to research. J Gerontol Geriatr. 2019;67(1):39–45.
55. Han A, Bokshan S, Marcaccio S, DePasse J, Daniels A. Diagnostic criteria and clinical outcomes in sarcopenia research: a literature review. J Clin Med. 2018;7(4):70.
56. Robinson SM, Reginster JY, Rizzoli R, Shaw SC, Kanis JA, Bautmans I, et al. Does nutrition play a role in the prevention and management of sarcopenia? Clin Nutr. 2018;37(4):1121–32.
57. Malafarina V, Reginster JY, Cabrerizo S, Bruyère O, Kanis JA, Alfredo Martinez J, et al. Nutritional status and nutritional treatment are related to outcomes and mortality in older adults with hip fracture. Nutrients. 2018;10(5):1–26.
58. Ohkura Y, Haruta S, Tanaka T, Ueno M, Udagawa H. Effectiveness of postoperative elemental diet (Elental®) in elderly patients after gastrectomy. World J Surg Oncol [Internet]. 2016;14(1):1–6. https://doi.org/10.1186/s12957-016-1013-3.

59. Benton K, Thomson I, Isenring E, Mark Smithers B, Agarwal E. An investigation into the nutritional status of patients receiving an enhanced recovery after surgery (ERAS) protocol versus standard care following oesophagectomy. Support Care Cancer. 2018;26(6):2057–62.
60. Roberts HC, Lim SER, Cox NJ, Ibrahim K. The challenge of managing undernutrition in older people with frailty. Nutrients. 2019;11(4):1–17.
61. Volkert D, Beck AM, Cederholm T, Cruz-Jentoft A, Goisser S, Hooper L, et al. ESPEN guideline on clinical nutrition and hydration in geriatrics. Clin Nutr. 2019;38(1):10–47. https://doi.org/10.1016/j.clnu.2018.05.024.
62. Vlisides P, Avidan M. Recent advances in preventing and managing postoperative delirium. F1000Res. 2019;8:1–10.
63. Aldecoa C, Bettelli G, Bilotta F, Sanders RD, Audisio R, Borozdina A, et al. European Society of Anaesthesiology evidence-based and consensus-based guideline on postoperative delirium. Eur J Anaesthesiol. 2017;34(4):192–214.
64. Mosk CA, van Vugt JLA, de Jonge H, Witjes CDM, Buettner S, Ijzermans JNM, et al. Low skeletal muscle mass as a risk factor for postoperative delirium in elderly patients undergoing colorectal cancer surgery. Clin Interv Aging. 2018;13:2097–106.
65. Hempenius L, Slaets JPJ, van Asselt DZB, Schukking J, de Bock GH, T., van Wiggers BL. Interventions to prevent postoperative delirium in elderly cancer patients should be targeted at those undergoing nonsuperficial surgery with special attention to the cognitive impaired patients. Eur J Surg Oncol. 2015;41(1):28–33.
66. Evered LA, Silbert BS. Postoperative cognitive dysfunction and noncardiac surgery. Anesth Analg. 2018;127(2):496–505.
67. Mrkobrada M, Chan MTV, Cowan D, Campbell D, Wang CY, Torres D, et al. Perioperative covert stroke in patients undergoing non-cardiac surgery (NeuroVISION): a prospective cohort study. Lancet. 2019;394(10203):1022–9.
68. Nair S, Oliver D, Cracknell A. Meeting the needs of older patients. [Internet]. In J North (Author), M McKee, S Merkur, N Edwards, E Nolte (Eds), The changing role of the hospital in European Health Systems (European Observatory on Health Systems and PoliciesACN Bold Voices. Cambridge: Cambridge University Press; 2020. 85–119 p. Available from: http://search.ebscohost.com/login.aspx?direct=true&db=c8h&AN=119171688&lang=pt-br&site=ehost-live
69. England N. Hospital discharge service: Policy Operating Model. 2020.
70. Harari D, Hopper A, Dhesi J, Babic-Illman G, Lockwood L, Martin F. Proactive care of older people undergoing surgery ('POPS'): designing, embedding, evaluating and funding a comprehensive geriatric assessment service for older elective surgical patients. Age Ageing. 2007;36(2):190–6.
71. Partridge J, Sbai M, Dhesi J. Proactive care of older people undergoing surgery. Aging Clin Exp Res. 2018;30(3):253–7. https://doi.org/10.1007/s40520-017-0879-4.
72. Braude P, Goodman A, Elias T, Babic-Illman G, Challacombe B, Harari D, et al. Evaluation and establishment of a ward-based geriatric liaison service for older urological surgical patients: proactive care of older people undergoing surgery (POPS)-urology. BJU Int. 2017;120(1):123–9.
73. Partridge JSL, Collingridge G, Gordon AL, Martin FC, Harari D, Dhesi JK. Where are we in perioperative medicine for older surgical patients? A UK survey of geriatric medicine delivered services in surgery. Age Ageing. 2014;43(5):721–4.
74. Dhesi JK, Swart M. Specialist pre-operative assessment clinics. Anaesthesia. 2016;71:3–8.
75. Durrand J, Singh SJ, Danjoux G. CMJv19n6-Durrand.indd. Clin Med (Northfield, IL). 2017;17(6):458–64.
76. Dhesi J. Setting up a proactive service to make surgery safer for older people. 2013;1–6.
77. Rogerson A, Partridge JS, Dhesi JK. Perioperative medicine for older people. Ann Acad Med Singap. 2019;48(11):376–81.

78. Partridge JSL, Harari D, Martin FC, Dhesi JK. The impact of pre-operative comprehensive geriatric assessment on postoperative outcomes in older patients undergoing scheduled surgery: a systematic review. Anaesthesia. 2014;69(suppl 1):8–16.
79. Pędziwiatr M, Mavrikis J, Witowski J, Adamos A, Major P, Nowakowski M, et al. Current status of enhanced recovery after surgery (ERAS) protocol in gastrointestinal surgery. Med Oncol. 2018;35(6):1–8. https://doi.org/10.1007/s12032-018-1153-0.
80. Melnyk M, Casey RG, Black P, Koupparis AJ. Enhanced recovery after surgery (eras) protocols: time to change practice? J Can Urol Assoc. 2011;5(5):342–8.
81. Paton F, Chambers D, Wilson P, Eastwood A, Craig D, Fox D, et al. Effectiveness and implementation of enhanced recovery after surgery programmes: a rapid evidence synthesis. BMJ Open. 2014;4(7):e005015.
82. Jones C, Kelliher L. Enhanced recovery after surgery: past, present and future. Dig Med Res. 2019;2:19.
83. Bettelli G, Maggi S. Decision-making about surgery in the elderly. Aging Clin Exp Res. 2018;30(3):225–7. https://doi.org/10.1007/s40520-018-0915-z.

Chapter 14
Radiotherapy and Systemic Anti-Cancer Treatment in Older Adults with Cancer and Frailty

Anita O'Donovan, Capucine Baldini, and Nicolò Matteo Luca Battisti

Introduction

Cancer is a disease of older individuals [1]. Nonetheless, they are less likely to receive standard anticancer treatments compared with younger adults [2, 3]. Concerns involve the higher prevalence of frailty with increased risk of adverse events, morbidity and mortality, although patient and physician preferences are also important drivers [4]. Chronological age is a poor descriptor of the complexity of older adults with cancer, as they are a highly heterogeneous population [5]. Treatment benefits, toxicities and their impact on quality of life (QoL) and functional status should be considered in the context of patient preferences, estimated life expectancy, age-related organ function decline and competing risks of morbidity and mortality.

Frailty is a consequence of age-related decline in many physiological systems and vulnerability to stressors [6]. Age-related changes in organ function, along with alterations in drug absorption, distribution and excretion, increase the risk of adverse outcomes from treatment in older adults [7, 8]. Moreover, comorbidities are

A. O'Donovan (✉)
Applied Radiation Therapy Trinity (ARTT), School of Medicine, Trinity College Dublin, Dublin, Ireland
e-mail: anita.odonovan@tcd.ie

C. Baldini
Drug Development Department (DITEP), Gustave Roussy, Université Paris-Saclay, Villejuif, France
e-mail: Capucine.BALDINI@gustaveroussy.fr

N. M. L. Battisti
Department of Medicine, The Royal Marsden NHS Foundation Trust, Sutton, London, UK

Breast Cancer Research Division, The Institute of Cancer Research, Sutton, London, UK
e-mail: Nicolo.Battisti@rmh.nhs.uk

F. Gomes (ed.), *Frailty in Older Adults with Cancer*,
https://doi.org/10.1007/978-3-030-89162-6_14

prevalent in this age group and may affect the prognosis and risk of toxicity of anti-cancer therapies. Older adults, particularly those with frailty, are underrepresented in clinical trials [9]. In fact, even when older patients are included, the results may not be extrapolated to the entire age group, as those with significant comorbidities, functional problems and renal, hepatic or bone marrow impairment are usually excluded. Thus, the applicability of existing data and guidelines is questionable [10].

There is no accepted standard definition of frailty and several measurement tools exist. Multiple factors impact frailty, functional status and physiologic reserve among older adults, while age, comorbidities and disability may be associated with frailty but do not necessarily establish it as a diagnosis [11]. Nonetheless, fitness is a continuum, whereby at one end fit individuals with no functional limitations can benefit from standard treatments, while those with severe frailty have limited ability to withstand cancer treatment. A comprehensive geriatric assessment (CGA) is the standard of care to address the unique complexity of this population [12–14].

CGA is a multidisciplinary diagnostic process evaluating domains relevant to the wellbeing of older adults, such as comorbidities, functional status, cognition, nutrition, mood, social support, polypharmacy and geriatric syndromes [15]. There are a range of benefits from using CGA in older patients with cancer, including predicting functional decline, estimating survival, assisting treatment decisions, detecting issues neglected by routine assessments, improving mental health, symptom control and communication [16–21]. Recent randomised clinical trials have demonstrated the CGA's positive impact on chemotherapy toxicity, QoL, hospitalisations and completion of advanced directives [22–25]. A key benefit is the ability to predict complications and side effects from anticancer treatments [26–32].

The focus of this chapter is on the role and safety of radiation therapy (RT) and systemic anticancer therapies, in the context of older cancer patients with frailty.

Radiation Therapy

General Considerations

Approximately 50% of all cancer patients require RT as part of their disease management [33]. The use of RT in older adults should be discussed, based on the risks and benefits of treatment, the patient's level of fitness or frailty and personal preferences [34]. RT is an effective, albeit underutilised [2, 3], treatment for cancer in older adults with frailty, especially for those deemed surgically inoperable or for whom systemic therapy poses too great a risk [35]. Its underutilisation is exacerbated by a relative paucity of research in older patients with frailty undergoing RT [36], and therefore toxicity data are limited. Compared to other treatment modalities, there is often a significant burden of additional travel involved in order to receive RT, which is a consideration for those who are socially frail. Often, travel to regional centres is required over a period of weeks, depending on the treatment regime. Another requirement is that patients have the ability to lie still for treatment each day, which can be a challenge for those with moderate or advanced dementia. In such cases, the RT environment can be very distressing and the patient can often become very agitated. Detailed guidelines on how to best adapt care for people with dementia in the RT setting have been produced in recent years, reflecting a growing need to address such care needs in clinical practice [37].

As RT is a localised treatment, its effects are specific to the site that is treated [38–40]. Conventional external beam RT uses high energy X-rays to deliver as high a dose as possible to the tumour/treatment area, in a carefully targeted manner, in order to spare as much surrounding normal tissue as possible. This balance is referred to as the "therapeutic ratio" and is considerably enhanced with modern day RT techniques. While RT leads to cellular DNA damage of both tumour cells and normal tissue, tumour cells have less ability to repair and recover, compared to normal tissue. The total RT dose is delivered over a number of daily sessions (Monday to Friday usually), known as fractions. The purpose of fractionation is to allow recovery of normal tissue between successive treatments [15].

In clinical practice, the therapeutic ratio is achieved by giving the greatest possible dose to the tumour (or surgical bed/area at risk of recurrence), while keeping the dose to the surrounding normal tissue as low as possible [41]. This is often a delicate balance when treating areas adjacent to sensitive structures, but it is more achievable using modern RT technology. Depending on the treatment area, different structures have varying tolerances to radiation. The structure of tissues and organs plays a critical role in the response to RT, and this response may depend on the existing reserve capacity of the organ in question, which is a consideration in those patients with frailty and poor reserve capacity.

Factors Determining RT Toxicity

Toxicity depends on various factors, including the overall dose delivered, the dose per fraction, the overall treatment time, treatment volume and site irradiated, additional treatments such as surgery or chemotherapy, as well as individual patient factors, i.e. individual radiosensitivity and certain genetic conditions. The patient's own physiologic reserve capacity and/or frailty is also a consideration for compliance with RT treatment schedules. However, the evidence base supporting the influence of patient frailty in RT is much less robust, as it has not been studied extensively [42]. Ultimately, there are no conclusive data to suggest frailty impacts RT toxicity.

The side effects of RT may be acute (up to 90 days following the start of RT) or late (>90 days after the onset of RT). The inflammatory response during RT causes acute effects, which occur in rapidly proliferating tissues, such as the gastrointestinal tract, skin and the haematopoietic system [43]. It is important to note that the latency period, or time of clinical manifestation of acute side effects varies, depends on tissue type and the time required for precursor cells to proliferate and form mature cells [44]. This latency period can be 7–10 days after the initiation of RT and it has a cumulative effect up to and in the immediate aftermath of RT completion.

For a patient with frailty, this might require additional support in the community, but often general physicians are ill-equipped to deal with RT-related toxicity [45, 46].

Acute toxicity depends on overall treatment duration, therefore gaps in treatment may be introduced for some cancer sites [47–49], usually 2–3 weeks, especially for patients with frailty to help cope with toxicity. However, this may compromise tumour control in certain sites e.g., a squamous cell carcinoma of head and neck. This is often recognised as a necessary trade-off in terms of the risk-benefit ratio of the patient's overall management. Ultimately, acute reactions of RT are not to be underestimated for their impact on patients with frailty.

Late toxicity, on the other hand, depends on the dose per fraction delivered, with higher doses contributing more damage to underlying tissue [50]. Late side effects are irreversible, and thus may have a substantial impact on the patient's long-term QOL. Therefore, due consideration is given to these in the planning phase of RT, and there are evidence-based dose constraints applied, in order to mitigate their effect on patients.

Toxicity During RT

Fatigue is a significant issue for patients undergoing RT [51] and can result in a reduction in usual activities. This may further exacerbate existing frailty and lead to physical deconditioning due to a lack of exercise [52, 53]. The benefits of physical activity are especially relevant in an older population at high risk for functional decline, and recent research has focused on the importance of exercise prescription [54–56]. Fatigue may also result from travel to RT each day, especially if patients are required to travel long distances to access care. In general, acute toxicity eases within 3–4 weeks of treatment completion, however fatigue may be more long-lasting.

RT is a localised treatment and therefore the side effects are dependent on the site irradiated, in combination with the factors mentioned previously in relation to individual and dosimetric factors [57].

Skin reactions or radiation dermatitis with modern day RT techniques are often mild, but can be more severe in superficial sites, e.g. anal and vulvar cancer, head and neck cancer, particularly when RT is combined with systemic therapies. Topical skin agents are commonly employed for prophylaxis and management during treatment [58, 59], with more specialised dressings required in cases of high-grade dermatitis.

Mucositis and dry mouth can result from RT to the head and neck region, and patients may also develop an altered sense of taste which can decrease appetite and reduced nutritional input. Also, there is an increased risk of mucositis in older patients [60], which can lead to considerable pain and discomfort. Other side effects include secondary dysphagia and odynophagia, thus nutritional monitoring is especially vital for those at risk of malnutrition, particularly older patients with frailty.

For CNS treatments, alopecia in the irradiated area, lethargy, somnolence and headache are common side effects of RT. For thoracic irradiation, pneumonitis, oesophagitis and dyspnoea are relatively common. Gastrointestinal effects include nausea, vomiting, proctitis and diarrhoea for those receiving radiation to the lower abdomen and pelvis. Older patients with frailty, in particular, need to be closely monitored during treatment, as untreated diarrhoea can lead to dehydration and electrolyte disturbance quite quickly. Genitourinary side effects include urinary frequency, dysuria and nocturia. Those with poor existing reserve capacity may experience more discomfort from RT, e.g. those with chronic respiratory conditions may experience worse thoracic side effects during RT. However, overall, RT appears to be well tolerated [38].

Late toxicity manifests much later, sometimes years after treatment has ended and is irreversible. Yet, this may not be an important factor in decision-making for those older cancer patients with frailty and a limited life expectancy [57].

Modern RT Techniques and Their Role in Patients with Frailty

The manner in which toxicity may be reduced, for those who have frailty, is by targeting the specific factors mentioned previously, i.e. volume of tissue irradiated, dose/fractionation and additional therapies, and aiming to mitigate their effects through the use of specific technologies or techniques. In reality, RT has a whole host of mechanisms at its disposal to enhance its toxicity profile or make treatment more accessible to those with frailty.

Dose Fractionation

Hypofractionated RT, i.e. the use of larger doses per fraction than the conventional 2Gy, with less fractions overall, can be particularly useful to reduce the overall length of treatment. It is increasingly considered in older patients with frailty who have difficulties with transportation, particularly those with social frailty. It is also commonly employed in palliative care [61] or for those with dementia in order to limit the upheaval to daily routine [62]. A higher dose per fraction can increase the risk of late effects, which, as previously mentioned, are irreversible. However, there are certain sites, e.g. breast cancer [63] and prostate cancer [64], where its use has been proven to be efficacious for all patients, without significant toxicity. Hypofractionation can limit the additional burden of travel to the RT department and offer greater convenience. There are many examples of its use in those who are older and with frailty, many of which were adopted during the COVID-19 pandemic [65, 66], e.g. glioblastoma multiforme (GBM). A treatment regime of 25 Gy in 5 treatments has been shown to be non-inferior to 40Gy in 15 treatments [67]. Other examples include the use of short course RT (1 week) over long course chemoradiation in locally advanced resectable rectal cancer [68], the FAST-forward regime, of

26 Gy in 5 fractions (1 week), for early breast cancer [63], moderate (20 fractions) [64] and ultra (5 fractions) [69] hypofractionation in prostate cancer. More detailed information on potentially useful regimes are discussed in the COVID-19 literature review of guidelines by Thomson et al. [70].

Looking to the future, recent RT studies incorporating frailty assessment have allocated patients to RT treatment arms based on CGA. The ELAN RT trial is currently investigating the non-inferiority of hypofractionated RT compared to standard RT for unfit patients with head and neck cancer [71], based on CGA allocation. These studies have the potential to change practice, as patients with head and neck cancer are known to have more frailty than those with other cancers [72].

Intensity Modulated RT and Volumetric Modulated Arc Therapy

Modern day RT typically includes Intensity Modulated RT (IMRT) and Volumetric Modulated Arc Therapy (VMAT). IMRT and VMAT are techniques that allow more conformal treatment planning than traditional "3D conformal RT", its predecessor, with differing dose intensities across the target volume. These have greatly improved the ability to maximise the therapeutic ratio, and for those who have frailty, reduce the burden of toxicity making RT more tolerable [73, 74]. There is now a strong evidence base for the use of IMRT in reducing xerostomia in patients with head and neck cancer, in particular [75]. VMAT has reduced time on the couch for many treatments, again especially useful for those who have frailty and find it difficult to tolerate longer times.

Image-Guided RT

Older RT techniques necessitated the addition of additional safety margins during treatment planning, to allow for patient movement, the most significant of which occurs internally due to physiological changes within the body, e.g. breathing and rectal/bladder filling. This made it difficult to accurately reproduce the patient's treatment position each day, based on the initial planning scan, taken at a fixed time-point. However, newer technology has allowed more sophisticated on-treatment imaging to identify and correct for daily changes in physiology, to ensure more targeted treatment and to reduce the necessity of additional margins which result in more damage to surrounding normal tissue. This is called "image-guided RT" (IGRT), which combined with IMRT and VMAT offers an enhanced treatment for the person with frailty by reducing acute and late toxicity.

IGRT has also allowed the development of "adaptive RT". This takes into account of tumour shrinkage and internal changes during a course of RT and adapts the treatment plan accordingly, guided by on-treatment imaging, using a variety of approaches [76]. It is particularly useful in sites such as bladder cancer [77].

Brachytherapy

Brachytherapy is used alone or in combination with external beam RT to treat a variety of cancers including gynaecological cancers, prostate cancer, rectal cancer and skin cancer [74, 78]. Brachytherapy is also a very localised treatment, whereby a radioactive source is applied adjacent to (intracavitary) or directly into (interstitial) tissue (sometimes feasible under local anaesthetic). The benefits of brachytherapy include its steep dose gradient, with a sharp reduction in radiation dose from the tumour to surrounding normal tissue. Therefore, much higher doses can be delivered, without additional toxicity. Again, the benefit for older patients with frailty is that the course of treatment is much shorter.

Stereotactic RT

Alternatively, patients with frailty may benefit from stereotactic body RT (SBRT), also called stereotactic ablative body radiotherapy (SABR), with fewer hospital visits and potentially less toxicity [79]. SBRT allows a very high radiation dose to be precisely delivered to a well-defined area, in a very short overall treatment duration (ultra-hypofractionation). It is a suitable alternative to surgery in those with early-stage NSCLC [80]. The use of SBRT is especially useful for those with frailty, in view of the limited number of fractions required, compared to conventional courses of RT and has revolutionised the care of this group who are often excluded from surgical approaches. Comparison of outcomes with surgical series is difficult given the selection bias, since SBRT candidates more often are frail, but it is known to be effective and well tolerated in older adults [81]. Good local control and similar toxicity has been demonstrated with SBRT in both patients with frailty and those without it [82, 83].

Magnetic Resonance-Guided Therapy

More recently, the magnetic resonance (MR)-linac has been introduced into clinical practice in some centres, which is a combination of a linear accelerator and an MR scanner [84]. MR-guided RT is an enhanced form of IGRT using MR, considered superior to the traditional CT-based IGRT, due to its better soft tissue visualisation and diagnostic quality image production during treatment delivery [85]. Its introduction has also allowed the possibility of daily adaption of RT fields, i.e. selecting the best treatment plan, from a number of options, which best suit the patient's internal anatomy on any particular day [86]. However, treatment times are longer than standard treatments, which may prove difficult for patients with frailty and caution must be exercised for those with pacemakers in place. Moreover, the clinical availability of MR-guided external beam RT is limited at present.

Proton Therapy

Proton therapy is a type of RT that uses protons rather than the standard X-rays (photon beams). Protons are positively charged particles that have several advantages over conventional photon beam RT, namely their so-called spread out Bragg peak characteristics, which, in contrast to conventional RT, facilitates a much lower exit dose [87]. This allows the deposition of dose precisely at the disease site, with a very well-defined range of penetration and rapid fall-off in dose in adjacent normal tissue. Studies estimate proton therapy could deliver approximately half of the RT dose to surrounding normal tissue, compared to photon beams [88], thus greatly enhancing the toxicity profile which is especially attractive for those older patients with frailty [89]. However, proton therapy centres are scarce in supply and expensive, limiting accessibility for most patients [90, 91]. The distance to the proton therapy centre, often entailing travel to another country, may be an even more significant deterrent for those older patients with frailty.

Systemic Therapy

Chemotherapy

There is much variation in the use of chemotherapy in older patients with cancer and the risk of under- and overtreatment is considerable [92]. Older adults with frailty present specific challenges that may substantially impact the efficacy and toxicity of cytotoxics. The aging process correlates with a gradual decline in the function of multiple organs which may reduce their physiologic reserve and affect the pharmacokinetics and pharmacodynamic systemic agents [7, 8]. A decline in the hepatic volume and blood flow may increase the drug concentrations for longer periods of time, although this usually requires dose adjustments only in the context of concurrent hepatic impairment due to the tumour or comorbidities. The glomerular filtration rate also diminishes with age, which increases the risk of dehydration and challenges the role of routine renal function measurements such as creatinine in this age group. However, this decline can also increase the peak drug levels and exposure to chemotherapy agents. The gradual decline in bone marrow reserve can also increase the chances of haematological toxicity and may frequently require dose modifications. The distribution of chemotherapy agents is also affected by a different body composition in older/frail individuals, including an increasing fat content and a decreasing intracellular water, although this does not usually require dose adjustments. Changes in the gastrointestinal motility and atrophy of the intestinal mucosa may also impact the absorption of drugs.

Comorbidities involving the functional reserve of kidneys, liver, bone marrow and cardiovascular system may also impact tolerance to chemotherapy in this population. Their presence frequently requires dose modifications or the use of primary prophylaxis with haematopoietic growth factors to minimise the risk of side effects

[93, 94]. For example, cardiovascular disease is more prevalent in older individuals and may amplify the risk of heart failure on anthracyclines or coronary artery vasospasm on fluoropyrimidines. Comorbid conditions are also associated with the risk of polypharmacy and harmful drug interactions, particularly via the cytochrome P450 system [95]. Potential toxicities of the different chemotherapy agents are listed in Table 14.1.

Concerns with QoL are also key aspects of decision-making for older adults with cancer, where they may well be more relevant compared with survival outcomes. Nonetheless, there is a substantial lack of evidence on the impact of chemotherapy on QoL. A recent study of older patients with early-stage breast cancer evaluated with baseline geriatric assessments documented a significant but temporary impact of chemotherapy on QoL domains [96].

Models based upon CGA have been developed to predict chemotherapy toxicity in this population (Table 14.2). Whilst none of these predictive tools have formally incorporated a frailty assessment, there are several other measured that may be surrogates of frailty. The Cancer and Aging Research Group (CARG) model includes age, type of cancer, the proposed chemotherapy regimen, renal and haematologic function, hearing and activity levels from the CGA (ability to take medications, physical activity, social activity) [29]. This approach was shown to be significantly better than clinician assessment of performance status for predicting chemotherapy toxicity. In an independent validation cohort including 250 patients ≥65 years, CARG score correlated with frequency of toxicities, with 37% of patients with low CARG scores experiencing chemotherapy-related toxicities versus 62% of those with medium and 70% of those with high CARG scores [28]. A specific chemotherapy toxicity tool for older patients with early-stage breast cancer has also been developed [97].

Investigators at the Moffitt Cancer Center developed a Chemotherapy Risk Assessment Scale for High age (CRASH) score to predict the risk of chemotherapy-related hematologic and nonhaematologic toxicity in older persons [26]. This model takes into account the specific chemotherapy regimen to be used, as well as laboratory parameters (creatinine, albumin, haemoglobin, lactate dehydrogenase, liver function tests) and assessments of functional, mental and nutritional status.

Recent trials have confirmed the positive impact of CGA specifically on chemotherapy toxicity. The GAP 70 cluster randomised study enrolled 718 patients aged ≥70 years with stage III-IV cancer and more than 1 impaired CGA domain other than polypharmacy and due to start a new chemotherapy regimen in 41 private oncology practices [25]. Recommendations based on geriatric assessment were sent to the primary oncologist by the investigators and outcomes compared versus usual care. The study documented a reduction in the rate of severe toxicities in the experimental arm compared with the standard arm (50.1% versus 71.0%), along with a reduction in non-haematological toxicities (31.8% versus 51.8%). The GAIN study enrolled 600 patients aged 65 years and older with solid tumours of any stage and due to initiate a new line of chemotherapy [22]. Patients were randomised to usual care plus geriatric assessment-driven interventions led by a nurse practitioner versus standard care following a baseline CGA. The investigators documented a reduction

Table 14.1 Chemotherapy toxicities according to class of agents

Class of agents	Organ/system	Toxicities
Anthracyclines	Bone marrow	Anaemia Neutropenia Thrombocytopenia
	Gastrointestinal	Emesis Mucositis
	Cardiovascular	LV systolic dysfunction
Taxanes	Bone marrow	Anaemia Neutropenia Thrombocytopenia
	Nervous	Sensory neuropathy
	Lungs	Pneumonitis
	Liver	Hepatotoxicity (increased ALP, AST, ALT)
	Musculoskeletal	Myalgia Arthralgia
Fluoropyrimidines	Bone marrow	Anaemia Neutropenia Thrombocytopenia
	Gastrointestinal	Emesis Mucositis Diarrhoea
	Skin	Hand-foot syndrome
	Cardiovascular	Coronary artery vasospasm
Platinum compounds	Bone marrow	Anaemia Neutropenia Thrombocytopenia
	Gastrointestinal	Emesis Mucositis Diarrhoea
	Kidney	Acute kidney injury Electrolyte disturbances
	Nervous	Sensory neuropathy Ototoxicity
Vinca alkaloids	Bone marrow	Anaemia Neutropenia Thrombocytopenia
	Gastrointestinal	Emesis Diarrhoea
	Nervous	Sensory neuropathy

in the rate of grade 3–5 chemotherapy-related toxicities (50% versus 60.4%). The INTEGERATE study enrolled 154 patients aged over 70 years with solid tumours or diffuse large B cell lymphoma, due to receive chemotherapy, targeted therapy or immunotherapy [23]. Patients were randomised to integrated oncogeriatric care involving a geriatrician-led CGA and guided management versus usual care. The study showed an improvement in QoL, along with less frequent emergency

Table 14.2 Chemotherapy toxicity prediction tools

A) Cancer and Aging Research Group (CARG) tool

Risk factors	**Points**			
	0	**1**	**2**	**3**
Age	<72 years		≥72 years	
Cancer type	Other		GI or GU	
Chemotherapy dose	Dose reduced		Standard dose	
No. of chemotherapy drugs	Mono-chemotherapy		Polychemotherapy	
Haemoglobin	≥11 g/dL (male) ≥10 g/dL (female)			<11 g/dL (male) <10 g/dL (female)
Creatinine clearance (Jeliffe, ideal weight)	≥34 mL/min			<34 mL/min
Hearing (with hearing aid, if needed)	Excellent or good		Fair, poor or totally deaf	
No. of falls in last 6 months	None			≥1
IADL: taking medications	Without help	With some help or completely unable		
MOS: Walking 1 block	Not limited at all		Limited a little or limited a lot	
MOS: Decreased social activity because of physical/emotional health	A little of the time or none of the time	Some of the time, Most of the time, or all the time		
TOTAL SCORE				
Jeliffe formula	$CrCl\left(\frac{mL}{min} \times 1.73m^2\right) = \frac{98 - 16 \times \left(\frac{age - 20}{20}\right)}{serum\ creatinine\left(\frac{mg}{dL}\right)}$ *CrCl is multiplied by 0.9 for female patients*			

Total Risk Score		**% risk of grade 3-5 adverse events**
Low	**0-3**	25%
	4-5	32%
Medium	**6-7**	50%
	8-9	54%
High	**10-11**	77%
	12-19	89%

(continued)

Tab. 14.2 (continued)

B) Chemotherapy Risk Assessment Scale for High-Age Patients (CRASH) Score

Chemotherapy risk (see CRASH points table)		
Haematologic risk factors		
Diastolic blood pressure (>72 = 1)		
IADL (<26 = 1)		
LDH (>459 = 1)		
Non-haematologic risk factors		
ECOG PS (1-2 = 1; 3-4 = 2)		
Mini Mental State Examination (<30 = 2)		
Mini Nutritional Assessment (<28 = 2)		
Haeme score		
Non-haeme score		
Combined score		

CRASH points		
0	**1**	**2**
Capecitabine 2g	Capecitabine 2.5g	5FU/LV (Roswell Park)
Cisplatin/pemetrexed	Carboplatin/gemcitabine AUC 4-6/1g d1,d8	5FU/LV (Mayo)
Dacarbazine	Carboplatin/pemetrexed	5FU/LV and bevacizumab
Docetaxel weekly	Carboplatin/paclitaxel q3w	CAF
FOLFIRI	Cisplatin/gemcitabine d1,d8	Carboplatin/docetaxel q3w
Gemcitabine 1g 3/4 wk	ECF	CHOP
Gemcitabine 1.25g 3/4 wk	Fludarabine	Cisplatin/docetaxel 75/75
Paclitaxel weekly	FOLFOX 85mg	Cisplatin/etoposide
Pemetrexed	Gemcitabine 7/8 wk then 3/4 wk	Cisplatin/gemcitabine d1,d8,d15
	Gemcitabine/irinotecan	Cisplatin/paclitaxel 135-24h q3w
	PEG doxorubicin 50mg q4w	CMF classic
	Topotecan weekly	Doxorubicin q3w
	XELOX	FOLFOX 100-130mg
		Gemcitabine/pemetrexed d8
		Irinotecan q3w
		Paclitaxel q3w
		Docetaxel q3w
		Topotecan monthly

CRASH score						
Heme subscore		**Non-Heme subscore**		**Combined score**		**Risk category**
0-1	7%	**0-2**	33%	**0-3**	50%	**Low**
2-3	23%	**3-4**	46%	**4-6**	58%	**Intermediate-Low**
4-5	54%	**5-6**	67%	**7-9**	77%	**Intermediate-High**
>5	100%	**>6**	93%	**>9**	79%	**High**

presentations (−39%), unplanned hospitalisations (−41%), unplanned hospital overnight bed-days (−24%) and lower early treatment discontinuations in the absence of any differences in treatment reduction, escalation and delay.

Chemotherapy regimens may be adapted based on treatment goals and setting, patients' preferences and available evidence on predicted benefits and safety profile. Especially in the palliative setting, the use of single-agent chemotherapy is favoured over combinations that are associated with a substantially higher risk of severe toxicities in this population [28, 29]. On the other hand, where indicated the use of upfront dose reduction may be an appropriate strategy to assess tolerance and may not necessarily have a detrimental impact on efficacy outcomes in patients with advanced disease as shown in the GAP 70 study [25]. Finally, the use of primary granulocyte-colony stimulating factor prophylaxis on cytotoxics is standard of care in older patients as recommended by international guidelines [94].

Targeted Therapies

Targeted therapies are an approach involving the use of agents to target specific genes and proteins key to the growth and survival of cancer cells. Targeted agents are now included in the routine management of a number of malignancies. Similarly to chemotherapy, as older cancer patients with frailty have reduced organ function, higher prevalence of comorbidities and polypharmacy and reduced overall functional status, they may ultimately have sub-optimal tolerability and treatment benefit.

In breast cancer, monoclonal antibodies targeting the human epidermal growth factor receptor 2 (HER2) are standard of care for the management of HER2-positive breast cancer both in the curative and in the palliative setting. Although their benefit is similar regardless of age, older individuals with frailty may have a higher risk of left ventricular dysfunction, especially in the context of cardiovascular comorbidities [98, 99]. Compared with younger patients, de-escalation strategies involving shorter courses of treatment in the adjuvant setting, or a different chemotherapy companion in the curative or palliative setting, might represent safer alternative systemic treatment options based on the individual risk profile.

Cyclin-dependent kinase 4/6 inhibitors are also an effective and well-tolerated treatment option in older patients with advanced oestrogen receptor (ER)-positive, HER2-negative breast cancer enrolled according to the findings of the relevant pivotal trials [100, 101] and their pooled analysis documenting similar progression free survival and slightly higher rates of grade 3–4 adverse events (mostly neutropenia, diarrhoea and increased serum creatinine) [102]. Therefore, they should be considered standard of care in this setting [103].

In colorectal cancer, evidence on the efficacy and safety of antibodies targeting the epidermal growth factor receptor (EGFR) or the vascular endothelial growth factor A (VEGF-A) in older individuals with frailty is sparse. Pre-existing registration trials did not document any differences in outcomes compared with younger patients [104], although this cohort was highly selected. The anti-EGFR agent cetuximab is considered safe and effective, regardless of age [105, 106]. On the other hand, the risk of thromboembolism is a major concern when using bevacizumab in this age group. Alternative regimens, incorporating the anti-VEGF antibody bevacizumab with capecitabine, may offer a safer therapeutic choice [107, 108].

In lung cancer, tyrosine kinase inhibitors (TKI) usually represent a safe systemic treatment option for older patients with EGFR mutation-driven non-small cell lung cancer [109]. The registration trials of erlotinib, gefitinib and afatinib have not documented any differential benefit and safety according to age [110–112]. Nonetheless, the risk of gastrointestinal, cardiac and neurologic toxicity and drug interactions on TKIs targeting EGFR and anaplastic lymphoma kinase (ALK) requires additional caution in individuals with frailty, and dose modifications may be required [113].

Immunotherapy

In recent years, immunotherapy has become one of the cornerstones of cancer treatment. Several immune checkpoint blockers (ICB) such as anti-programmed cell death 1 (PD-1), anti-programmed cell death ligand 1 (PD-L1) and anti-cytotoxic T-lymphocyte-associated protein 4 (CTLA-4) have now been approved in various tumour types [114]. Some concerns have emerged regarding efficacy and toxicity of these targeted agents in older patients considering changes in the immune system called immunosenescence [115–119]. Both the innate and the adaptive immunity are affected by this phenomenon [120–125]. One of the most important hallmarks of this senescence is the lower number and frequency of naïve CD8+ lymphocyte T cells in the peripheral blood, and a slightly lower frequency of naïve CD4+ lymphocyte T cells compared to younger individuals. This is most likely due to the conversion of naïve cells to memory cells over a lifetime of exposures to immune challenges (mainly infections but also cancer neoantigens) [126]. As there is little or no continued production of naïve cells because of thymic involution at puberty, reserves of naïve cells are depleted over the life course, with increasing susceptibility to exposure to previously un-encountered neoantigens. Concomitantly an increasing number of CD8+ memory T cells is commonly seen, but recently it has become clear that their accumulation is mostly the result of persistent antigenic stimulation caused by infection with viruses, particularly Cytomegalovirus (CMV) [127, 128]. Another typical aspect of the immunosenescence process is a low-grade proinflammatory state, with an increase in serum inflammatory mediators, such as IL-6, IL-1RA, TNF-a, IL-1 and C-reactive protein (CRP) [129, 130]. This low-grade inflammatory state named "inflammaging" is associated with a diminished ability to produce efficient immune responses during the aging process [130].

Despite all these theoretical concerns about immunosenescence and the possible impact on efficacy and tolerability of ICB, several studies have now been published regarding efficacy in older patients suggesting that they derive similar benefit from ICB in clinical trials but also in real life cohorts [131–145].

Using ICB in older patients with frailty is an attractive option considering the low rate of immune-related adverse events (irAEs) observed in pivotal studies (10% grade 3–4 irAEs) [146, 147]. Classic autoimmune diseases have known clinical risk factors including age, gender and seasonality, but the clinical factors that lead to irAEs are not well-defined. The toxicity spectrum of irAEs is presented in Fig. 14.1.

Several sub-analyses of prospective randomised trials showed no difference in terms of occurrence of irAEs between older and younger patients with various thresholds, i.e. 65, 70 or 75 years old [148–151]. However, data in pooled analysis of randomised trials shows conflicting results [152–154]. In the United States Food and Drug Administration (FDA) subset analysis of registration trials evaluating nivolumab, 1030 patients were treated for lung cancer, renal cancer and melanoma with ICB. There were more grade 3–5 AEs (any cause) in patients aged ≥70 years

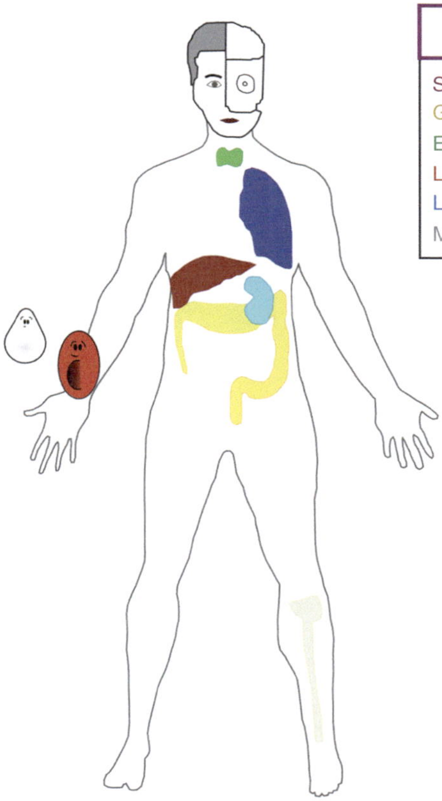

ICB	
Skin toxicity	10-50%
GI toxicity	4-24%
Endocrine toxicity	10-20%
Liver toxicity	2-10%
Lung toxicity	4-6%
Musculoskeletal toxicity	0-6%

Fig. 14.1 Toxicity spectrum of immune-related adverse events (irAEs) in older patients, any grade

(72% compared to 58% in patients <65 years old) and a trend towards a higher incidence of irAEs requiring treatment with immune-modulating medication (52% versus 42%) [152]. However, the pooled analysis of the KEYNOTE trials in melanoma, lung cancer, head and neck cancers, urothelial carcinoma and Hodgkin's lymphoma with pembrolizumab did not report increased high-grade irAEs in patients aged 75 years old (9% versus 7%) [154]. In real life cohorts, irAEs incidence varied drastically between cohorts and age thresholds (Table 14.3) [140, 148, 155–159]. Interestingly, one study reported a significant increase of multitoxicities of grade ≥ 2 in older patients (32% versus 18%; $p = 0.037$) [159].

Table 14.3 Toxicity profile in older and younger patients with immune checkpoint blockers in monotherapy

Study	Sample size and number of older patients	Tumour type	ICB(s) type	irAEs incidence (any grade)	Type of irAE (any grade)
Sattar 2019	Total: 78 65–74 years: 26 (33%) ≥75 years: 23 (30%)	Melanoma NSCLC Renal cell carcinoma	Ipilimumab Nivolumab Pembrolizumab	<65 years: 41% 65–74 years: 58% ≥75 years: 61%	GI toxicity <65 years: 30% 65–74 years: 50% ≥75 years: 20% Skin toxicity <65 years: 21% 65–74 years: 29% ≥75 years: 50% Endocrine toxicity <65 years: 40% 65–74 years: 40% ≥75 years: 20%
Chiarion Sileni 2014	Total: 855 >70 years: 193 (23%)	Melanoma	Ipilimumab	≤70 years: 46% >70 years: 50%	GI toxicity ≤70 years: 8% >70 years: 5% Skin toxicity ≤70 years: 7% >70 years: 10% Liver toxicity ≤70 years: 2% >70 years: 2%
Leroy 2019	Total: 52 < 80 yo: 29 (56%) ≥80 years: 23 (44%)	Melanoma	Ipilimumab	<80 years: 52% ≥80 years: 65%	GI toxicity <80 years: 9% ≥80 years: 9% Skin toxicity <80 years: 44% ≥80 years: 24% Liver toxicity <80 years: 0% ≥80 years: 9%

(continued)

Table 14.3 (continued)

Study	Sample size and number of older patients	Tumour type	ICB(s) type	irAEs incidence (any grade)	Type of irAE (any grade)
Freeman 2015	Total: 148 ≥ 65 years: 52 (35%)	Melanoma	Nivolumab	≤70 years: 46% > 70 years: 50%	GI toxicity < 65 years: 30% ≥65 years: 21% Skin toxicity <65 years: 39% ≥65 years: 40% Liver toxicity ≤70 years: 2% >70 years: 2%
Betof 2017	Total: 254 65–74 years: 65 (26%) ≥75 years: 47 (19%)	Melanoma	Anti PD-(L)1	50–64 years: 44% 65–74 years: 49% ≥75 years: 40%	GI toxicity: 50–64 years: 12% 65–74 years: 11% ≥75 years: 11% Skin toxicity 50–64 years: 15% 65–74 years: 9% ≥75 years: 13% Arthritis 50–64 years: 2% 65–74 years: 11% ≥75 years: 4% Liver toxicity 50–64 years: 11% 65–74 years: 3% ≥75 years: 4% Lung toxicity 50–64 years: 7% 65–74 years: 5% ≥75 years: 9% Endocrine toxicity 50–64 years: 5% 65–74 years: 12% ≥75 years: 17%
Muchnik 2019	Total: 75 <80 years: 58 (77%) ≥80 years: 17 (23%)	NSCLC	Nivolumab Pembrolizumab	Any age: 28 (37%)	GI toxicity <80 years: 3 (5%) ≥80 years: 4 (24%) Skin toxicity <80 years: 5 (9%) ≥80 years: 2 (12%) Lung toxicity <80 years: 8 (14%) ≥80 years: 1 (6%) Musculoskeletal toxicity <80 years: 2 (3%) ≥80 years: 0 (0%)

(continued)

Table 14.3 (continued)

Study	Sample size and number of older patients	Tumour type	ICB(s) type	irAEs incidence (any grade)	Type of irAE (any grade)
Baldini 2020	Total:603 <70 years: 412 (68%) ≥70 years: 191 (32%)	Melanoma NSCLC Urothelial Renal cell carcinoma	Anti PD-(L)1	<70 years: 25% ≥70 years: 33%	GI toxicity <70 years: 15% ≥70 years: 8% Skin toxicity <70 years: 28% ≥70 years: 49% Liver toxicity ≤70 years: 3% >70 years: 10% Endocrine toxicity ≤70 years: 25% >70 years: 14%
Gomes 2021	Total: 140 <70 years: 70 (50%) ≥70 years: 70 (50%)	Melanoma NSCLC	Anti PD-(L)1	<70 years: 51% ≥70 years: 60% Grade 3–5 <70 years: 13% ≥70 years: 19%	Any grade: n/a GI toxicity Grade 3–5 <70 years: 3% ≥70 years: 4% Skin toxicity Grade 3–5 <70 years: 3% ≥70 years: 0% Liver toxicity Grade 3–4 <70 years: 3% ≥70 years: 4% Lung toxicity Grade 3–4 <70 years: 0% ≥70 years: 4%

ICB immune checkpoint blocker; *irAEs* immune related adverse events; *n/a* not available; *NSCLC* non small cell lung cancer; *PD-(L)1* programmed death-(ligand) 1; *y* years old

There is still limited data about the impact of frailty on irAEs, their incidence and severity. Among the few studies that analysed associations between frailty and irAEs, no CGA domains impacted toxicity [160–162]. However, the cohorts of patients were small, thus limiting any formal conclusions being made. One small retrospective study of patients with various solid tumours highlighted a correlation between frailty and toxicity. Frailty was associated with an increased risk of irAE: OR 3.03 (95% CI 1.36–6.74; $p = 0.006$) [163]. Nevertheless, the prospective ELDERS study comparing older and younger patients receiving single-agent ICB for patients with advanced lung cancer or melanoma showed no significant increase in grade 3–5 irAEs incidence in older patients (18.6% versus 12.9%; $p = 0.35$) [164]. Importantly, this study incorporated geriatric assessment and 50% of patients within the older cohort were screened as frail based on Geriatric 8 (G8) screening tool. Here, frailty was not associated with increased irAEs incidence, but it played a role in how patients coped with AEs, being associated with higher risk of hospital admission [164].

Combination strategies with ICB are now the gold standard in many tumour types [165–168]. In randomised clinical trials evaluating chemotherapy and immunotherapy, and presenting subgroup analysis of older patients with a threshold of 65 years old in lung cancer, all patients benefited from combination therapy [169–171]. In the subgroup analysis of CheckMate 227 assessing the survival benefit of nivolumab and ipilimumab in the first line setting in NSCLC, hazard ratios (HR) were not significant in patients aged 75 years old or over [168]. Similar results were presented for this combination in advanced renal cell carcinoma [166]. Regarding combination therapy of anti-angiogenic agents and immunotherapy, benefit was similar irrespective of age [165, 172].

One of the major concerns with combination therapy in older patients with frailty is safety. Balaji et al. showed that anti PD-(L)1 combination based therapy and age were associated with an increased risk of irAE admission [173]. Myocarditis and pneumonitis were more frequent in older adults treated with the anti PD-1 therapy and anti CTLA4 association in the study by Shah and colleagues [174]. Ultimately, to better select older patients for combination therapy, prospective clinical trials or real life cohorts of patients are needed, as well as predictive factors for toxicity. CGA can help in the decision-making process (Fig. 14.2) but older cancer patients with frailty should receive monotherapy ICB whenever possible.

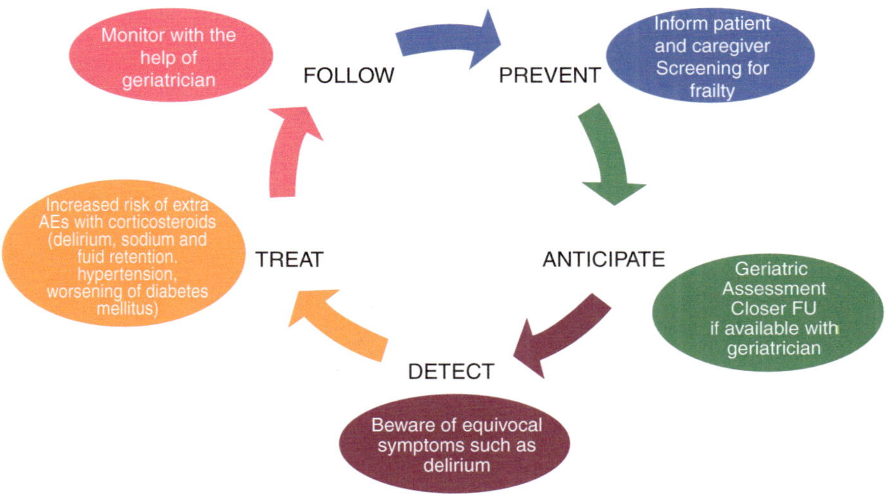

Fig. 14.2 The cycle of management of immune-related adverse events (irAEs) in older patients

Conclusion

The management of older cancer patients with frailty remains a challenge. Maintaining efficacy and limiting toxicities are the ultimate goal. The toxicity spectrum varies substantially between treatment modality and patients. Identifying frailty is paramount and CGA has clear benefits for patients to reduce severe toxicities, unplanned hospitalisations, emergency presentations and early treatment discontinuation [22, 23]. It should therefore be implemented in the care of all older patients. The substantive changes operating in the last decades in technologies, techniques and innovative treatments support better QoL and preservation of functional status. Multidimensional and tailored approaches using CGA oriented interventions could help improve tolerability, while preserving efficacy [175]. However clinical trials are the key to try to develop efficient tailored approaches. Efforts should continue to develop dedicated clinical trials as older cancer patients, particularly with frailty, are still largely excluded from participation [176].

References

1. Ries EM, Kosary CL, Hankey BF. SEER Cancer Statistics Review: 1975–2000. In: Institute NC, editor. Bethesda, MD.
2. Derks MGM, Bastiaannet E, Kiderlen M, Hilling DE, Boelens PG, Walsh PM, et al. Variation in treatment and survival of older patients with non-metastatic breast cancer in five European countries: a population-based cohort study from the EURECCA Breast Cancer Group. Br J Cancer. 2018;119(1):121–9. https://doi.org/10.1038/s41416-018-0090-1.
3. Claassen YHM, Vermeer NCA, Iversen LH, van Eycken E, Guren MG, Mroczkowski P, et al. Treatment and survival of rectal cancer patients over the age of 80 years: a EURECCA international comparison. Br J Cancer. 2018;119(4):517–22. https://doi.org/10.1038/s41416-018-0215-6.
4. Elkin EB, Kim SH, Casper ES, Kissane DW, Schrag D. Desire for information and involvement in treatment decisions: elderly cancer patients' preferences and their physicians' perceptions. J Clin Oncol. 2007;25(33):5275–80. https://doi.org/10.1200/jco.2007.11.1922.
5. Soto-Perez-de-Celis E, Li D, Yuan Y, Lau YM, Hurria A. Functional versus chronological age: geriatric assessments to guide decision making in older patients with cancer. Lancet Oncol. 2018;19(6):e305–e16. https://doi.org/10.1016/s1470-2045(18)30348-6.
6. Clegg A, Young J, Iliffe S, Rikkert MO, Rockwood K. Frailty in elderly people. Lancet. 381(9868):752–62. https://doi.org/10.1016/S0140-6736(12)62167-9.
7. Sawhney R, Sehl M, Naeim A. Physiologic aspects of aging: impact on cancer management and decision making, part I. Cancer J. 2005;11(6):449–60. https://doi.org/10.1097/00130404-200,511,000-00004.
8. Sehl M, Sawhney R, Naeim A. Physiologic aspects of aging: impact on cancer management and decision making, part II. Cancer J. 2005;11(6):461–73. https://doi.org/10.1097/00130404-200,511,000-00005.
9. Scher KS, Hurria A. Under-representation of older adults in cancer registration trials: known problem, little progress. J Clin Oncol. 2012;30(17):2036–8. https://doi.org/10.1200/jco.2012.41.6727.

10. Battisti NML, Sehovic M, Extermann M. Assessment of the external validity of the National Comprehensive Cancer Network and European Society for Medical Oncology guidelines for non-small-cell lung cancer in a population of patients aged 80 years and older. Clin Lung Cancer. 2017;18(5):460–71. https://doi.org/10.1016/j.cllc.2017.03.005.
11. Hamerman D. Toward an understanding of frailty. Ann Intern Med. 1999;130(11):945–50. https://doi.org/10.7326/0003-4819-130-11-199,906,010-00022.
12. Mohile SG, Dale W, Somerfield MR, Hurria A. Practical assessment and management of vulnerabilities in older patients receiving chemotherapy: ASCO guideline for geriatric oncology summary. J Oncol Pract. 2018;14(7):442–6. https://doi.org/10.1200/jop.18.00180.
13. Wildiers H, Heeren P, Puts M, Topinkova E, Janssen-Heijnen ML, Extermann M, et al. International Society of Geriatric Oncology consensus on geriatric assessment in older patients with cancer. J Clin Oncol. 2014;32(24):2595–603. https://doi.org/10.1200/jco.2013.54.8347.
14. Decoster L, Van Puyvelde K, Mohile S, Wedding U, Basso U, Colloca G, et al. Screening tools for multidimensional health problems warranting a geriatric assessment in older cancer patients: an update on SIOG recommendations. Ann Oncol. 2015;26(2):288–300. https://doi.org/10.1093/annonc/mdu210.
15. Loh KP, Soto-Perez-de-Celis E, Hsu T, de Glas NA, Battisti NML, Baldini C, et al. What every oncologist should know about geriatric assessment for older patients with cancer: Young International Society of Geriatric Oncology Position Paper. J Oncol Pract. 2018;14(2):85–94. https://doi.org/10.1200/jop.2017.026435.
16. Kenis C, Decoster L, Bastin J, Bode H, Van Puyvelde K, De Greve J, et al. Functional decline in older patients with cancer receiving chemotherapy: a multicenter prospective study. J Geriatr Oncol. 2017;8(3):196–205. https://doi.org/10.1016/j.jgo.2017.02.010.
17. Shahrokni A, Vishnevsky BM, Jang B, Sarraf S, Alexander K, Kim SJ, et al. Geriatric assessment, not ASA physical status, is associated with 6-month postoperative survival in patients with cancer aged ≥75 years. J Natl Compr Cancer Netw. 2019;17(6):687–94. https://doi.org/10.6004/jnccn.2018.7277.
18. Kenis C, Bron D, Libert Y, Decoster L, Van Puyvelde K, Scalliet P, et al. Relevance of a systematic geriatric screening and assessment in older patients with cancer: results of a prospective multicentric study. Ann Oncol. 2013;24(5):1306–12. https://doi.org/10.1093/annonc/mds619.
19. Hamaker ME, Prins MC, Stauder R. The relevance of a geriatric assessment for elderly patients with a haematological malignancy: a systematic review. Leuk Res. 2014;38(3):275–83. https://doi.org/10.1016/j.leukres.2013.12.018.
20. Extermann M, Meyer J, McGinnis M, Crocker TT, Corcoran MB, Yoder J, et al. A comprehensive geriatric intervention detects multiple problems in older breast cancer patients. Crit Rev Oncol Hematol. 2004;49(1):69–75. https://doi.org/10.1016/s1040-8428(03)00099-4.
21. Rao AV, Hsieh F, Feussner JR, Cohen HJ. Geriatric evaluation and management units in the care of the frail elderly cancer patient. J Gerontol A Biol Sci Med Sci. 2005;60(6):798–803.
22. Li D, Sun CL, Kim H, Soto-Perez-de-Celis E, Chung V, Koczywas M, et al. Geriatric Assessment-Driven Intervention (GAIN) on Chemotherapy-Related Toxic Effects in Older Adults With Cancer: A Randomized Clinical Trial. JAMA Oncol. 2021;7(11):e214158. https://doi.org/10.1001/jamaoncol.2021.4158. Epub 2021 Nov 18. PMID: 34591080; PMCID: PMC8485211.
23. Soo W-K, King M, Pope A, Parente P, Darzins P, Davis ID. Integrated geriatric assessment and treatment (INTEGERATE) in older people with cancer planned for systemic anticancer therapy. J Clin Oncol. 2020;38(15 suppl):12011. https://doi.org/10.1200/JCO.2020.38.15_suppl.12011.
24. Qian CL, Knight HP, Ferrone CR, Kunitake H, Castillo CF, Lanuti M, et al. Randomized trial of a perioperative geriatric intervention for older adults with cancer. J Clin Oncol. 2020;38(15 suppl):12012. https://doi.org/10.1200/JCO.2020.38.15_suppl.12012.
25. Mohile SG, Mohamed MR, Xu H, Culakova E, Loh KP, Magnuson A, et al. Evaluation of geriatric assessment and management on the toxic effects of cancer treatment (GAP70+):

a cluster-randomised study. Lancet. 2021;398(10314):1894–904. https://doi.org/10.1016/S0140-6736(21)01789-X. Epub 2021 Nov 3. PMID: 34741815; PMCID: PMC8647163.
26. Extermann M, Boler I, Reich RR, Lyman GH, Brown RH, DeFelice J, et al. Predicting the risk of chemotherapy toxicity in older patients: the Chemotherapy Risk Assessment Scale for High-Age Patients (CRASH) score. Cancer. 2012;118(13):3377–86. https://doi.org/10.1002/cncr.26646.
27. Extermann M, Bonetti M, Sledge GW, O'Dwyer PJ, Bonomi P, Benson AB 3rd. MAX2: a convenient index to estimate the average per patient risk for chemotherapy toxicity; validation in ECOG trials. Eur J Cancer. 2004;40(8):1193–8. https://doi.org/10.1016/j.ejca.2004.01.028.
28. Hurria A, Mohile S, Gajra A, Klepin H, Muss H, Chapman A, et al. Validation of a prediction tool for chemotherapy toxicity in older adults with cancer. J Clin Oncol. 2016;34(20):2366–71. https://doi.org/10.1200/jco.2015.65.4327.
29. Hurria A, Togawa K, Mohile SG, Owusu C, Klepin HD, Gross CP, et al. Predicting chemotherapy toxicity in older adults with cancer: a prospective multicenter study. J Clin Oncol. 2011;29(25):3457–65. https://doi.org/10.1200/jco.2011.34.7625.
30. Freyer G, Geay JF, Touzet S, Provencal J, Weber B, Jacquin JP, et al. Comprehensive geriatric assessment predicts tolerance to chemotherapy and survival in elderly patients with advanced ovarian carcinoma: a GINECO study. Ann Oncol. 2005;16(11):1795–800. https://doi.org/10.1093/annonc/mdi368.
31. Ramjaun A, Nassif MO, Krotneva S, Huang AR, Meguerditchian AN. Improved targeting of cancer care for older patients: a systematic review of the utility of comprehensive geriatric assessment. J Geriatr Oncol. 2013;4(3):271–81. https://doi.org/10.1016/j.jgo.2013.04.002.
32. Corre R, Greillier L, Le Caër H, Audigier-Valette C, Baize N, Bérard H, et al. Use of a comprehensive geriatric assessment for the management of elderly patients with advanced non-small-cell lung cancer: the Phase III Randomized ESOGIA-GFPC-GECP 08–02 Study. J Clin Oncol. 2016;34(13):1476–83. https://doi.org/10.1200/JCO.2015.63.5839.
33. Slotman BJ, Cottier B, Bentzen SM, Heeren G, Lievens Y, van den Bogaert W. Overview of national guidelines for infrastructure and staffing of radiotherapy. ESTRO-QUARTS: Work package 1. Radiother Oncol. 2005;75(3):349. https://doi.org/10.1016/j.radonc.2004.12.005.
34. Wildes TM, O'Donovan A, Colloca GF, Cheung K-L. Tumour boards in geriatric oncology. Age Ageing. 2017;47(2):168–70. https://doi.org/10.1093/ageing/afx171.
35. O'Hanlon S, O'Donovan A, Cree A. Geriatric oncology: assessing the needs of older people with cancer. Br J Hosp Med (Lond). 2019;80(5):252–7. https://doi.org/10.12968/hmed.2019.80.5.252.
36. Szumacher E, Sattar S, Neve M, Do K, Ayala AP, Gray M, et al. Use of comprehensive geriatric assessment and geriatric screening for older adults in the radiation oncology setting: a systematic review. Clin Oncol. 2018;30(9):578–88. https://doi.org/10.1016/j.clon.2018.04.008.
37. Society and College of Radiographers Practice Guideline Document. Caring for people with dementia: a clinical practice guideline for the radiography workforce (imaging and radiotherapy). 2020. Available from https://www.sor.org/getmedia/db2b70ad-2771-42f1-a204-009fde177071/sor_dementia_academic_doc_llv2.pdf
38. Mohile SG, Heckler C, Fan L, Mustian K, Jean-Pierre P, Usuki K, et al. Age-related differences in symptoms and their interference with Quality of Life in 903 Cancer Patients Undergoing Radiation Therapy. J Geriatr Oncol. 2011;2(4):225–32. https://doi.org/10.1016/j.jgo.2011.08.002.
39. Jilani OK, Singh P, Wernicke AG, Kutler DI, Kuhel W, Christos P, et al. Radiation therapy is well tolerated and produces excellent control rates in elderly patients with locally advanced head and neck cancers. J Geriatr Oncol. 2012;3(4):337–43. https://doi.org/10.1016/j.jgo.2012.05.001.
40. Pignon T, Scalliet P. 193Age related morbidity in radiotherapy(RT): EORTC database survey. Radiother Oncol. 1996;40:S51. https://doi.org/10.1016/S0167-8140(96)80202-7.
41. Joiner M, Avd K. Basic clinical radiobiology. 4th ed. London: Hodder Arnold; 2009.

42. Whelehan S, Lynch O, Treacy N, Gleeson C, Oates A, O'Donovan A. Optimising clinical trial design in older cancer patients. Geriatrics (Basel, Switzerland). 2018;3(3) https://doi.org/10.3390/geriatrics3030034.
43. Hall EJ. Radiobiology for the radiologist. 4th ed. Philadelphia: J.B. Lippincott; 1994.
44. Kim JH, Jenrow KA, Brown SL. Mechanisms of radiation-induced normal tissue toxicity and implications for future clinical trials. Radiat Oncol J. 2014;32(3):103–15. https://doi.org/10.3857/roj.2014.32.3.103.
45. Samant R, Malette M, Tucker T, Lightfoot N. Radiotherapy education among family physicians and residents. J Cancer Educ. 2001;16(3):134–8. https://doi.org/10.1080/08858190109528754.
46. Ben Mustapha S, Meijnders P, Jansen N, Lakosi F, Coucke P. The status of radiation oncology (RO) teaching to medical students in Europe. Clin Transl Radiat Oncol. 2019;17:40–6. https://doi.org/10.1016/j.ctro.2019.04.010.
47. Bird T, Michael M, Bressel M, Chu J, Chander S, Cooray P, et al. FOLFOX and intensified split-course chemoradiation as initial treatment for rectal cancer with synchronous metastases. Acta Oncol. 2017;56(5):646–52. https://doi.org/10.1080/0284186X.2017.1296584.
48. Bledsoe TJ, Noble AR, Reddy CA, Burkey BB, Greskovich JF, Nwizu T, et al. Split-course accelerated hypofractionated radiotherapy (SCAHRT): a safe and effective option for head and neck cancer in the elderly or infirm. Anticancer Res. 2016;36(3):933–9.
49. Vrouvas J, Dodwell D, Ash D, Probst H. Split course radiotherapy for bladder cancer in elderly unfit patients. Clin Oncol. 1995;7(3):193–5.
50. Brush J, Lipnick SL, Phillips T, Sitko J, McDonald JT, McBride WH. Molecular mechanisms of late normal tissue injury. Seminars in radiation oncology. New York: Elsevier; 2007. p. 121–30.
51. Muszalik M, Kołucka-Pluta M, Kędziora-Kornatowska K, Robaczewska J. Quality of life of women with breast cancer undergoing radiotherapy using the functional assessment of chronic illness therapy-fatigue questionnaire. Clin Interv Aging. 2016;11:1489–94. https://doi.org/10.2147/CIA.S113530.
52. Furmaniak AC, Menig M, Markes MH. Exercise for women receiving adjuvant therapy for breast cancer. Cochrane Database Syst Rev. 2016;9:Cd005001. https://doi.org/10.1002/14651858.CD005001.pub3.
53. Hojan K, Kwiatkowska-Borowczyk E, Leporowska E, Gorecki M, Ozga-Majchrzak O, Milecki T, et al. Physical exercise for functional capacity, blood immune function, fatigue, and quality of life in high-risk prostate cancer patients during radiotherapy: a prospective, randomized clinical study. Eur J Phys Rehab Med. 2016;52(4):489–501.
54. Katz PP, Pate R. Exercise as medicine. Ann Intern Med. 2016;165(12):880–1. https://doi.org/10.7326/M16-2086.
55. Gill TM, Guralnik JM, Pahor M, et al. Effect of structured physical activity on overall burden and transitions between states of major mobility disability in older persons: secondary analysis of a randomized trial. Ann Intern Med. 2016;165(12):833–40. https://doi.org/10.7326/M16-0529.
56. Horgan S, O'Donovan A. The impact of exercise during radiation therapy for prostate cancer on fatigue and quality of life: a systematic review and meta-analysis. J Med Imaging Radiat Sci. 2018;49(2):207–19. https://doi.org/10.1016/j.jmir.2018.02.056.
57. O'Donovan A, Leech M, Gillham C. Assessment and management of radiotherapy induced toxicity in older patients. J Geriatr Oncol. 2017;8(6):421–7. https://doi.org/10.1016/j.jgo.2017.07.001.
58. Salvo N, Barnes E, van Draanen J, Stacey E, Mitera G, Breen D, et al. Prophylaxis and management of acute radiation-induced skin reactions: a systematic review of the literature. Curr Oncol. 2010;17(4):94–112.
59. O'Donovan A, Coleman M, Harris R, Herst P. Prophylaxis and management of acute radiation-induced skin toxicity: a survey of practice across E urope and the USA. Eur J Cancer Care. 2015;24(3):425–35.

60. de Castro G Jr, Guindalini RS. Supportive care in head and neck oncology. Curr Opin Oncol. 2010;22(3):221–5.
61. O'Donovan A, Morris L. Palliative radiation therapy in older adults with cancer: age-related considerations. Clin Oncol. 2020; https://doi.org/10.1016/j.clon.2020.06.011.
62. Flood J, O'Hanlon S, Gibb M, O'Donovan A. Caring for patients with dementia undergoing radiation therapy: a national audit. J Geriatr Oncol. 2019;10(5):811–8. https://doi.org/10.1016/j.jgo.2019.04.003.
63. Murray Brunt A, Haviland JS, Wheatley DA, Sydenham MA, Alhasso A, Bloomfield DJ, et al. Hypofractionated breast radiotherapy for 1 week versus 3 weeks (FAST-Forward): 5-year efficacy and late normal tissue effects results from a multicentre, non-inferiority, randomised, phase 3 trial. Lancet. 2020;395(10237):1613–26. https://doi.org/10.1016/S0140-6736(20)30932-6.
64. Dearnaley D, Syndikus I, Mossop H, Khoo V, Birtle A, Bloomfield D, et al. Conventional versus hypofractionated high-dose intensity-modulated radiotherapy for prostate cancer: 5-year outcomes of the randomised, non-inferiority, phase 3 CHHiP trial. Lancet Oncol. 2016;17(8):1047–60. https://doi.org/10.1016/S1470-2045(16)30102-4.
65. Simcock R, Thomas TV, Estes C, Filippi AR, Katz MS, Pereira IJ, et al. COVID-19: global radiation oncology's targeted response for pandemic preparedness. Clin Transl Radiat Oncol. 2020;22:55–68. https://doi.org/10.1016/j.ctro.2020.03.009.
66. Battisti NML, Mislang AR, Cooper L, O'Donovan A, Audisio RA, Cheung K-L, et al. Adapting care for older cancer patients during the COVID-19 pandemic: recommendations from the International Society of Geriatric Oncology (SIOG) COVID-19 Working Group. J Geriatr Oncol. 2020; https://doi.org/10.1016/j.jgo.2020.07.008.
67. Roa W, Kepka L, Kumar N, Sinaika V, Matiello J, Lomidze D, et al. International atomic energy agency randomized phase III study of radiation therapy in elderly and/or frail patients with newly diagnosed glioblastoma multiforme. J Clin Oncol. 2015; https://doi.org/10.1200/jco.2015.62.6606.
68. Marijnen CAM, Peters FP, Rödel C, Bujko K, Haustermans K, Fokas E, et al. International expert consensus statement regarding radiotherapy treatment options for rectal cancer during the COVID 19 pandemic. Radiother Oncol. 2020;148:213–5. https://doi.org/10.1016/j.radonc.2020.03.039.
69. Widmark A, Gunnlaugsson A, Beckman L, Thellenberg-Karlsson C, Hoyer M, Lagerlund M, et al. Ultra-hypofractionated versus conventionally fractionated radiotherapy for prostate cancer: 5-year outcomes of the HYPO-RT-PC randomised, non-inferiority, phase 3 trial. Lancet. 2019;394(10196):385–95.
70. Thomson DJ, Yom SS, Saeed H, El Naqa I, Ballas L, Bentzen SM, et al. Radiation fractionation schedules published during the COVID-19 pandemic: a systematic review of the quality of evidence and recommendations for future development. Int J Radiat Oncol Biol Phys. https://doi.org/10.1016/j.ijrobp.2020.06.054.
71. Ortholan C, Auperin A, Mertens C, Le Caer H, Guigay J. Radiothérapie hypofractionnée des cancers ORL chez le sujet âgé. Cancer/Radiothérapie. 2018;22(6):640–3. https://doi.org/10.1016/j.canrad.2018.06.008.
72. Bras L, Driessen DAJJ, de Vries J, Festen S, van der Laan BFAM, van Leeuwen BL, et al. Patients with head and neck cancer: are they frailer than patients with other solid malignancies? Eur J Cancer Care. 2020;29(1):e13170. https://doi.org/10.1111/ecc.13170.
73. Straube C, Pigorsch SU, Scherb H, Wilkens JJ, Bier H, Combs SE. Reduced volume SIB-IMRT/IGRT to head and neck cancer in elderly and frail patients: outcome and toxicity. Radiat Oncol. 2016;11(1):133. https://doi.org/10.1186/s13014-016-0711-x.
74. Hammer L, Laufer M, Dotan Z, Leibowitz-Amit R, Berger R, Felder S, et al. Accelerated hypofractionated radiation therapy for elderly frail bladder cancer patients unfit for surgery or chemotherapy. Am J Clin Oncol. 2019;42(2):179–83. https://doi.org/10.1097/coc.0000000000000491.

75. Nutting CM, Morden JP, Harrington KJ, Urbano TG, Bhide SA, Clark C, et al. Parotid-sparing intensity modulated versus conventional radiotherapy in head and neck cancer (PARSPORT): a phase 3 multicentre randomised controlled trial. Lancet Oncol. 2011;12(2):127–36. https://doi.org/10.1016/S1470-2045(10)70290-4.
76. Jaffray D, Kupelian P, Djemil T, Macklis RM. Review of image-guided radiation therapy. Expert Rev Anticancer Ther. 2007;7(1):89–103.
77. Hafeez S, McDonald F, Lalondrelle S, McNair H, Warren-Oseni K, Jones K, et al. Clinical outcomes of image guided adaptive hypofractionated weekly radiation therapy for bladder cancer in patients unsuitable for radical treatment. Int J Radiat Oncol Biol Phys. 2017;98(1):115–22. https://doi.org/10.1016/j.ijrobp.2017.01.239.
78. Guinot JL, Rembielak A, Perez-Calatayud J, Rodríguez-Villalba S, Skowronek J, Tagliaferri L, et al. GEC-ESTRO ACROP recommendations in skin brachytherapy. Radiother Oncol. 2018;126(3):377–85. https://doi.org/10.1016/j.radonc.2018.01.013.
79. Palma D, Visser O, Lagerwaard FJ, Belderbos J, Slotman BJ, Senan S. Impact of introducing stereotactic lung radiotherapy for elderly patients with stage I non–small-cell lung cancer: a population-based time-trend analysis. J Clin Oncol. 2010;28(35):5153–9.
80. Schneider BJ, Daly ME, Kennedy EB, Antonoff MB, Broderick S, Feldman J, et al. Stereotactic body radiotherapy for early-stage non-small-cell lung cancer: American Society of Clinical Oncology Endorsement of the American Society for Radiation Oncology evidence-based guideline. J Clin Oncol. 2018;36(7):710–9. https://doi.org/10.1200/jco.2017.74.9671.
81. Chang JY, Senan S, Paul MA, Mehran RJ, Louie AV, Balter P, et al. Stereotactic ablative radiotherapy versus lobectomy for operable stage I non-small-cell lung cancer: a pooled analysis of two randomised trials. Lancet Oncol. 2015;16(6):630–7. https://doi.org/10.1016/s1470-2045(15)70168-3.
82. Franco I, Chen Y-H, Chipidza F, Agrawal V, Romano J, Baldini E, et al. Use of frailty to predict survival in elderly patients with early stage non-small-cell lung cancer treated with stereotactic body radiation therapy. J Geriatr Oncol. 2018;9(2):130–7.
83. Raghavan G, Shaverdian N, Chan S, Chu F-I, Lee P. Comparing Outcomes of Patients With Early-Stage Non–Small-Cell Lung Cancer Treated With Stereotactic Body Radiotherapy Based on Frailty Status. Clin Lung Cancer. 2018;19(5):e759–e66. https://doi.org/10.1016/j.cllc.2018.05.008.
84. Kerkmeijer LGW, Fuller CD, Verkooijen HM, Verheij M, Choudhury A, Harrington KJ, et al. The MRI-linear accelerator consortium: evidence-based clinical introduction of an innovation in radiation oncology connecting researchers, methodology, data collection, quality assurance, and technical development. Front Oncol. 2016;6:215. https://doi.org/10.3389/fonc.2016.00215.
85. Lagendijk JJ, Raaymakers BW, Raaijmakers AJ, Overweg J, Brown KJ, Kerkhof EM, et al. MRI/linac integration. Radiother Oncol. 2008;86(1):25–9. https://doi.org/10.1016/j.radonc.2007.10.034.
86. Pollard JM, Wen Z, Sadagopan R, Wang J, Ibbott GS. The future of image-guided radiotherapy will be MR guided. Br J Radiol. 2017;90(1073):20160667. https://doi.org/10.1259/bjr.20160667.
87. Liu H, Chang JY. Proton therapy in clinical practice. Chin J Cancer. 2011;30(5):315–26. https://doi.org/10.5732/cjc.010.10529.
88. De Laney TF, Kooy HM. Proton and charged particle radiotherapy. Philadelphia: Lippincott Williams & Wilkins; 2008.
89. Thariat J, Sio T, Blanchard P, Patel S, Demizu Y, Ampil F, et al. Using proton beam therapy in the elderly population: a snapshot of current perception and practice. Int J Radiat Oncol Biol Phys. 2017;98(4):840–2. https://doi.org/10.1016/j.ijrobp.2017.01.007.
90. Goozner M. The proton beam debate: are facilities outstripping the evidence? J Natl Cancer Inst. 2010;102(7):450–3. https://doi.org/10.1093/jnci/djq112.

91. Bekelman JE, Asch DA, Tochner Z, Friedberg J, Vaughn DJ, Rash E, et al. Principles and reality of proton therapy treatment allocation. Int J Radiat Oncol Biol Phys. 2014;89(3):499–508. https://doi.org/10.1016/j.ijrobp.2014.03.023.
92. Battisti NML, Wallington M, Ring A, Payne S, Birch R, Bomb M, et al. Is age a barrier to chemotherapy? Rates of treatment in older patients treated with breast, colon and lung cancer in England in 2014: a national registry study. Ann Oncol. 2018;29:viii562. https://doi.org/10.1093/annonc/mdy297.
93. Smith TJ, Khatcheressian J, Lyman GH, Ozer H, Armitage JO, Balducci L, et al. 2006 update of recommendations for the use of white blood cell growth factors: an evidence-based clinical practice guideline. J Clin Oncol. 2006;24(19):3187–205. https://doi.org/10.1200/jco.2006.06.4451.
94. NCCN. Clinical practice guidelines in oncology. Older adult oncology.
95. Tam-McDevitt J. Polypharmacy, aging, and cancer. Oncology (Williston Park). 2008;22(9):1052–5.
96. Battisti NML, Reed MW, Herbert E, Morgan JL, Collins KA, Ward SE, et al. Bridging the age gap in breast cancer: impact of chemotherapy on quality of life in older women with early breast cancer. Eur J Cancer. 2020;144:269–80.
97. Magnuson A, Sedrak MS, Gross CP, Tew WP, Klepin HD, Wildes TM, et al. Development and validation of a risk tool for predicting severe toxicity in older adults receiving chemotherapy for early-stage breast cancer. J Clin Oncol. 2021;39:608.
98. Brollo J, Curigliano G, Disalvatore D, Marrone BF, Criscitiello C, Bagnardi V, et al. Adjuvant trastuzumab in elderly with HER-2 positive breast cancer: a systematic review of randomized controlled trials. Cancer Treat Rev. 2013;39(1):44–50. https://doi.org/10.1016/j.ctrv.2012.03.009.
99. Owusu C, Klepin HD, Kimmick GG, Sutton L, Brufsky A. Safety and efficacy of single-agent adjuvant trastzumab in older women with breast cancer. J Clin Oncol. 2011;29(15 suppl):TPS109. https://doi.org/10.1200/jco.2011.29.15_suppl.tps109.
100. Freedman RA, Tolaney SM. Efficacy and safety in older patient subsets in studies of endocrine monotherapy versus combination therapy in patients with HR+/HER2- advanced breast cancer: a review. Breast Cancer Res Treat. 2018;167(3):607–14. https://doi.org/10.1007/s10549-017-4560-6.
101. Rugo HS, Turner NC, Finn RS, Joy AA, Verma S, Harbeck N, et al. Palbociclib plus endocrine therapy in older women with HR+/HER2-advanced breast cancer: a pooled analysis of randomised PALOMA clinical studies. Eur J Cancer. 2018;101:123–33. https://doi.org/10.1016/j.ejca.2018.05.017.
102. Howie LJ, Singh H, Bloomquist E, Wedam S, Amiri-Kordestani L, Tang S, et al. Outcomes of older women with hormone receptor-positive, human epidermal growth factor receptor-negative metastatic breast cancer treated with a CDK4/6 inhibitor and an aromatase inhibitor: an FDA pooled analysis. J Clin Oncol. 2019;37(36):3475–83. https://doi.org/10.1200/jco.18.02217.
103. Battisti NML, De Glas N, Sedrak MS, Loh KP, Liposits G, Soto-Perez-de-Celis E, et al. Use of cyclin-dependent kinase 4/6 (CDK4/6) inhibitors in older patients with ER-positive HER2-negative breast cancer: Young International Society of Geriatric Oncology review paper. Ther Adv Med Oncol. 2018;10:1758835918809610. https://doi.org/10.1177/1758835918809610.
104. Papamichael D, Audisio RA, Glimelius B, de Gramont A, Glynne-Jones R, Haller D, et al. Treatment of colorectal cancer in older patients: International Society of Geriatric Oncology (SIOG) consensus recommendations 2013. Ann Oncol. 2015;26(3):463–76. https://doi.org/10.1093/annonc/mdu253.
105. Bouchahda M, Macarulla T, Spano JP, Bachet JB, Lledo G, Andre T, et al. Cetuximab efficacy and safety in a retrospective cohort of elderly patients with heavily pretreated metastatic colorectal cancer. Crit Rev Oncol Hematol. 2008;67(3):255–62. https://doi.org/10.1016/j.critrevonc.2008.02.003.

106. Jehn CF, Boning L, Kroning H, Possinger K, Luftner D. Cetuximab-based therapy in elderly comorbid patients with metastatic colorectal cancer. Br J Cancer. 2012;106(2):274–8. https://doi.org/10.1038/bjc.2011.554.
107. Cunningham D, Lang I, Marcuello E, Lorusso V, Ocvirk J, Shin DB, et al. Bevacizumab plus capecitabine versus capecitabine alone in elderly patients with previously untreated metastatic colorectal cancer (AVEX): an open-label, randomised phase 3 trial. Lancet Oncol. 2013;14(11):1077–85. https://doi.org/10.1016/s1470-2045(13)70154-2.
108. Feliu J, Safont MJ, Salud A, Losa F, Garcia-Giron C, Bosch C, et al. Capecitabine and bevacizumab as first-line treatment in elderly patients with metastatic colorectal cancer. Br J Cancer. 2010;102(10):1468–73. https://doi.org/10.1038/sj.bjc.6605663.
109. Losanno T, Gridelli C. Recent advances in targeted advanced lung cancer therapy in the elderly. Expert Rev Anticancer Ther. 2017;17(9):787–97. https://doi.org/10.1080/14737140.2017.1348232.
110. Inoue Y, Inui N, Asada K, Karayama M, Matsuda H, Yokomura K, et al. Phase II study of erlotinib in elderly patients with non-small cell lung cancer harboring epidermal growth factor receptor mutations. Cancer Chemother Pharmacol. 2015;76(1):155–61. https://doi.org/10.1007/s00280-015-2784-x.
111. Wu YL, Sequist LV, Tan EH, Geater SL, Orlov S, Zhang L, et al. Afatinib as first-line treatment of older patients with EGFR mutation-positive non-small-cell lung cancer: subgroup analyses of the LUX-Lung 3, LUX-lung 6, and LUX-lung 7 trials. Clin Lung Cancer. 2018;19(4):e465–e79. https://doi.org/10.1016/j.cllc.2018.03.009.
112. Takeyasu YG, Morita R, Sato J, Murakami S, Horinouchi H, Fujiwara Y, Kanda S, Yamamoto N, Ohe Y. Efficacy and safety of Epidermal Growth Factor Receptor (EGFR) - Tyrosine Kinase Inhibitors (TKI) in elderly patients with EGFR mutation-positive NSCLC. European Society for Medical Oncology Asia 2018 Congress. Singapore.
113. Miyamoto S, Azuma K, Ishii H, Bessho A, Hosokawa S, Fukamatsu N, et al. Low-dose Erlotinib treatment in elderly or frail patients with EGFR mutation-positive non-small cell lung cancer: a multicenter phase 2 trial. JAMA Oncol. 2020;6(7):e201250. https://doi.org/10.1001/jamaoncol.2020.1250.
114. Hirsch L, Zitvogel L, Eggermont A, Marabelle A. PD-Loma: a cancer entity with a shared sensitivity to the PD-1/PD-L1 pathway blockade. Br J Cancer. 2019;120(1):3–5.
115. Candore G, Grimaldi M, Listi F, Ferlazzo V, Colonna-Romano G, Motta M, et al. Prevalence of non organ-specific autoantibodies in healthy centenarians. Arch Gerontol Geriatr. 2002;35:75–80.
116. Pawelec G, Derhovanessian E, Larbi A. Immunosenescence and cancer. Crit Rev Oncol Hematol. 2010;75(2):165–72. https://doi.org/10.1016/j.critrevonc.2010.06.012.
117. Nagele EP, Han M, Acharya NK, DeMarshall C, Kosciuk MC, Nagele RG. Natural IgG autoantibodies are abundant and ubiquitous in human sera, and their number is influenced by age, gender, and disease. PLoS One. 2013;8(4):e60726.
118. Gavazzi G, Krause K-H. Ageing and infection. Lancet Infect Dis. 2002;2(11):659–66. https://doi.org/10.1016/s1473-3099(02)00437-1.
119. Ramos-Casals M, Brito-Zerón P, López-Soto A, Font J. Systemic autoimmune diseases in elderly patients: atypical presentation and association with neoplasia. Autoimmun Rev. 2004;3(5):376–82. https://doi.org/10.1016/j.autrev.2003.12.002.
120. Thomas R, Wang W, Su D-M. Contributions of age-related thymic involution to immunosenescence and inflammaging. Immun Ageing. 2020;17(1):1–17.
121. Fülöp T, Larbi A, Witkowski JM. Human inflammaging. Gerontology. 2019;65(5):495–504.
122. Ventura MT, Casciaro M, Gangemi S, Buquicchio R. Immunosenescence in aging: between immune cells depletion and cytokines up-regulation. Clin Mol Allergy. 2017;15(1):1–8.
123. Aiello A, Farzaneh F, Candore G, Caruso C, Davinelli S, Gambino CM, et al. Immunosenescence and its hallmarks: how to oppose aging strategically? A review of potential options for therapeutic intervention. Front Immunol. 2019;10:2247.

124. Oishi Y, Manabe I. Macrophages in age-related chronic inflammatory diseases. NPJ Aging Mech Dis. 2016;2(1):1–8.
125. Xu W, Larbi A. Markers of T cell senescence in humans. Int J Mol Sci. 2017;18(8):1742.
126. Pawelec G. Hallmarks of human "immunosenescence": adaptation or dysregulation? Immunity Ageing. 2012;9:15.
127. Pawelec G. Immunosenenescence: role of cytomegalovirus. Exp Gerontol. 2014;54:1–5.
128. Di Benedetto S, Derhovanessian E, Steinhagen-Thiessen E, Goldeck D, Müller L, Pawelec G. Impact of age, sex and CMV-infection on peripheral T cell phenotypes: results from the Berlin BASE-II Study. Biogerontology. 2015;16(5):631–43.
129. Franceschi C, Campisi J. Chronic inflammation (inflammaging) and its potential contribution to age-associated diseases. J Gerontol A Biol Sci Med Sci. 2014;69(Suppl 1):S4–9. https://doi.org/10.1093/gerona/glu057.
130. Franceschi C, Bonafè M, Valensin S, Olivieri F, De Luca M, Ottaviani E, et al. Inflamm-aging. An evolutionary perspective on immunosenescence. Ann N Y Acad Sci. 2000;908:244–54. https://doi.org/10.1111/j.1749-6632.2000.tb06651.x.
131. Nishijima TF, Muss HB, Shachar SS, Moschos SJ. Comparison of efficacy of immune checkpoint inhibitors (ICIs) between younger and older patients: a systematic review and meta-analysis. Cancer Treat Rev. 2016;45:30–7.
132. Elias R, Giobbie-Hurder A, McCleary NJ, Ott P, Hodi FS, Rahma O. Efficacy of PD-1 & PD-L1 inhibitors in older adults: a meta-analysis. J Immunother Cancer. 2018;6(1):1–8.
133. Ferrara R, Mezquita L, Auclin E, Chaput N, Besse B. Immunosenescence and immunecheckpoint inhibitors in non-small cell lung cancer patients: does age really matter? Cancer Treat Rev. 2017;60:60–8.
134. Hodi FS, O'Day SJ, McDermott DF, Weber RW, Sosman JA, Haanen JB, et al. Improved survival with ipilimumab in patients with metastatic melanoma. N Engl J Med. 2010;363(8):711–23.
135. Herin H, Aspeslagh S, Castanon E, Dyevre V, Marabelle A, Varga A, et al. Immunotherapy phase I trials in patients older than 70 years with advanced solid tumours. Eur J Cancer. 2018;95:68–74.
136. Elkrief A, Richard C, Malo J, Cvetkovic L, Florescu M, Blais N, et al. Efficacy of immune checkpoint inhibitors in older patients with non-small cell lung cancer: real-world data from multicentric cohorts in Canada and France. J Geriatr Oncol. 2020;11(5):802–6.
137. Gettinger S, Rizvi NA, Chow LQ, Borghaei H, Brahmer J, Ready N, et al. Nivolumab monotherapy for first-line treatment of advanced non–small-cell lung cancer. J Clin Oncol. 2016;34(25):2980.
138. Spigel DR, McCleod M, Jotte RM, Einhorn L, Horn L, Waterhouse DM, et al. Safety, efficacy, and patient-reported health-related quality of life and symptom burden with nivolumab in patients with advanced non-small cell lung cancer, including patients aged 70 years or older or with poor performance status (CheckMate 153). J Thorac Oncol. 2019;14(9):1628–39.
139. Grossi F, Crinò L, Logroscino A, Canova S, Delmonte A, Melotti B, et al. Use of nivolumab in elderly patients with advanced squamous non-small-cell lung cancer: results from the Italian cohort of an expanded access programme. Eur J Cancer. 2018;100:126–34.
140. Betof AS, Nipp RD, Giobbie-Hurder A, Johnpulle RA, Rubin K, Rubinstein SM, et al. Impact of age on outcomes with immunotherapy for patients with melanoma. Oncologist. 2017;22(8):963.
141. Robert C, Long GV, Brady B, Dutriaux C, Maio M, Mortier L, et al. Nivolumab in previously untreated melanoma without BRAF mutation. N Engl J Med. 2015;372(4):320–30.
142. Sileni VC, Pigozzo J, Ascierto PA, Grimaldi AM, Maio M, Di Guardo L, et al. Efficacy and safety of ipilimumab in elderly patients with pretreated advanced melanoma treated at Italian centres through the expanded access programme. J Exp Clin Cancer Res. 2014;33(1):1–7.
143. Balar AV, Castellano D, O'Donnell PH, Grivas P, Vuky J, Powles T, et al. First-line pembrolizumab in cisplatin-ineligible patients with locally advanced and unresectable or metastatic

urothelial cancer (KEYNOTE-052): a multicentre, single-arm, phase 2 study. Lancet Oncol. 2017;18(11):1483–92.
144. Bellmunt J, De Wit R, Vaughn DJ, Fradet Y, Lee J-L, Fong L, et al. Pembrolizumab as second-line therapy for advanced urothelial carcinoma. N Engl J Med. 2017;376(11):1015–26.
145. Johnpulle RA, Conry RM, Sosman JA, Puzanov I, Johnson DB. Responses to immune checkpoint inhibitors in nonagenarians. Oncoimmunology. 2016;5(11):e1234572.
146. Borghaei H, Paz-Ares L, Horn L, Spigel DR, Steins M, Ready NE, et al. Nivolumab versus docetaxel in advanced nonsquamous non-small-cell lung cancer. N Engl J Med. 2015;373(17):1627–39. https://doi.org/10.1056/NEJMoa1507643.
147. Brahmer J, Reckamp KL, Baas P, Crinò L, Eberhardt WE, Poddubskaya E, et al. Nivolumab versus docetaxel in advanced squamous-cell non-small-cell lung cancer. N Engl J Med. 2015;373(2):123–35. https://doi.org/10.1056/NEJMoa1504627.
148. Freeman M, Weber J. Subset analysis of the safety and efficacy of nivolumab in elderly patients with metastatic melanoma. J Immunother Cancer. 2015;3(2):P133. https://doi.org/10.1186/2051-1426-3-S2-P133.
149. Popat S, Ardizzoni A, Ciuleanu T, Cobo Dols M, Laktionov K, Szilasi M, et al. Nivolumab in previously treated patients with metastatic squamous NSCLC: results of a European single-arm, phase 2 trial (CheckMate 171) including patients aged ≥70 years and with poor performance status. Ann Oncol. 2017;28:v463. https://doi.org/10.1093/annonc/mdx380.006.
150. Alkharabsheh O, Kannarkatt P, Kannarkatt J, Karapetyan L, Laird-Fick HS, Al-Janadi A. An overview of the toxicities of checkpoint inhibitors in older patients with cancer. J Geriatr Oncol. 2018;9(5):451–8. https://doi.org/10.1016/j.jgo.2018.02.002.
151. Gomes F, Wong M, Battisti NML, Kordbacheh T, Kiderlen M, Greystoke A, et al. Immunotherapy in older patients with non-small cell lung cancer: Young International Society of Geriatric Oncology position paper. Br J Cancer. 2020; https://doi.org/10.1038/s41416-020-0986-4.
152. Singh H, Kim G, Maher VE, Beaver JA, Pai-Scherf LH, Balasubramaniam S, et al. FDA subset analysis of the safety of nivolumab in elderly patients with advanced cancers. J Clin Oncol. 2016;34(15 suppl):10010. https://doi.org/10.1200/JCO.2016.34.15_suppl.10010.
153. Nishijima TF, Shachar SS, Nyrop KA, Muss HB. Safety and tolerability of PD-1/PD-L1 inhibitors compared with chemotherapy in patients with advanced cancer: a meta-analysis. Oncologist. 2017;22(4):470–9. https://doi.org/10.1634/theoncologist.2016-0419.
154. Nosaki K, Saka H, Hosomi Y, Baas P, de Castro G, Reck M, et al. Safety and efficacy of pembrolizumab monotherapy in elderly patients with PD-L1-positive advanced non-small-cell lung cancer: Pooled analysis from the KEYNOTE-010, KEYNOTE-024, and KEYNOTE-042 studies. Lung Cancer. 2019;135:188–95. https://doi.org/10.1016/j.lungcan.2019.07.004.
155. Sattar J, Kartolo A, Hopman WM, Lakoff JM, Baetz T. The efficacy and toxicity of immune checkpoint inhibitors in a real-world older patient population. J Geriatr Oncol. 2019;10(3):411–4. https://doi.org/10.1016/j.jgo.2018.07.015.
156. Chiarion Sileni V, Pigozzo J, Ascierto PA, Grimaldi AM, Maio M, Di Guardo L, et al. Efficacy and safety of ipilimumab in elderly patients with pretreated advanced melanoma treated at Italian centres through the expanded access programme. J Exp Clin Cancer Res. 2014;33(1):30. https://doi.org/10.1186/1756-9966-33-30.
157. Leroy V, Gerard E, Dutriaux C, Prey S, Gey A, Mertens C, et al. Adverse events need for hospitalization and systemic immunosuppression in very elderly patients (over 80 years) treated with ipilimumab for metastatic melanoma. Cancer Immunol Immunother. 2019;68(4):545–51. https://doi.org/10.1007/s00262-019-02298-9.
158. Muchnik E, Loh KP, Strawderman M, Magnuson A, Mohile SG, Estrah V, et al. Immune checkpoint inhibitors in real-world treatment of older adults with non-small cell lung cancer. J Am Geriatr Soc. 2019;67(5):905–12. https://doi.org/10.1111/jgs.15750.
159. Baldini C, Martin Romano P, Voisin AL, Danlos FX, Champiat S, Laghouati S, et al. Impact of aging on immune-related adverse events generated by anti-programmed death (ligand) PD-(L)1 therapies. Eur J Cancer. 2020;129:71–9. https://doi.org/10.1016/j.ejca.2020.01.013.

160. Welaya K, Loh KP, Messing S, Szuba E, Magnuson A, Mohile SG, et al. Geriatric assessment and treatment outcomes in older adults with cancer receiving immune checkpoint inhibitors. J Geriatr Oncol. 2020;11(3):523–8. https://doi.org/10.1016/j.jgo.2019.05.021.
161. Sbrana A, Antognoli R, Pasqualetti G, Linsalata G, Okoye C, Calsolaro V, et al. Effectiveness of Multi-Prognostic Index in older patients with advanced malignancies treated with immunotherapy. J Geriatr Oncol. 2020;11(3):503–7. https://doi.org/10.1016/j.jgo.2019.09.010.
162. Archibald WJ, Victor AI, Strawderman MS, Maggiore RJ. Immune checkpoint inhibitors in older adults with melanoma or cutaneous malignancies: the Wilmot Cancer Institute experience. J Geriatr Oncol. 2020;11(3):496–502. https://doi.org/10.1016/j.jgo.2019.07.005.
163. Silva CC, Herchenhorn D. Treating the elderly with immune checkpoint inhibitors: Real life experience from a large Brazilian center. J Clin Oncol. 2018;36(15 suppl):e15077. https://doi.org/10.1200/JCO.2018.36.15_suppl.e15077.
164. Gomes F, Lorigan P, Woolley S, Foden P, Burns K, Yorke J, et al. A prospective cohort study on the safety of checkpoint inhibitors in older cancer patients – the ELDERS study. ESMO Open. 2021;6(1):100042. https://doi.org/10.1016/j.esmoop.2020.100042.
165. Rini BI, Plimack ER, Stus V, Gafanov R, Hawkins R, Nosov D, et al. Pembrolizumab plus Axitinib versus sunitinib for advanced renal-cell carcinoma. N Engl J Med. 2019;380(12):1116–27. https://doi.org/10.1056/NEJMoa1816714.
166. Motzer RJ, Tannir NM, McDermott DF, Arén Frontera O, Melichar B, Choueiri TK, et al. Nivolumab plus Ipilimumab versus sunitinib in advanced renal-cell carcinoma. N Engl J Med. 2018;378(14):1277–90. https://doi.org/10.1056/NEJMoa1712126.
167. Gandhi L, Rodríguez-Abreu D, Gadgeel S, Esteban E, Felip E, De Angelis F, et al. Pembrolizumab plus chemotherapy in metastatic non-small-cell lung cancer. N Engl J Med. 2018;378(22):2078–92. https://doi.org/10.1056/NEJMoa1801005.
168. Hellmann MD, Paz-Ares L, Bernabe Caro R, Zurawski B, Kim SW, Carcereny Costa E, et al. Nivolumab plus Ipilimumab in advanced non-small-cell lung cancer. N Engl J Med. 2019;381(21):2020–31. https://doi.org/10.1056/NEJMoa1910231.
169. Paz-Ares L, Luft A, Vicente D, Tafreshi A, Gümüş M, Mazières J, et al. Pembrolizumab plus chemotherapy for squamous non-small-cell lung cancer. N Engl J Med. 2018;379(21):2040–51.
170. Nishio M, Barlesi F, West H, Ball S, Bordoni R, Cobo M, et al. Atezolizumab plus chemotherapy for first-line treatment of non-squamous non-small cell lung cancer: results from the randomized Phase III IMpower132 Trial. J Thorac Oncol. 2020.
171. West H, McCleod M, Hussein M, Morabito A, Rittmeyer A, Conter HJ, et al. Atezolizumab in combination with carboplatin plus nab-paclitaxel chemotherapy compared with chemotherapy alone as first-line treatment for metastatic non-squamous non-small-cell lung cancer (IMpower130): a multicentre, randomised, open-label, phase 3 trial. Lancet Oncol. 2019;20(7):924–37.
172. Motzer RJ, Penkov K, Haanen J, Rini B, Albiges L, Campbell MT, et al. Avelumab plus Axitinib versus sunitinib for advanced renal-cell carcinoma. N Engl J Med. 2019;380(12):1103–15. https://doi.org/10.1056/NEJMoa1816047.
173. Balaji A, Zhang J, Wills B, Marrone KA, Elmariah H, Yarchoan M, et al. Immune-related adverse events requiring hospitalization: spectrum of toxicity, treatment, and outcomes. J Oncol Pract. 2019;15(9):e825–e34. https://doi.org/10.1200/jop.18.00703.
174. Shah KP, Song H, Ye F, Moslehi JJ, Balko JM, Salem JE, et al. Demographic factors associated with toxicity in patients treated with anti-programmed cell death-1 therapy. Cancer Immunol Res. 2020;8(7):851–5. https://doi.org/10.1158/2326-6066.Cir-19-0986.
175. Macaire P, Morawska K, Vincent J, Quipourt V, Marilier S, Ghiringhelli F, et al. Therapeutic drug monitoring as a tool to optimize 5-FU-based chemotherapy in gastrointestinal cancer patients older than 75 years. Eur J Cancer. 2019;111:116–25. https://doi.org/10.1016/j.ejca.2019.01.102.
176. Abbasi J. Older patients (still) left out of cancer clinical trials. JAMA. 2019;322:1751–3. https://doi.org/10.1001/jama.2019.17016.

Chapter 15
Palliative Care in Older Adults with Cancer and Frailty

Arvindselvan Mohanaselvan, Rex Paulino, Lily Wieland, Ishwaria Subbiah, and Holly M. Holmes

Introduction

Palliative care is an approach that addresses and improves the quality of life (QoL) of patients and their family members by early recognition of pain and other distress symptoms, integrating psychological and spiritual aspects of patient care, and using a team approach to cater to the needs of the patient and family members [1]. Supportive care is an all-encompassing service providing care from diagnosis to bereavement, which includes palliative care with symptom management during cancer treatment [2]. The Center to Advance Palliative Care defines the methods of palliative medicine as "focused on providing patients with relief from the symptoms, pain, and stress of a serious illness-whatever the diagnosis or prognosis." The American Society of Clinical Oncology (ASCO) Provisional Clinical Opinion defines that palliative care is "focused on relief of suffering, in all of its dimensions." [3].

A. Mohanaselvan · R. Paulino · H. M. Holmes (✉)
Joan and Stanford Alexander Division of Geriatric and Palliative Medicine, McGovern Medical School, Houston, TX, USA
e-mail: arvindselvan.mohanaselvan@uth.tmc.edu; rexalvin.d.paulino@uth.tmc.edu; holly.m.holmes@uth.tmc.edu

L. Wieland
Rice University, Houston, TX, USA
e-mail: lcw4@rice.edu

I. Subbiah
Department of Palliative, Rehabilitation and Integrative Medicine, Division of Cancer Medicine, University of Texas MD Anderson Cancer Center, Houston, TX, USA
e-mail: isubbiah@mdanderson.org

F. Gomes (ed.), *Frailty in Older Adults with Cancer*,
https://doi.org/10.1007/978-3-030-89162-6_15

Hospice is a multidisciplinary team-based approach comprising routine home care, general inpatient care, continuous care and respite care according to the National Hospice and Palliative Care Organization [4]. Cicely Saunders, who founded the modern hospice movement, defined hospice care as having four pillars of support—medical, psychological, spiritual, and social care [5]. The Irish Hospice Foundation defines this as helping people with illness that is no longer curable, relieving the physical symptoms of the patients while equally addressing spiritual and emotional needs, supporting the family and helping with bereavement [6]. Countries in which resources are scarcer also may define their hospice and palliative care based on the services provided by oncology nurses to the patient and family [7].

The role of palliative care is increasing as the global population is aging and the life expectancy of a human being is slowly increasing, currently at a peak of 86 in Japan [8]. This is particularly marked in developed countries, where the number of people >65 years of age will double in the coming 30 years [9]. With the increasing numbers of older adults, the number of people affected with cancer will also increase. As of 2012, 22% of the United States (US) population is >65 years, and 28% of those >75 years are affected with cancer [10]. Moreover, with the increase in age, there is a significant decline in physiological reserve, increased development of acute and chronic illness, and acquisition of functional deficits [11]. Thus, older people face a significant burden of multimorbidity, disability, and geriatric syndromes [12]. As a result of cumulative deficits associated with advancing age, older people are more much likely to be frail. Frailty is also described as a syndrome of weakness, weight loss, low energy, and poor nutrition. Older patients with frailty are more susceptible to adverse effects of treatment and less capable to cope with cancer-related symptoms [13, 14]. Therefore, the role of palliative care is particularly crucial in this subgroup of patients.

A key step to inform decision-making for older adults with cancer is to use geriatric assessment to help determine whether a patient is fit, vulnerable, or frail. This helps to guide clinicians and patients about non-cancer prognosis compared to prognosis with cancer [15]. For those older patients with frailty and a poor prognosis (due primarily to cancer or frailty), palliative care has an important role with early provision of multidisciplinary care focused on improving QoL and preserving function as much as possible. Palliative care also plays an important role in the management of toxicities of cancer therapy, providing supportive care measures that could help patients with frailty to complete treatment. For patients whose cancer and frailty preclude active cancer therapy, the provision of primarily palliative care to alleviate cancer symptom burden may be the primary strategy.

This chapter will discuss the availability of palliative care, the ease of access in older adults, the benefits of early integration of palliative care in oncology treatments, pharmacological considerations in older adults, and a special focus on the specifics of care in older cancer patients with frailty.

Palliative Care Availability and Access

Palliative care availability, ease of access and the use of hospice care in older adults exist as a varied spectrum in different countries across the globe. This is best provided with an interprofessional team consisting of physicians, surgeons, palliative care trained nurses, dieticians, occupational therapists, pharmacists, social workers to begin with. Palliative care is the fastest-growing medical specialty in the United States. However, there is significant variation by region with respect to palliative medicine availability. According to the State-by-State Report Card on Access to Palliative Care published by the Center to Advance Palliative Care (CAPC), three-quarters of the states now have a grade of A or B with regard to access, meaning that 60% or more of the hospitals have palliative care [16].

Broadly, the provision of palliative care relies on a close collaboration between trained professionals and a volunteer community to help care for chronically ill and dying patients. In India and Tanzania, for example, the volunteers in the community, with the help of trained professionals, help with taking care of chronically ill and dying patients and integrate palliative care capacity to home-based care programs. In Romania, providers are getting palliative care training from purpose-built hospice/palliative training centers so that patients, both adults and children, get the necessary care needed. In Vietnam, the government-run hospital system is integrating palliative care training to interested medical staff members with the help of Harvard Medical School Center for Palliative Care (HMSCPC) and with those trained physicians opened up a department for palliative care with inpatient, outpatient, and consultation services. In Argentina, there is a not-for-profit non-governmental organization that has helped in providing palliative care in the acute care setting [17].

An important step in providing palliative care is to screen the patient for the need for it. However, traditionally, oncologists have only screened patients for their overall fitness by using performance status scales like the Karnofsky Performance Scale (KPS), Australia modified Karnofsky Performance Scale (AKPS) and the Eastern Cooperative Oncology Group Performance Status (ECOG-PS) [18, 19]. Geriatric assessments are a key step to effectively screen for frailty and the appropriateness of the treatment plan and also to identify key deficits that could be improved to provide the best supportive care [20]. Moreover, symptom screening instruments like the Edmonton Symptom Assessment Scale (ESAS) are useful to look for pain, fatigue, nausea, depression, anxiety, drowsiness, appetite, well-being, and shortness of breath. Failure to screen patients on any of the domains mentioned previously using the available screening tests is the first major obstacle in a patient getting the care they need resulting in underutilization of palliative care [21].

Another reason for the underutilization of palliative care is the failure to understand what it is and acceptance of what it pertains to. Providers and patients alike think of palliative care as "focusing on terminal pain," "managing actively dying patients," and the families perceive them as "providers giving up hope" or "pulling the plug." The study by Rodriguez et al. confirmed this and also found that a sizeable contribution to the barriers of early integration of palliative care came in the form of not understanding the complete range of palliative care services available as well as the physicians' concern about the loss of autonomy. There were also concerns about the reputation of the institutions, lawsuits, beliefs, and perceptions of the patients and economic constraints [22]. Even as multiple studies have shown that early integration of palliative care shows better outcomes, not all places where patients with cancer receive care have adequate access to palliative care and to hospice care [23].

Palliative Care Integration in Oncology

Early integration of palliative care is associated with symptom relief, improved mood, reduced depressive symptoms, improved QoL and survival, overall satisfaction with treatment outcomes, and reduced cost of care [5]. The most exhaustive review of the early integration of palliative care found evidence for overall improvement in QOL, decrease in symptom intensity, and improved mood and explained the growing support for the utilization of early integration of palliative care early [24]. Hui et al. recommended that successful early collaboration between the two fields could be facilitated by structural elements (presence of inpatient palliative care team and outpatient clinic) and clinical processes (interdisciplinary team, routine symptom screening, routine documentation of advanced care planning, and early referral) [25].

Efforts to integrate palliative care into the routine care delivery models have evolved out of compelling findings from clinical studies demonstrating the impact of palliative care on multiple domains of person's well-being. Several studies explored the impact of palliative care on the global symptom burden of persons with cancer [26–28]. Higginson and Evans in 2010 reviewed 32 studies, 8 of which were randomized controlled trials, which studied the impact of integrating palliative care versus standard oncological care on symptom control and hospital use. The review found that palliative care significantly improved all of these domains [26].

The study by Temel et al. in 2010 is widely considered the landmark trial that supports the benefits of early integration of palliative care. In this study, 151 patients with newly diagnosed non-small cell lung cancer (NSCLC) with an initial ECOG <2 and metastatic disease were enrolled to receive multidisciplinary palliative care concurrent with cancer care. The study included symptom assessment and provided early palliative care assessments to the intervention arm of the patients. Outcome measures included QoL metrics, assessments of depression and anxiety. Notably, they also evaluated overall survival. The median survival of patients receiving early palliative care was 11.6 months compared to patients without early integration, who had a median survival of 8.9 months. Combined care showed the greatest improvement in QoL, with improvements in depression, survival, and lower aggressiveness of care [29]. Another study from the same author showed more patients who received palliative care came to understand their prognosis accurately and received less chemotherapy at the end-of-life [30]..

Similarly, Zimmerman et al. investigated the impact of early integration of a palliative care team in conjunction with usual oncologic care versus usual oncologic care in 461 patients with advanced cancer in a cluster randomized, controlled study [31]. At 4 months, patients in the combination arm demonstrated improvement in the measures of their QoL, QoL at the end-of-life, symptom intensity/severity, as well as satisfaction with care. Rabow et al. studied patients with advanced cancer, chronic obstructive pulmonary disease, and congestive heart failure in a prospective, randomized, and controlled study with 90 participants [32]. Patients in the palliative care arm (as opposed to standard care) experienced improved symptoms, specifically dyspnea and anxiety, as well as improved spiritual well-being. Scibeta et al. showed that early palliative care at 6months (94-363 days) showed a statistically significant decrease in inpatient admission, intensive care unit admission and cost of care [33]. A study in 2012 by Wentlandt et al. showed that 42% of physicians considered the ideal time to refer to palliative care to be the time of diagnosis of incurable cancer, and 34% felt the ideal time was with an estimated 1–6 months survival, and 21% thought the best time for referral was when the prognosis was 6–12 months [34]. Reyes-Ortiz et al. showed that in hospitalized frail older adult patients, early palliative care consultations, i.e., within 3 days of admission, showed a statistically significant decrease in the length of stay, reduced long-term acute care admissions, and increased hospice care discharges [35].

These consistent findings across multiple advanced illnesses, including cancer, have led to consensus opinions among societies on the early integration of palliative care. Within oncology, the 2012 American Society of Clinical Oncology (ASCO) Provisional Clinical Opinion recommends combining standard oncologic care and palliative care at initial diagnosis based on substantial evidence from randomized, controlled trials showing that such combined care results in improved symptom control, QoL, and satisfaction for both patients and caregivers [3]. The 2016 ASCO updated guidelines emphasize the importance of integrating palliative care with standard oncological care at the onset of diagnosis for improved QoL, symptom control, survival, and patient and caregiver satisfaction [3].

Bakitas et al. conducted a randomized controlled trial of 322 patients with advanced cancer randomized to receive either standard oncologic care or standard care integrated with a palliative care psychoeducational intervention [36]. The multidisciplinary intervention named Project ENABLE (Educate, Nurture, Advise, Before Life Ends) consists of 4 weekly educational sessions followed by monthly sessions until study completion or death, all led by advanced practice nurses. Overall, those patients in the intervention arm demonstrated favorably better scores for mood and QoL when compared to the standard care arm but no statistically significant differences in symptom intensity or days in hospital or visits to the emergency center.

Hanks et al. conducted a randomized controlled trial of 261 patients in either a full multidisciplinary specialist palliative care team or a limited telephone advice palliative care team [28]. The patients in the full multidisciplinary care arm experienced better symptom relief, QoL, and mood than the more limited telephone care arm, though both groups had high satisfaction with care.

Trials comparing standard care with integrated or early integrated palliative care have shown improvements in QoL, depression, less chemotherapy use, improved communication, improved relationships, better psychosocial elements of illness, greater satisfaction, lower distress, and lower symptoms burden [26, 28–31].

Ultimately, by improving clinical outcomes with the integration of palliative care, this may also result in a more cost-effective model of care. Cassell et al. examined the cost of integrating palliative care for patients and for hospitals and concluded that it resulted in an overall cost reduction, providing the ten principles that made the "business case for palliative care" [37]. These principles include palliative care's tendency to reduce avoidable utilization of expensive health services and to improve symptoms, which reduces further admissions costs. Smith et al. examined 46 articles on the economic impacts of palliative care [38]. The review found that palliative care reduces direct costs for patients in most cases but provides the disclaimer that many studies did not examine informal care or out-of-pocket costs. The Brumley et al. study of 238 terminally ill patients also reported that those patients randomized to an integrated palliative care model (versus standard care) had a lower mean cost of care by almost $8000 [26]. Similarly, the previously described Gade et al. randomized trial of 512 seriously ill patients reported that the patients in the integrated palliative care arm had fewer intensive care unit stays and lower mean cost of care by almost $7000 compared to the control arm [39].

Palliative Care for Older Cancer Patients with Frailty

Patients with frailty may need modified treatment plans, greater symptom palliation and more intensive supportive care interventions to be able to receive cancer therapy. Often it is the frailty primarily, not cancer, that determines the cancer treatment strategy, limiting curative-intent strategies or even any active cancer treatment. Overall, the palliative care has a role in two major settings in older cancer patients with frailty:

1. By supporting these patients through their active cancer treatment, either palliative- or radical/curative-intent treatment, although usually with a bigger role in the first.
2. By supportive these patients when active cancer treatment in not appropriate but patients are symptomatic, a strategy described as "best supportive care only."

Caring for older cancer patients with frailty present many challenges to a healthcare provider. Issues such as concurrent comorbidities and diminished physiologic reserve coupled with a complex psychological, social, emotional, and spiritual situation make this responsibility more daunting. There can be a substantial difference between the biological age and chronological age of a person, resulting in a significant heterogeneity in the anticipated life expectancy for older adults who have the same chronological age [40]. The differences in survival may go undetected by traditional tools such as performance status and can equally lead to overtreatment and undertreatment in older adults with cancer, particularly those with frailty. Using geriatric assessment as a key tool to "stage the aging" of a patient with cancer can greatly assist in the decision-making process and to help guide when patients should have primarily a palliative-focused care [41]. A study by Schiphortst et al. showed that >90% of patients referred for geriatric consultation by an oncologist had at least one underlying geriatric syndrome, and 49% of the patients were previously undiagnosed [42, 43]. Knowing how fit or frail an older patient is before determining cancer therapy can help guide therapy to lower intensity, to provide additional supportive care or social interventions that make treatment more feasible and can improve communication between the oncology team and the patient and caregiver [14, 44].

The palliative care needs in older adults are an often under assessed domain and patients' symptoms, particularly pain, are often undertreated [45]. When such patients also have frailty, this increases the susceptibility to adverse outcomes, the rate of functional decline and the chances of a decline in QoL and physical status [46]. The way palliative care in older adults with frailty differs from non-frail older adults is that patients with frailty are more likely to have multiple deficits in domains of physical and psychological function and may benefit even more from a thorough and holistic approach. This approach includes identifying and treating reversible causes of decline, forming individualized treatment plans, screening for weight loss, pain, depression, insomnia, and assessing for the severity of frailty and communicating with the patient and family/caregivers about the prognostic implications of frailty [47]. Advanced Care Planning also plays a major role, especially in older adults with frailty. It is important to address these conversations early, as the patient might need time to process the information about their condition and the necessity to make advanced care planning [47]. Pain management as part of palliative care needs for frail older adults with cancer is also a challenge due to the higher risks of adverse events in frail older adults [48]. An example would be an older cancer patient with frailty having poorly controlled severe pain from bone metastasis, which then have a direct impact on functional status, mental health, treatment tolerability, among other impacts on QoL.

Another important consideration in palliative care is polypharmacy, which can be approached by using specific tools, such as the STOPP and START criteria [49], or even STOPPFrail, which is the STOPP criteria modified for frailty.

Serious illness in older adults is often associated with a high prevalence of untreated symptoms which could result in progressive functional decline and loss of independence, both of which negatively impact their QoL [50]. Family caregivers also play a vital role in caring for these individuals. Changes in roles and employment as well as disruption in schedules need to be accounted for when creating a treatment plan [51]. Recognizing the value of an older adults' social support is also essential since involving the caregiver in the treatment decision-making process facilitates compliance [50]. Appropriate utilization of a Palliative Care-led multidisciplinary approach to care in older cancer patients with frailty places emphasis on QoL, maintaining independence, minimizing symptom burden, and optimizing emotional and spiritual health.

At the end-of-life, marked progression of frailty in older adults with cancer is common. A cohort analysis looking at self- or proxy-reported physical function within the last year of life and predicted activities of daily living (ADL) dependency prior to death demonstrated that those with frailty were relatively more disabled in their final year (and especially dependent during their last month) when compared to patients with sudden death, cancer, and organ failure decedents. Older adults with frailty were more than eight times more likely than sudden death patients to be ADL dependent [52]. As such, it is not surprising that older adults with cancer at the end-of-life suffer from significant frailty-related complications. Terminally ill patients with advanced cancer could have as high as 42% prevalence of presumed infection at the final phase of care [53]. Data from the 2007 National Home and Hospice Care Survey reported 27% of hospice patients received an antibiotic during the last week of their life [54]. Wound prevalence studies of hospice patients report wound rates up to 47%, half of which are pressure related and directly related to immobility [55]. Cachexia at the end-of-life contributes to persistent weight loss and progressive functional decline. The inability to eat or drink, along with changes in body image, contribute to emotional distress among patients and caregivers [56]. These complications often lead to a shorter life expectancy with poor QoL. Clinicians need to clarify goals of care and practice shared decision-making to address these issues and ultimately determine which interventions contribute to an older adult's QoL.

Pharmacological Considerations

Older patients with cancer and frailty must have special considerations for safe medication use, particularly as palliative care implies the use of most often multiple drugs (on top of the usual patient medication and cancer treatment-related medication). Age-related changes in physiology may lead to altered pharmacokinetics and pharmacodynamics, which can result in more drug toxicities and ultimately higher incidence of morbidity and mortality. It is imperative to be mindful of these changes when considering treatment options to minimize complications.

Regarding pharmacokinetics, *Absorption* can be influenced by various gastrointestinal factors, including reduced motility, reduced gastric emptying time, reduced digestive enzyme activity, reduced splanchnic blood flow, and diminished mucosal integrity [57, 58]. Hepatic metabolism after gastrointestinal tract absorption is responsible for the wide range of opioid bioavailability. These factors altogether determine the bioavailability of an ingested drug which may be altered with advanced age, especially in octogenarians and older [57]. Volume of *distribution* (Vd) can be significantly higher for lipophilic drugs in patients with frailty due to higher relative body fat and reduced lean muscle mass, and decreased intracellular water [58]. In consequence, lipophilic drugs such as opioids distribute faster across the blood-brain barrier and, as such, tend to have a more rapid onset and shorter duration of action [59]. *Metabolism* is further complicated by age-related physiologic changes. Codeine, hydrocodone, and tramadol are mostly controlled by CYP 2D6 enzymes, whereas fentanyl, oxycodone, and methadone are metabolized by CYP 3A4 enzymes [60]. Phase II metabolism includes conjugation reactions mainly involving UDP-glucuronosyltransferase (UGT) to produce water-soluble substances which are excreted in the bile and urine [58]. Substrates are drugs that are metabolized by specific enzymes, e.g., CYP 450. When opioids are administered, they are considered substrates for that particular system. Concomitantly taking opioids with enzyme inhibitors or inducers can lead to opioid overactivity or inadequate analgesia, respectively (Table 15.1) [61]. In addition, age-related physiologic changes may inherently contribute to altered metabolism in the older individual. Hepatic function declines with age: decreased hepatic blood flow of around 1% annually beyond the age of 25 years and reduced liver size by a quarter to almost half between ages 20–80 years [58, 62], resulting in reduced hepatic drug clearance. The overall combination of all these factors heavily impacts effective analgesia. Age-related changes in renal *excretion* may impact drug dosing in the older individual. Renal function declines approximately 10% per decade after the second decade of life [58]. Reduced muscle mass in older adults results in age-related reduction in creatinine clearance (CrCl) which may not be proportional to a relatively normal serum creatinine [63] and should routinely be considered when formulating a treatment plan. Majority of opioid metabolites are excreted through the kidneys with one exception being Methadone which is primarily excreted through the bile [64]. Overall, these changes determine a drug's half-life that clinicians need to be mindful of when titrating opioids to effect.

Regarding pharmacodynamic considerations, such changes have not been well studied in the context of aging. Age-related changes in older adults can, for example, increase the sensitivity to opioids which suggests an altered intrinsic potency [65] and translates into an even narrower therapeutic window. Despite these challenges, the clinical implications of the aforementioned mechanisms are more straightforward to manage, for example, by example starting opioids at lower doses and with about 25–50% of the usual dose to account for higher sensitivity; also titrating slowly to allow for longer circulation times and anticipate longer duration of action due to reduced clearance.

Table 15.1 Cytochrome P450 3A4 and 2D6 Substrates, Inhibitors, and Inducers; drugs mentioned under inhibitors and inducers have the most clinically significant interaction with opioids (Adapted from [60, 61])

Enzyme	Substrates	Inhibitors	Inducers
CYP 3A4	Fentanyl, oxycodone, methadone, tramadol	Amiodarone, clarithromycin, diltiazem, erythromycin, fluconazole, itraconazole, ketoconazole, verapamil, voriconazole	Phenytoin, rifampin, troglitazone
CYP 2D6	Codeine, hydrocodone, tramadol, oxycodone[a], methadone[b]	Amiodarone, fluoxetine, mibefradil, paroxetine, quinidine, terbinafine, thioridazine	None reported

[a]Minor metabolic pathway
[b]Undergoes varying degrees of metabolism with CYP 2B6, CYP 2C8, CYP 2C19, and CYP 2C9

Conclusion

Palliative care and supportive care both address quality of life, symptom management and holistic well-being in a patient with life-limiting illness. Older patients with cancer and frailty need supportive care strategies in particular, due to underlying vulnerabilities that make treatment exceptionally challenging. In some cases, a primarily palliative approach is the best treatment strategy for an older cancer patient with frailty. Increasing numbers of studies show the benefits of palliative care and of early integration of this multidisciplinary approach to cancer treatment. Some symptoms may be more common or may even be unique in older adults with cancer and frailty, and a focus on unique toxicities and on caregiver support are essential, in addition to multidisciplinary care. Pharmacological considerations are essential to provide safe care in older patients with frailty and cancer. As always, an approach to a patient with frailty requires attention to the very delicate balance between overtreatment and undertreatment, which can more easily occur in older patients with cancer.

References

1. World Health Organization. WHO Definition for Palliative Care. Available at: https://www.who.int/cancer/palliative/definition/en/. Accessed October 23, 2020.
2. Hui D, De La Cruz M, Mori M, Parsons HA, Kwon JH, Torres-Vigil I, et al. Concepts and definitions for "supportive care," "best supportive care," "palliative care," and "hospice care" in the published literature, dictionaries, and textbooks. Support Care Cancer. 2013 Mar;21(3):659–85.
3. Ferrell BR, Temel JS, Temin S, Alesi ER, Balboni TA, Basch EM, et al. Integration of palliative care into standard oncology care: American Society of Clinical Oncology Clinical Practice Guideline Update. J Clin Oncol. 2017 Jan;35(1):96–112.
4. National Hospice and Palliative Care : Hopsice Care Overview for Professionals. 2020.; Available at https://www.nhpco.org/hospice-care-overview/hospice-faqs/. Accessed 25 October 2020.
5. Saunders DCM, Clark D. Cicely Saunders: selected writings 1958-2004. Oxford: Oxford University Press; 2006.
6. Irish Hospice Foundation. What is Hospice Care. 2020; Available at: https://hospicefoundation.ie/aboutus/hospice-palliative-and-end-of-life-care/what-is-hospice-care/. Accessed 25 October 2020.
7. Walker DK, Edwards RL, Bagcivan G, Bakitas MA. Cancer and palliative care in the United States, Turkey, and Malawi: developing global collaborations. Asia Pac J Oncol Nurs. 2017 Jul–Sep;4(3):209–19.
8. Kanasi E, Ayilavarapu S, Jones J. The aging population: demographics and the biology of aging. Periodontol 2000. 2016;72(1):13–8.
9. Trends G. Public health and aging: trends in aging—United States and worldwide. Public Health. 2003;347:921–5.
10. Blackwell DL, Lucas JW, Clarke TC. Summary health statistics for U.S. adults: national health interview survey, 2012. Vital Health Stat. 2014 Feb;260:1–161.
11. López-Otín C, Blasco MA, Partridge L, Serrano M, Kroemer G. The hallmarks of aging. Cell. 2013;153(6):1194–217.

12. American Geriatrics Society Expert Panel on the Care of Older Adults with Multimorbidity. Guiding principles for the care of older adults with multimorbidity: an approach for clinicians. J Am Geriatr Soc. 2012;60(10):E1–E25.
13. Rockwood K, Song X, MacKnight C, Bergman H, Hogan DB, McDowell I, et al. A global clinical measure of fitness and frailty in elderly people. CMAJ. 2005 Aug;173(5):489–95.
14. Mohile SG, Epstein RM, Hurria A, Heckler CE, Canin B, Culakova E, et al. Communication with older patients with cancer using geriatric assessment: a cluster-randomized clinical trial from the National Cancer Institute Community Oncology Research Program. JAMA Oncol. 2020 Feb 1;6(2):196–204.
15. National Comprehensive Cancer Network. National Comprehensive Cancer Network Guidelines in Oncology - Older Adult Oncology. 2020. Available at https://www.nccn.org/professionals/physician_gls/pdf/senior.pdf. Accessed 3 Nov 2020.
16. Morrison RS, Augustin R, Souvanna P, Meier DE. America's care of serious illness: a state-by-state report card on access to palliative care in our nation's hospitals. J Palliat Med. 2011;14(10):1094–6.
17. WHO. Global Atlas of Palliative care at the end of life. Geneva: WHO; 2014.
18. Chapman M, Le B, Gorelik A, Schwarz J. Prognostic factors in the elderly: a profile and outcomes study of a community palliative care service. Intern Med J. 2012;42(9):1046–9.
19. Young J, Badgery-Parker T, Dobbins T, Jorgensen M, Gibbs P, Faragher I, et al. Comparison of ECOG/WHO performance status and ASA score as a measure of functional status. J Pain Symptom Manag. 2015;49(2):258–64.
20. Loh KP, Soto-Perez-de-Celis E, Hsu T, de Glas NA, Battisti NML, Baldini C, et al. What every oncologist should know about geriatric assessment for older patients with cancer: young international society of geriatric oncology position paper. J Oncol Pract. 2018;14(2):85–94.
21. Abernethy AP, Wheeler JL, Currow DC. Utility and use of palliative care screening tools in routine oncology practice. Cancer J. 2010;16(5):444–60.
22. Rodriguez KL, Barnato AE, Arnold RM. Perceptions and utilization of palliative care services in acute care hospitals. J Palliat Med. 2007;10(1):99–110.
23. Hui D, Elsayem A, De La Cruz M. Cancer centers availability and integration of palliative Care at US. JAMA. 2010;303:1054–61.
24. Holmenlund K, Sjøgren P, Nordly M. Specialized palliative care in advanced cancer: what is the efficacy? A systematic review. Palliat Support Care. 2017;15(6):724.
25. Hui D, Bansal S, Strasser F, Morita T, Caraceni A, Davis M, et al. Indicators of integration of oncology and palliative care programs: an international consensus. Ann Oncol. 2015;26(9):1953–9.
26. Higginson IJ, Evans CJ. What is the evidence that palliative care teams improve outcomes for cancer patients and their families? Cancer J. 2010 Sep–Oct;16(5):423–35.
27. Ferrell B, Sun V, Hurria A, Cristea M, Raz DJ, Kim JY, et al. Interdisciplinary palliative care for patients with lung cancer. J Pain Symptom Manag. 2015;50(6):758–67.
28. Hanks G, Robbins M, Sharp D, Forbes K, Done K, Peters T, et al. The imPaCT study: a randomised controlled trial to evaluate a hospital palliative care team. Br J Cancer. 2002;87(7):733–9.
29. Temel J, Greer J, Pirl W. Early palliative care in non-small-cell lung cancer. N Engl J Med. 2010;363(23):2264–5.
30. Temel JS, Greer JA, Admane S, Gallagher ER, Jackson VA, Lynch TJ, et al. Longitudinal perceptions of prognosis and goals of therapy in patients with metastatic non–small-cell lung cancer: Results of a randomized study of early palliative care. J Clin Oncol. 2011;29(17):2319–26.
31. Zimmermann C, Swami N, Krzyzanowska M, Hannon B, Leighl N, Oza A, et al. Early palliative care for patients with advanced cancer: a cluster-randomised controlled trial. Lancet. 2014;383(9930):1721–30.
32. Rabow MW, Dibble SL, Pantilat SZ, McPhee SJ. The comprehensive care team: a controlled trial of outpatient palliative medicine consultation. Arch Intern Med. 2004;164(1):83–91.

33. Scibetta C, Kerr K, Mcguire J, Rabow MW. The costs of waiting: implications of the timing of palliative care consultation among a cohort of decedents at a comprehensive cancer center. J Palliat Med. 2016;19(1):69–75.
34. Wentlandt K, Krzyzanowska MK, Swami N, Rodin GM, Le LW, Zimmermann C. Referral practices of oncologists to specialized palliative care. J Clin Oncol. 2012;30(35):4380–6.
35. Reyes-Ortiz CA, Williams C, Westphal C. Comparison of early versus late palliative care consultation in end-of-life care for the hospitalized frail elderly patients. Am J Hospice Palliat Med. 2015;32(5):516–20.
36. Bakitas M, Lyons KD, Hegel MT, Balan S, Brokaw FC, Seville J, et al. Effects of a palliative care intervention on clinical outcomes in patients with advanced cancer: the Project ENABLE II randomized controlled trial. JAMA. 2009;302(7):741–9.
37. Cassel JB, Kerr KM, Kalman NS, Smith TJ. The business case for palliative care: translating research into program development in the US. J Pain Symptom Manag. 2015;50(6):741–9.
38. Smith S, Brick A, O'Hara S, Normand C. Evidence on the cost and cost-effectiveness of palliative care: a literature review. Palliat Med. 2014;28(2):130–50.
39. Gade G, Venohr I, Conner D, McGrady K, Beane J, Richardson RH, et al. Impact of an inpatient palliative care team: a randomized controlled trial. J Palliat Med. 2008;11(2):180–90.
40. Walter L, Schonberg M, Francisco S, Medical H, Israel B, Medical D. Screening mammography in older women: a review. JAMA. 2014;311:1336–47.
41. Wildiers H, Heeren P, Puts M, Topinkova E, Janssen-Heijnen ML, Extermann M, et al. International Society of Geriatric Oncology consensus on geriatric assessment in older patients with cancer. J Clin Oncol. 2014 Aug;32(24):2595–603.
42. Schiphorst A, Ten Bokkel HD, Breumelhof R, Burgmans J, Pronk A, Hamaker M. Geriatric consultation can aid in complex treatment decisions for elderly cancer patients. Eur J Cancer Care. 2016;25(3):365–70.
43. Sattar S, Alibhai SM, Spoelstra SL, Fazelzad R, Puts MT. Falls in older adults with cancer: a systematic review of prevalence, injurious falls, and impact on cancer treatment. Support Care Cancer. 2016;24(10):4459–69.
44. Mohile SG, Mohamed MR, Culakova E, Xu H, Loh KP, Magnuson A, et al. A geriatric assessment (GA) intervention to reduce treatment toxicity in older patients with advanced cancer: a University of Rochester Cancer Center NCI community oncology research program cluster randomized clinical trial (CRCT). J Clin Oncol. 2020;38(15):12009.
45. Davies E, Higginson IJ, World Health Organization. Better palliative care for older people. 2004.
46. Fried LP, Tangen CM, Walston J, Newman AB, Hirsch C, Gottdiener J, et al. Frailty in older adults: evidence for a phenotype. J Gerontol A Biol Sci Med Sci. 2001;56(3):M146–57.
47. Pal LM, Manning L. Palliative care for frail older people. Clin Med (Lond). 2014 Jun;14(3):292–5.
48. Koller K, Rockwood K. Frailty in older adults: implications for end-of-life care. Cleve Clin J Med. 2013 Mar;80(3):168–74.
49. Gallagher P, Baeyens J, Topinkova E, Madlova P, Cherubini A, Gasperini B, et al. Inter-rater reliability of STOPP (Screening Tool of Older Persons' Prescriptions) and START (Screening Tool to Alert doctors to Right Treatment) criteria amongst physicians in six European countries. Age Ageing. 2009;38(5):603–6.
50. Alexander K, Goldberg J, Korc-Grodzicki B. Palliative care and symptom management in older patients with cancer. Clin Geriatr Med. 2016;32(1):45–62.
51. Haley WE. Family caregivers of elderly patients with cancer: understanding and minimizing the burden of care. J Support Oncol. 2003 Nov–Dec;1(4 Suppl 2):25–9.
52. Lunney JR, Lynn J, Foley DJ, Lipson S, Guralnik JM. Patterns of functional decline at the end of life. JAMA. 2003;289(18):2387–92.
53. Nagy-Agren S, Haley HB. Management of infections in palliative care patients with advanced cancer. J Pain Symptom Manag. 2002;24(1):64–70.

54. Albrecht JS, McGregor JC, Fromme EK, Bearden DT, Furuno JP. A nationwide analysis of antibiotic use in hospice care in the final week of life. J Pain Symptom Manag. 2013;46(4):483–90.
55. Kelechi TJ, Prentice M, Madisetti M, Brunette G, Mueller M. Palliative care in the management of pain, odor, and exudate in chronic wounds at the end of life: a cohort study. J Hospice Palliat Nurs. 2017;19(1):17–25.
56. Hui D, Dev R, Bruera E. The last days of life: symptom burden and impact on nutrition and hydration in cancer patients. Curr Opin Support Palliat Care. 2015;9(4):346.
57. Lichtman SM. Guidelines for the treatment of elderly cancer patients. Cancer Control. 2003;10(6):445–53.
58. Baker SD, Grochow LB. Pharmacology of cancer chemotherapy in the older person. Clin Geriatr Med. 1997;13(1):169–83.
59. Agrawal A, Asthana V, Sharma JP, Gupta V. Efficacy of lipophilic vs lipophobic opioids in addition to hyperbaric bupivacaine for patients undergoing lower segment caeserean section. Anesth Essays Res. 2016 Sep–Dec;10(3):420–4.
60. Smith HS. Opioid metabolism. Mayo Clinic Proc. 2009;84(7):613–24.
61. Overholser BR, Foster DR. Opioid pharmacokinetic drug-drug interactions. Am J Manag Care. 2011 Sep;17(Suppl 11):S276–87.
62. Ilene Browner MD. Applications in Geriatric Oncology. 2020; Available at: https://www.hopkinsmedicine.org/gec/series/cancer_aging.html. Accessed 23 August 2020.
63. Weinstein JR, Anderson S. The aging kidney: physiological changes. Adv Chronic Kidney Dis. 2010;17(4):302–7.
64. Pruskowski J, Arnold RM. Opioid pharmacokinetics# 307. J Palliat Med. 2016;19(6):668–70.
65. Malec M, Shega JW. Pain management in the elderly. Med Clin North Am. 2015 Mar;99(2):337–50.

Chapter 16
Frailty Research: The Present and the Future

Martine Puts, Alastair Greystoke, and Supriya Mohile

Introduction

As the population is aging worldwide, the number of older adults with frailty will increase and it is important that they are included in studies to provide evidence on how to deliver the best care to account for their increased vulnerability to stressors, both from disease and therapy. Older adults with cancer, and particularly the frailer subjects, are underrepresented in clinical trials [1, 2].

Research on older adults with frailty can be more challenging, due to visual and hearing impairments, mobility limitations, cognitive impairments and dependency on a caregiver. Barriers to study participation can exist at the study level (characteristics of the study design and procedures such as weekly visits to the hospital), at the clinician level (thinking the patient is too frail to participate in the study), and at the individual patient level (not seeing the benefit of participating, not being able to complete all the study visits due to mobility impairment or financial impairments, or not wanting to be randomized) [3, 4].

This chapter will highlight the key actions required to improve research recruitment in this patient group and provide examples of large research projects

M. Puts (✉)
Lawrence S. Bloomberg Faculty of Nursing, University of Toronto, Toronto, ON, Canada
e-mail: martine.puts@utoronto.ca

A. Greystoke
Newcastle University Centre for Cancer, Newcastle upon Tyne, UK
e-mail: alastair.greystoke@newcastle.ac.uk

S. Mohile
University of Rochester Medical Center, Rochester, NY, USA
e-mail: Supriya_Mohile@urmc.rochester.edu

F. Gomes (ed.), *Frailty in Older Adults with Cancer*,
https://doi.org/10.1007/978-3-030-89162-6_16

impacting daily clinical practice. This will be followed by an overview of research on frailty biomarkers and the top research priorities for older cancer patients with frailty.

Improving the Recruitment of Older Cancer Patients with Frailty in Research

A recent review written by Lui et al. [5] highlighted 5 necessary actions to improve recruitment of older adults with frailty in research. Lui et al. recommended the need to (1) broaden eligibility criteria, (2) measure relevant endpoints, (3) expand standard trial designs, (4) increase resources (e.g., institutional support, interdisciplinary care, and telehealth), and (5) develop targeted interventions (e.g., behavioural interventions to promote patient enrolment).

Broaden the Eligibility Criteria

Many older adults have multimorbidity. Multimorbidity refers to the simultaneous occurrence of several medical conditions, functional limitations, and/or geriatric syndromes in one person [6]. Organ dysfunction, multimorbidity, and frailty are common reasons for exclusion from clinical studies [7, 8]. The American Society of Clinical Oncology (ASCO) and Friends of Cancer Research established a working group and made recommendations for increased inclusiveness of patients with organ dysfunction, prior or concurrent malignancies, and comorbidities in clinical trials to enhance representativeness of the study populations [9, 10]. A French multicentre cohort study enrolling all older adults aged 65 years and over with colorectal cancer found that only 27% of 577 older adults were eligible for a clinical trial, 20% were not eligible due to performance status (>2 or 1 depending on trial), 14% due to comorbidities, 14% due to inappropriate haematologic, hepatic, or renal biomarker profile, and 10% due to age limitations [11].

In addition, incorporating comprehensive geriatric assessment (CGA) in all clinical studies can help the clinicians determine how fit or frail the older adult is in order to guide shared decision-making with the patient and their family caregiver about what the best treatment approach is, including participating in clinical trials. The American Society of Clinical Oncology and the International Society of Geriatric Oncology recommend a CGA for all older adults for whom cancer treatment is considered [12, 13]. By using the CGA a better assessment of the potential risks and benefits of treatment can be made and this information can be used to share decision-making with the patients.

Relevant Endpoints Need to Be Selected for Clinical Studies

While many studies focus on the endpoints of progression-free survival and treatment toxicity, it is important to include outcomes that are important to older adults, such as health-related quality of life, independence and maintenance of functional status both in short-term and long-term [14]. Stakeholders such as patient partners can help with selecting patient-reported outcomes that reflect relevant endpoints for clinical studies in addition to traditional endpoints such as survival. In addition, a minimum geriatric dataset has been developed [15] but requires full validation. This will ensure that a measure of frailty is included in future studies to improve representation of frailer older adults and allow comparison of populations between studies. Lastly, opportunities should be taken to include exploratory endpoints within clinical studies, such as biological markers of aging, to study how cancer and its treatment impact the aging process [5].

Expand Standard Trial Designs

Using alternative study designs to help recruit more older adults in studies that are less burdensome may aid in generating evidence for older adults with frailty. Lui et al. [5] developed examples of alternative study designs that could be considered in geriatric oncology (Table 16.1). These include the development of pragmatic randomized studies which study the intervention/treatment effectiveness in real-world settings rather than an idealized setting [16] and thus they tend to have more broad inclusion criteria and allow inclusion of a more heterogeneous population [17] and utilize endpoints that are routinely collected and relevant for patients and physicians [18]. In addition, cluster randomization by geographical area or medical practice can be used in such studies where individual randomization is challenging or not possible [19].

Another type of study design that is commonly used in educational and health policy intervention studies is the stepped-wedge design. Here, the intervention is delivered to the cluster after an observation period so the cluster serves as their own control; each cluster crosses over to the intervention at a given time and there is fixed amount of time between the clusters crossing over (step) [20–22] until all clusters have received intervention. This design reduces the sample size requirement compared to a randomized design using parallel clusters and could be relevant for geriatric oncology in evaluating the introduction of policy changes in clinical practice. Other types of modifications to the standard parallel arms randomized controlled trial design include the use of the preference based trial design in which the participant chooses the arm they want to be in (intervention or control) [23]. This can be used to address the issue of refusal to be randomized. Allowing participants to choose the arm they want to be in can reduce the attrition that can occur

Table 16.1 Overview research designs and examples for geriatric oncology research (Adapted from [5])

Study design	Description	Potential objectives and outcomes	Advantages	Limitations	Examples in geriatric oncology
Pragmatic trial	Intervention is delivered in everyday clinical practice and participants are included using more inclusive inclusion criteria. Typically the centres are randomized using cluster randomization instead of individual patient randomization	To determine the effectiveness of the intervention in everyday clinical practice	– More inclusive due to less restrictive inclusion criteria – More accessible for participants – Study burden is lower as typically majority of data is collected as part of routine clinical care – Outcomes more relevant to stakeholders	– The selection of the comparator can be challenging due to treatment preferences – Non-adherence and loss to follow-up may be higher – Not all centres may document the same information as part of routine care – Due to more heterogeneous population poorer internal validity may limit the ability to determine effects – Require large samples	– An educational intervention for patients and their caregivers can be implemented in some centres in routine care and not in other centres using cluster randomization – A stepped-wedge design may be used to study, for example, a new clinical intervention in a geriatric oncology clinic so that each participant is their own control reducing sample size requirements and objections against receiving placebo
Randomized controlled trial	– Participants are randomly assigned to intervention or control treatment – The population can be limited, for example, to only include older patients – Enrolment can be stratified based on age – Adaptive designs are possible where modifications to the study design are made based on interim analysis	To determine efficacy of the treatment compared to one or more comparators – Considered the gold standard of testing interventions	– Direct comparison of two or more treatments – Least risk of bias – Minimizes confounding – Generalizable to the population included in the study	– Require large samples – Costly and time-consuming – Recruitment can be slow due to study burden to participants – More frail older adults are not included or more like to drop out due to study burden	– A randomized controlled trial to compare a comprehensive geriatric assessment and management model compared to usual oncology care. – A randomized trial of a new treatment previously tested and found effective in younger subjects, now evaluated in a study recruiting only older adults

Prospective cohort study	– Assessment of an clearly defined exposure that can be an existing treatment, a relatively new intervention that is in use but has not been tested in older adults. – Clear inclusion criteria are needed to define the inception. – Observational study, no randomization	– To determine associations between an exposure and outcomes, such as level of frailty and subsequent emergency department use – To understand trajectories over time, for example trajectories in functional status after surgery	– Findings are generalizable – Multiple exposures and outcomes can be studied simultaneously – No randomization is needed and thus may appeal to patients who object to being randomized – Can be used to examine incidence of outcomes	– Large samples are needed to be followed often for years – Can be expensive and time-consuming – If differential loss to follow-up may lead to selection bias – If time between follow-up is long, changes in outcomes and exposures may not always be captured	– Following older adults from the moment of diagnosis to examine how much physical activity they perform each week to examine the association of physical activity and tolerance to treatment during systemic treatment – Examining those older adults with no caregiver support how well they manage during systemic treatment compared to those with significant available support
Extended trial	Addition of cohort of older patients to the superior treatment arm	Determine tolerability in older adults	– Trial infrastructure already established – Existing data on treatment efficacy will make accrual easier	– Lack of data on the inferior treatment arm in older adults	– Can be done with any new cancer treatment where there was low enrolment of older adults
Embedded study (Correlative Study or Ancillary study or Sub-study)	Includes additional measures of interest in the infrastructure of a parent study	Describe a cohort or determine the relationship in more detail in a subgroup	– Better understand the characteristics in an older population – Identification of predictors of outcomes in a sub sample	– In studies not limited to older adults, the sample of older adults may limit analyses	– Implement additional measures such as geriatric assessment tools, for example, physical performance tests in a new treatment trial
N-of-1 (Single Subject trial)	To determine the optimal therapy for a single patient	Determine the best intervention for an individual patient using objective criteria	– Patient-centred care – To understand the Effectiveness of treatment among different patients	– Carryover effects possible – Wash-out period needed – Blinding is not possible	– Start of a new intervention to address insomnia, compare different medications and sleep hygiene

when participants are randomized to an arm they find unacceptable [24]. Table 16.1 provides an overview of research designs and examples for geriatric oncology research.

Increase Resources Such as Institutional Support, Interdisciplinary Care, and Telehealth

For smaller centres, it may not be feasible to complete clinical trials in a timely manner with sufficient older adult enrolment. Therefore, to enhance geriatric oncology research, it is important for researchers across centres to work together to design clinical studies to improve patient care. Examples of large collaborations in geriatric oncology include the Belgium multicentre cohort study examining the benefits of implementing geriatric assessment [25] and the French prospective study ONCOdage that validated the G8 questionnaire [26]. Examples from North America include the validation of the Cancer and Aging Research Group Prediction of Chemotherapy Toxicity Tool [27] and in Canada the 5C intervention study that is using a randomized controlled trial to assess the clinical and cost-effectiveness of implementing geriatric assessment and management in 8 hospitals in 3 provinces in 2 languages [28]. Furthermore, research with older adults is more complex due to multimorbidity and can best be conducted by an interdisciplinary team. A recently developed framework by Bowling et al. [29] called the 5Ts: Target population, Team, Tools, Time, and Tips to Accommodate was developed to complement the 5Ms model for geriatric care and to increase enrolment of more older adults with frailty in research. Their recommendation is to include geriatricians and other aging experts as well as patients and caregivers in the development of studies, so they are relevant and more feasible for older adults [29]. In addition, using technology can facilitate study participation by using virtual visits. However, older adults with frailty may be less able to access and use telehealth due to cognitive impairment, sensory impairment or no device available or not able to use it [30]. During the COVID-19 pandemic research has demonstrated access barriers for older adults with frailty [31].

Develop Targeted Interventions to Increase Enrolment

There may be financial barriers for older adults with cancer to enrol in clinical studies due to increased costs from extra hospital visits and other procedures [3]. Providing home visits may reduce the study burden particularly for older adults with frailty who are dependent on caregivers for transportation to the hospital [32, 33]. Financial incentives to compensate for time can also increase recruitment and retention [34]. The 5T framework recommends budgeting for transportation as well the use of pocket talkers and designing visuals in patient facing materials that can appeal to older adults (large font, high contrast print) to allow informed consent and study participation [29].

Interventional Research Studies Impacting Daily Clinical Practice

A large, cluster-randomized, multisite study of community oncology practices recently demonstrated that the use of CGA tailored to deficits in aging-related conditions improves communication about aging-related issues as well as patient and caregiver satisfaction [35]. A large, single arm study of patients aged ≥70 with cancer in Belgium evaluated a model of care where geriatric expertise was brought to patients [36]. Overall, 710 patients were evaluable and a median of two CGA management recommendations were provided per patient. However, only 35% of all CGA management recommendations were performed, with the most frequent being dietician, social work, and psychologist referrals. Smaller, randomized pilot studies have also been conducted to evaluate the feasibility of delivering CGA [15, 37]. These have shown variable implementation of known evidence-based CGA-guided management recommendations for older cancer patients with frailty.

The first three large recent randomized trials (RCTs) used CGA implemented in different ways but all had positive impacts on decreasing treatment toxicity and improving quality of life [38–40]. In the INTEGERATE study by Soo et al. [40] patients received a CGA performed by a geriatrician followed by interventions to address the issues identified with follow-up at 12 and 24 weeks. The primary endpoint was the Elderly Functional Index (ELFI) which is a composite measure of the European Organisation of Research and Treatment of Cancer (EORTC) Quality of Life Questionnaire (EORTC QLQ C30) and the EORTC QLQ C30 Elderly Subscale (QLQ ELD-14). The participants in the intervention group had significantly higher ELFI scores at 12, 18, and 24 weeks, lower admission to hospital rates, less emergency department visits, and lower treatment discontinuation rates due to side effects.

In the second recently completed cluster RCT by Mohile et al. [39], the participant ($n = 718$) completed the CGA and the oncologist received management recommendations; primary outcome was grade 3–5 toxicity graded using the National Cancer Institute Common Toxicity Criteria for Adverse Events (CTCAE). The relative risk reduction of the intervention of grade 3–5 toxicity was 0.74 (95% CI: 0.63–0.87; $p = 0.0002$); with the difference mostly driven by non-haematological toxicities (RR 0.73; 95% CI: 0.53–1.0, $p < 0.05$). More participants in intervention group received reduced intensity treatment at cycle 1 (49% vs 35%, RR 0.81, $p = 0.01$) and overall survival was not significantly different.

The GAIN study by Li et al. [38] (Geriatric assessment-driven intervention (GAIN) on chemotherapy toxicity in older adults with cancer) was an RCT that enrolled 600 patients aged 65 and over starting a new chemotherapy regimen. Participants in the intervention group had 9.9% less grade 3–5 toxicities compared to the control group ($p < 0.05$) and were significantly more likely to have completed an advance care directive (24.1% vs 10.4%).

A search for ongoing randomized studies examining the benefits of CGA in the ClinicalTrials.gov registry on August 18, 2020 showed that are currently 81 randomized studies underway so in coming years there will be more data on the potential benefits of CGA for older adults and the optimal method of delivering the intervention.

In the area of prehabilitation (defined as the process of enhancing an individual's functional capacity to enable them to withstand a forthcoming stressor), several studies have been completed, but so far with mixed outcomes. A recent review of prehabilitation interventions for older adults with frailty found 3 studies that used a unimodal approach of an exercise program; 2 studies had no significant benefit and in one small RCT the intervention had a positive impact on postoperative recovery [41]. The review identified 4 RCTs of multimodal interventions including exercise, nutritional support, education, and psychological support [41]. The populations were different and the studies had mixed results, but the multimodal interventions may be effective improving postoperative functional recovery with larger RCTs needed. These are currently underway with 50 prehabilitation intervention studies in the oncology surgical setting on the Clinicaltrials.gov registry on August 18, 2020.

Many new eHealth interventions are currently being developed and examples include computer-guided CGA and interventions which can support health care providers in seeing more older adults as well as identifying those who have frailty and need more support [42–48]. Using an electronic pre-operative fitness assessment followed by inpatient geriatric co-management compared to usual surgical care, Shahrokni et al. [49] demonstrated in 1009 patients that adjusted rates of 90-day mortality was lower in geriatric co-management group compared to the surgical group (4.3% and 9.2%, p-value < 0.0001). While this was not an RCT, it shows the potential of eHealth interventions combined with geriatric care in older adults with frailty. A recent review of eHealth interventions to support healthy aging also showed the benefits of physical activity interventions [50]. Furthermore, the importance of loneliness and lack of social support and the additional detrimental effect it has on the health of older adults and frailty has been shown in older community-dwelling adults [51–53], but this has not been studied in geriatric oncology context. eHealth interventions can foster social connections and this could be potentially very useful for geriatric oncology to incorporate support mechanisms when developing eHealth tools.

There is increasing interest in the use of activity monitors to supplement clinical assessment of functional status. This is in part due to improvements in technology and their routine integration into devices in common use such as smartphones. These can not only give information as to activity undertaken including intensity, but other key parameters as to a patient's health including sleep quality [54], sedentary time [55], average heart rate, and recovery time from exertion. These have been shown to be able to accurately gauge a patient's fitness and may eliminate any bias between younger and older patients [56]. However, the routine use of smartphones or activity trackers does decrease with age, and they may be less acceptable in the older population. All activity trackers are less accurate when gait is slow, with decreased arm swing as is common in patients with frailty [57]. The range of monitors initially available has led to potential issues with validation, although this situation is now stabilizing with most studies using those made by one of 5 main manufacturers and a recent survey found Fitbit is registered in ClinicalTrials studies 10 times as often as other brands [58].

Important points to consider when using these monitors are to assess physical activity in real life over a period of several days and weeks and to determine the type of activity performed during non-wear time and reasons for non-wear of the devices [59]. Whilst a number of studies have been done to show the feasibility of using these activity monitors in cancer patients, most have concentrated on their utility to enable prehabilitation programmes or improve fitness and quality of life in cancer survivors (reviewed in Beg et al. [60] and Peddle et al. [61]) who have been found to have low activity levels and long periods of sedentary behaviour [62]. In a small study in patients with pleural effusions activity was associated with poor performance status and survival [63], whilst in a study of 100 patients with treatment naïve cancer activity correlated (although weakly) with performance status. However, in this study only 25 patients were over 65 [56].

Lastly, recent systematic reviews and meta-analyses of interventions to reduce frailty in community-dwelling older adults demonstrate that multimodal interventions may be effective in reducing frailty [64–67] and that the combination of physical activity and nutritional intervention may be the most effective.

Use of Biomarkers in Frailty Research

The rationale to investigate biomarkers of frailty includes:

1. Improved identification of patients who are at risk.
2. Identification of surrogate measures that may be able to monitor response to therapy in interventional studies.
3. Greater understanding of the development of frailty in response to cancer and its treatments.
4. The ability to individualize intervention on the basis of the patient's deficits.

Assessment of Muscle Function

Cancer patients suffer from muscle loss, both through sarcopenia (age-related loss in muscle bulk) and cachexia (cytokine mediated degradation of muscle), although much of the research in this area in cancer patients does not distinguish between the two processes [68]. Simple measures of muscle strength and physical fitness can be routinely integrated into the clinic and include grip strength or timed exertions such as Get up and Go, arm curls, or shuttle walks [69]. However, these may be adversely impacted by cancer related pain, nerve damage due to the cancer or therapy, and myopathy (e.g., secondary to steroid use). A number of tools exist to evaluate muscle mass including measurement of mid-arm muscle circumference, dual-energy X-ray absorptiometry, and body impedance [70]. However, given the frequent Computerized Tomography (CT) scans that most cancer patients have, particularly in the metastatic setting, to assess therapeutic response, this can give valuable information as to muscle bulk and composition. Most publications concentrate on skeletal muscle area from the third lumbar vertebra region which includes the psoas, paraspinal muscles and the abdominal wall muscles [71]. Voluming the muscles and assessment over several CT slices can decrease inter- and intra-observer variability and increase the utility of this tool [72]. Using this technique in large meta-analysis of 38 studies the incidence of sarcopenia was estimated at between 11% and 74% (using a range of cut-points for defining sarcopenia) and was associated with poor survival across tumour sites and stages [73]. Importantly sarcopenia is also associated with complications of therapy including surgery, chemotherapy, and targeted therapies [74–76]. The quality of muscle may be as important as actual muscle bulk and can be assessed by measurement of the muscle radio-density which assesses myosteatosis (infiltration of muscle by fat) [75, 77].

Recovery time from exercise and skeletal muscle mitochondrial function can be measured in a relatively non-invasive manner by assessment of phosphocreatine using localized phosphorus (P31) magnetic resonance spectroscopy after a short period of defined exercise and correlates with clinical frailty in a cohort of subjects without cancer [78]. Overall integration of radiological assessments such as those described above with functional strength measures, such as grip strength, may be the most sensitive way to pick up abnormalities [68].

The use of blood tests to investigate aspects of frailty is appealing due to ease of sampling, ready acceptance by both patients and clinicians, and ability to perform multiple assessments over time to allow a dynamic picture of the patient's condition. Work has been done to identify blood-borne biomarkers of frailty; given that frailty is normally an age-related condition, candidate biomarkers have been chosen based on genes and pathways that become disturbed in aging or age-related diseases [79]. In particular these have concentrated on the changes in immune function, metabolism, and epigenetics that occur in the older patient. However no fully validated and qualified biomarkers of frailty exist [80], perhaps reflecting the complexity of the underlying processes and the heterogeneity between patients. One of the most comprehensive attempts at validation was performed in the Newcastle 85+ study, a longitudinal population-based study; participants were recruited in the year that they turned 85 and only a minority had a history of cancer. Frailty status and biomarkers were analysed at baseline to assess their association, and a panel of 21 biomarkers identified that predicted the presence of frailty and subsequent survival [81]. Selected biomarkers are discussed with the other evidence below but the differences in age group when compared to cancer patients and the potential impact of the cancer on these biomarkers should be considered when considering them for use in studies.

Inflammation and the Immune System

One of the main areas of frailty biomarker identification has been measures of inflammation and the changes in the immune system that are seen in the older person. These are some of the more reproducible changes seen with aging and are readily amenable to assessment on a blood sample. In the older person, a large number of studies have demonstrated the presence of non-specific low-grade inflammation, commonly referred to as "inflammaging" [82]. The levels of inflammation can be assessed through cytokines such as interleukin-6, Tumour Necrosis Factor-Alpha and Transforming Growth Factor-Beta, or circulating levels of acute phase proteins such as C-reactive Protein and fibrinogen. High levels of CRP and TGF-beta but not IL-6 or TNF-alpha were associated with survival in the Newcastle 85+ frailty panel. [81]

Marked changes are seen in both the innate and adaptive immune systems with increasing age possibly in response to chronic antigen challenge. This is termed "immunosenescence", although this term is likely to be an over-simplification of the complex changes involved in this process. Overall there is reduced chemotaxis, phagocytosis and generation of reactive oxygen species by monocytes and macrophages, and reduced proliferation and cytokine production by effector T lymphocytes in response to antigen challenge [83, 84]. Higher levels of immune suppressive cells such as myeloid derived suppressor cells and T-regulatory (T_{reg}) cells are also seen [85, 86]. Senescent immune cells also increase secretion of pro-inflammatory cytokines such as IL-6 contribution to the inflammaging described above. Changes in cell receptor status such as the loss of the CD28 co-stimulatory receptor or the development of the senescent phenotype demonstrated by expression of p16 ^{INK4a} can be assessed on peripheral blood mono-nuclear cells by flow cytometry or RNA expression [87]. In a study of patients who had received chemotherapy for breast cancer an increase in p16 ^{INK4a} was seen which was calculated by the authors to be equivalent to a 14.7-year increase in chronological age [87] but whether this had any functional consequences is unclear. A low CD4:CD8 ratio in T lymphocytes, and higher proportions of memory:naïve T lymphocytes but not the presence of senescent CD4 T lymphocytes were associated with survival in the Newcastle 85+ frailty panel [81].

The problem with these biomarkers of inflammation and the immune system in patients with cancer is that many of them will be affected by the presence of cancer. The Systemic Inflammatory Response is frequently activated in patients with cancer and associated with a poor prognosis [88]. It leads to high levels of CRP and low levels of albumin which have been suggested as potential biomarkers of frailty in the non-cancer population [79]; whether the relationship still holds true in patients with cancer has not been established, although it has been found to be associated with quality of life [89]. In addition these biomarkers may be impacted by therapies used to treat the cancer [90], particularly with the growing use of immunotherapies such as the checkpoint inhibitors across a range of tumour types.

Metabolism

As people age there is a reduction in lean muscle mass and an increase in both visceral and intra-abdominal fat [91]. This is associated with a change in key hormones such as growth hormone and insulin like growth factor (IGF-1), resistance to insulin and increased production of adipokines such as adiponectin and leptin [81]. Adiponectin levels may be particularly challenging to interpret as whilst high levels are associated with frailty in a number of papers including the Newcastle 85+ frailty panel [81], levels are also higher in healthy centenarians [92], and in a cohort of patients with lung cancer low levels were associated with a poor prognosis [93].

The bio-availability of IGF-1and its association with different binding proteins may be as important as absolute levels [94]. Low levels of IGF-1 and high levels of the main binding protein IFGBP 3 (which will reduce active IGF-1) are associated with metabolic resistance and adverse cardiovascular outcomes, whilst the alternative binding protein IGFBP1 has been associated with improved outcomes. However higher levels of IGFBP-1 have been associated with frailty [94] and were associated with poor survival in the Newcastle 85+ frailty panel [81] whilst IFGBP 3 was not.

The impact of the weight loss and cachexia on these biomarkers is uncertain but likely to be profound. In addition some cancer therapies such as the m-TOR inhibitors impact on IGF signalling and lead to perturbations in this system which will limit utility in patients taking these agents.

Biological Clocks

Changes in protein transcription and translation as people age are controlled epigenetically by modifications to DNA and the associated histone proteins (such as methylation and acetylation) and by non-coding RNAs such as micro-RNAs and long non-coding RNAs [95]. A number of methylation assays exist that can be utilized across a range of tissue types including in the blood. Increasing methylation at the specified loci has been associated with a number of different disorders from dementia to cardiovascular disease [95], and the subsequent development of cancer in a number of studies. They associate with frailty in cross-sectional cohorts but have been unable to predict subsequent deterioration over time [96, 97]. Whilst there has been considerable interest in the non-coding RNAs as potential circulating biomarkers of aging, and these track changes in age and with calorie restriction in animal models, their utility in humans has yet to be fully assessed [98].

In general, as can be seen there have been a number of studies that have assessed links between clinical frailty, putative circulating biomarkers and outcomes in subjects without cancer. Some work has been performed as to validation and qualification in cancer patients but in general studies have not looked to assess links with clinical frailty scales and outcomes of interest such as survival, tolerability of therapy or health-related quality of life.

Research Priorities for the Next 5 Years

There are several limitations to the current guidelines for addressing frailty in geriatric oncology [99–101]. There is a lack of robust data on prevalence of frailty and impact on outcomes for older adults undergoing other systemic therapies (e.g., immunotherapy and targeted agents) [102–105]. In addition, while guidelines recommend specific CGA domains and tools, it does not provide practical information on who should be performing these assessments or how the CGA can be done. With advances in technology, there is a need to evaluate how to best utilize electronic medical records and mobile health to facilitate the administration and delivery of CGA-guided interventions for frailty [45, 47, 106]. While current guidelines provide recommendations on how to conduct the CGA and which relevant tools and assessments to use [100] implementation in daily oncology practice remains poor due in part to practice/institutional availability, lack of resources, and need for integration into clinical trials that define the standards of care for this population. Pragmatic study designs utilizing the CGA for older patients with cancer to address frailty may enhance implementation and warrant further exploration.

Despite significant improvements in cancer outcomes over the past two decades, older adults with cancer, especially those with frailty, continue to have worse outcomes than their younger counterparts. Managing cancer is challenging because of competing health and age-related conditions that can influence treatment decision-making and affect outcomes. More research is needed to identify patients at most at risk for poor outcomes with cancer treatment and assist in better allocating treatment for these patients. Implementation of evidence-based management strategies to address and manage aging-related conditions may improve clinical outcomes in this population. Clinical trials are currently underway to further determine the impact of the geriatric assessment with management interventions on cancer outcomes. This section summarizes and prioritizes research directions to address frailty in older patients with cancer.

Understanding Cancer Incidence and Mortality in Older Adults with Cancer with Aging-Related Conditions and Frailty

While there has been significant scientific progress in research to address frailty in older patients with cancer, the benefits have not been equally distributed [107]. There continue to be disparities based on age, gender, and race [108, 109]. Adults aged 85+ (compared to age 65–84) and older adults with frailty and/or aging-related conditions are diagnosed at later stages, are less likely to receive guideline-concordant care including surgery, and often receive inadequate treatment, including supportive care interventions [110]. Further inequities exist in cancer incidence and mortality for older adults globally. Low to middle income countries in regions such as Latin America, Africa, and India have the highest cancer incidence and mortality [111, 112]. Limited participation of older adults and racial minorities in clinical research leave patients vulnerable to poor outcomes from frailty. As an example from therapeutic clinical trials, there were significant age-related disparities, with the median age of participants in these trials being 6.5 years younger than the median age of the general population [113]. The inequity in clinical trial participation is more profound in racial and ethnic minorities and this gap has been steadily widening over the past decade and extends into behavioural, cancer care delivery, and cancer control interventions [114, 115]. Clinical research to address frailty in older patients with cancer should ensure appropriate representation of ages, sexes, and races of participants. In addition, research that addresses the needs of older adults with cancer in low to middle income countries is needed. Innovative mechanisms to recruit, retain, and evaluate outcomes of older adults with cancer who may have frailty should be developed by a diverse group of stakeholders (patients, caregivers, researchers) in the context of the cultural and societal needs of those patients where they live and globally.

Understanding the Measurement and Impact of Aging-Related Conditions and Frailty in Older Patients with Cancer

Comorbidity is highly prevalent in the cancer population and increases with age [116]. In older adults with cancer, the prevalence of comorbidity appears to differ within patients who have different cancer types [108, 117, 118]. For example, patients with lung and colorectal cancer have a higher prevalence and burden of comorbidity compared to patients with breast or prostate cancer [108, 118]. Risk factors such as smoking or health habits which contribute to both cancer and to other chronic conditions may account for these differences and requires further study, as these may be amenable to risk prevention strategies. Geriatric syndromes do not fit into discreet disease categories and are caused by several underlying factors involving multiple organ systems that make older adults "vulnerable to situational challenges [119]". Furthermore, research is needed to understand how biomarkers (e.g., cell counts, markers of inflammation) may aid in the identification of which older adults with cancer may be at risk for future adverse outcomes from frailty. Defined studies in patients with cancer are required as impact of the disease and its therapy on some of the putative biomarkers could affect both potential utility and threshold values associated with increased risk of frailty. Moving forward, frailty biomarkers should meet the following criteria (1) correlating with clinical outcomes (2) adding information to clinical frailty scales and (3) reflecting dynamic changes in the patients' clinical condition.

Several age-related conditions that are known to increase risk of adverse outcomes (e.g., polypharmacy, cognitive impairment, malnutrition) are common in vulnerable and frail older adults. However, the relative contribution of how each index condition contributes to frailty and increases the risk of adverse outcomes (e.g., toxicity, functional decline, institutionalization, hospitalization) due to cancer and its treatment should be prioritized in future research as there remain gaps in knowledge. Understanding the relative contribution of different aging-related conditions can help to guide the development of interventions to prevent or address frailty in older patients with cancer.

Understanding How to Intervene on Age-Related Conditions and Frailty in Older Patients with Cancer

High-priority interventions for each CGA domain have been identified through two Delphi consensus studies [120, 121] and these results were recently incorporated into the American Society of Clinical Oncology guidelines [100] Future research on how to implement aging-sensitive models of care that identify and address frailty in older patients with cancer across different clinical settings is needed. Future research should examine how specific interventions (e.g., prehabilitation, exercise) can modify functional trajectories for older patients with cancer who have aging-related conditions and/or frailty.

Conclusion

Older adults with cancer, particularly those with frailty, are underrepresented in clinical research and improvements are needed to guide treatment and care for this growing population. Therefore, there is a need to broaden the inclusion criteria so that more older adults are eligible to participate, as well as using different types of study designs including pragmatic study designs, to reduce the study burden for participants and allow the inclusion of real-world patients. Moreover, it is important to expand the outcomes included in clinical studies to ensure that those that matter to older adults, such as independence and maintained cognition, are captured. More support and resources for studies with older adults with cancer are needed to ensure these are feasible to recruit and retain them by accommodating their needs.

The 5T framework described many relevant recommendations for geriatric oncology researchers, such as including a team member with geriatric expertise to ensure the study is feasible and relevant to the population. Recently, the publication of several large randomized controlled trials implementing geriatric assessment and management for older adults with cancer confirmed their value in predicting treatment toxicity (in addition to helping optimize treatment decisions), reducing treatment toxicity, improving QoL for older adults with cancer, and reducing unplanned hospital admissions.

Another key aspect is the use of biomarkers in frailty research, which should be included: (a) to improve identification of patients who are at high risk; (b) to identify surrogate measures that may be able to monitor response to therapy in interventional studies; (c) to develop our understanding of the development of frailty in response to cancer and its treatments; and d) to individualize interventions on the basis of the patient's deficits and needs. Biomarkers currently studied include muscle mass, markers of inflammation and inflammaging, changes in metabolism and biological clocks.

Lastly, research priorities for the next 5 years include ensuring study populations have appropriate representation of ages, sexes, and races. Furthermore, there is a need to better understand the relative contribution of different aging-related conditions to outcomes to help guiding the development of interventions to prevent or address frailty in older patients with cancer.

References

1. Scher KS, Hurria A. Under-representation of older adults in cancer registration trials: known problem, little progress. J Clin Oncol. 2012;30(17):2036–8.
2. Outlaw D, Williams GR. Is the lack of evidence in older adults with cancer compromising safety? Expert Opin Drug Saf. 2020;19:1059–61.
3. Nipp RD, Hong K, Paskett ED. Overcoming barriers to clinical trial enrollment. Am Soc Clin Oncol Educ Book. 2019;39:105–14.
4. Townsley CA, Chan KK, Pond GR, Marquez C, Siu LL, Straus SE. Understanding the attitudes of the elderly towards enrolment into cancer clinical trials. BMC Cancer. 2006;6:34.
5. Liu J, Gutierrez E, Tiwari A, Padam S, Li D, Dale W, et al. Strategies to improve participation of older adults in cancer research. J Clin Med. 2020;9(5):1571.
6. Warner DF, Schiltz NK, Stange KC, Given CW, Owusu C, Berger NA, et al. Complex multimorbidity and health outcomes in older adult cancer survivors. Fam Med Community Health. 2017;5(2):129–38.
7. Hamaker ME, Stauder R, van Munster BC. Exclusion of older patients from ongoing clinical trials for hematological malignancies: an evaluation of the National Institutes of Health Clinical Trial Registry. Oncologist. 2014;19(10):1069–75.
8. Unger JM, Cook E, Tai E, Bleyer A. The role of clinical trial participation in cancer research: barriers, evidence, and strategies. Am Soc Clin Oncol Educ Book. 2016;35:185–98.
9. Kim ES, Bruinooge SS, Roberts S, Ison G, Lin NU, Gore L, et al. Broadening eligibility criteria to make clinical trials more representative: American Society of Clinical Oncology and Friends of Cancer Research Joint Research Statement. J Clin Oncol. 2017;35(33):3737–44.
10. Lichtman SM, Harvey RD, Damiette Smit MA, Rahman A, Thompson MA, Roach N, et al. Modernizing clinical trial eligibility criteria: recommendations of the American Society of Clinical Oncology-Friends of Cancer Research Organ Dysfunction, Prior or Concurrent Malignancy, and Comorbidities Working Group. J Clin Oncol. 2017;35(33):3753–9.
11. Canouï-Poitrine F, Lièvre A, Dayde F, Lopez-Trabada-Ataz D, Baumgaertner I, Dubreuil O, et al. Inclusion of older patients with cancer in clinical trials: the SAGE Prospective Multicenter Cohort Survey. Oncologist. 2019;24(12):e1351–e9.
12. Mohile SG, Dale W, Somerfield MR, Hurria A. Practical assessment and management of vulnerabilities in older patients receiving chemotherapy: ASCO guideline for geriatric oncology summary. J Oncol Pract. 2018;14(7):442–6.
13. Sattar S, Alibhai SM, Wildiers H, Puts MT. How to implement a geriatric assessment in your clinical practice. Oncologist. 2014;19(10):1056–68.

14. Puts MT, Tapscott B, Fitch M, Howell D, Monette J, Wan-Chow-Wah D, et al. A systematic review of factors influencing older adults' decision to accept or decline cancer treatment. Cancer Treat Rev. 2015;41(2):197–215.
15. Magnuson A, Lemelman T, Pandya C, Goodman M, Noel M, Tejani M, et al. Geriatric assessment with management intervention in older adults with cancer: a randomized pilot study. Support Care Cancer. 2018;26(2):605–13.
16. Zuidgeest MGP, Goetz I, Groenwold RHH, Irving E, van Thiel G, Grobbee DE. Series: pragmatic trials and real world evidence: Paper 1. Introduction. J Clin Epidemiol. 2017;88:7–13.
17. Oude Rengerink K, Kalkman S, Collier S, Ciaglia A, Worsley SD, Lightbourne A, et al. Series: pragmatic trials and real world evidence: Paper 3. Patient selection challenges and consequences. J Clin Epidemiol. 2017;89:173–80.
18. Welsing PM, Oude Rengerink K, Collier S, Eckert L, van Smeden M, Ciaglia A, et al. Series: pragmatic trials and real world evidence: Paper 6. Outcome measures in the real world. J Clin Epidemiol. 2017;90:99–107.
19. Nipp RD, Yao NA, Lowenstein LM, Buckner JC, Parker IR, Gajra A, et al. Pragmatic study designs for older adults with cancer: report from the U13 conference. J Geriatr Oncol. 2016;7(4):234–41.
20. Hemming K, Haines TP, Chilton PJ, Girling AJ, Lilford RJ. The stepped wedge cluster randomised trial: rationale, design, analysis, and reporting. BMJ. 2015;350:h391.
21. Hussey MA, Hughes JP. Design and analysis of stepped wedge cluster randomized trials. Contemp Clin Trials. 2007;28(2):182–91.
22. Tugwell P, Knottnerus JA. Stepped wedge designs are coming of age in clinical epidemiology. J Clin Epidemiol. 2019;107:vi–viii.
23. Delevry D, Le QA. Effect of treatment preference in randomized controlled trials: systematic review of the literature and meta-analysis. Patient. 2019;12(6):593–609.
24. Sidani S, Fox M, Epstein D. Conducting a two-stage preference trial: utility and challenges. Int J Nurs Stud. 2015;52(5):1017–24.
25. Kenis C, Decoster L, Flamaing J, Debruyne PR, De Groof I, Focan C, et al. Adherence to geriatric assessment-based recommendations in older patients with cancer: a multicenter prospective cohort study in Belgium. Ann Oncol. 2018;29(9):1987–94.
26. Soubeyran P, Bellera C, Goyard J, Heitz D, Curé H, Rousselot H, et al. Screening for vulnerability in older cancer patients: the ONCODAGE prospective multicenter cohort study. PLoS One. 2014;9(12):e115060.
27. Hurria A, Mohile S, Gajra A, Klepin H, Muss H, Chapman A, et al. Validation of a prediction tool for chemotherapy toxicity in older adults with cancer. J Clin Oncol. 2016;34(20):2366–71.
28. Puts MTE, Hsu T, Mariano C, Monette J, Brennenstuhl S, Pitters E, et al. Clinical and cost-effectiveness of a comprehensive geriatric assessment and management for Canadian elders with cancer-the 5C study: a study protocol for a randomised controlled phase III trial. BMJ Open. 2019;9(5):e024485.
29. Bowling CB, Whitson HE, Johnson TM 2nd. The 5Ts: preliminary development of a framework to support inclusion of older adults in research. J Am Geriatr Soc. 2019;67(2):342–6.
30. Narasimha S, Madathil KC, Agnisarman S, Rogers H, Welch B, Ashok A, et al. Designing telemedicine systems for geriatric patients: a review of the usability studies. Telemed J E Health. 2017;23(6):459–72.
31. Lam K, Lu AD, Shi Y, Covinsky KE. Assessing telemedicine unreadiness among older adults in the united states during the COVID-19 pandemic JAMA. Intern Med. 2020;180(10):1389–91.
32. Mody L, Miller DK, McGloin JM, Freeman M, Marcantonio ER, Magaziner J, et al. Recruitment and retention of older adults in aging research. J Am Geriatr Soc. 2008;56(12):2340–8.
33. Provencher V, Mortenson WB, Tanguay-Garneau L, Bélanger K, Dagenais M. Challenges and strategies pertaining to recruitment and retention of frail elderly in research studies: a systematic review. Arch Gerontol Geriatr. 2014;59(1):18–24.

34. Brueton V, Stenning SP, Stevenson F, Tierney J, Rait G. Best practice guidance for the use of strategies to improve retention in randomized trials developed from two consensus workshops. J Clin Epidemiol. 2017;88:122–32.
35. Mohile SG, Epstein RM, Hurria A, Heckler CE, Canin B, Culakova E, et al. Communication with older patients with cancer using geriatric assessment: a cluster-randomized clinical trial from the National Cancer Institute Community Oncology Research Program JAMA. Oncol. 2019;6(2):196–204.
36. Baitar A, Kenis C, Moor R, Decoster L, Luce S, Bron D, et al. Implementation of geriatric assessment-based recommendations in older patients with cancer: a multicentre prospective study. J Geriatr Oncol. 2015;6(5):401–10.
37. Puts MTE, Sattar S, Kulik M, MacDonald ME, McWatters K, Lee K, et al. A randomized phase II trial of geriatric assessment and management for older cancer patients. Support Care Cancer. 2018;26(1):109–17.
38. Li D, Sun CL, Kim H, Chung V, Koczywas M, Fakih M, et al. Geriatric assessment-driven intervention (GAIN) on chemotherapy toxicity in older adults with cancer: a randomized controlled trial. JAMA Oncol. 30:e214158.
39. Mohile SG, Mohamed MR, Culakova E, Xu H, Loh KP, Magnuson A, et al. A geriatric assessment (GA) intervention to reduce treatment toxicity in older patients with advanced cancer: a University of Rochester Cancer Center NCI community oncology research program cluster randomized clinical trial (CRCT). 2020.
40. Soo WJ, King M, Pope A, Parente P, Darzins P, Davis IA. Integrated geriatric assessment and treatment (INTEGERATE) in older people with cancer planned for systemic anticancer therapy. Lancet. 2020.
41. Norris CM, Close JCT. Prehabilitation for the frailty syndrome: improving outcomes for our most vulnerable patients. Anesth Analg. 2020;130(6):1524–33.
42. Shahrokni A, Alexander K. What will perioperative geriatric assessment for older cancer patients look like in 2025? Advantages and limitations of new technologies in geriatric assessment. Eur J Surg Oncol. 2020;46(3):305–9.
43. Shahrokni A, Loh KP, Wood WA. Toward modernization of geriatric oncology by digital health technologies. Am Soc Clin Oncol Educ Book. 2020;40:1–7.
44. Shahrokni A, Maggiore RJ, Ghassemzadeh H. New technologies in geriatric oncology care. J Geriatr Oncol. 2018;9(6):687–9.
45. Shahrokni A, Tin A, Downey RJ, Strong V, Mahmoudzadeh S, Boparai MK, et al. Electronic rapid fitness assessment: a novel tool for preoperative evaluation of the geriatric oncology patient. J Natl Compr Canc Netw. 2017;15(2):172–9.
46. Shahrokni A, Vishnevsky BM, Jang B, Sarraf S, Alexander K, Kim SJ, et al. Geriatric assessment, not ASA physical status, is associated with 6-month postoperative survival in patients with cancer aged ≥75 years. J Natl Compr Canc Netw. 2019;17(6):687–94.
47. Loh KP, Ramsdale E, Culakova E, Mendler JH, Liesveld JL, O'Dwyer KM, et al. Novel mHealth app to deliver geriatric assessment-driven interventions for older adults with cancer: pilot feasibility and usability study. JMIR Cancer. 2018;4(2):e10296.
48. Haase KR, Drury A, Puts M. Supportive care and ehealth: a narrative review of technologies, interventions, and Opportunities for Optimizing Care in Patients With Cancer. Clin J Oncol Nurs. 2020;24(3):32–41.
49. Shahrokni A, Tin A, Sarraf S, Alexander K, Kim SJ, Yulico H, et al. Reduced 90-day post-operative mortality through geriatric comanagement after cancer surgery. J Clin Oncol. 2019;37(15 suppl):11512.
50. Buyl R, Beogo I, Fobelets M, Deletroz C, Van Landuyt P, Dequanter S, et al. e-Health interventions for healthy aging: a systematic review. Syst Rev. 2020;9(1):128.
51. Bunt S, Steverink N, Olthof J, van der Schans CP, Hobbelen JSM. Social frailty in older adults: a scoping review. Eur J Ageing. 2017;14(3):323–34.
52. Fritz H, Cutchin MP, Gharib J, Haryadi N, Patel M, Patel N. Neighborhood characteristics and frailty: a scoping review. Gerontologist. 2020;60(4):e270–e85.

53. Maltby J, Hunt SA, Ohinata A, Palmer E, Conroy S. Frailty and social isolation: comparing the relationship between frailty and unidimensional and multifactorial models of social isolation. J Aging Health. 2020;2020:898264320923245.
54. Chen D, Yin Z, Fang B. Measurements and status of sleep quality in patients with cancers. Support Care Cancer. 2018;26(2):405–14.
55. Swain CTV, Nguyen NH, Eagles T, Vallance JK, Boyle T, Lahart IM, et al. Postdiagnosis sedentary behavior and health outcomes in cancer survivors: a systematic review and meta-analysis. Cancer. 2020;126(4):861–9.
56. Broderick JM, Hussey J, Kennedy MJ, DM OD. Patients over 65 years are assigned lower ECOG PS scores than younger patients, although objectively measured physical activity is no different. J Geriatr Oncol. 2014;5(1):49–56.
57. Ehrler F, Weber C, Lovis C. Influence of pedometer position on pedometer accuracy at various walking speeds: a comparative study. J Med Internet Res. 2016;18(10):e268.
58. Henriksen A, Haugen Mikalsen M, Woldaregay AZ, Muzny M, Hartvigsen G, Hopstock LA, et al. Using fitness trackers and smartwatches to measure physical activity in research: analysis of consumer wrist-worn wearables. J Med Internet Res. 2018;20(3):e110.
59. Reichert M, Giurgiu M, Koch E, Wieland LM, Lautenbach S, Neubauer AB, et al. Ambulatory assessment for physical activity research: state of the science, best practices and future directions. Psychol Sport Exerc. 2020;50:101742.
60. Beg MS, Gupta A, Stewart T, Rethorst CD. Promise of wearable physical activity monitors in oncology practice. J Oncol Pract. 2017;13(2):82–9.
61. Peddle-McIntyre CJ, Cavalheri V, Boyle T, McVeigh JA, Jeffery E, Lynch BM, et al. A review of accelerometer-based activity monitoring in cancer survivorship research. Med Sci Sports Exerc. 2018;50(9):1790–801.
62. Sweegers MG, Boyle T, Vallance JK, Chinapaw MJ, Brug J, Aaronson NK, et al. Which cancer survivors are at risk for a physically inactive and sedentary lifestyle? Results from pooled accelerometer data of 1447 cancer survivors. Int J Behav Nutr Phys Act. 2019;16(1):66.
63. Jeffery E, Lee YG, McVeigh J, Straker L, Wooding T, Newton RU, et al. Feasibility of objectively measured physical activity and sedentary behavior in patients with malignant pleural effusion. Support Care Cancer. 2017;25(10):3133–41.
64. Negm AM, Kennedy CC, Thabane L, Veroniki AA, Adachi JD, Richardson J, et al. Management of frailty: a systematic review and network meta-analysis of randomized controlled trials. J Am Med Dir Assoc. 2019;20(10):1190–8.
65. Apóstolo J, Cooke R, Bobrowicz-Campos E, Santana S, Marcucci M, Cano A, et al. Effectiveness of interventions to prevent pre-frailty and frailty progression in older adults: a systematic review. JBI Database System Rev Implement Rep. 2018;16(1):140–232.
66. Travers J, Romero-Ortuno R, Bailey J, Cooney MT. Delaying and reversing frailty: a systematic review of primary care interventions. Br J Gen Pract. 2019;69(678):e61–e9.
67. Gielen E, Beckwée D, Delaere A, De Breucker S, Vandewoude M, Bautmans I. Nutritional interventions to improve muscle mass, muscle strength, and physical performance in older people: an umbrella review of systematic reviews and meta-analyses. Nutr Rev. 2020;79(2):121–47.
68. Peterson SJ, Mozer M. Differentiating sarcopenia and cachexia among patients with cancer. Nutr Clin Pract. 2017;32(1):30–9.
69. Simcock R, Wright J. Beyond Performance Status. Clin Oncol (R Coll Radiol). 2020;32(9):553–61.
70. Cruz-Jentoft AJ, Baeyens JP, Bauer JM, Boirie Y, Cederholm T, Landi F, et al. Sarcopenia: European consensus on definition and diagnosis: report of the European Working Group on sarcopenia in older people. Age Ageing. 2010;39(4):412–23.
71. Shen W, Punyanitya M, Wang Z, Gallagher D, St-Onge MP, Albu J, et al. Total body skeletal muscle and adipose tissue volumes: estimation from a single abdominal cross-sectional image. J Appl Physiol (1985). 2004;97(6):2333–8.

72. Perthen JE, Ali T, McCulloch D, Navidi M, Phillips AW, Sinclair RCF, et al. Intra- and interobserver variability in skeletal muscle measurements using computed tomography images. Eur J Radiol. 2018;109:142–6.
73. Shachar SS, Williams GR, Muss HB, Nishijima TF. Prognostic value of sarcopenia in adults with solid tumours: a meta-analysis and systematic review. Eur J Cancer. 2016;57:58–67.
74. Shachar SS, Deal AM, Weinberg M, Nyrop KA, Williams GR, Nishijima TF, et al. Skeletal muscle measures as predictors of toxicity, hospitalization, and survival in patients with metastatic breast cancer receiving taxane-based chemotherapy. Clin Cancer Res. 2017;23(3):658–65.
75. Xiao J, Caan BJ, Cespedes Feliciano EM, Meyerhardt JA, Peng PD, Baracos VE, et al. Association of low muscle mass and low muscle radiodensity with morbidity and mortality for colon cancer surgery. JAMA Surg. 2020;155(10):942–9.
76. Mir O, Coriat R, Blanchet B, Durand JP, Boudou-Rouquette P, Michels J, et al. Sarcopenia predicts early dose-limiting toxicities and pharmacokinetics of sorafenib in patients with hepatocellular carcinoma. PLoS One. 2012;7(5):e37563.
77. Kroenke CH, Prado CM, Meyerhardt JA, Weltzien EK, Xiao J, Cespedes Feliciano EM, et al. Muscle radiodensity and mortality in patients with colorectal cancer. Cancer. 2018;124(14):3008–15.
78. Varadhan R, Russ DW, Gabr RE, Huang J, Kalyani RR, Xue QL, et al. Relationship of physical frailty to phosphocreatine recovery in muscle after mild exercise stress in the oldest-old women. J Frailty Aging. 2019;8(4):162–8.
79. Cardoso AL, Fernandes A, Aguilar-Pimentel JA, de Angelis MH, Guedes JR, Brito MA, et al. Towards frailty biomarkers: Candidates from genes and pathways regulated in aging and age-related diseases. Ageing Res Rev. 2018;47:214–77.
80. Kane AE, Sinclair DA. Frailty biomarkers in humans and rodents: current approaches and future advances. Mech Ageing Dev. 2019;180:117–28.
81. Mitnitski A, Collerton J, Martin-Ruiz C, Jagger C, von Zglinicki T, Rockwood K, et al. Age-related frailty and its association with biological markers of ageing. BMC Med. 2015;13:161.
82. Ferrucci L, Corsi A, Lauretani F, Bandinelli S, Bartali B, Taub DD, et al. The origins of age-related proinflammatory state. Blood. 2005;105(6):2294–9.
83. Hazeldine J, Lord JM. Innate immunesenescence: underlying mechanisms and clinical relevance. Biogerontology. 2015;16(2):187–201.
84. Weng NP, Akbar AN, Goronzy J. CD28(-) T cells: their role in the age-associated decline of immune function. Trends Immunol. 2009;30(7):306–12.
85. Verschoor CP, Johnstone J, Millar J, Dorrington MG, Habibagahi M, Lelic A, et al. Blood CD33(+)HLA-DR(-) myeloid-derived suppressor cells are increased with age and a history of cancer. J Leukoc Biol. 2013;93(4):633–7.
86. Lages CS, Suffia I, Velilla PA, Huang B, Warshaw G, Hildeman DA, et al. Functional regulatory T cells accumulate in aged hosts and promote chronic infectious disease reactivation. J Immunol. 2008;181(3):1835–48.
87. Sanoff HK, Deal AM, Krishnamurthy J, Torrice C, Dillon P, Sorrentino J, et al. Effect of cytotoxic chemotherapy on markers of molecular age in patients with breast cancer. J Natl Cancer Inst. 2014;106(4):dju057.
88. Dolan RD, McSorley ST, Horgan PG, Laird B, McMillan DC. The role of the systemic inflammatory response in predicting outcomes in patients with advanced inoperable cancer: systematic review and meta-analysis. Crit Rev Oncol Hematol. 2017;116:134–46.
89. Laird BJ, Fallon M, Hjermstad MJ, Tuck S, Kaasa S, Klepstad P, et al. Quality of life in patients with advanced cancer: differential association with performance status and systemic inflammatory response. J Clin Oncol. 2016;34(23):2769–75.
90. Weber JS, Hamid O, Chasalow SD, Wu DY, Parker SM, Galbraith S, et al. Ipilimumab increases activated T cells and enhances humoral immunity in patients with advanced melanoma. J Immunother. 2012;35(1):89–97.

91. Beaufrère B, Morio B. Fat and protein redistribution with aging: metabolic considerations. Eur J Clin Nutr. 2000;54(Suppl 3):S48–53.
92. Arai Y, Kamide K, Hirose N. Adipokines and aging: findings from centenarians and the very old. Front Endocrinol (Lausanne). 2019;10:142.
93. Wyatt N, Hogarth L, Turner D, Patterson M, Jamieson D, Black F, et al. P2.01-070 circulating biomarkers of frailty are associated with a poor prognosis in patients with advanced Non-Small Cell Lung Cancer (NSCLC): topic: marker for prognosis. J Thoracic Oncol. 2017;12(1):S829–S30.
94. Yeap BB, Chubb SA, Ho KK, Setoh JW, McCaul KA, Norman PE, et al. IGF1 and its binding proteins 3 and 1 are differentially associated with metabolic syndrome in older men. Eur J Endocrinol. 2010;162(2):249–57.
95. Horvath S, Raj K. DNA methylation-based biomarkers and the epigenetic clock theory of ageing. Nat Rev Genet. 2018;19(6):371–84.
96. Gale CR, Marioni RE, Harris SE, Starr JM, Deary IJ. DNA methylation and the epigenetic clock in relation to physical frailty in older people: the Lothian Birth Cohort 1936. Clin Epigenetics. 2018;10(1):101.
97. Marioni RE, Shah S, McRae AF, Ritchie SJ, Muniz-Terrera G, Harris SE, et al. The epigenetic clock is correlated with physical and cognitive fitness in the Lothian Birth Cohort 1936. Int J Epidemiol. 2015;44(4):1388–96.
98. Dhahbi JM. Circulating small noncoding RNAs as biomarkers of aging. Ageing Res Rev. 2014;17:86–98.
99. Wildiers H, Heeren P, Puts M, Topinkova E, Janssen-Heijnen ML, Extermann M, et al. International Society of Geriatric Oncology consensus on geriatric assessment in older patients with cancer. J Clin Oncol. 2014;32(24):2595–603.
100. Mohile SG, Dale W, Somerfield MR, Schonberg MA, Boyd CM, Burhenn PS, et al. Practical assessment and management of vulnerabilities in older patients receiving chemotherapy: ASCO guideline for geriatric oncology. J Clin Oncol. 2018;36(22):2326–47.
101. Decoster L, Van Puyvelde K, Mohile S, Wedding U, Basso U, Colloca G, et al. Screening tools for multidimensional health problems warranting a geriatric assessment in older cancer patients: an update on SIOG recommendations. Ann Oncol. 2015;26(2):288–300.
102. Welaya K, Loh KP, Messing S, Szuba E, Magnuson A, Mohile SG, et al. Geriatric assessment and treatment outcomes in older adults with cancer receiving immune checkpoint inhibitors. J Geriatr Oncol. 2019;11(3):523–8.
103. Muchnik E, Loh KP, Strawderman M, Magnuson A, Mohile SG, Estrah V, et al. Immune checkpoint inhibitors in real-world treatment of older adults with non-small cell lung cancer. J Am Geriatr Soc. 2019;67(5):905–12.
104. Xue DD, Cheng Y, Wu M, Zhang Y. Comprehensive geriatric assessment prediction of postoperative complications in gastrointestinal cancer patients: a meta-analysis. Clin Interven Aging. 2018;13:723–36.
105. Szumacher E, Sattar S, Neve M, Do K, Ayala AP, Gray M, et al. Use of comprehensive geriatric assessment and geriatric screening for older adults in the radiation oncology setting: a systematic review. Clin Oncol (R Coll Radiol). 2018;30(9):578–88.
106. Hurria A, Akiba C, Kim J, Mitani D, Loscalzo M, Katheria V, et al. Reliability, validity, and feasibility of a computer-based geriatric assessment for older adults with cancer. J Oncol Pract. 2016;12(12):e1025–e34.
107. Siegel RL, Jemal A, Wender RC, Gansler T, Ma J, Brawley OW. An assessment of progress in cancer control. CA Cancer J Clin. 2018;68(5):329–39.
108. Edwards BK, Noone AM, Mariotto AB, Simard EP, Boscoe FP, Henley SJ, et al. Annual report to the Nation on the status of cancer, 1975-2010, featuring prevalence of comorbidity and impact on survival among persons with lung, colorectal, breast, or prostate cancer. Cancer. 2014;120(9):1290–314.
109. Jemal A, Thun MJ, Ries LA, Howe HL, Weir HK, Center MM, et al. Annual report to the nation on the status of cancer, 1975-2005, featuring trends in lung cancer, tobacco use, and tobacco control. J Natl Cancer Inst. 2008;100(23):1672–94.

110. DeSantis CE, Miller KD, Dale W, Mohile SG, Cohen HJ, Leach CR, et al. Cancer statistics for adults aged 85 years and older, 2019. CA Cancer J Clin. 2019;69(6):452–67.
111. Ashing KT, Soto-Perez-de-Celis E. Disparities within a disparity: global health and health equity in geriatric oncology. J Geriatr Oncol. 2019;11:200–2.
112. Soto-Perez-de-Celis E, de Glas NA, Hsu T, Kanesvaran R, Steer C, Navarrete-Reyes AP, et al. Global geriatric oncology: achievements and challenges. J Geriatr Oncol. 2017;8(5):374–86.
113. Ludmir EB, Mainwaring W, Lin TA, Miller AB, Jethanandani A, Espinoza AF, et al. Factors associated with age disparities among cancer clinical trial participants. JAMA Oncol. 2019;5(12):1769–73.
114. Duma N, Vera Aguilera J, Paludo J, Haddox CL, Gonzalez Velez M, Wang Y, et al. Representation of minorities and women in oncology clinical trials: review of the past 14 years. J Oncol Pract. 2018;14(1):e1–e10.
115. Murthy VH, Krumholz HM, Gross CP. Participation in cancer clinical trials: race-, sex-, and age-based disparities. JAMA. 2004;291(22):2720–6.
116. Healthy aging at a glance, 2011: helping people to live long and productive lives and enjoy a good quality of life. In: Prevention CfDCa, editor. 2011.
117. Services CfMaM. Chronic Conditions among Medicare Beneficiaries, Chartbook, 2017 Edition. https://www.cms.gov/research-statistics-data-and-systems/statistics-trends-and-reports/chronic-conditions/downloads/2012chartbook.pdf.2012
118. Cho H, Mariotto AB, Mann BS, Klabunde CN, Feuer EJ. Assessing non-cancer-related health status of US cancer patients: other-cause survival and comorbidity prevalence. Am J Epidemiol. 2013;178(3):339–49.
119. Tinetti ME, Inouye SK, Gill TM, Doucette JT. Shared risk factors for falls, incontinence, and functional dependence. Unifying the approach to geriatric syndromes. JAMA. 1995;273(17):1348–53.
120. Mohile SG, Velarde C, Hurria A, Magnuson A, Lowenstein L, Pandya C, et al. Geriatric assessment-guided care processes for older adults: a Delphi consensus of geriatric oncology experts. J Natl Compr Canc Netw. 2015;13(9):1120–30.
121. O'Donovan A, Mohile SG, Leech M. Expert consensus panel guidelines on geriatric assessment in oncology. Eur J Cancer Care (Engl). 2015;24(4):574–89.

Part III
Frailty and the Treatment of Common Cancer Types

Chapter 17
Breast Cancer in Older Adults with Frailty

Lissandra Dal Lago, Alex de Caluwe, Cindy Borghgraef, Laura Dumont, and Thierry Pepersack

Introduction

Despite the high incidence of breast cancer and its related mortality in an aged population, the knowledge about optimal treatment for older patients with cancer is far from adequate, particularly for those also living with frailty. By 2040, patients older than 65 will account for more than 70% of all new cancer diagnoses [1] and many will have frailty. Since older adults have more competing mortality risks, treatment decisions should consider not just the risk of cancer recurrence, but also the risk of dying of other causes, which is strongly affected by the patients' frailty.

Older patients with breast cancer and frailty are still underrepresented in clinical trials, however recent guidelines proposed extended eligibility criteria [2] which might increase the number of older patients enrolled in clinical trials. Moreover, a new generation of clinical trials are including other global health/fitness assessments, including for example the Charlson comorbidity index and scales for activities of daily living, as factors within the eligibility criteria.

Whilst older patients present more often with larger breast cancer tumours, they also present with more favourable biologic characteristics compared to their younger counterparts [3]. These include a higher prevalence of mucinous sub-type, a higher degree of hormone receptor expression and less peri-tumoural vascular invasion [3].

L. D. Lago (✉) · C. Borghgraef · L. Dumont · T. Pepersack
Department of Medicine, Institut Jules Bordet, Université Libre de Bruxelles, Brussels, Belgium
e-mail: lissandra.dallago@bordet.be; cindy.borghgraef@bordet.be; laura.dumont@bordet.be; Thierry.Pepersack@bordet.be

A. de Caluwe
Department of Radiation Oncology, Institut Jules Bordet, Université Libre de Bruxelles, Brussels, Belgium
e-mail: alex.decaluwe@bordet.be

F. Gomes (ed.), *Frailty in Older Adults with Cancer*,
https://doi.org/10.1007/978-3-030-89162-6_17

Moreover, despite the proportion of luminal tumours increasing with age and the percentage of basal-like tumours decreasing, older patients still have a substantial proportion of high-risk tumour subtypes [4–6]. And in several countries, older patients are diagnosed with breast cancer at a later stage with more advanced disease [7]. In order to guide the management of breast cancer in older patients, the International Society of Geriatric Oncology (SIOG) published in collaboration with the European Society of Breast Cancer Specialists updated recommendations [8].

Lastly, considerations about breast cancer screening in older patients are complex. Whilst screening mammography in patients aged 70–75 years could be of benefit to some of these patients, particularly if life expectancy is 10 years or more. For those older than that, screening is unlikely to be beneficial due to a considerable risk of overdiagnoses. For older breast cancer survivors, surveillance is generally recommended for women aged up to 80 years. In any case, more than chronological age, the decision for older patients should be individualised and based on risks and benefits, patient preference, physiological age, comorbidity, frailty and life expectancy, with several expert groups considering stopping screening or surveillance when life expectancy is under 5–10 years [8–10]. Nonetheless, the focus of this chapter will be on reviewing the current evidence regarding the treatment of breast cancer in older patients with frailty, from an early stage to a metastatic setting.

Management of Early-Stage and Locally Advanced Breast Cancer

Clinicians facing older breast cancer patients with frailty have available some decision-support tools to weigh risks and benefits of surgical or adjuvant treatment to support a shared decision-making.

Accurate estimation of life expectancy is essential in selecting treatment for older adults with cancer, especially for those patients also living with frailty for whom the potential survival benefit of, for example, adjuvant chemotherapy may be nullified by competing medical comorbidities. Several validated online tools are available that enable accurate estimates of mortality risk to be made, and which may incorporate geriatric assessment variables in addition to demographic and clinical data (e.g., https://eprognosis.ucsf.edu/calculators) [11].

Regarding toxicity prediction, when a surgery is considered, the American College of Surgeons National Surgical Quality Improvement Program (ACS NSQIP) Surgical Risk Calculator provides patient-specific postoperative risks [12]. By using 20 variables, including the type of planned surgical intervention, this web-based tool estimates expected length of stay and patient's risk of having any of 18 different outcomes within the first 30 days following surgery (e.g., post-surgery infection, renal failure, readmission, discharge to nursing, sepsis, death). When (neo)adjuvant chemotherapy is being considered, another relevant tool is the Cancer and Aging Research Group—Breast Cancer (CARG-BC) tool. This was developed to identify older patients with operable breast cancer who are at higher risk of developing toxicity associated with (neo)adjuvant chemotherapy. This risk score was validated in patients aged 65 years and older with stage I–III breast cancer and derives from the main CARG-Score, which was specifically developed to identify grade 3–5 chemotherapy toxicity risk. The CARG-BC consists of eight independent predictors of toxicity: tumour stage, use of anthracycline, planned treatment duration, liver function, anaemia, lack of social support, limited mobility and falls. Each risk factor is assigned a score and when scores are summed, patients are categorized as low risk (0–5 points), intermediate risk (6–9 points) and high risk (10–19 points) [13].

Regarding survival prediction, several other tools have been developed to aid decision-making in the selection of treatment plans. The Adjuvant! Online prediction tool was developed in a patient population aged 69 years or younger and when its validity in older patients was investigated in a large cohort of unselected older patients, it did not accurately predict overall survival and recurrence in that subgroup of patients [14]. The PREDICT Breast Cancer [15, 16] is another online tool dedicated to women who had surgery for early invasive breast cancer and for whom an adjuvant treatment is being discussed. This tool estimates overall survival, breast cancer survival with no adjuvant treatment and how different treatments (endocrine therapy, chemotherapy, trastuzumab, and bisphosphonates) may improve survival rates up to 15 years after diagnosis. The PREDICT model considers several variables known to affect average survival including, age at diagnosis, menopausal status, oestrogen receptor, HER2, Ki67, tumour size, presence of positives lymph nodes and micrometastases. However, differently to Adjuvant! Online it does not include comorbidity burden. The development of PREDICT included almost 1800 women aged 65 years or over and it is more accurate than Adjuvant! Online for older patients. It accurately predicts 5-year overall survival in older patients with breast cancer. However, the 10-year overall survival is overestimated in this older sub-group and it is not reliable in the presence of comorbidities and age over 80 years [17]. Nonetheless, as the tool lacks factors such as comorbidity and frailty, its applicability in the sub-group of older patients with frailty is less clear. Yet, other prediction tools have been developed in that setting. The online Age Gap decision tool was developed specifically to optimise the management of older women with operable breast cancer aged 70 and above, reducing the age-related gap in cancer outcomes seen between older and younger women. This online tool was developed as part of the bridging the age gap study based on survival data from the United Kingdom cancer registry, adjusted for comorbidities and frailty. This tool is promising and requires prospective validation but its use alongside booklets and brief decision aids facilitates shared decision-making and alters treatment selection for this sub-group of patients [18]. The recently published PORTRET-tool was also developed to predict recurrence, survival and other-cause mortality in older patients aged 65 and over with breast cancer based on data from the Netherlands. This model includes geriatric assessments and considers competing risks for survival outcomes in this complex sub-group of patients [19].

Therefore, the use of these tools promotes a more suitable and personalized risk assessment for older patients with frailty in order to appropriately guide treatment decision-making.

Surgery

Surgery is the primary component of curative therapy for early-stage breast cancer. Appropriately selected older women tolerate breast surgery well. Perioperative morbidity is low, and mortality rates range from 0% to 2%, more correlated to comorbidity and frailty than chronological age. The above-described ACS NSQIP Surgical Risk Calculator is particularly helpful to support this decision-making process [12]. Older women often prefer breast-conserving surgery over mastectomy since it is associated with better quality of life. However, when considering surgery, women should be informed that the adverse effects on quality of life are seen in the first few months after surgery, but by 24 months these have largely resolved [20].

Overall the SIOG recommendations propose that most women older than 70 years of age should be offered similar surgical options and axilla sampling as younger women, yet completion of axillary clearance is not always needed [8]. For those with significant comorbid illnesses or frailty, surgery under local anaesthesia may be better tolerated than general anaesthesia. Another important consideration for older patients undergoing general anaesthesia, unlike younger patients, is the higher risk to experience short-term cognitive impairment [21]. But ultimately, in many cases of older patients with significant frailty, surgical procedures may not be appropriate and alternative options such as primary endocrine therapy (if hormone receptor-positive) or radiotherapy may be considered.

For those older patients with locally advanced disease, surgery upfront may be particularly challenging in order to achieve clear margins and neo-adjuvant strategies should be considered in fit patients [8]. However, in the context of an older patient with frailty and a higher risk of adverse events, such strategies are rarely appropriate. If operable, surgery upfront is recommended, otherwise most patients with significant frailty and locally advanced breast cancer will be alternatively better served with primary endocrine therapy (if hormone receptor-positive) or radiotherapy.

Radiotherapy

Postoperative whole-breast radiotherapy remains the standard of care for most patients treated by breast-conserving surgery, irrespective of age and other risk factors [22]. The PRIME II trial investigated breast conservative surgery with or without post-operative irradiation in women aged 65 years or older with hormone-receptor positive breast cancer [23]. This trial demonstrated a very low risk of local recurrence after breast-conserving surgery and adjuvant endocrine treatment in women allocated to whole-breast radiotherapy. The latest update at the 2020 San Antonio Breast Cancer Symposium reported outcomes at 10 years and although local recurrence was greater in the group without radiation therapy (9.8% vs 0.9%), there was no difference in contra-lateral recurrence, distant metastasis and overall survival. Therefore, for older women with frailty and an early stage hormone receptor-positive node-negative breast cancer ($\leq$3 cm at the longest dimension) after breast-conserving surgery, adjuvant endocrine treatment alone is a reasonable therapeutic option.

Regarding the delivery of postoperative radiotherapy, the FAST-Forward investigated hypofractionation in patients with low absolute risk of local tumour relapse, using 26 Gy in 5 fractions over 1 week versus 40 Gy in 15 fractions over 3 weeks. This hypofractionated schedule over 1 week was non-inferior in terms of ipsilateral breast tumour recurrence with a good safety profile. Therefore, this may be a good alternative for patients to reduce the duration of treatment for older patients with frailty [24].

Radiotherapy may also be an alternative to axillary lymph node dissection for older patients with significant frailty and positive sentinel lymph nodes, as described by the AMAROS trial [25]. Lastly, as this sub-group of patients is often not eligible for any surgical procedures, primary radiotherapy may be an option. In one large series of more than 450 breast cancer patients treated with radiation alone at doses of 70–80 Gy, the 3-year local control rates were 81%, 71%, 61% and 36% for tumours less than 4 cm, 4–6 cm, 6–8 cm and greater than 8 cm, respectively. In general, doses higher than 60 Gy are needed to achieve durable local control in the absence of surgical excision [26].

Luminal Breast Cancer

As previously described, this represents the most common sub-type of breast cancer in older patients [4–6].

Upfront surgery rather than primary endocrine therapy is the preferred treatment in older patients with hormone-receptor positive breast cancer [27]. However, in patients with significant frailty, when general anaesthesia is contraindicated or the surgical procedure cannot be done by local anaesthesia, primary endocrine therapy is offered. Most data on the role of primary endocrine therapy derive from retrospective studies with acceptable response rates and similar time to progression in those receiving tamoxifen or aromatase inhibitors [28, 29].

In the adjuvant setting, older patients with luminal-type tumours and frailty are better treated with endocrine therapy. In fact, adjuvant chemotherapy has a survival benefit primarily limited to older women with hormone receptor-negative breast cancer [30–32]. There is however some contradictory evidence suggesting that older patients with hormone receptor-positive tumours may have a survival benefit, particularly in the presence of other high risk characteristics such as positive nodal disease

[33]. Ultimately, the added benefit of adjuvant chemotherapy decreases in this group of older women with frailty considering the competing risks of morbidity and mortality, particularly for those with hormone-receptor positive breast cancer [34].

Moreover, there is insufficient evidence regarding the value of genomic testing to categorise prognosis and predict treatment benefit in older patients. One retrospective study from SEER database [35] demonstrated that the Oncotype DX recurrence score was less likely to be used in older patients (aged 70 or older). For those assessed, older patients had a similar distribution in terms of recurrence risk as compared to younger patients. Whilst high-risk was prognostic in older patients, chemotherapy was not associated with improved survival. Other tests such as MammaPrint in the MINDACT trial [36] only included fit patients up to 70 years of age. However, the ongoing ASTER70 study (NCT01564056) is investigating the role of adjuvant chemotherapy based on genomic testing in older women over 70 years of age [37].

Therefore, it is recommended that [8, 38] adjuvant endocrine therapy should be offered to all women with hormone-receptor positive breast tumours >0.5 cm, regardless of age, provided there is no contra-indication for medical therapy. The administration of an aromatase inhibitor is preferred because of its benefits in the adjuvant setting compared with tamoxifen, as well as avoidance of the thromboembolic risks and endometrial thickening/bleeding associated with tamoxifen. However, for women at risk for cardiovascular complications or bone loss, and those unable to tolerate an aromatase inhibitor due to toxicity, tamoxifen is a reasonable alternative. Data from toxicity from ATAC and MA.17 trials are not conclusive regarding risk of bone fractures, but provided that patients with frailty might be at higher risk, careful monitoring of bone mineral density, calcium and vitamin D supplementation, and osteoporosis treatment should be offered to minimize the risk of these complications [39]. Regarding the use of tamoxifen, attention should be given to the administration of concomitant drugs that inhibit CYP2D6, for example, certain selective serotonin reuptake inhibitors that may potentially alter the metabolism of the drug.

The treatment duration of five years for endocrine therapy should be considered standard for older women with frailty. Longer durations up to 10 years might be appropriate in selected patients with higher-risk tumour features (e.g., nodal involvement), but this should be discussed in the perspective of other comorbidities and mortality risk [40]. Lower compliance with endocrine therapy is seen in the oldest patients treated for breast cancer, which is potentially related to side effects. The switch method where oral adjuvant endocrine therapy is switched at some point between tamoxifen and aromatase inhibitors demonstrated a better tolerance and adherence in older breast cancer patients, compared with giving only tamoxifen or aromatase inhibitor for the all duration of endocrine therapy [41].

Lastly, there is a growing interest in the use of bisphosphonates in the adjuvant setting with the aim to reduce the relapse risk, and to decrease the risk of therapy-induced osteoporotic fractures [42]. However, there is no age-specific data and attention should be given as renal function declines with age, and the dose of zoledronic acid needs to be adjusted to renal function.

Triple Negative Breast Cancer

Triple negative breast cancer represents approximately 10% of breast cancer patients over 65 years of age and it is a distinct phenotype of breast cancer characterized by rapid tumour growth, a relapse rate that peaks in the first 2–3 years after diagnosis [43]. The treatment of triple-negative breast cancer is challenging, given that chemotherapy is the only available adjuvant systemic therapy after surgery for these patients, and it can be associated with significant toxicity. Therefore, its management is challenging in older patients with frailty.

As described in the previous sub-section, the benefit of adjuvant chemotherapy in older patients seems to be particularly limited to the hormone-receptor negative tumours, irrespective of nodal status [30–32]. But the use of chemotherapy should not be guided by chronological age alone and frailty plays a significant role in determining tolerability [8]. Therefore, appropriate patient selection is key and the previous described CARG-BC tool to predict chemotherapy toxicity is useful to support decision-making [13].

Regarding the choice of chemotherapy, third-generation regimens that include both anthracyclines and taxanes yield better survival outcomes than first-generation regimens in older patients but are not generally recommended in patients with frailty, particularly because of the risk of cardiotoxicity [44, 45]. Therefore, the more reasonable options to consider in selected patients with frailty, if eligible to any, are the second-generation taxotere-cyclophosphamide (TC) or doxorubicin-cyclophosphamide or single-agent weekly paclitaxel if unfit for polychemotherapy [8, 46]. Overall, TC can be given and completed in >90% of older patients (aged 70+), recovering from a slight decline in quality of life and functionality after 1 year of follow-up [47]. However frailty impacts these outcomes and administration of granulocyte growth factors is necessary to reduce the risk of febrile neutropenia and another concern is the development of taxane-related neuropathy, which even mild can be clinically significant in older patients with frailty. Therefore, clinicians should also consider the other alternatives, including single-agent strategy. In any case, whenever considering chemotherapy, its negative impact on the quality of life is significant at 6 months but resolves by 18 months, which is crucial information to guide decision-making for older patients contemplating chemotherapy [48].

HER2 Positive Breast Cancer

In patients with human epidermal growth factor receptor 2 (HER2)-positive breast cancer, the benefit of adding trastuzumab to adjuvant chemotherapy is essentially independent of age for fit patients without cardiac dysfunction in adjuvant clinical trials [49].

Trastuzumab may be added to the adjuvant chemotherapy regimens described in the previous sub-section [8]. The preference here is also to avoid combinations with anthracyclines, and although it could be combined with docetaxel–cyclophosphamide, in older patients with frailty the combination of paclitaxel and trastuzumab represents an appropriate regimen. This preserves quality of life while achieving excellent outcomes for patients with stage I breast cancer [50]. An effort to minimize toxicity is the trastuzumab treatment in combination with navelbine according to FinHER trial [51]. Since trastuzumab is associated with cardiotoxicity, another alternative for patients with frailty with a higher risk of cardiotoxicity is the short duration of trastuzumab according to PERSEPHONE trial. In this study, 6 months of adjuvant trastuzumab was non-inferior to 12 months [52]. Lastly, a trastuzumab regimen without chemotherapy in the case of hormone receptor-positive tumours in older patients (aged 70+) might be an option for patients with frailty, according to the RESPECT trial results [53]. Although trastuzumab-only may result in a reduction in overall survival at 3 years of about 1 month in comparison with its combination with chemotherapy; in light of less toxicity and a better quality of life profile, trastuzumab-only may be an alternative for older patients with frailty not suitable for chemotherapy. This trial has recently reported that the detrimental effects of adjuvant chemotherapy on global quality of life lasted for at least 12 months, which further supports a potential preference for trastuzumab-only in this sub-group of older patients with frailty [54].

Management of Advanced Metastatic Breast Cancer

In the context of advanced metastatic disease, it is key to consider not just to prolong survival but also, and often more importantly, an improvement in symptoms, function and quality of life. Although clinical trials designed specifically for the management of older women are scarce, there are evidence-based guidelines that provide a framework for clinical teams [8].

Chemotherapy

Any decision on the administration of chemotherapy in older women should be individualized, based on their tumour and the potential benefits and risks of treatment. Chemotherapy should be considered in the first-line setting if life-threatening or rapidly progressive visceral disease with end-organ dysfunction, particularly if triple negative breast cancer.

When chemotherapy is being considered, the use of toxicity prediction models such as the CARG and CRASH scores can be useful when weighing risks and benefits of chemotherapy with an older patient with frailty [55, 56].

Particular care should be paid to avoiding treatment-related toxicities, this can include selecting less toxic options and adjusting treatment schedules. A choice between the available chemotherapy agents should be based on the patient's clinical status, comorbidities, and careful consideration of the agents, their schedule of administration, and specific toxicities [57]. For older patients with frailty, sequential single-agent therapy rather than combination chemotherapy should be preferred [8]. However, there is no optimal or preferred sequence of agents. Lastly, recent studies have suggested the use of single drug nab-paclitaxel and eribulin could be good options for this sub-group of patients, for being well-tolerated and preserving quality of life and function [58, 59].

Endocrine and Targeted Therapies

Endocrine therapy is the first line standard of care for hormone receptor-positive tumours, with the previously described exception of visceral crisis [8]. Although there are no age-specific data on the role of palliative endocrine therapy, particularly in patients with frailty, this is an attractive systemic therapy option for these patients considering its tolerability profile. There are however several considerations in the selection of the endocrine therapy for older adults, as described in a previous section.

The scope for endocrine therapy can be enhanced by its combination with other agents, such as cyclin-dependent kinase 4/6 (CDK4/6) inhibitors and mammalian target of rapamycin (mTOR) inhibitors.

The CDK4/6 inhibitors were a significant breakthrough in the management of hormone receptor-positive HER2-negative tumours. These may be an attractive option in the context of their efficacy, safety profile and impact on quality of life [60–62]. But decision-making should consider patient preferences and the different safety profiles of the different CDK4/6 inhibitors, in fact frequent adjustments are needed. For example, there is more myelosuppression with palbociclib and ribociclib, whilst there is more gastro-intestinal toxicity with abemaciclib. But there is a lack of data in older patients with frailty and if these combinations are not tolerated, endocrine therapy alone is a reasonable option.

Lastly, the mTOR inhibitor everolimus combined with endocrine therapy improved treatment efficacy and is relatively well tolerated in older patients but it has a worse safety profile compared to CDK4/6 inhibitors. It requires careful monitoring and appropriate dose reductions or interruptions for the management of adverse events [63, 64]. Therefore, this may not be an appropriate option for older patients with frailty and its use should be approached with caution and on a case-by-case basis.

Anti-HER2 Therapy

Older patients with HER2-positive breast cancer should receive a HER2-directed agent as part of their treatment regimen, unless contraindicated by impaired left ventricular ejection fraction [8].

The monoclonal antibody pertuzumab targets a different HER2 epitope than trastuzumab, blocks HER2 dimerization, and in combination with trastuzumab results in a dual HER2 blockade. The combination of trastuzumab and pertuzumab with docetaxel on the CLEOPATRA trial identified the new standard of care for fit patients. Although a pre-defined sub-analysis of this trial showed that survival benefits were similar for older and younger patients, data were less conclusive after 75 years of age [65, 66]. Also, the combination of this double blockade with docetaxel is not an appropriate option for the majority of older patients with frailty because of its side effects. In older patients not suitable for taxanes, capecitabine or vinorelbine can be considered. Moreover, the EORTC 75111 trial combined the dual HER2 blockade with metronomic chemotherapy (cyclophosphamide) which might offer a good alternative and better tolerated for selected older patients with frailty [67]. Single-agent trastuzumab may also suit those older patients with frailty with hormone receptor-negative tumours if chemotherapy is contraindicated. However, it is less active alone than with chemotherapy [68].

Tyrosine kinase inhibitors anti-HER2 are also available, such as lapatinib, neratinib and tucatinib. Lapatinib can be used in combination with chemotherapy, but a head-to-head comparison suggested inferiority to trastuzumab-based treatment [69]. Moreover, the toxicity profile of these tyrosine kinase inhibitors, in particular gastro-intestinal toxicity with lapatinib, means these are unlikely to be an appropriate option for older patients with frailty.

TDM1 is a stable conjugate of trastuzumab with DM1, a microtubule inhibitor, allowing targeted delivery of the cytotoxic to HER2-positive cells and potentially improving the therapeutic index. EMILIA [70] and TH3RESA [71] trials showed improved progression-free survival and overall survival in the latter trial. KAMILLA safety study included only 20% of patients more than 65 and only 3% over 75. Treatment discontinuation was 14.3% in patients older than 65 vs 9.5% in younger ones, and the overall rate of adverse events was higher [72]. Though relevant in fit older patients, further investigation in patients with frailty is warranted.

For those also with hormone receptor-positive breast cancer, the combination of trastuzumab and endocrine therapy in the TAnDEM trial showed a significant improvement in progression free survival, compared to endocrine therapy alone [73]. The combination of endocrine plus anti-HER2 approach (without chemotherapy) is reasonable in older patients with strongly hormone receptor-positivity with low volume/slowly progressive disease, and in the vulnerable and those with frailty. The dual HER2 blockade with trastuzumab and pertuzumab with endocrine therapy in the PERTAIN trial is also an attractive option for older patients with frailty without cardiac contra-indication [74]. The combination of lapatinib to letrozole for hormone receptor-positive metastatic breast cancer led to an improvement in progression-free survival irrespective of age [75]. Although this may be appropriate for older patients, its toxicity profile can be problematic for those with significant frailty and since data is lacking, its use should be approached with caution and on a case-by-case basis. Lastly, the ALTERNATIVE trial showed that dual HER2 blockade with lapatinib and trastuzumab with endocrine therapy has superior efficacy to endocrine therapy-only and is a safe chemotherapy-sparing alternative treatment regimen. However, there are no conclusive data on older patients with frailty and this may be less appropriate due to the lapatinib toxicity profile [76].

Novel Treatments

Novel treatment strategies in breast cancer are evolving, such as PDL-1 inhibitors in combination with chemotherapy for the treatment of triple-negative metastatic breast cancer in patients whose tumours express the PD-L1 protein [77]. However, there is no available data for older patients with frailty.

Conclusion

Breast cancer management in older patients with frailty should consider risk of relapse, life expectancy, expected tolerability and patient preference. Many older women may have frailty and not be candidates for chemotherapy. It is important to recognize, however, that omission of therapy may significantly alter outcomes for older women with high-risk disease, particularly in adjuvant treatment. In these women, it may be increasingly important to have accurate staging information in order to make decisions around adjuvant therapy.

Following initial screening and preferably a geriatric assessment, management of the older patients with frailty and breast cancer can be divided into four steps: (1) determine whether the medical goal of treatment is to improve the chance for cure or palliation and convey this information to the patient and family; (2) query the patient as to what is important to her and what her goals are for being treated; (3) use geriatric assessment-based data and appropriate tools and models, including estimates of life expectancy for the individual patient, calculate the risks and benefits of treatment and (4) present these risks-and-benefits data to the patient and family using shared decision-making and in language that they can understand, to finalize the care plan [78, 79].

References

1. Bluethmann SM, Mariotto AB, Rowland JH. Anticipating the “Silver Tsunami”: prevalence trajectories and comorbidity burden among older cancer survivors in the United States. Cancer Epidemiol Biomarkers Prev. 2016;25(7):1029–36.
2. Lichtman SM, Harvey RD, Damiette Smit MA, Rahman A, Thompson MA, Roach N, et al. Modernizing clinical trial eligibility criteria: recommendations of the American Society of Clinical Oncology-Friends of Cancer Research Organ Dysfunction, Prior or Concurrent Malignancy, and Comorbidities Working Group. J Clin Oncol. 2017;35(33):3753–9.

3. Gennari R, Curigliano G, Rotmensz N, Robertson C, Colleoni M, Zurrida S, et al. Breast carcinoma in elderly women: features of disease presentation, choice of local and systemic treatments compared with younger postmenopasual patients. Cancer. 2004;101(6):1302–10.
4. Jenkins EO, Deal AM, Anders CK, Prat A, Perou CM, Carey LA, et al. Age-specific changes in intrinsic breast cancer subtypes: a focus on older women. Oncologist. 2014;19(10):1076–83.
5. Partridge AH, Hughes ME, Warner ET, Ottesen RA, Wong YN, Edge SB, et al. Subtype-dependent relationship between young age at diagnosis and breast cancer survival. J Clin Oncol. 2016;34(27):3308–14.
6. Diab SG, Elledge RM, Clark GM. Tumor characteristics and clinical outcome of elderly women with breast cancer. J Natl Cancer Inst. 2000;92(7):550–6.
7. Cabrera-Galeana P, Soto-Perez-de-Celis E, Reynoso-Noverón N, Villarreal-Garza C, Arce-Salinas C, Matus-Santos J, et al. Clinical characteristics and outcomes of older women with breast cancer in Mexico. J Geriatr Oncol. 2018;9(6):620–5.
8. Biganzoli L, Battisti NML, Wildiers H, McCartney A, Colloca G, Kunkler IH, et al. Updated recommendations regarding the management of older patients with breast cancer: a joint paper from the European Society of Breast Cancer Specialists (EUSOMA) and the International Society of Geriatric Oncology (SIOG). Lancet Oncol. 2021;22(7):e327–e40.
9. Walter LC, Schonberg MA. Screening mammography in older women: a review. JAMA. 2014;311(13):1336–47.
10. Freedman RA, Minami CA, Winer EP, Morrow M, Smith AK, Walter LC, et al. Individualizing surveillance mammography for older patients after treatment for early-stage breast cancer: multidisciplinary expert panel and international society of geriatric oncology consensus statement. JAMA Oncol. 2021;7(4):609–15.
11. Yourman LC, Lee SJ, Schonberg MA, Widera EW, Smith AK. Prognostic indices for older adults: a systematic review. JAMA. 2012;307(2):182–92.
12. Bilimoria KY, Liu Y, Paruch JL, Zhou L, Kmiecik TE, Ko CY, et al. Development and evaluation of the universal ACS NSQIP surgical risk calculator: a decision aid and informed consent tool for patients and surgeons. J Am Coll Surg. 2013;217(5):833–42 e1-3.
13. Magnuson A, Sedrak MS, Gross CP, Tew WP, Klepin HD, Wildes TM, et al. Development and validation of a risk tool for predicting severe toxicity in older adults receiving chemotherapy for early-stage breast cancer. J Clin Oncol. 2021;39(6):608–18.
14. de Glas NA, van de Water W, Engelhardt EG, Bastiaannet E, de Craen AJM, Kroep JR, et al. Validity of Adjuvant! Online program in older patients with breast cancer: a population-based study. Lancet Oncol. 2014;15(7):722–9.
15. National Health Service UK. PREDICT tool version 2.0: breast cancer overall survival.
16. Wishart GC, Azzato EM, Greenberg DC, Rashbass J, Kearins O, Lawrence G, et al. PREDICT: a new UK prognostic model that predicts survival following surgery for invasive breast cancer. Breast Cancer Res. 2010;12(1):R1.
17. de Glas NA, Bastiaannet E, Engels CC, de Craen AJM, Putter H, van de Velde CJH, et al. Validity of the online PREDICT tool in older patients with breast cancer: a population-based study. Br J Cancer. 2016;114(4):395–400.
18. Wyld L, Reed MWR, Collins K, Burton M, Lifford K, Edwards A, et al. Bridging the age gap in breast cancer: cluster randomized trial of two decision support interventions for older women with operable breast cancer on quality of life, survival, decision quality, and treatment choices. Br J Surg. 2021;108(5):499–510.
19. van der Plas-Krijgsman W, Giardiello D, Putter H, Steyerberg EW, Bastiaannet E, Stiggelbout AM, et al. Abstract PS6-08: the PORTRET-tool: a prediction tool for older patients with breast cancer that predicts recurrence, survival and other-cause mortality. Cancer Res. 2021;81(4 Suppl):PS6–08.
20. Morgan JL, Shrestha A, Reed MWR, Herbert E, Bradburn M, Walters SJ, et al. Bridging the age gap in breast cancer: impact of omission of breast cancer surgery in older women with oestrogen receptor-positive early breast cancer on quality-of-life outcomes. Br J Surg. 2021;108(3):315–25.

21. Audisio RA. The surgical risk of elderly patients with cancer. Surg Oncol. 2004;13(4):169–73.
22. Smith BD, Bellon JR, Blitzblau R, Freedman G, Haffty B, Hahn C, et al. Radiation therapy for the whole breast: Executive summary of an American Society for Radiation Oncology (ASTRO) evidence-based guideline. Pract Radiat Oncol. 2018;8(3):145–52.
23. Kunkler IH, Williams LJ, Jack WJ, Cameron DA, Dixon JM, investigators PI. Breast-conserving surgery with or without irradiation in women aged 65 years or older with early breast cancer (PRIME II): a randomised controlled trial. Lancet Oncol. 2015;16(3):266–73.
24. Brunt AM, Haviland JS, Sydenham M, Agrawal RK, Algurafi H, Alhasso A, et al. Ten-year results of FAST: a randomized controlled trial of 5-fraction whole-breast radiotherapy for early breast cancer. J Clin Oncol. 2020;38(28):3261–72.
25. Donker M, van Tienhoven G, Straver ME, Meijnen P, van de Velde CJ, Mansel RE, et al. Radiotherapy or surgery of the axilla after a positive sentinel node in breast cancer (EORTC 10981-22023 AMAROS): a randomised, multicentre, open-label, phase 3 non-inferiority trial. Lancet Oncol. 2014;15(12):1303–10.
26. Arriagada R, Mouriesse H, Sarrazin D, Clark RM, Deboer G. Radiotherapy alone in breast cancer. I. Analysis of tumor parameters, tumor dose and local control: the experience of the Gustave-Roussy Institute and the Princess Margaret Hospital. Int J Radiat Oncol Biol Phys. 1985;11(10):1751–7.
27. Hind D, Wyld L, Beverley CB, Reed MW. Surgery versus primary endocrine therapy for operable primary breast cancer in elderly women (70 years plus). Cochrane Database Syst Rev. 2006;1:CD004272.
28. Balakrishnan A, Ravichandran D. Early operable breast cancer in elderly women treated with an aromatase inhibitor letrozole as sole therapy. Br J Cancer. 2011;105(12):1825–9.
29. Wink CJ, Woensdregt K, Nieuwenhuijzen GA, van der Sangen MJ, Hutschemaekers S, Roukema JA, et al. Hormone treatment without surgery for patients aged 75 years or older with operable breast cancer. Ann Surg Oncol. 2012;19(4):1185–91.
30. Elkin EB, Hurria A, Mitra N, Schrag D, Panageas KS. Adjuvant chemotherapy and survival in older women with hormone receptor–negative breast cancer: assessing outcome in a population-based, observational cohort. J Clin Oncol. 2006;24(18):2757–64.
31. Ring A, Battisti NML, Reed MWR, Herbert E, Morgan JL, Bradburn M, et al. Bridging The Age Gap: observational cohort study of effects of chemotherapy and trastuzumab on recurrence, survival and quality of life in older women with early breast cancer. Br J Cancer. 2021;125(2):209–19.
32. Giordano SH, Duan Z, Kuo Y-F, Hortobagyi GN, Goodwin JS. Use and outcomes of adjuvant chemotherapy in older women with breast cancer. J Clin Oncol. 2006;24(18):2750–6.
33. Tamirisa N, Lin H, Shen Y, Shaitelman SF, Sri Karuturi M, Giordano SH, et al. Association of chemotherapy with survival in elderly patients with multiple comorbidities and estrogen receptor-positive, node-positive breast cancer. JAMA Oncol. 2020;6(10):1548–54.
34. Battisti NML, McCartney A, Biganzoli L. The conundrum of the association of chemotherapy with survival outcomes among elderly patients with curable luminal breast cancer. JAMA Oncol. 2020;6(10):1535–7.
35. Kizy S, Altman AM, Marmor S, Denbo JW, Jensen EH, Tuttle TM, et al. 21-gene recurrence score testing in the older population with estrogen receptor-positive breast cancer. J Geriatr Oncol. 2019;10(2):322–9.
36. Cardoso F, van't Veer LJ, Bogaerts J, Slaets L, Viale G, Delaloge S, et al. 70-gene signature as an aid to treatment decisions in early-stage breast cancer. N Engl J Med. 2016;375(8):717–29.
37. Brain E, Girre V, Rollot F, Bonnetain F, Debled M, Lacroix M, et al. ASTER 70s: benefit of adjuvant chemotherapy for estrogen receptor-positive HER2-negative breast cancer in women over 70 according to genomic grade—A French GERICO/UCBG UNICANCER multicenter phase III trial. J Clin Oncol. 2012;30(15_suppl):TPS667-TPS.
38. Burstein HJ, Curigliano G, Loibl S, Dubsky P, Gnant M, Poortmans P, et al. Estimating the benefits of therapy for early-stage breast cancer: the St. Gallen International Consensus Guidelines for the primary therapy of early breast cancer 2019. Ann Oncol. 2019;30(10):1541–57.

39. Lee SY, Seo JH. Current strategies of endocrine therapy in elderly patients with breast cancer. Biomed Res Int. 2018;2018:6074808.
40. Goldvaser H, Barnes TA, Seruga B, Cescon DW, Ocana A, Ribnikar D, et al. Toxicity of extended adjuvant therapy with aromatase inhibitors in early breast cancer: a systematic review and meta-analysis. J Natl Cancer Inst. 2018;110(1)
41. Meng-Ting P, Shin-Cheh C, When-Chi S, Yubg-Chang L, Hsien-Kun C. The adherence and tolerance of adjuvant endocrine therapy in geriatric breast cancer patients. J Cancer Res Pract. 2016;3(3)
42. Hadji P, Coleman RE, Wilson C, Powles TJ, Clezardin P, Aapro M, et al. Adjuvant bisphosphonates in early breast cancer: consensus guidance for clinical practice from a European Panel. Ann Oncol. 2016;27(3):379–90.
43. Howlader N, Altekruse SF, Li CI, Chen VW, Clarke CA, Ries LA, et al. US incidence of breast cancer subtypes defined by joint hormone receptor and HER2 status. J Natl Cancer Inst. 2014;106(5)
44. Freedman RA, Seisler DK, Foster JC, Sloan JA, Lafky JM, Kimmick GG, et al. Risk of acute myeloid leukemia and myelodysplastic syndrome among older women receiving anthracycline-based adjuvant chemotherapy for breast cancer on Modern Cooperative Group Trials (Alliance A151511). Breast Cancer Res Treat. 2017;161(2):363–73.
45. Muss HB, Berry DA, Cirrincione C, Budman DR, Henderson IC, Citron ML, et al. Toxicity of older and younger patients treated with adjuvant chemotherapy for node-positive breast cancer: the Cancer and Leukemia Group B Experience. J Clin Oncol. 2007;25(24):3699–704.
46. Jones S, Holmes FA, O'Shaughnessy J, Blum JL, Vukelja SJ, McIntyre KJ, et al. Docetaxel with cyclophosphamide is associated with an overall survival benefit compared with doxorubicin and cyclophosphamide: 7-year follow-up of us oncology research trial 9735. J Clin Oncol. 2009;27(8):1177–83.
47. Brouwers B, Hatse S, Dal Lago L, Neven P, Vuylsteke P, Dalmasso B, et al. The impact of adjuvant chemotherapy in older breast cancer patients on clinical and biological aging parameters. Oncotarget. 2016;7(21):29977–88.
48. Battisti NML, Reed MWR, Herbert E, Morgan JL, Collins KA, Ward SE, et al. Bridging the age gap in breast cancer: impact of chemotherapy on quality of life in older women with early breast cancer. Eur J Cancer. 2021;144:269–80.
49. Brain E, Caillet P, de Glas N, Biganzoli L, Cheng K, Lago LD, et al. HER2-targeted treatment for older patients with breast cancer: an expert position paper from the International Society of Geriatric Oncology. J Geriatr Oncol. 2019;10(6):1003–13.
50. Tolaney SM, Barry WT, Dang CT, Yardley DA, Moy B, Marcom PK, et al. Adjuvant paclitaxel and trastuzumab for node-negative, HER2-positive breast cancer. N Engl J Med. 2015;372(2):134–41.
51. Joensuu H, Bono P, Kataja V, Alanko T, Kokko R, Asola R, et al. Fluorouracil, epirubicin, and cyclophosphamide with either docetaxel or vinorelbine, with or without trastuzumab, as adjuvant treatments of breast cancer: final results of the FinHer Trial. J Clin Oncol. 2009;27(34):5685–92.
52. Earl HM, Hiller L, Vallier AL, Loi S, McAdam K, Hughes-Davies L, et al. 6 versus 12 months of adjuvant trastuzumab for HER2-positive early breast cancer (PERSEPHONE): 4-year disease-free survival results of a randomised phase 3 non-inferiority trial. Lancet. 2019;393(10191):2599–612.
53. Sawaki M, Saito T, Baba S, Kobayashi K, Kawashima H, Tsuneizumi M, et al. Evaluation of trastuzumab without chemotherapy as a postoperative adjuvant therapy in HER2-positive elderly breast cancer patients: Randomized controlled trial (RESPECT). J Clin Oncol. 2018;36(15_suppl):510.
54. Taira N, Sawaki M, Uemura Y, Saito T, Baba S, Kobayashi K, et al. Health-related quality of life with trastuzumab monotherapy versus trastuzumab plus standard chemotherapy as adjuvant therapy in older patients with HER2-positive breast cancer. J Clin Oncol. 2021;39(22):2452–62.

55. Hurria A, Togawa K, Mohile SG, Owusu C, Klepin HD, Gross CP, et al. Predicting chemotherapy toxicity in older adults with cancer: a prospective multicenter study. J Clin Oncol. 2011;29(25):3457–65.
56. Extermann M, Boler I, Reich RR, Lyman GH, Brown RH, DeFelice J, et al. Predicting the risk of chemotherapy toxicity in older patients: the Chemotherapy Risk Assessment Scale for High-Age Patients (CRASH) score. Cancer. 2012;118(13):3377–86.
57. Aapro M, Monfardini S, Jirillo A, Basso U. Management of primary and advanced breast cancer in older unfit patients (medical treatment). Cancer Treat Rev. 2009;35(6):503–8.
58. Leo S, Arnoldi E, Repetto L, Coccorullo Z, Cinieri S, Fedele P, et al. Eribulin mesylate as third or subsequent line chemotherapy for elderly patients with locally recurrent or metastatic breast cancer: a multicentric observational study of GIOGer (Italian Group of Geriatric Oncology)-ERIBE. Oncologist. 2019;24(6):e232–e40.
59. Biganzoli L, Cinieri S, Berardi R, Pedersini R, McCartney A, Minisini AM, et al. EFFECT: a randomized phase II study of efficacy and impact on function of two doses of nab-paclitaxel as first-line treatment in older women with advanced breast cancer. Breast Cancer Res. 2020;22(1):83.
60. Battisti NML, De Glas N, Sedrak MS, Loh KP, Liposits G, Soto-Perez-de-Celis E, et al. Use of cyclin-dependent kinase 4/6 (CDK4/6) inhibitors in older patients with ER-positive HER2-negative breast cancer: Young International Society of Geriatric Oncology review paper. Ther Adv Med Oncol. 2018;10:1758835918809610.
61. Howie LJ, Singh H, Bloomquist E, Wedam S, Amiri-Kordestani L, Tang S, et al. Outcomes of older women with hormone receptor-positive, human epidermal growth factor receptor-negative metastatic breast cancer treated with a CDK4/6 inhibitor and an aromatase inhibitor: an FDA pooled analysis. J Clin Oncol. 2019;37(36):3475–83.
62. Rugo HS, Turner NC, Finn RS, Joy AA, Verma S, Harbeck N, et al. Palbociclib plus endocrine therapy in older women with HR+/HER2- advanced breast cancer: a pooled analysis of randomised PALOMA clinical studies. Eur J Cancer. 2018;101:123–33.
63. Pritchard KI, Burris HA 3rd, Ito Y, Rugo HS, Dakhil S, Hortobagyi GN, et al. Safety and efficacy of everolimus with exemestane vs. exemestane alone in elderly patients with HER2-negative, hormone receptor-positive breast cancer in BOLERO-2. Clin Breast Cancer. 2013;13(6):421–32.e8.
64. Freedman RA, Tolaney SM. Efficacy and safety in older patient subsets in studies of endocrine monotherapy versus combination therapy in patients with HR+/HER2− advanced breast cancer: a review. Breast Cancer Res Treat. 2018;167(3):607–14.
65. Miles D, Baselga J, Amadori D, Sunpaweravong P, Semiglazov V, Knott A, et al. Treatment of older patients with HER2-positive metastatic breast cancer with pertuzumab, trastuzumab, and docetaxel: subgroup analyses from a randomized, double-blind, placebo-controlled phase III trial (CLEOPATRA). Breast Cancer Res Treat. 2013;142(1):89–99.
66. Swain SM, Miles D, Kim S-B, Im Y-H, Im S-A, Semiglazov V, et al. Pertuzumab, trastuzumab, and docetaxel for HER2-positive metastatic breast cancer (CLEOPATRA): end-of-study results from a double-blind, randomised, placebo-controlled, phase 3 study. Lancet Oncol. 2020;21(4):519–30.
67. Wildiers H, Tryfonidis K, Dal Lago L, Vuylsteke P, Curigliano G, Waters S, et al. Pertuzumab and trastuzumab with or without metronomic chemotherapy for older patients with HER2-positive metastatic breast cancer (EORTC 75111-10114): an open-label, randomised, phase 2 trial from the Elderly Task Force/Breast Cancer Group. Lancet Oncol. 2018;19(3):323–36.
68. Vogel CL, Cobleigh MA, Tripathy D, Gutheil JC, Harris LN, Fehrenbacher L, et al. Efficacy and safety of trastuzumab as a single agent in first-line treatment of HER2-overexpressing metastatic breast cancer. J Clin Oncol. 2002;20(3):719–26.
69. Gelmon KA, Boyle FM, Kaufman B, Huntsman DG, Manikhas A, Di Leo A, et al. Lapatinib or trastuzumab plus taxane therapy for human epidermal growth factor receptor 2-positive advanced breast cancer: final results of NCIC CTG MA.31. J Clin Oncol. 2015;33(14):1574–83.

70. Verma S, Miles D, Gianni L, Krop IE, Welslau M, Baselga J, et al. Trastuzumab emtansine for HER2-positive advanced breast cancer. N Engl J Med. 2012;367(19):1783–91.
71. Dieras V, Harbeck N, Budd GT, Greenson JK, Guardino AE, Samant M, et al. Trastuzumab emtansine in human epidermal growth factor receptor 2-positive metastatic breast cancer: an integrated safety analysis. J Clin Oncol. 2014;32(25):2750–7.
72. Montemurro F, Ellis P, Anton A, Wuerstlein R, Delaloge S, Bonneterre J, et al. Safety of trastuzumab emtansine (T-DM1) in patients with HER2-positive advanced breast cancer: primary results from the KAMILLA study cohort 1. Eur J Cancer. 2019;109:92–102.
73. Kaufman B, Mackey JR, Clemens MR, Bapsy PP, Vaid A, Wardley A, et al. Trastuzumab plus anastrozole versus anastrozole alone for the treatment of postmenopausal women with human epidermal growth factor receptor 2-positive, hormone receptor-positive metastatic breast cancer: results from the randomized phase III TAnDEM study. J Clin Oncol. 2009;27(33):5529–37.
74. Rimawi M, Ferrero JM, de la Haba-Rodriguez J, Poole C, De Placido S, Osborne CK, et al. First-line trastuzumab plus an aromatase inhibitor, with or without pertuzumab, in human epidermal growth factor receptor 2-positive and hormone receptor-positive metastatic or locally advanced breast cancer (PERTAIN): a randomized, open-label phase II trial. J Clin Oncol. 2018;36(28):2826–35.
75. Schwartzberg LS, Franco SX, Florance A, O'Rourke L, Maltzman J, Johnston S. Lapatinib plus letrozole as first-line therapy for HER-2+ hormone receptor-positive metastatic breast cancer. Oncologist. 2010;15(2):122–9.
76. Johnston SRD, Hegg R, Im S-A, Park IH, Burdaeva O, Kurteva G, et al. Phase III, randomized study of dual human epidermal growth factor receptor 2 (HER2) blockade with lapatinib plus trastuzumab in combination with an aromatase inhibitor in postmenopausal women with HER2-positive, hormone receptor–positive metastatic breast cancer: updated results of alternative. J Clin Oncol. 2020;39(1):79–89.
77. Schmid P, Adams S, Rugo HS, Schneeweiss A, Barrios CH, Iwata H, et al. Atezolizumab and nab-paclitaxel in advanced triple-negative breast cancer. N Engl J Med. 2018;379(22):2108–21.
78. Shachar SS, Jolly TA, Jones E, Muss HB. Management of triple-negative breast cancer in older patients: how is it different? Oncology (Williston Park). 2018;32(2):58–63.
79. National comprehensive cancer network. Accessed September 1st, 2020. https://www.nccn.org/professionals/physician_gls/pdf/senior.pdf2020

Chapter 18
Non-Small Cell Lung Cancer in Older Adults with Frailty

Fabio Gomes, Kathryn Banfill, Andrea Bille, Stephanie Fraser, and Giuseppe Banna

Introduction

Lung cancer is the leading cause of cancer death worldwide, accounting for an estimated 1.8 million deaths in 2018 [1]. Non-small cell lung cancer (NSCLC) is the most frequent lung tumour subtype, accounting for 85% of patients with lung cancer [2]. More than half of all patients with NSCLC are aged 70 years or above, with about 10% aged 80 years or above [2]. Older patients have a higher prevalence of frailty, which has implications regarding decision-making for cancer management [3].

Frailty is a state of diminished physiological reserves that results in increased vulnerability to stressors (e.g., cancer, treatments) and a higher risk of adverse events (e.g., complications, dependency, death) [4]. The prevalence of frailty in patients with NSCLC referred to a specialist cancer centre in the United Kingdom is in the region of 40% [5], suggesting a higher proportion of patients with frailty at presentation. Frailty is associated with comorbidity, impairments in mobility, function, nutrition, mood, cognition and social vulnerability [4]. Ultimately, frailty can

F. Gomes (✉)
Medical Oncology Department, The Christie NHS Foundation Trust, Manchester, UK
e-mail: fabio.gomes2@nhs.net

K. Banfill
Clinical Oncology Department, The Christie NHS Foundation Trust, Manchester, UK
e-mail: kathryn.banfill@nhs.net

A. Bille · S. Fraser
Thoracic Surgery Department, Guy's and St Thomas NHS Foundation Trust, Manchester, UK
e-mail: Andrea.Bille@gstt.nhs.uk; StephanieFlorence.Fraser@gstt.nhs.uk

G. Banna
Medical Oncology Department, Portsmouth Hospitals University NHS Trust, Portsmouth, UK
e-mail: giuseppe.banna@nhs.net

F. Gomes (ed.), *Frailty in Older Adults with Cancer*,
https://doi.org/10.1007/978-3-030-89162-6_18

impact the patient tolerability to anti-cancer treatments, quality of life and survival [5]. Therefore, older patients with lung cancer should be screened for frailty and further geriatric assessments should be incorporated in clinical practice.

A study using the Surveillance, Epidemiology, and End Results (SEER)-Medicare database (2002–2007) found that only 45% of patients aged 65 and above received treatment concordant with guidelines [6]. The likelihood of receiving guideline-concordant care significantly decreased with increasing age, non-white race, higher comorbidity score and lower income. Over the last decade, clinical teams saw a marked increase in the number of treatment options available. In fact, the management of NSCLC, particularly with advanced/metastatic disease, has been revolutionised following the implementation of targeted therapies in patients harbouring oncogene-driven tumours and the introduction of immune-checkpoint inhibitors (ICIs). Yet, older patients continue to be underrepresented in the pivotal clinical trials [7], with patients recruited to the ICIs trials being about 10 years younger than the median age of NSCLC diagnosis in the United Kingdom [8]. These recent and extensive changes in the treatment pathways alongside the more recent combinations of several anti-cancer treatments pose a challenge regarding an increasingly complex patient-treatment selection [9]. Ultimately, with more treatment options available there is an increasing need for an appropriate patient assessment, multidisciplinary working and a shared decision-making with patients and their families, in order to find the right management plan for each individual patient.

This chapter outlines the management of an older patient with frailty through the different stages of NSCLC and summarises the available evidence to guide decision-making in this patient group.

Management of Early-Stage and Locally Advanced NSCLC

Surgery

Surgery plays a key role in this setting but whilst older patients should be considered for lung resection, those with or at high risk of frailty require careful assessments to determine their eligibility as this may not be an appropriate option for a considerable proportion of these patients.

Surgery can be safely performed in octogenarians without a significant increase in morbidity and, when compared to younger patients, post-operative quality of life can be maintained [10]. Therefore, chronological age is not a contra-indication for thoracic surgery, but teams need to assess the patient eligible for surgery and frailty plays a significant role. Frailty is associated with poor recovery from the stressors of surgery, particularly due to factors such as impaired cardiac physiology [11], impaired renal function [12], cognitive impairment [13], comorbidity burden and polypharmacy. From a respiratory perspective, alongside reduced reserve and respiratory drive, reduced skeletal muscle density is associated with poor cough, retained secretions and adverse post-operative outcomes [14]. Consequently, patients with frailty have more morbidity and mortality with surgery [15].

The pre-operative assessment of these patients is paramount, not just to determine patient eligibility for surgery but also to determine the appropriate support needed throughout the peri-operative period. Modifiable risk factors should be addressed including management and optimisation of anaemia, diabetic control, electrolyte imbalances, chronic obstructive pulmonary disease and polypharmacy [16]. Assessment of physical fitness using a 6-min walk test or cardiopulmonary exercise testing may also help to identify those patients who are more likely to develop post-operative complications [17].

For those patients eligible for surgery, prehabilitation with a tailored exercise programme focusing on increasing the patient's physical activity, building muscle and training their inspiratory muscles should be considered. Structured exercise programs have been shown to improve cardiovascular and respiratory function and lower post-operative complication [18].

Regarding surgical options, surgeons need to carefully consider all tools and techniques in their surgical armamentarium to offer older patients with frailty the best available treatment. Minimally invasive surgery is associated with lower mortality in older patients and should always be considered [19]. Segmentectomy is associated with comparable early outcomes to lobectomy [20] and on-going work is investigating whether there is an improvement in long-term pulmonary function and quality of life [21]. Mediastinal lymph node dissection in older patients is associated with increased cardiac morbidity and mortality rates [22] and surgeons may choose to avoid extensive lymphadenectomy in selected cases. Lastly, pneumectomy is a very extensive surgery which can significantly reduce the quality of life of these patients and therefore it is rarely considered [23].

Alongside the discussion of operative options, surgeons should initiate conversations regarding advanced care planning to ensure patients' wishes are respected and their dignity maintained. Enhanced recovery plans should be made with early involvement of thoracic anaesthetists to assess potentially difficult airways and consider a multimodal analgesia plan with the aim of reducing the total opiate consumption [24]. In the post-operative period, medical and outreach teams should be utilised alongside good nurse training to try and improve the rates of 'rescue' from complications, by early detection and management [25].

In conclusion, anatomical lung resections should be considered in selected older patients with frailty, but involvement of the whole thoracic multidisciplinary team is essential to support the shared decision-making and provide the necessary peri-operative care and prehabilitation. Although surgical options may not appropriate for a large proportion of these older patients with frailty, surgery is more likely appropriate in the setting of early-stage NSCLC, compared to locally advanced NSCLC where these patients unlikely to tolerate a multimodality strategy.

Post-operative (Adjuvant) Systemic Treatment

Adjuvant chemotherapy with a cisplatin-based doublet following surgery for NSCLC confers a 5-year survival benefit of 5.4% with the clearer benefit seen in patients with stage 2 and 3 [26]. The median age of all patients included in this meta-analysis was 60 years and the benefit for older patients was less clear. Moreover, in the small group of patients with performance status 2 for whom outcome data was available, sub-group analysis showed no benefit of adjuvant chemotherapy on either overall or disease-free survival. Of note, the incidence of grade 3–4 toxicity was 66% across the whole population. Another pooled analysis using data from the clinical trials that formed the basis of the previous analysis focused on the effect of age [27]. Median age was still 60 years with 29% of patients aged 65 or above and only 9% aged 70 or above. The overall survival benefit in the small group aged 70+ was not confirmed (HR 0.90; 95% CI 0.70–1.16). However, significantly more patients in this older group died from non-lung cancer-related causes. The incidence of severe toxicity was similar regardless of age, but the group aged 70+ received lower chemotherapy doses and completed less cycles.

A more recent study focused on a real-world population and it also investigated the effect of age in the efficacy of adjuvant chemotherapy [28]. From a sample of about 7500 patients, 38% were aged 70+ or older. The proportion of older patients receiving adjuvant chemotherapy was half compared to younger patients (15.3% vs 31.6%; $p < 0.0001$). Moreover, carboplatin-based doublets were used in 65% of cases, instead of cisplatin-based. Older patients derived a similar magnitude of survival benefit as younger patients (HR 0.81; 95% CI 0.71–0.92 versus HR 0.79; 95% CI 0.72–0.86). Several other studies confirmed a survival benefit from adjuvant chemotherapy of similar magnitude between patients older and younger patients [29, 30].

However, looking beyond age, comorbidity has been shown to impact the outcomes of older patients on adjuvant chemotherapy. One study showed that older patients (65+) have significantly more comorbidities (measured using the Charlson comorbidity index ≥1) than younger patients (42% vs 26%; $P < 0.0001$) and that the presence of a higher comorbidity index (≥1) was associated with worse survival [31]. Another study focused on the risk factor for early mortality (within 6 months) in patients undergoing adjuvant chemotherapy. Patients aged 70+, those with higher comorbidity scores (measured using Charlson comorbidity index ≥2) and those with a prolonged length of post-operative stay (over 6 days), were all associated with a higher earlier mortality risk [32].

Ultimately, older cancer patients are underrepresented in most adjuvant trials and there is a clear lack of data regarding those with frailty. If an older patient with frailty underwent surgery, that already indicates this is a pre-selected patient with likely mild frailty. Nonetheless, that does not mean the patient is eligible for chemotherapy. There is a reasonable concern regarding the tolerability and the survival benefit for these patients, who often may already have had a longer post-operative recovery period. Therefore, whilst adjuvant chemotherapy may be considered in selected older patients with frailty, this may not be an appropriate option for the majority, even considering the use of carboplatin-based regimens instead of cisplatin-based regimens.

Looking beyond chemotherapy, the recently published ADAURA trial investigated the use of a targeted treatment Osimertinib, which targets the epidermal growth factor receptor (EGFR) in those tumours with sensitising EGFR mutations

[33]. Whilst the overall survival data is still awaited, the impressive improvement in disease-free survival makes this a very promising option. At 24 months, 89% of patients in the Osimertinib group versus 52% of patients in the placebo group were alive and disease-free. Targeted treatments have a better toxicity profile, as described in a subsequent section, and although there is a lack of data regarding older patients with frailty in this adjuvant setting, this is a potential good option for this sub-group of patients with EGFR mutations.

Stereotactic Ablative Body Radiotherapy (SABR)

In early-stage NSCLC, stereotactic ablative body radiotherapy (SABR) is an effective treatment in which an ablative dose of radiotherapy is delivered to a tumour over a small number of fractions. This is suitable for tumours ≤5 cm with no nodal involvement that do not about the trachea, lobar bronchi, heart or great vessels. Patients with tumours close to these central structures receive more fractionated courses of radiotherapy.

Access to SABR has been found to reduce the number of patients over the age of 75 who do not receive any treatment for early-stage lung cancer [34] as it provides a viable alternative for patients who are not suitable for surgery, such as older patients with frailty. Consequently, the patients in trials of SABR are on average above 70 years of age [35]. SABR achieves 3-year local control rates of about 90% with minimal toxicity [36]. Toxicities following SABR vary depending on tumour location and dose delivered; the more common toxicities are dyspnoea, pneumonitis, chest pain and fatigue. The risk of pneumonitis grade 3 or higher is about 3% [35]. The incidence of chest wall pain grade 2 or higher is 6.2% and the incidence of rib fracture is 6.4%, rising to 12.5% in patients aged 75 and over. The risk of both chest wall pain and rib fracture increase with increasing chest wall dose and in cases where the tumour is less than 25 mm from the chest wall [37].

Comparing surgery to SABR in early-stage NSCLC through prospective clinical trials has proven difficult. Recruitment is challenging as both the multidisciplinary teams and the patients may have a treatment preference avoiding a randomisation in this setting [38]. Therefore, most of the data comparing surgery and SABR comes from retrospective databases. But these real-world data is often biased as SABR is most often reserved to older patients and those not eligible for surgery. One of the largest studies with 76,623 patients from the American National Cancer Database found that SABR was associated with significantly better 30- and 90-day mortality rates compared to surgery, especially in patients over the age of 70 [39]. Although SABR has a lower immediate post-procedure mortality than surgery, the longer-term survival of patients who have SABR is lower than those who have surgery. There is however no difference in lung cancer specific survival in patients over the age of 75 who have SABR compared to surgery [40]. This can be justified by the previously mentioned pre-selection bias, as in fact patients offered SABR have high rates of non-cancer related death [41]. A study incorporated a modified frailty index assessment in a cohort of older patients (median age 74 years) undergoing SABR to investigate its correlation with overall survival and non-cancer related death. Patients with frailty had a lower overall survival at 3 years (37.3% vs 74.7%, $p = 0.003$), yet they were also more likely to die of causes unrelated to the lung cancer [42].

Therefore, SABR is an appropriate and the preferred treatment option for the majority of older patients with frailty, particularly those with a significant risk of post-operative morbidity and mortality.

Multimodality Treatments

In locally advanced NSCLC there are several possible treatment options, such as surgery, chemotherapy and radiotherapy, which may be used in different combinations. Selecting the right treatment strategy can be challenging and there is limited evidence from trials regarding multimodality treatments in older patients with frailty, as these patients are often excluded from trials in this setting due to overall poor fitness and pre-existing conditions [43, 44].

Regarding the role of surgery in locally advanced disease, an upfront decision must be done if the locally advanced tumour is resectable and if the patient is a surgical candidate. A meta-analysis investigated the role of surgery or radiotherapy following induction chemotherapy or chemo-radiotherapy [45]. The hazard ratio of death in patients randomised to surgery after chemotherapy was 1.01 (95% CI 0.82 to 1.23; $p = 0.954$) whereas for patients randomised to surgery after chemo-radiotherapy was 0.87 (0.75 to 1.01; $p = 0.068$). Moreover, other trials comparing chemo-radiotherapy followed by surgery with chemo-radiotherapy alone have not demonstrated a superiority with the trimodality treatment [46, 47]. Therefore, all these options can in principle be considered in case of upfront resectable disease.

However, when considering older patients with frailty, this trimodality strategy is not appropriate due to the high toxicity burden. These patients should instead be considered for either upfront surgery (if resectable and patient eligible) or a bimodality strategy with chemotherapy and radiotherapy. Alternatively, depending on the severity of frailty and comorbidity burden, treatment with definitive radiotherapy alone may be the only appropriate curative-intent option.

A bimodality strategy combining chemotherapy and radiotherapy can see these treatments delivered either concurrently or sequentially. A Cochrane meta-analysis found that adding chemotherapy before radiotherapy improved the 2-year overall survival by 8% compared to radiotherapy alone. And that the use of chemo-radiotherapy concurrently improved the 2-year overall survival by 13% yet causing more grade 3 oesophagitis [48]. Hence that for unresectable or medically inoperable locally advanced NSCLC, concurrent chemo-radiotherapy is considered a standard treatment. Despite these results, concurrent chemo-radiotherapy is still only used in a minority of patients with locally advanced disease [49]. Moreover, this evidence is based on relatively fit and younger patients.

A real-world retrospective study reviewed the use of concurrent chemo-radiotherapy, sequential chemo-radiotherapy and radiotherapy alone in older patients (70+) with locally advanced NSCLC [50]. In this study, patients received concurrent treatment in 33% of cases, sequential treatment in 24% of cases, definitive radiotherapy alone in 16% and no curative treatment in 27% of cases. Comorbidity and performance status were the most common reasons to omit concurrent treatment. For those treated with a curative intent, there were no significant survival differences between the three modalities. Even though only the fittest older patients were offered concurrent chemo-radiotherapy, their tolerability was worse compared with the other options, especially for those with severe comorbidity.

Another large comparative effectiveness study investigated chemo-radiotherapy (sequential or concurrent) versus definitive radiotherapy alone in older patients (70+) [51]. Whilst chemo-radiotherapy resulted in a survival advantage compared with definitive radiotherapy alone. Sequential chemo-radiotherapy was superior to concurrent in older patients.

Several other retrospective subset analyses of patients ≥70 years from trials involving chemo-radiotherapy have conflicting results. An analysis combining all patients ≥70 years from six RTOG trials found that the addition of chemotherapy to radiotherapy did not improve survival outcomes and resulted in increased toxicity [52]. Other sub-group analyses of older patients in trials of concurrent chemo-radiotherapy have shown equivalent survival to younger patients. However, older patients had increased rates of grade 3+ toxicity (pneumonitis, haematological toxicity or oesophagitis) and were less likely to complete the full course of treatment [53]. A phase 2 trial evaluated the ability of a CGA to select older patients who may potentially benefit from concurrent chemo-radiotherapy [54]. Although this was a small study with no control arm, this proved to be a good method to better select eligible older patients. Another study, the ELDAPT trial (Elderly With Locally Advanced Lung Cancer: Deciding Through Geriatric Assessment on the Optimal Treatment Strategy) is a phase 3 randomised trial currently on-going (NCT02284308) which is investigating a screening tool to identify which patients aged 75+ with stage 3 NSCLC are eligible for chemo-radiotherapy, and then randomised them to either concurrent or sequential chemo-radiotherapy. The primary endpoint is quality of life and secondary endpoints include toxicity, survival and the degree of independence following treatment [55]. This will provide important information to guide decision-making in this setting for this complex patient group.

A more recent breakthrough in the field of locally advanced NSCLC resulted from the PACIFIC trial which changed clinical practice, further promoting the use of concurrent chemo-radiotherapy. This study defined the gold standard treatment for unresectable locally advanced NSCLC of concurrent chemo-radiotherapy followed by 1 year of adjuvant treatment with the checkpoint inhibitor durvalumab. However, there was not a standard definition of resectable disease. In this trial the 24 months overall survival rate was 66.3% in those who received durvalumab compared to 55.6% for those who did not. Progression free survival also improved with durvalumab (17.2 months v 5.6 months) [56]. In pre-planned sub-group analyses, the progression free survival benefit of adjuvant durvalumab for patients aged 65 and over was less than in younger patients (HR 0.74; 95%CI 0.54-1.01 versus HR 0.43; 95% CI 0.32-0.057) [56]. Moreover, this is a highly selected trial population and there is no evidence for patients with frailty.

Ultimately, whilst concurrent chemo-radiotherapy may be considered in selected older patients with frailty, this is not appropriate for the majority of these patients, depending on the severity of frailty and comorbidities. Therefore, a sequential strategy of chemo-radiotherapy, or even the use of definitive radiotherapy alone, should be considered as more appropriate alternatives.

Management of Advanced/Metastatic NSCLC

Radiotherapy

Radiotherapy has an important role in the palliation of symptoms in the setting of advanced/metastatic disease, and for some older patients with severe frailty, this may be the only treatment appropriate even in a non-metastatic setting.

Chest radiotherapy is effective for palliation of cough, haemoptysis, chest pain and dyspnoea. A number of trials have compared different radiotherapy dose/fractionations and have shown that for patients with poor performance status a 10 Gy single fraction is effective at improving symptoms [57]. Patients with good performance status benefit from longer dose fractionations of 30–39 Gy in 10–13 fractions [58]. Moreover, in the emergency setting, radiotherapy can be used to treat malignant spinal cord compression and superior vena cava obstruction (SVCO). A trial of patients with cord compression from any primary tumour, in which 19% of patients had lung cancer, found that 69.3% were ambulatory 8 weeks after treatment with a single 8 Gy fraction [59]. Radiotherapy can improve symptoms of SVCO in 64% of patients with the best symptom response after 3 weeks. However, this is longer than the relief of symptoms within 48 h with a SVC stent [60].

Chemotherapy

Chemotherapy was the only standard systemic anti-cancer treatment available for patients with advanced NSCLC until the more recent introduction of targeted treatments soon followed by immunotherapy with checkpoint inhibitors. The eligibility assessment for chemotherapy and the choice of the most appropriate regimen for older patients with frailty can be challenging. Age alone should not dictate this decision-making. The assessment of frailty, comorbidity and the risk of chemotherapy toxicity [61], ideally within the context of a Comprehensive Geriatric Assessment (CGA), should instead support this decision-making process [62, 63].

The phase 3 randomised ESOGIA-GFPC-GECP 08-02 study [64] focused on older patients (aged 70+) investigated the integration of CGA for the selection of first line chemotherapy compared to a selection on the basis of age and performance status. Whilst the study was negative for its primary endpoint of treatment failure free survival, patients in the CGA arm experienced slightly less any grade toxicity (85.6% v 93.4%; $p = 0.015$) and fewer treatment failures because of toxicity (4.8% v 11.8%; $p = 0.007$).

Whilst there have been several chemotherapy clinical trials specifically designed for older patients, a significant amount of data derives from sub-group analysis from other large trials, such as SWOG 9509 [65], ECOG 5592 [66], ECOG 1594 [67], CALGB 9730 [68] and ECOG 4599 [69]. These trials did not observe clear differences in the chemotherapy efficacy between younger and older patients with advanced NSCLC. However, older patients were underrepresented. Moreover, beyond treatment efficacy, their tolerability is a key consideration in older patients.

In this setting, there are several key clinical trials focusing on the older population. The ELVIS trial [70] was a phase 3 randomised trial which confirmed the superiority, in terms of survival and quality of life, of single-agent intravenous vinorelbine over best supportive care in patients aged over 70 years. The MILES trial [71] was another randomised phase 3 trial in the same older population and it confirmed that the combination of vinorelbine plus gemcitabine was not more effective than single-agent vinorelbine or gemcitabine. This resulted in the wider use of single-agent chemotherapy as the standard of care for older patients, particularly those less fit. In this context, other studies concluded that metronomic oral vinorelbine was also a safe and active option [72–74]. Moreover, this option prolonged the median progression free survival without grade 4 toxicity compared to the weekly oral schedule [75]. However, subsequent further attempts at using combination chemotherapy in this population led to the phase 3 randomised trial ICFT-0501 [76] which demonstrated a longer survival with platinum-based doublets versus single-agent vinorelbine or gemcitabine (HR 0.64, 95%CI 0.52–0.78; $p < 0.0001$), despite more toxicity, in an older population aged 70–89 years with performance status 0–2. Furthermore, the ABOUND.70+ phase 4 trial [77] assessed the safety and efficacy of nab-paclitaxel and carboplatin given continuously or with a 1-week break in between cycles in older patients aged 70+. The regimen with 1-week break resulted in improved progression free survival and objective response rate but no significant changes in overall survival or toxicity profile. Lastly, the MILES-3 and MILES-4 trials were jointly analysed [78] to explore the role of a cisplatin-based versus single-agent gemcitabine or pemetrexed in older patients aged 70 or older with performance status 0–1. Whilst the addition of cisplatin improved progression free survival and objective response rate, there was no improvement in overall survival, and cisplatin resulted in significantly more toxicity.

Ultimately, whilst non-platinum single-agent chemotherapy is the most appropriate option for the majority of older patients with frailty, the use of carboplatin doublets should be considered in selected patients, depending on the severity of frailty and comorbidity burden.

Targeted Treatments

Genetic alterations such as epidermal growth factor receptor (*EGFR*) mutations and anaplastic lymphoma kinase (*ALK*) represent the two most common oncogene-driven subtypes with available targeted treatments and will be covered in this section. However, several other targetable yet less common genomic abnormalities have been identified, such as ROS1, BRAF, MET, RET, NTRK. All these genomic abnormalities are usually mutually exclusive.

EGFR mutations are found in about 12% of western patients with an adenocarcinoma NSCLC [79]. The first generation of EGFR-tyrosine kinase inhibitors (TKIs) gefitinib and erlotinib, the second generation afatinib and dacomitinib and the third generation osimertinib are currently approved for the treatment of EGFR-mutant advanced NSCLC. Several phase 3 clinical trials comparing platinum-based chemotherapy with the different EGFR-TKIs confirmed the superiority of the latter in terms of efficacy, safety and quality of life for those with sensitising EGFR mutations [80]. Overall, these pivotal trials did not find inferior survival outcomes for older patients. However, these trials enrolled primarily younger patients with only a minority aged 65 years and above [81–91]. Moreover, these studies did not report on tolerability between age groups.

There are however several studies reporting on older and more vulnerable patients. Gefitinib has shown a strong antitumour activity and an acceptable toxicity profile in older patients with a poor performance status of 2–4, resulting in improvements not just in survival but also in the baseline performance status in 80% of these patients [92, 93]. Erlotinib was assessed in a large phase 4 study, which confirmed that its efficacy and tolerability in older patients was similar to their younger counterparts [94]. Another real-world study focused on older patients enrolled 25% of patients with a performance status of 2 and above, reporting a comparable efficacy and safety profile to previous studies [95]. Moreover, patients unsuitable for chemotherapy, often because of poor performance status or comorbidity burden, have also tolerated treatment with erlotinib [96]. Nonetheless, older patients may require more dose reductions [97]. Whilst there are no comparative toxicity analyses showing a clear higher incidence of TKI-related toxicity in older patients, the potential occurrence of more acute toxicity in the older population can be explained by differences in pharmacokinetics due to, for example, changes in body composition, with the mean concentration of erlotinib reported being 1.5-fold higher in patients aged $\geq$75 and even 2.0-fold higher in those aged $\geq$80 [98]. Afatinib is overall associated with more toxicity than the other EGFR-TKIs but the toxicity profile is similar between older and younger patients, alongside its efficacy profile [99]. Osimertinib was initially approved in subsequent lines after prior EGFR-TKIs but it also proved its superiority in the first line treatment, and apart from an improvement in progression free survival and overall survival, its toxicity profile is also overall better than the other TKIs [89, 100].

Overall, whilst the incidence of toxicity with EGFR-TKIs may not increase in older patients with frailty, their tolerability is more limited and therefore, whilst these TKIS are mostly well tolerated, at times dose reductions are necessary. Lastly, their efficacy is overall maintained in older patients and a meta-analysis confirmed these agents improved progression free survival (HR 0.44, 95% CI 0.28–0.69; $p = 0.0004$) in EGFR-mutated NSCLC patients, with a benefit even more pronounced in older patients (HR 0.39; $p = 0.008$) compared to their younger counterparts (HR 0.48; $P = 0.04$) [101].

ALK translocations are found in up to 5% of western patients with an adenocarcinoma NSCLC [102]. Whilst crizotinib was the first ALK-TKI available, multiple other agents have become available since, such as ceritinib, alectinib, brigatinib and lorlatinib [103–107]. Similar evidence to that described for EGFR-mutants also comes from patients harbouring ALK translocations, with the relevant difference being that these patients are generally younger than the EGFR-mutant population. But the available evidence shows that older patients have similar progression free survival compared to younger patients, with some data suggesting a possibly even better outcome in older patients with crizotinib or alectinib [103, 108]. Similar to the data from EGFR-TKIs, these treatments are beneficial also in patients with poor performance status [103]. However, one analysis on the toxicity profile of crizotinib in older patients [109] suggested that the rate of grade 3–4 events could be higher in older patients (15% vs. 7%), albeit this was not statistically significant. Similarly to the EGFR-TKIs, the latest generation of ALK-TKIs, apart from an improved progression free survival, showed in the overall population a better toxicity profile than crizotinib, with less frequent grade 3–5 adverse events [110, 111].

In summary, these TKIs targeting genomic abnormalities such as EGFR and ALK are appropriate treatments for the majority of older patients with frailty. Therefore, the molecular profiling of this sub-group of patients with advanced/metastatic NSCLC is appropriate and should be part of standard clinical practice, particularly for those with adenocarcinoma subtype.

Immunotherapy

The checkpoint inhibitors currently in clinical practice target the cytotoxic T-lymphocyte-associated antigen 4 (CTLA-4) and the programmed death receptor-1 (PD-1) and its ligand (PD-L1). Similarly to targeted treatments, checkpoint inhibitors have a largely more favourable safety profile compared with chemotherapy [112]. Whilst checkpoint inhibitors are revolutionising the care for many patients with cancer, older patients and particularly those with frailty remain underrepresented in trials [113]. Older adults with NSCLC represent the largest subset of older cancer patients treated with checkpoint inhibitors. Yet, the proportion of older adults in the pivotal phase 3 trials accounts for less than half of enrolled patients, resulting in a selected trial population which is about 10 years younger than the median age of NSCLC diagnosis [8]. Older patients not only have a higher prevalence of frailty and comorbidity, which may impact treatment tolerability, but also the physiological remodelling of the immune-system associated with the ageing process (immunosenescence) [114] may ultimately influence the patient/treatment interaction.

Regarding single-agent checkpoint inhibitors, for untreated advanced/metastatic NSCLC, a phase 3 randomised trial with pembrolizumab confirmed its superiority in terms of overall survival versus platinum-based chemotherapy in high PD-L1 expressers (≥50%) [115, 116]. A pooled analysis of several trials confirmed this survival benefit with pembrolizumab in older adults (HR 0.40, 95% CI 0.25–0.64) [117]. For pre-treated patients, multiple phase 3 trials demonstrated the overall survival benefit of pembrolizumab, nivolumab and atezolizumab versus docetaxel [112, 118–122]. Whilst the sub-group analysis showed a benefit for patients aged 65 years and older, data on patients aged 75 years and older was very limited. Following the success of single-agent checkpoint inhibitors, the next step in the clinical trials was their combination with chemotherapy. Two key phase 3 trials in patients untreated for advanced/metastatic NSCLC demonstrated the overall survival superiority of pembrolizumab in combination with chemotherapy [123, 124]. These trials enrolled a considerable number of adults aged 65 years and older (49–55%), but this sub-group of patients had a smaller magnitude of benefit, particularly in the squamous subtype. Another trial added atezolizumab to chemotherapy and bevacizumab (an anti-angiogenic) also confirming its benefit, which was similar in older and younger patients, however only 10% of patients were aged 75 years and older [125, 126]. More recently, combinations of different checkpoint inhibitors, nivolumab plus ipilimumab, with or without chemotherapy have also been investigated, all confirming improvements in overall survival [127, 128].

While a large meta-analysis of multiple trials with PD-(L)1 inhibitors found comparable efficacy among older and younger patients [129], an important limitation of these pivotal trials is the highly selected population resulting in the exclusion of less fit older adults, such as those with frailty, which represent a significant part of the real-world clinical practice. A large multicentre retrospective study in the United Kingdom with over 2000 patients, of which 20% were aged over 75 years, documented that older patients were less likely to receive combination treatments but had a similar overall survival compared with younger patients [130]. Another study focused on evaluating the impact of performance status (0–1 vs 2) on the checkpoint inhibitors and found that a poor performance status was associated with lower disease control rate, progression free survival and overall survival [131]. However, the single-arm phase 2 PePS2 trial assessed the role of pembrolizumab in patients with performance status 2, suggesting that the efficacy outcomes were similar to those with performance status 0–1 [132].

Regarding toxicity with checkpoint inhibitors, these can cause immune-related adverse events (irAEs) by damaging normal healthy tissues/organs. Virtually any tissue/organ is at risk but the most frequently affected are the endocrine system, skin, colon, liver and lung. Importantly, the incidence of high grade irAEs (grade 3+) is only 14% with PD-(L)1 inhibitors [133], which are the most commonly used for NSCLC. Whilst few studies have focused specifically on older adults, the toxicity profile seems to be similar in incidence and severity to younger adults. The

CheckMate-153 is the largest prospective trial focusing on nivolumab safety within a North America population with a pre-planned analysis for older patients undergoing treatment with nivolumab [134]. Among 1426 patients enrolled, a total of 556 (39%) were aged 70 years and above. This study confirmed the good tolerability of single-agent nivolumab. The CheckMate-171 trial evaluated the safety of nivolumab in a European population of pre-treated patients with squamous NSCLC and reported a similar tolerability for older patients and for those with performance status 2 [135]. In the real-world setting, the previously mentioned large multicentre retrospective study in the United Kingdom with over 2000 patients documented no difference in high grade irAEs (grade 3+) [130]. One study of patients with NSCLC who were treated with PD-(L)1 inhibitors also found no difference in the incidence of irAEs, hospitalisations or steroid use according to age [136]. Reassuringly, another study of older adults with NSCLC receiving checkpoint inhibitors reported that the irAEs incidence did not differ with age, comorbidity or performance status [137]. Moreover, the previously reported study investigating the impact of performance status (0–1 vs 2) in treatment efficacy and safety found no difference in the incidence of irAEs for patients with performance status 2 [131]. However, in the event of irAEs, a meta-analysis did find that older age is a risk factor for fatal toxicities [138]. This may be justified by a higher prevalence of comorbidities and other geriatric syndromes, such as frailty. Lastly, the recently published ELDERS study is one of the first prospective studies designed primarily to investigate the safety of checkpoint inhibitors in older adults [139]. Patients with advanced NSCLC or malignant melanoma starting single-agent treatment were enrolled into two age-based cohorts (≥70 y and <70 y). Half of the older patients were screened positive for frailty based on the Geriatric-8 (G8) screening tool. This superiority study was negative for its primary endpoint with no significant difference in the incidence of grade 3–5 irAEs between older and younger adults (18.6% vs 12.9%; OR 1.55, 95% CI 0.61–3.89; $p = 0.35$). Frailty and geriatric assessments were implemented in the study design. Older adults with a positive G8 screening had a higher risk of hospital admissions ($p = 0.03$) and death ($p = 0.01$), but not a higher incidence or severity of irAEs [139].

But the tolerability of combination regimens in older patients, particularly those with frailty, is uncertain due to lack of data but is reasonable to assume that it is associated with higher risks. In this context, the phase 2 Alliance A171901 trial (NCT04533451), also designed specifically for older adults, is investigating the toxicity, quality of life and overall survival in older patients aged 70 and older treated with first line pembrolizumab with or without chemotherapy based on oncologist's/ patient's choice. This is therefore a more inclusive trial design that does not determine access to treatment based on performance status, which will result in a more generalisable older patient sample.

Regarding the management of irAEs in older adults, this is identical to younger patients. But as older adults may have poorer functional reserve and multiple comorbidities compared to their younger counterparts, this may increase their risk of poor outcomes in case of irAEs, therefore a timely intervention is key [140, 141]. Another important consideration is that the treatment of irAEs in older adults, particularly with corticosteroids, should be tailored considering their pre-existing comorbidities. The use of corticosteroids can cause a wide range of other complications, such as significantly worsen diabetes, osteoporosis or even trigger delirium.

Ultimately, based on the available evidence regarding the use of checkpoint inhibitors in older patients with frailty, single-agent treatment may be an appropriate option for patients with mild frailty as more data emerges. Regarding the use of combination regimens in this group of patients, there is no evidence but considering the higher risk of toxicity, this should be avoided.

Conclusion

Older patients with NSCLC represent one of the largest populations of older cancer patients. This poses a challenge in daily clinical practice as older patients are widely underrepresented in clinical trials. Therefore, to guide a well-informed shared decision-making process, clinical teams should incorporate frailty and geriatric assessments, ideally within the setting of a CGA. The recent revolution in the treatment pathways of NSCLC, particularly for those with advanced/metastatic disease has brought new opportunities with the use of targeted treatments and checkpoint inhibitors, but also new challenges in terms of patient selection. The presence of frailty in these older patients, often associated with significant comorbidity means that these new developments are not appropriate for all of them. In the case of immunotherapy with checkpoint inhibitors, more research is needed to improve our ability to estimate the risk of toxicity, similarly to the tools developed to predict the toxicity risk with chemotherapy. Moreover, the definition of toxicity particularly in older patients should include quality of life and functional status. But ultimately, the prospects for these patients have improved significantly and although more dedicated research is needed, clinical teams have a growing armamentarium of cancer treatments, non-cancer specific interventions and supportive measures to improve the care of this complex sub-group of NSCLC patients.

References

1. Bray F, Ferlay J, Soerjomataram I, et al. Global cancer statistics 2018: GLOBOCAN estimates of incidence and mortality worldwide for 36 cancers in 185 countries. CA Cancer J Clin. 2018;68:394–424.
2. SEER cancer statistics factsheets: lung and bronchus cancer. In NCI (ed). https://seer.cancer.gov/statfacts/html/lungb.html; 2019.
3. Soto-Perez-de-Celis E, Li D, Yuan Y, et al. Functional versus chronological age: geriatric assessments to guide decision making in older patients with cancer. Lancet Oncol. 2018;19:e305–16.
4. Morley JE, Vellas B, van Kan GA, et al. Frailty consensus: a call to action. J Am Med Dir Assoc. 2013;14:392–7.

5. Gomes F, Baker K, Woods J, et al. MA19.09 Assessing clinical frailty in advanced lung cancer patients – an opportunity to improve patient outcomes? J Thorac Oncol. 2019;14:S329.
6. Nadpara PA, Madhavan SS, Tworek C, et al. Guideline-concordant lung cancer care and associated health outcomes among elderly patients in the United States. J Geriatr Oncol. 2015;6:101–10.
7. Tang M, Pearson S-A, Schaffer AL, et al. Are clinical trial eligibility criteria representative of older patients with lung cancer? A population-based data linkage study. J Geriatr Oncol. 2021;12:930–6.
8. Gomes F, Wong M, Battisti NML, et al. Immunotherapy in older patients with non-small cell lung cancer: Young International Society of Geriatric Oncology position paper. Br J Cancer. 2020;123:874–84.
9. Decoster L, Schallier D. Treatment of older patients with advanced non-small cell lung cancer: a challenge. J Geriatr Oncol. 2019;10:528–33.
10. Asemota N, Saftic I, Tsitsias T et al. Quality of life in octogenarians after lung resection compared to younger patients. Clin Lung Cancer; 2021.
11. Shinmura K. Cardiac senescence, heart failure, and frailty: a triangle in elderly people. Keio J Med. 2016;65:25–32.
12. Roderick PJ, Atkins RJ, Smeeth L, et al. Detecting chronic kidney disease in older people; what are the implications? Age Ageing. 2008;37:179–86.
13. Borges MK, Canevelli M, Cesari M, Aprahamian I. Frailty as a predictor of cognitive disorders: a systematic review and meta-analysis. Front Med (Lausanne). 2019;6:26.
14. Williams GR, Deal AM, Muss HB, et al. Frailty and skeletal muscle in older adults with cancer. J Geriatr Oncol. 2018;9:68–73.
15. Shinall MC Jr, Arya S, Youk A, et al. Association of preoperative patient frailty and operative stress with postoperative mortality. JAMA Surg. 2019;155:e194620.
16. Gagné S, McIsaac DI. Modifiable risk factors for patients undergoing lung cancer surgery and their optimization: a review. J Thorac Dis. 2018;10:S3761–s3772.
17. Ha D, Mazzone PJ, Ries AL, et al. The utility of exercise testing in patients with lung cancer. J Thorac Oncol. 2016;11:1397–410.
18. Wynter-Blyth V, Moorthy K. Prehabilitation: preparing patients for surgery. BMJ. 2017;358:j3702.
19. Hristov B, Eguchi T, Bains S, et al. Minimally invasive lobectomy is associated with lower noncancer-specific mortality in elderly patients: a propensity score matched competing risks analysis. Ann Surg. 2019;270:1161–9.
20. Suzuki K, Saji H, Aokage K, et al. Comparison of pulmonary segmentectomy and lobectomy: Safety results of a randomized trial. J Thorac Cardiovasc Surg. 2019;158:895–907.
21. Yang F, Sui X, Chen X, et al. Sublobar resection versus lobectomy in Surgical Treatment of Elderly Patients with early-stage non-small cell lung cancer (STEPS): study protocol for a randomized controlled trial. Trials. 2016;17:191.
22. Chida M, Minowa M, Karube Y, et al. Worsened long-term outcomes and postoperative complications in octogenarians with lung cancer following mediastinal lymph-node dissection. Interact Cardiovasc Thorac Surg. 2009;8:89–92.
23. Balduyck B, Hendriks J, Lauwers P, et al. Quality of life evolution after lung cancer surgery in septuagenarians: a prospective study. Eur J Cardiothorac Surg. 2009;35:1070–5. discussion 1075
24. Thompson C, French DG, Costache I. Pain management within an enhanced recovery program after thoracic surgery. J Thorac Dis 10 (Suppl 32) (November 2018): J Thorac Dis (Enhanced recovery: the evidence supporting best perioperative care in thoracic surgery); 2018.
25. Sheetz KH, Waits SA, Krell RW, et al. Improving mortality following emergent surgery in older patients requires focus on complication rescue. Ann Surg. 2013;258:614–7. discussion 617–618
26. Pignon JP, Tribodet H, Scagliotti GV, et al. Lung adjuvant cisplatin evaluation: a pooled analysis by the LACE Collaborative Group. J Clin Oncol. 2008;26:3552–9.

27. Fruh M, Rolland E, Pignon JP, et al. Pooled analysis of the effect of age on adjuvant cisplatin-based chemotherapy for completely resected non-small-cell lung cancer. J Clin Oncol. 2008;26:3573–81.
28. Ganti AK, Williams CD, Gajra A, Kelley MJ. Effect of age on the efficacy of adjuvant chemotherapy for resected non-small cell lung cancer. Cancer. 2015;121:2578–85.
29. Cuffe S, Booth CM, Peng Y, et al. Adjuvant chemotherapy for non-small-cell lung cancer in the elderly: a population-based study in Ontario, Canada. J Clin Oncol. 2012;30:1813–21.
30. Wisnivesky JP, Smith CB, Packer S, et al. Survival and risk of adverse events in older patients receiving postoperative adjuvant chemotherapy for resected stages II-IIIA lung cancer: observational cohort study. BMJ. 2011;343:d4013.
31. Asmis TR, Ding K, Seymour L, et al. Age and comorbidity as independent prognostic factors in the treatment of non small-cell lung cancer: a review of National Cancer Institute of Canada Clinical Trials Group trials. J Clin Oncol. 2008;26:54–9.
32. Morgensztern D, Samson PS, Waqar SN, et al. Early mortality in patients undergoing adjuvant chemotherapy for non-small cell lung cancer. J Thorac Oncol. 2018;13:543–9.
33. Wu Y-L, Tsuboi M, He J, et al. Osimertinib in resected EGFR-mutated non-small-cell lung cancer. N Engl J Med. 2020;383:1711–23.
34. Palma D, Visser O, Lagerwaard FJ, et al. Impact of introducing stereotactic lung radiotherapy for elderly patients with stage I non-small-cell lung cancer: a population-based time-trend analysis. J Clin Oncol. 2010;28:5153–9.
35. Bayman N, Alam N, Faivre-Finn C. Radiotherapy for lung cancer in the elderly. Lung Cancer. 2010;68:129–36.
36. Simone CB II, Wildt B, Haas AR, et al. Stereotactic body radiation therapy for lung cancer. Chest. 2013;143:1784–90.
37. Ma JT, Liu Y, Sun L, et al. Chest wall toxicity after stereotactic body radiation therapy: a pooled analysis of 57 studies. Int J Radiat Oncol Biol Phys. 2019;103:843–50.
38. Franks KN, McParland L, Webster J et al. SABRTOOTH: a randomised controlled feasibility study of Stereotactic Ablative Radiotherapy (SABR) with surgery in paTients with peripheral stage I nOn-small cell lung cancer (NSCLC) cOnsidered To be at Higher risk of complications from surgical resection. Eur Respir J; 2020.
39. Stokes WA, Bronsert MR, Meguid RA, et al. Post-treatment mortality after surgery and stereotactic body radiotherapy for early-stage non-small-cell lung cancer. J Clin Oncol. 2018;36:642–51.
40. Shirvani SM, Jiang J, Chang JY, et al. Lobectomy, sublobar resection, and stereotactic ablative radiotherapy for early-stage non-small cell lung cancers in the elderly. JAMA Surg. 2014;149:1244–53.
41. Spencer KL, Kennedy MPT, Lummis KL, et al. Surgery or radiotherapy for stage I lung cancer? An intention-to-treat analysis. Eur Respir J. 2019;53:1801568.
42. Franco I, Chen Y-H, Chipidza F, et al. Use of frailty to predict survival in elderly patients with early stage non-small-cell lung cancer treated with stereotactic body radiation therapy. J Geriatr Oncol. 2018;9:130–7.
43. De Ruysscher D, Botterweck A, Dirx M, et al. Eligibility for concurrent chemotherapy and radiotherapy of locally advanced lung cancer patients: a prospective, population-based study. Ann Oncol. 2009;20:98–102.
44. Firat S, Pleister A, Byhardt RW, Gore E. Age is independent of comorbidity influencing patient selection for combined modality therapy for treatment of stage III nonsmall cell lung cancer (NSCLC). Am J Clin Oncol. 2006;29:252–7.
45. McElnay PJ, Choong A, Jordan E, et al. Outcome of surgery versus radiotherapy after induction treatment in patients with N2 disease: systematic review and meta-analysis of randomised trials. Thorax. 2015;70:764–8.
46. Albain KS, Swann RS, Rusch VW, et al. Radiotherapy plus chemotherapy with or without surgical resection for stage III non-small-cell lung cancer: a phase III randomised controlled trial. Lancet. 2009;374:379–86.
47. Eberhardt WE, Pöttgen C, Gauler TC, et al. Phase III study of surgery versus definitive concurrent chemoradiotherapy boost in patients with resectable stage IIIA(N2) and selected IIIB

non-small-cell lung cancer after induction chemotherapy and concurrent chemoradiotherapy (ESPATUE). J Clin Oncol. 2015;33:4194–201.
48. O'Rourke N, Roqué IFM, Farré Bernadó N, Macbeth F. Concurrent chemoradiotherapy in non-small cell lung cancer. Cochrane Database Syst Rev 2010; Cd002140.
49. Evison M, on behalf of AstraZeneca UKL. The current treatment landscape in the UK for stage III NSCLC. Br J Cancer. 2020;123:3–9.
50. Driessen EJ, Bootsma GP, Hendriks LE, et al. Stage III non-small cell lung cancer in the elderly: patient characteristics predictive for tolerance and survival of chemoradiation in daily clinical practice. Radiother Oncol. 2016;121:26–31.
51. Miller ED, Fisher JL, Haglund KE, et al. The addition of chemotherapy to radiation therapy improves survival in elderly patients with stage III non-small cell lung cancer. J Thorac Oncol. 2018;13:426–35.
52. Movsas B, Scott C, Sause W, et al. The benefit of treatment intensification is age and histology-dependent in patients with locally advanced non-small cell lung cancer (NSCLC): a quality-adjusted survival analysis of radiation therapy oncology group (RTOG) chemoradiation studies. Int J Radiat Oncol Biol Phys. 1999;45:1143–9.
53. Cardenal F, Nadal E, Jové M, Faivre-Finn C. Concurrent systemic therapy with radiotherapy for the treatment of poor-risk patients with unresectable stage III non-small-cell lung cancer: a review of the literature. Ann Oncol. 2015;26:278–88.
54. Locher C, Pourel N, Le Caer H, et al. Impact of a comprehensive geriatric assessment to manage elderly patients with locally advanced non-small-cell lung cancers: an open phase II study using concurrent cisplatin-oral vinorelbine and radiotherapy (GFPC 08-06). Lung Cancer. 2018;121:25–9.
55. Driessen EJM, Janssen-Heijnen MLG, Maas HA, et al. Study protocol of the NVALT25-ELDAPT trial: selecting the optimal treatment for older patients with stage III non-small-cell lung cancer. Clin Lung Cancer. 2018;19:e849–52.
56. Antonia SJ, Villegas A, Daniel D, et al. Overall survival with durvalumab after chemoradiotherapy in stage III NSCLC. N Engl J Med. 2018;379:2342–50.
57. Bleehen NM, Girling DJ, Machin D, et al. A Medical Research Council (MRC) randomised trial of palliative radiotherapy with two fractions or a single fraction in patients with inoperable non-small-cell lung cancer (NSCLC) and poor performance status. Br J Cancer. 1992;65:934–41.
58. Medical Research Council Lung Cancer Working P, Macbeth FR, Bolger JJ, et al. Randomized trial of palliative two-fraction versus more intensive 13-fraction radiotherapy for patients with inoperable non-small cell lung cancer and good performance status. Clin Oncol. 1996;8:167–75.
59. Hoskin PJ, Hopkins K, Misra V, et al. Effect of single-fraction vs multifraction radiotherapy on ambulatory status among patients with spinal canal compression from metastatic cancer: the SCORAD randomized clinical trial. JAMA. 2019;322:2084–94.
60. Rowell NP, Gleeson FV. Steroids, radiotherapy, chemotherapy and stents for superior vena caval obstruction in carcinoma of the bronchus. Cochrane Database Syst Rev. 2015.
61. Hurria A, Togawa K, Mohile SG, et al. Predicting chemotherapy toxicity in older adults with cancer: a prospective multicenter study. J Clin Oncol. 2011;29:3457–65.
62. Almodovar T, Teixeira E, Barroso A, et al. Elderly patients with advanced NSCLC: the value of geriatric evaluation and the feasibility of CGA alternatives in predicting chemotherapy toxicity. Pulmonology. 2019;25:40–50.
63. Extermann M, Aapro M, Bernabei R, et al. Use of comprehensive geriatric assessment in older cancer patients: recommendations from the task force on CGA of the International Society of Geriatric Oncology (SIOG). Crit Rev Oncol Hematol. 2005;55:241–52.
64. Corre R, Greillier L, Le Caër H, et al. Use of a comprehensive geriatric assessment for the management of elderly patients with advanced non-small-cell lung cancer: the phase III randomized ESOGIA-GFPC-GECP 08-02 study. J Clin Oncol. 2016;34:1476–83.
65. Kelly K, Crowley J, Bunn PA Jr, et al. Randomized phase III trial of paclitaxel plus carboplatin versus vinorelbine plus cisplatin in the treatment of patients with advanced non--small-cell lung cancer: a Southwest Oncology Group trial. J Clin Oncol. 2001;19:3210–8.

66. Johnson DH. Phase III trial (E5592) comparing cisplatin plus etoposide with cisplatin plus paclitaxel at two dose levels for treatment of advanced non-small-cell lung cancer. Eastern Cooperative Oncology Group. J Natl Cancer Inst Monogr. 1995;61–63.
67. Treat JA, Gonin R, Socinski MA, et al. A randomized, phase III multicenter trial of gemcitabine in combination with carboplatin or paclitaxel versus paclitaxel plus carboplatin in patients with advanced or metastatic non-small-cell lung cancer. Ann Oncol. 2010;21:540–7.
68. Lilenbaum RC, Herndon JE II, List MA, et al. Single-agent versus combination chemotherapy in advanced non-small-cell lung cancer: the cancer and leukemia group B (study 9730). J Clin Oncol. 2005;23:190–6.
69. Tyagi P. Bevacizumab, when added to paclitaxel/carboplatin, prolongs survival in previously untreated patients with advanced non-small-cell lung cancer: preliminary results from the ECOG 4599 trial. Clin Lung Cancer. 2005;6:276–8.
70. Gridelli C. The ELVIS trial: a phase III study of single-agent vinorelbine as first-line treatment in elderly patients with advanced non-small cell lung cancer. Elderly Lung Cancer Vinorelbine Italian Study. Oncologist. 2001;6(Suppl 1):4–7.
71. Gridelli C, Perrone F, Gallo C, et al. Chemotherapy for elderly patients with advanced non-small-cell lung cancer: the Multicenter Italian Lung Cancer in the Elderly Study (MILES) phase III randomized trial. J Natl Cancer Inst. 2003;95:362–72.
72. Banna GL, Camerini A, Bronte G, et al. Oral metronomic vinorelbine in advanced non-small cell lung cancer patients unfit for chemotherapy. Anticancer Res. 2018;38:3689–97.
73. Camerini A, Banna GL, Cinieri S, et al. Metronomic oral vinorelbine for the treatment of advanced non-small cell lung cancer: a multicenter international retrospective analysis. Clin Transl Oncol. 2019;21:790–5.
74. Pujol JL, Coffy A, Camerini A, et al. An individual patient-data meta-analysis of metronomic oral vinorelbine in metastatic non-small cell lung cancer. PLoS One. 2019;14:e0220988.
75. Camerini A, Morabito A, Montanino A, et al. Metronomic oral vinorelbine in previously untreated advanced non-small-cell lung cancer patients unfit for platinum-based chemotherapy: results of the randomized phase II Tempo Lung trial. ESMO Open. 2021;6:100051.
76. Quoix E, Zalcman G, Oster JP, et al. Carboplatin and weekly paclitaxel doublet chemotherapy compared with monotherapy in elderly patients with advanced non-small-cell lung cancer: IFCT-0501 randomised, phase 3 trial. Lancet. 2011;378:1079–88.
77. Langer CJ, Kim ES, Anderson EC, et al. nab-paclitaxel-based therapy in underserved patient populations: the ABOUND.70+ study in elderly patients with advanced NSCLC. Front Oncologia. 2018;8:262.
78. Gridelli C, Morabito A, Cavanna L, et al. Cisplatin-based first-line treatment of elderly patients with advanced non-small-cell lung cancer: joint analysis of MILES-3 and MILES-4 phase III trials. J Clin Oncol. 2018;36:2585–92.
79. Midha A, Dearden S, McCormack R. EGFR mutation incidence in non-small-cell lung cancer of adenocarcinoma histology: a systematic review and global map by ethnicity (mutMapII). Am J Cancer Res. 2015;5:2892–911.
80. Gomes F, Tay R, Chiramel J, Califano R. The role of targeted agents and immunotherapy in older patients with non-small cell lung cancer. Drugs Aging. 2018;35:819–34.
81. Zhou C, Wu YL, Chen G, et al. Erlotinib versus chemotherapy as first-line treatment for patients with advanced EGFR mutation-positive non-small-cell lung cancer (OPTIMAL, CTONG-0802): a multicentre, open-label, randomised, phase 3 study. Lancet Oncol. 2011;12:735–42.
82. Wu YL, Zhou C, Liam CK, et al. First-line erlotinib versus gemcitabine/cisplatin in patients with advanced EGFR mutation-positive non-small-cell lung cancer: analyses from the phase III, randomized, open-label, ENSURE study. Ann Oncol. 2015;26:1883–9.
83. Rosell R, Carcereny E, Gervais R, et al. Erlotinib versus standard chemotherapy as first-line treatment for European patients with advanced EGFR mutation-positive non-small-cell lung cancer (EURTAC): a multicentre, open-label, randomised phase 3 trial. Lancet Oncol. 2012;13:239–46.

84. Mitsudomi T, Morita S, Yatabe Y, et al. Gefitinib versus cisplatin plus docetaxel in patients with non-small-cell lung cancer harbouring mutations of the epidermal growth factor receptor (WJTOG3405): an open label, randomised phase 3 trial. Lancet Oncol. 2010;11:121–8.
85. Maemondo M, Inoue A, Kobayashi K, et al. Gefitinib or chemotherapy for non-small-cell lung cancer with mutated EGFR. N Engl J Med. 2010;362:2380–8.
86. Mok TS, Wu YL, Thongprasert S, et al. Gefitinib or carboplatin-paclitaxel in pulmonary adenocarcinoma. N Engl J Med. 2009;361:947–57.
87. Sequist LV, Yang JC, Yamamoto N, et al. Phase III study of afatinib or cisplatin plus pemetrexed in patients with metastatic lung adenocarcinoma with EGFR mutations. J Clin Oncol. 2013;31:3327–34.
88. Wu YL, Zhou C, Hu CP, et al. Afatinib versus cisplatin plus gemcitabine for first-line treatment of Asian patients with advanced non-small-cell lung cancer harbouring EGFR mutations (LUX-Lung 6): an open-label, randomised phase 3 trial. Lancet Oncol. 2014;15:213–22.
89. Soria JC, Ohe Y, Vansteenkiste J, et al. Osimertinib in untreated EGFR-mutated advanced non-small-cell lung cancer. N Engl J Med. 2018;378:113–25.
90. Mok TS, Wu YL, Ahn MJ, et al. Osimertinib or platinum-pemetrexed in EGFR T790M-positive lung cancer. N Engl J Med. 2017;376:629–40.
91. Wu YL, Cheng Y, Zhou X, et al. Dacomitinib versus gefitinib as first-line treatment for patients with EGFR-mutation-positive non-small-cell lung cancer (ARCHER 1050): a randomised, open-label, phase 3 trial. Lancet Oncol. 2017;18:1454–66.
92. Morikawa N, Minegishi Y, Inoue A, et al. First-line gefitinib for elderly patients with advanced NSCLC harboring EGFR mutations. A combined analysis of North-East Japan Study Group studies. Expert Opin Pharmacother. 2015;16:465–72.
93. Inoue A, Kobayashi K, Usui K, et al. First-line gefitinib for patients with advanced non-small-cell lung cancer harboring epidermal growth factor receptor mutations without indication for chemotherapy. J Clin Oncol. 2009;27:1394–400.
94. Yoshioka H, Komuta K, Imamura F, et al. Efficacy and safety of erlotinib in elderly patients in the phase IV POLARSTAR surveillance study of Japanese patients with non-small-cell lung cancer. Lung Cancer. 2014;86:201–6.
95. Brueckl WM, Achenbach HJ, Ficker JH, Schuette W. Erlotinib treatment after platinum-based therapy in elderly patients with non-small-cell lung cancer in routine clinical practice - results from the ElderTac study. BMC Cancer. 2018;18:333.
96. Lee SM, Khan I, Upadhyay S, et al. First-line erlotinib in patients with advanced non-small-cell lung cancer unsuitable for chemotherapy (TOPICAL): a double-blind, placebo-controlled, phase 3 trial. Lancet Oncol. 2012;13:1161–70.
97. Yamada K, Azuma K, Takeshita M, et al. Phase II trial of erlotinib in elderly patients with previously treated non-small cell lung cancer: results of the lung oncology group in Kyushu (LOGiK-0802). Anticancer Res. 2016;36:2881–7.
98. Bigot F, Boudou-Rouquette P, Arrondeau J, et al. Erlotinib pharmacokinetics: a critical parameter influencing acute toxicity in elderly patients over 75 years-old. Investig New Drugs. 2017;35:242–6.
99. Wu YL, Sequist LV, Tan EH, et al. Afatinib as first-line treatment of older patients with EGFR mutation-positive non-small-cell lung cancer: subgroup analyses of the LUX-Lung 3, LUX-Lung 6, and LUX-Lung 7 trials. Clin Lung Cancer. 2018;19:e465–79.
100. Ramalingam SS, Vansteenkiste J, Planchard D, et al. Overall survival with osimertinib in untreated, EGFR-mutated advanced NSCLC. N Engl J Med. 2020;382:41–50.
101. Roviello G, Zanotti L, Cappelletti MR, et al. Are EGFR tyrosine kinase inhibitors effective in elderly patients with EGFR-mutated non-small cell lung cancer? Clin Exp Med. 2018;18:15–20.
102. Chia PL, Mitchell P, Dobrovic A, John T. Prevalence and natural history of ALK positive non-small-cell lung cancer and the clinical impact of targeted therapy with ALK inhibitors. Clin Epidemiol. 2014;6:423–32.

103. Solomon BJ, Mok T, Kim DW, et al. First-line crizotinib versus chemotherapy in ALK-positive lung cancer. N Engl J Med. 2014;371:2167–77.
104. Mok T, Camidge DR, Gadgeel SM, et al. Updated overall survival and final progression-free survival data for patients with treatment-naive advanced ALK−positive non-small-cell lung cancer in the ALEX study. Ann Oncol. 2020;31:1056–64.
105. Soria JC, Tan DSW, Chiari R, et al. First-line ceritinib versus platinum-based chemotherapy in advanced ALK-rearranged non-small-cell lung cancer (ASCEND-4): a randomised, open-label, phase 3 study. Lancet. 2017;389:917–29.
106. Camidge DR, Kim HR, Ahn MJ, et al. Brigatinib versus crizotinib in advanced ALK inhibitor-naive ALK-positive non-small cell lung cancer: second interim analysis of the phase III ALTA-1L trial. J Clin Oncol. 2020;38:3592–603.
107. Shaw AT, Bauer TM, de Marinis F, et al. First-line lorlatinib or crizotinib in advanced ALK-positive lung cancer. N Engl J Med. 2020;383:2018–29.
108. Shaw AT, Kim DW, Nakagawa K, et al. Crizotinib versus chemotherapy in advanced ALK-positive lung cancer. N Engl J Med. 2013;368:2385–94.
109. Blackhall F, Shaw A, Jaenne P et al. Crizotinib safety profile in elderly and non-elderly patients (pts) with advanced ALK plus non-small cell lung cancer (NSCLC). Eur J Cancer. 2013;S821–S821.
110. Hida T, Nokihara H, Kondo M, et al. Alectinib versus crizotinib in patients with ALK-positive non-small-cell lung cancer (J-ALEX): an open-label, randomised phase 3 trial. Lancet. 2017;390:29–39.
111. Peters S, Camidge DR, Shaw AT, et al. Alectinib versus crizotinib in untreated ALK-positive non-small-cell lung cancer. N Engl J Med. 2017;377:829–38.
112. Gettinger S, Borghaei H, Brahmer J, et al. Five-year outcomes from the randomized, phase 3 trials CheckMate 017/057: nivolumab vs docetaxel in previously treated NSCLC. J Thorac Oncol. 2019;14:S244–5.
113. Sedrak MS, Freedman RA, Cohen HJ et al. Older adult participation in cancer clinical trials: a systematic review of barriers and interventions. CA Cancer J Clin; 2020.
114. Nikolich-Zugich J. The twilight of immunity: emerging concepts in aging of the immune system. Nat Immunol. 2018;19:10–9.
115. Reck M, Rodríguez-Abreu D, Robinson AG, et al. Pembrolizumab versus chemotherapy for PD-L1–positive non–small-cell lung cancer. N Engl J Med. 2016;375:1823–33.
116. Brahmer JR, Rodriguez-Abreu D, Robinson AG, et al. KEYNOTE-024 5-year OS update: first-line (1L) pembrolizumab (pembro) vs platinum-based chemotherapy (chemo) in patients (pts) with metastatic NSCLC and PD-L1 tumour proportion score (TPS) 50%. Ann Oncol. 2020;31:S1181–2.
117. Nosaki K, Saka H, Hosomi Y, et al. Safety and efficacy of pembrolizumab monotherapy in elderly patients with PD-L1-positive advanced non-small-cell lung cancer: pooled analysis from the KEYNOTE-010, KEYNOTE-024, and KEYNOTE-042 studies. Lung Cancer. 2019;135:188–95.
118. Herbst RS, Baas P, Kim DW, et al. Pembrolizumab versus docetaxel for previously treated, PD-L1-positive, advanced non-small-cell lung cancer (KEYNOTE-010): a randomised controlled trial. Lancet. 2016;387:1540–50.
119. Herbst RS, Garon EB, Kim DW et al. Long-term follow-up in the KEYNOTE-010 study of pembrolizumab (pembro) for advanced NSCLC, including in patients (pts) who completed 2 years of pembro and pts who received a second course of pembro. Ann Oncol. 2018;29.
120. Brahmer J, Reckamp KL, Baas P, et al. Nivolumab versus docetaxel in advanced squamous-cell non-small-cell lung cancer. N Engl J Med. 2015;373:123–35.
121. Borghaei H, Paz-Ares L, Horn L, et al. Nivolumab versus docetaxel in advanced nonsquamous non-small-cell lung cancer. N Engl J Med. 2015;373:1627–39.
122. Rittmeyer A, Barlesi F, Waterkamp D, et al. Atezolizumab versus docetaxel in patients with previously treated non-small-cell lung cancer (OAK): a phase 3, open-label, multicentre randomised controlled trial. Lancet. 2017;389:255–65.

123. Gandhi L, Rodriguez-Abreu D, Gadgeel S, et al. Pembrolizumab plus chemotherapy in metastatic non-small-cell lung cancer. N Engl J Med. 2018;378:2078–92.
124. Paz-Ares L, Luft A, Vicente D, et al. Pembrolizumab plus chemotherapy for squamous non-small-cell lung cancer. N Engl J Med. 2018;379:2040–51.
125. Socinski MA, Jotte RM, Cappuzzo F, et al. Atezolizumab for first-line treatment of metastatic nonsquamous NSCLC. N Engl J Med. 2018;378:2288–301.
126. Socinski MA, Jotte RM, Cappuzzo F, et al. Overall survival (OS) analysis of IMpower150, a randomized Ph 3 study of atezolizumab (atezo) + chemotherapy (chemo) ± bevacizumab (bev) vs chemo + bev in 1L nonsquamous (NSQ) NSCLC. J Clin Oncol. 2018;36:9002.
127. Hellmann MD, Paz-Ares L, Bernabe Caro R, et al. Nivolumab plus ipilimumab in advanced non-small-cell lung cancer. N Engl J Med. 2019;381:2020–31.
128. Reck M, Ciuleanu T-E, Dols MC, et al. Nivolumab (NIVO) + ipilimumab (IPI) + 2 cycles of platinum-doublet chemotherapy (chemo) vs 4 cycles chemo as first-line (1L) treatment (tx) for stage IV/recurrent non-small cell lung cancer (NSCLC): CheckMate 9LA. J Clin Oncol. 2020;38:9501.
129. Elias R, Giobbie-Hurder A, McCleary NJ, et al. Efficacy of PD-1 & PD-L1 inhibitors in older adults: a meta-analysis. J Immunother Cancer. 2018;6:26.
130. Olsson-Brown AC, Baxter M, Dobeson C, et al. Real-world outcomes in older adults treated with immunotherapy: a United Kingdom multicenter series of 2,049 patients. J Clin Oncol. 2021;39:–12026.
131. Lobefaro R, Viscardi G, Di Liello R, et al. Immunotherapy in advanced non-small cell lung cancer patients with poor performance status: the role of clinical-pathological variables and inflammatory biomarkers. Lung Cancer. 2021;152:165–73.
132. Middleton G, Brock K, Savage J, et al. Pembrolizumab in patients with non-small-cell lung cancer of performance status 2 (PePS2): a single arm, phase 2 trial. Lancet Respir Med. 2020;8:895–904.
133. Wang Y, Zhou S, Yang F, et al. Treatment-related adverse events of PD-1 and PD-L1 inhibitors in clinical trials: a systematic review and meta-analysis. JAMA Oncol. 2019;5:1008–19.
134. Spigel DR, McCleod M, Jotte RM, et al. Safety, efficacy, and patient-reported health-related quality of life and symptom burden with nivolumab in patients with advanced non-small cell lung cancer, including patients aged 70 years or older or with poor performance status (CheckMate 153). J Thorac Oncol. 2019;14:1628–39.
135. Felip E, Ardizzoni A, Ciuleanu T, et al. CheckMate 171: a phase 2 trial of nivolumab in patients with previously treated advanced squamous non-small cell lung cancer, including ECOG PS 2 and elderly populations. Eur J Cancer. 2020;127:160–72.
136. Lichtenstein MRL, Nipp RD, Muzikansky A, et al. Impact of age on outcomes with immunotherapy in patients with non-small cell lung cancer. J Thorac Oncol. 2019;14:547–52.
137. Muchnik E, Loh KP, Strawderman M, et al. Immune checkpoint inhibitors in real-world treatment of older adults with non-small cell lung cancer. J Am Geriatr Soc. 2019;67:905–12.
138. Wang DY, Salem JE, Cohen JV, et al. Fatal toxic effects associated with immune checkpoint inhibitors: a systematic review and meta-analysis. JAMA Oncol. 2018;4:1721–8.
139. Gomes F, Lorigan P, Woolley S, et al. A prospective cohort study on the safety of checkpoint inhibitors in older cancer patients - the ELDERS study. ESMO Open. 2021;6:100042.
140. van Holstein Y, Kapiteijn E, Bastiaannet E, et al. Efficacy and adverse events of immunotherapy with checkpoint inhibitors in older patients with cancer. Drugs Aging. 2019;36:927–38.
141. Johns A, Wei L, Grogan M, et al. Checkpoint inhibitor immunotherapy toxicity and overall survival among older adults with advanced cancer. J Geriatr Oncol. 2021;12(5):813–9.

Chapter 19
Colorectal Cancer in Older Adults with Frailty

Ana Ferreira, Louis J. Vitone, L. S. Prasad Kellati, Katie Ormston, and Hassan Shikhrakab

Introduction

Colorectal cancer is a disease primarily of older people, approximately 60% of new cases being diagnosed in individuals above 65 years of age [1]. Whilst increasing age is associated with a decline in physiological reserves and an increase in comorbidities and frailty, chronologic age is not equivalent to physiologic age. Approximately 40% of older cancer patients are reported to have frailty [2], but this depends on a variety of factors such as the tumour type and where the patient is within the cancer journey. In the context of colorectal cancer, a study focusing on patients aged 75 years and above screened all patients before chemotherapy with the Geriatric-8 (G8) tool [3]. Forty-five percent of patients had metastatic disease and about 80% had a positive G8 screening, suggesting frailty is very prevalent in this population.

Frailty and comorbidity are prognostic factors in patients with colorectal cancer. A systematic review and meta-analysis investigated the prognostic role of comorbidity and frailty in colorectal cancer [4]. Only a small number of studies incorporated measures of frailty but those patients with colorectal cancer and frailty had a higher

A. Ferreira (✉) · K. Ormston · H. Shikhrakab
Medical Oncology Department, East Lancashire Hospitals NHS Trust, Blackburn, UK
e-mail: Ana.Ferreira@elht.nhs.uk; Katie.Ormston@elht.nhs.uk; Hassan.Shikhrakab@elht.nhs.uk

L. J. Vitone
Surgery Department, East Lancashire Hospitals NHS Trust, Blackburn, UK
e-mail: Louis.Vitone@elht.nhs.uk

L. S. P. Kellati
Medical Oncology Department, Lancashire Teaching Hospitals NHS Foundation Trust, Preston, UK
e-mail: Prasad.Kellati@lthtr.nhs.uk

F. Gomes (ed.), *Frailty in Older Adults with Cancer*,
https://doi.org/10.1007/978-3-030-89162-6_19

overall mortality than patients without frailty (hazard ratio (HR) range: 2.60–3.39). Regarding comorbidity where there were more studies available, compared to patients without comorbidity, those with mild/moderate and severe comorbidity had, respectively, a higher risk of 30-day (odds ratio (OR) = 1.71; 95% confidence interval (CI): 1.26–2.31 and OR = 2.62; 95% CI: 1.97–3.47), overall (HR = 1.41; 95% CI: 1.23–1.62 and HR = 2.03; 95% CI: 1.76–2.34), and colorectal cancer-specific mortality (HR = 1.06; 95% CI: 1.02–1.10 and HR = 1.14; 95% CI: 1.04–1.23).

Therefore, risk assessment is essential to consider the potential risks and benefits at the time of treatment decision-making for older patients with colorectal cancer. The International Society of Geriatric Oncology (SIOG) recommends that a comprehensive geriatric assessment (CGA) is used to guide this decision-making [5]. A CGA is a multidimensional, interdisciplinary diagnostic approach to determine an older person's medical, psychosocial and functional capabilities and limitations in order to develop a holistic care plan [6].

The management of colorectal cancer is particularly challenging in older patients with frailty, but there are also important considerations earlier on, regarding bowel screening for colorectal cancer. Whilst screening is often recommended until 75 years of age, the evidence beyond that is conflicting and the decisions should be individualised [7]. A recent study [8] confirmed that screening endoscopy in patients aged 75 or over was associated with a lower risk of colorectal cancer incidence and related mortality. However, the reduction in mortality was not seen in patients with cardiovascular disease (HR 1.18, 95% CI 0.59–2.35) or with significant comorbidities (HR 1.17, 95% CI 0.57–2.43). Therefore, for most older patients with frailty, who have a reduced life expectancy and significant comorbidities, continuing screening for bowel cancer is more likely inappropriate leading to overdiagnosis.

The focus of this chapter is on reviewing the current evidence regarding the treatment of colorectal cancer in older patients with frailty, from an early stage to a metastatic setting

Management of Early-Stage and Locally Advanced Colorectal Cancer

Surgery

Surgery is the cornerstone in the treatment of early-stage and locally advanced colorectal cancer. Older patients represent a heterogeneous population so the risks and benefits of surgical intervention must be carefully considered on an individualised basis to reduce the risk of overtreating some patients and undertreating others.

A study documented that 30-day mortality after colorectal surgery vastly underestimated 1-year mortality (4.9% vs 12.4%), moreover several risk factors were identified for excess mortality, in particular patient with comorbidities (measured by Charlson score >1) [9]. Focusing on mortality within the first year after curative colorectal cancer surgery, another study confirmed that 1-year mortality increased with age, and older patients with comorbidity died more frequently due to complications [10]. In fact, regardless of the comorbidity tool used, results are consistent, with highest comorbidity burden being significantly associated with shorted survival after colorectal cancer surgery [11]. And in older patients, particularly those aged 75 and over, a German study reported a mean of five comorbidities at the time of colorectal cancer diagnosis [12]. Nonetheless, a large study in the United States demonstrated that older age (65+), even after controlling for comorbidities, was an independent prognostic factor for mortality after colorectal cancer surgery [13]. This highlights that there is a complex interplay in older patients that goes beyond comorbidity burden.

Frailty in these older patients plays a key role, and although is not an absolute contraindication to colorectal surgery, it limits the appropriateness of this approach in many of these patients. A systematic review examined the impact of frailty on post-operative outcomes in individuals aged 65+ who underwent elective surgery for colorectal cancer [14]. This showed that older individuals with frailty have a significantly higher risk of post-operative complications, longer length of hospital stay and a poorer long-term survival. There is however no consensus on how to best assess frailty in this context of older patients considered for colorectal cancer surgery [15]. A study compared an assessment of frailty based on CGA versus the Fried physical phenotype of frailty before colorectal cancer surgery, to analyse which best correlated with post-operative complications and survival [16]. The CGA-based frailty assessment being more holistic identified more patients with frailty (43% vs 13%). Whilst both measures predicted survival, only the CGA-based frailty measure predicted post-operative complications. Another well-established measure to predict outcomes is the cardiorespiratory fitness, which is an independent predictor of post-operative mortality, length of hospital stay and admission to critical care, providing significantly more accurate prognostic and predictive information than age alone [17]. Therefore, cardiopulmonary exercise testing (CPET) should be incorporated to aid the identification of high-risk older patients [18]. In order to further support some of these older patients undergoing colorectal cancer surgery, elective admission to critical care unit after the procedure, instead of standard surgical ward care, reduced cardiac events [19].

Advances in minimally invasive colorectal surgery pushed the boundaries of surgical eligibility, particularly for older patients with frailty. However, some colorectal surgeons remain reluctant to offer laparoscopic surgery in older patients for fear of their reduced physiological reserves and challenged cardiorespiratory physiology evoked by the nuances of a steep Trendelenburg position or carbon dioxide pneumoperitoneum giving rising to high intra-abdominal pressures [20]. In one of the largest meta-analyses to date, Antoniou et al. [21] reported a substantial benefit for older patients undergoing laparoscopic colorectal surgery in comparison with open surgery.

But when determining eligibility for surgery particularly for those older patients with mild frailty, it is important to consider their overall function and what a deterioration after surgery may mean for their daily life. A systemic review looked at the patients' functional status after colorectal surgery, in particular role and physical function [22]. This showed that physical function dropped by 10% in median (range −26% to −5%) at 3 months and this was still reduced by 5% at 12 months after surgery (Range −13% to +5%). This reduction was even more significant in the role function dropping by 18% (range −39% to −2%) at 3 months and still by 5% (−17% to +10%) at 12 months. Importantly, older patients were the ones who experienced the greatest and more persistent decline in function.

Overall, the outcomes following colorectal cancer surgery have improved due to a variety of factors, such as laparoscopic surgery, prehabilitation protocols, enhanced recovery protocols, reduced use of defunctioning stomas [23–25], as well as improved patient selection and support. Therefore, surgery may be an appropriate option for selected older patients with mild frailty. Beyond a holistic geriatric assessment, a robust multidisciplinary team approach to managing these patients is essential, with an open and clear discussion ensuring realistic expectations on the potential risks and benefits from surgery [25]. Lastly, an emphasis on morbidity over mortality may prove more important or relevant to a patient who already has a reduced life expectancy based on age and frailty.

Radiotherapy

Radiotherapy has a role in the management of rectal cancer, either preoperative (neoadjuvant) or palliative. And approximately one third of patients with colorectal cancer present with rectal disease [25].

The role of preoperative radiotherapy in rectal tumours is to reduce the risk of local recurrence after surgery and to down-stage inoperable tumours. It can be delivered as a short course or a long course [26]. The short course is usually given over a period of 1 week (5 fractions over 5 days) followed by either immediate curative surgery (within 1 week) or delayed curative surgery (within 4–8 weeks). The long course is delivered over a period of 5 weeks (25 fractions), ideally with chemotherapy for better outcomes, followed by surgery (within 4–8 weeks). The decision of short or long course radiotherapy (the latter with or without chemotherapy) is made after discussion in multidisciplinary team depending on tumour staging, location of tumour in rectum (upper, middle and lower), distance of tumour from circumferential resection margin and the overall fitness of patients, such as the existence of frailty.

In the context of an older patient with frailty, chemotherapy combined with radiotherapy for increased local cancer control is rarely used, nonetheless preoperative radiotherapy in older patients has been shown to improve local control [27]. Therefore, preoperative radiotherapy, most likely a short course, with delayed surgery can be a more appropriate option for this sub-group of patients, if considered for radical surgery [25]. An important consideration, treatment eligibility apart, is that often older patients are understandably keen to avoid a permanent stoma and may accept a higher risk of local recurrence in the future to achieve this, favouring function and quality of life [28]. However, as previously described, only a selected number of these patients are eligible for surgery, this consequently affects the use of preoperative radiotherapy, resulting in a higher proportion receiving palliative radiotherapy as an alternative.

Palliative radiotherapy treatment courses should be short and consider the patient circumstances in keeping with best practice. Palliative radiotherapy is very useful for palliation of symptoms from locally advanced rectal cancer like intermittent bleeding and pain. Reducing fractionation to single-fraction regimens, where appropriate, may be considered, or alternatively hypo-fractionated regimens may be suitable.

Lastly, when planning radiotherapy to treat a patient with frailty it is important to consider careful positioning and immobilisation, bearing in mind age-related considerations, such as arthritis, Parkinson's disease or other restrictions on range of motion. Moreover, certain geriatric syndromes, such as hearing impairment or cognitive impairments, which are common among older patients with frailty, may affect communication and compliance regarding radiotherapy treatment.

Chemotherapy

Adjuvant chemotherapy should be considered following curative surgery for high-risk stage 2 and stage 3 colorectal cancers with the aim of eradicating micro-metastatic disease, thereby reducing the risk of disease recurrence. The backbone of adjuvant chemotherapy is a fluoropyrimidine, either intravenous 5-fluorouracil (5-FU) or oral capecitabine.

For stage 2 colorectal cancer, some parameters are prognostic and inform the risk assessment, such as surgery with insufficient lymph node sampling (<12 nodes), tumour presented with obstruction or perforation at presentation, a large tumour (pT4), a high-grade tumour or a tumour with vascular/lymphatic/perineural invasion [29]. Therefore, in this context of high-risk stage 2 disease, adjuvant chemotherapy should be considered as it reduces the risk of death by 3–5% with fluoropyrimidines alone [29]. A small sub-group of these patients may have microsatellite instability (MSI), and these patients are at a very low risk of recurrence and may not benefit from this chemotherapy. However, in addition to the already marginal survival benefit in the context of high-risk stage 2 disease, there is controversial evidence of benefit in older patients, particularly those with frailty [25]. Hence this is not commonly used in this setting and may be omitted, but if it were to be considered in very selected cases it should consist of fluoropyrimidines alone.

For stage 3 colorectal cancer, adjuvant chemotherapy with fluoropyrimidines alone reduces the risk of death by 10–15%, with a further 4–5% improvement with the addition of oxaliplatin [29]. Whilst there is a stronger rationale to consider fluoropyrimidines in this context for selected older patients with frailty. The addition of oxaliplatin should be omitted for most of these patients. Evidence regarding fit older patients pooled from several randomised trials showed that the improvement in disease-free survival and overall survival with the combination was present, yet modestly attenuated in patients aged 70+ and in those with comorbidities. Moreover, older patients had more high-grade adverse events on treatment [30]. Therefore, it is reasonable to infer that most older patients with frailty will not be eligible for a combination strategy with oxaliplatin.

A sub-group analysis of the TOSCA trial, which was a phase 3 trial assessing different lengths of treatment with oxaliplatin-based combination chemotherapy, compared the younger with the older cohort (aged 70+) [31, 32]. Of note, the older cohort had worse performance status, more advanced tumours and more high-grade/poorly differentiated tumours. In patients over 70, there was a greater proportion of dose reductions (46.7% vs 41.4%, $p = 0.018$), treatment interruptions (26.1% vs 19.3%, $p < 0.001$) and a higher proportion of recurrences (24.2% vs 20.3%, $p = 0.033$).

Regarding the duration of adjuvant chemotherapy, this was traditionally delivered over 6 months, but several clinical trials have confirmed that a duration of 3 months can be reasonably considered for the combination of fluoropyrimidines with oxaliplatin [33, 34]. This development is particularly relevant for the small group of selected older patients with mild frailty that could be suitable for a combination strategy. However the duration of fluoropyrimidines alone is recommended for a 6-month period [29].

Lastly, regarding the delivery of fluoropyrimidines, oral capecitabine is at least equivalent to bolus 5-FU in patients aged 70+ years [35] with some variations in the toxicity profile but undeniably more convenient to patients [36]. The doses of fluoropyrimidines are often adjusted particularly in older patients with frailty. The dose of capecitabine may be capped at 1000 mg/m^2 when it is used on its own, or at 800 mg/m^2 when it is used in combination with oxaliplatin. Nonetheless, this group of patients are more likely to experience dose reduction or discontinuation. In this context, the GERICO study randomised older frail patients (aged 70+ with positive G8 screening) undergoing chemotherapy to receive CGA or standard care [37]. About 60% of patients were receiving chemotherapy in an adjuvant setting. More patients in the interventional arm completed the scheduled chemotherapy (45% vs. 28%, $P = 0.0366$). Moreover, quality of life also improved with a decreased burden of illness ($P = 0.048$) and improved mobility ($P = 0.008$). This highlights the need to further support these patients through the treatment plan.

Management of Advanced Metastatic Colorectal Cancer

The majority of patients who present with metastatic disease are not suitable for potentially curative resection and the treatment intent is palliative. However, in selected cases with initially unresectable disease in whom the metastases have a significant response to systemic anti-cancer treatment, resection may become an option. Moreover, despite the disease presentation, depending on the patient overall fitness the optimal treatment options may not be appropriate. Therefore, it is key to determine an upfront treatment plan.

Patients with advanced metastatic colorectal cancer can be categorised in four groups [38, 39]:

Group 0: The liver and/or lung metastasis are technically fully resectable. Typically, this group presents with limited metastases (in number and size), and there is a curative-intent to decrease the risk of relapse.

Group 1: The liver and/or lung metastasis are potentially resectable after response to induction chemotherapy. In this group, chemotherapy is offered aiming to downsize the tumour and allow a subsequent curative-intent surgery. This strategy is limited to patients fit enough to undergo not just major surgery but also more intensive chemotherapy to achieve maximum tumour shrinkage. Therefore, a chemotherapy doublet along with a targeted agent (e.g. bevacizumab) or even a chemotherapy triplet is considered in this setting.

Group 2: Disseminated metastatic disease with rapid tumour progression and/or tumour-related symptoms and/or risk of rapid deterioration. The aim is to use an intensive chemotherapy regimen to achieve significant tumour shrinkage with a palliative intent. However, there may be a possibility for subsequent tumour resection if there is a significant tumour shrinkage. Therefore, the strategy here is only appropriate to patients eligible to undergo an intensive chemotherapy regimen. A chemotherapy doublet in combination with a targeted agent is the preference. In patients responding to the initially selected treatment, reconsideration of the treatment options should be done in a multidisciplinary team.

Group 3: Disseminated metastatic disease with no option of resection and/or no major symptoms or risk of deterioration. This group also includes patients who are not eligible to the previous strategies due to severe comorbidity and frailty. Therefore, in this setting tumour shrinkage is less relevant and treatments with low toxicity are more relevant aiming to delay further cancer progression with a low toxicity risk. The treatment plan usually consists of treatment with either single-agent or a doublet chemotherapy with low toxicity. However best supportive care should also be considered.

Therefore, in the context of older patients with frailty, the majority of patients with advanced colorectal cancer will fit within group 3. Then, if a patient is suitable to undergo chemotherapy, this can be delivered for a fixed period of 3–6 months, a maintenance treatment after starting with an 'induction treatment' or treatment until progression or toxicity.

Systemic Treatment

Chemotherapy

Similarly to adjuvant chemotherapy, the backbone of first-line palliative chemotherapy consists of a fluoropyrimidine, either intravenous 5-FU or oral capecitabine. This can then be used in various combinations with oxaliplatin or irinotecan, resulting in the FOLFOX/CAPOX and FOLFIRI/XELIRI regimens, respectively. A triplet combination including both oxaliplatin and irinotecan with the fluoropyrimidine backbone comprises the FOLFOXIRI regimen. Moreover, chemotherapy can also be combined with other targeted agents.

An age-based study compared the multidisciplinary decision-making regarding chemotherapy [40]. In this palliative setting, the multidisciplinary team recommended chemotherapy in 98% of younger and 69% of older patients and 81% and 45%, respectively, subsequently received in fact chemotherapy. Beyond chronological age, comorbidity and the patient's physical condition were key reasons for withholding chemotherapy. When older patients did receive chemotherapy, reduced intensity regimens were often effectuated.

Regarding the selection of the chemotherapy options in these patients there are several important considerations: (1) the use of monotherapy or combinations; (2) the use of irinotecan- or oxaliplatin-based regimens; (3) the sequence of treatments; (4) the duration and schedule of treatments and (5) full dose or reduced-dose treatments.

Combination chemotherapy is often the preferred option with the intent of achieving maximum tumour response, despite the higher risk of toxicity compared to monotherapy. But the use of combination chemotherapy can be particularly challenging for many older patients with frailty. The MRC FOCUS trial challenged this assumption that, in the non-curative setting, maximum tolerable treatment is necessary upfront. This trial showed that combination chemotherapy was not superior to sequential treatment in terms of overall survival. Therefore, starting sequential therapy with fluoropyrimidine alone is a valid option in selected patients with frailty [41]. Similarly, the CAIRO trial investigated whether combination treatment was better than the sequential administration of the same drugs in patients with advanced colorectal cancer. There was no significant difference in overall survival [42]. The OPTIMOX-1 study demonstrated similar survival outcomes between younger and older patients using an approach of combination chemotherapy alternating with 5-FU monotherapy as maintenance [43]. This is therefore a reasonable strategy in selected older patients to minimise toxicity. Alternatively, the OPTIMOX-2 approach consisted of alternating between treatment and chemotherapy-free intervals. This resulted in worse survival outcomes, particularly in patients with poor prognosis [44]. However, chemotherapy-free intervals can be considered in selected patients particularly those with frailty.

The MCR FOCUS2 study recruited patients to 4 different arms investigating fluoropyrimidines only and combinations with oxaliplatin (FOLFOX and CAPOX) at either full- or reduced-dose which could be escalated if no toxicity [45]. This study also used a novel composite measure, overall treatment utility (OTU) which consisted of the clinician assessment of the treatment efficacy, the treatment toxicity and the patient feedback in hindsight regarding their experience of undergoing treatment. This study showed that the addition of oxaliplatin to fluoropyrimidine alone did not result in a significant change in progression free survival (median 5.8 months vs. 4.5 months; HR 0.84, 95% CI 0.69–1.01, $p = 0.07$). However, the use of oxaliplatin-based combinations was one of the strongest predictors of a good OTU at 3 months, in univariate analysis. The addition of oxaliplatin did not significantly increase grade ≥3 toxicities (38% vs. 32%; $p = 0.17$), this was higher with capecitabine than with 5-FU (40% vs. 30%; $p = 0.03$).

The NORDIC9 study investigated randomised older patients (aged 70+) who were not candidates for standard combination chemotherapy, to full dose fluoropyrimidine alone versus reduced-dose fluoropyrimidine with oxaliplatin [46]. This was a non-inferiority study with quality of life at 9 weeks as the primary endpoint. The investigators concluded that dose-reduced combination chemotherapy may be recommended in more vulnerable older patients. The FNCLCC/GERICO 02 study investigated the effect of oxaliplatin-based combination on the functional ability of older patients (aged 70+) and in 90% of patients their function ability for activities of daily living was maintained or improved after 3 cycles of treatment [47].

When selecting a chemotherapy drug, there is no evidence to support a certain sequence over another. But the toxicity profile, particularly for these older patients with frailty, is a key consideration in this selection. Irinotecan causes more alopecia, neutropenia and diarrhoea, whilst oxaliplatin is more associated with polyneuropathy which can significantly impact daily life activities.

Therefore, the incorporation of geriatric assessments can help guide the decision making for these complex patients. A study found that following geriatric assessments, those patients undergoing palliative chemotherapy with malnutrition and frailty had an increased mortality risk [48]. Another example is the previously described GERICO study which randomised older frail patients (aged 70+ with positive G8 screening) undergoing chemotherapy to receive comprehensive geriatric assessment or standard care [37]. About 40% of patients were receiving chemotherapy in the setting of metastatic disease. More patients in the interventional arm completed the scheduled chemotherapy (45% vs. 28%, $P = 0.0366$) and an improvement in different aspects of quality of life was also observed. This highlights the need to further support these patients through the treatment plan.

Overall, intense combination chemotherapy strategies may not be appropriate for older patients with frailty and a metastatic colorectal cancer. Therefore, monotherapy approaches and the use of doublets with low toxicity, potentially with adapted schedules and/or doses, are the most suitable options. Best supportive care should also be considered for patients not eligible for chemotherapy.

Biological Targeted Agents

Monoclonal antibodies (bevacizumab) or proteins (aflibercept) against vascular endothelial growth factor (VEGF) and the monoclonal antibody (cetuximab or panitumumab) against the epidermal growth factor receptor (EGFR) in combination with chemotherapy should be considered in patients with metastatic colorectal cancer to improve survival outcomes. Only trials with a combination of chemotherapy and a biological targeted treatment consistently reported a median overall survival exceeding 24 months [49].

Based on the available data, fluoropyrimidine-based monotherapy plus bevacizumab is currently considered a standard upfront treatment for older patients, irrespective of RAS (Rat sarcoma viral oncogene homolog) status, based on the result of the phase III open-label AVEX trial. Patients aged ≥70 years were randomised to receive capecitabine with or without bevacizumab. Among 280 randomised patients, the addition of bevacizumab improved progression free survival, the primary endpoint (9.1 versus 5.1 months; HR 0.53, 95% CI 0.41–0.69; $p < 0.0001$), as well as the overall response rate (19% versus 10%; $p = 0.04$); the difference in overall survival, a secondary end point, was not statistically significant (20.7 months versus 16.8 months; HR 0.79, 95% CI 0.57–1.09; $p = 0.18$) [50]. However, an increase in thromboembolic events is observed in patients >65 years [50, 51].

The anti-EGFR antibodies cetuximab and panitumumab are active in different lines of treatment and as a single agent or in various combinations. These are usually well tolerated and can be an appropriate option for the majority of older patients with frailty, since they are associated mainly with cutaneous toxicity which is easily managed and the concerns are primarily related with the chemotherapy component when delivered within combination regimens [52, 53]. Hypomagnesaemia is another class-related side effect which requires monitoring. Importantly, the data available of these agents from clinical trials does not reflect the general older patients nor those with frailty, since in 93% of these trials the median age of the included population was <65 years old with minimal comorbidities [54]. Cetuximab has a similar efficacy and safety profile for younger and older patients [55]. Moreover, its use in combination with chemotherapy in selected older patients is an effective therapy [56]. Panitumumab in the context of older patients was investigated in the PANDA phase 2 trial, which randomised older patients (aged 70+) to receive FOLFOX plus panitumumab or 5-FU plus panitumumab for up to 12 cycles followed by panitumumab maintenance until progressive disease [57]. Patients were stratified based on age (75 years cut-off), performance status and geriatric assessment with G8 tool. The primary endpoint was progression free survival which was similar in both arms (9.6 vs 9.1 months). However, there was more high-grade toxicity in the FOLFOX plus panitumumab arm. Therefore, 5-FU plus panitumumab followed by maintenance panitumumab is a more appropriate option for older patients with frailty. Lastly, single-agent panitumumab has also been shown to be an effective and well-tolerated first-line treatment for older patients with frailty deemed unfit for chemotherapy [58]. Nonetheless, the use of anti-EGFRs is limited to patients in whom a RAS mutation is excluded. Therefore, the knowledge of the RAS status is a prerequisite for the use of an anti-EGFR antibody.

There are other targeted agents available, however with limited data for older patients, particularly those with frailty. Aflibercept, a recombinant fusion protein, that blocks the activity of VEGF-A, VEGF-B and placenta growth factor, improves survival outcomes and response rates when combined in second line with FOLFIRI in oxaliplatin pre-treated patients, whether or not the patients were pre-treated with bevacizumab in first line [59, 60]. Regorafenib is an oral multitargeted multikinase inhibitor with dual antiproliferative and antiangiogenic activity. Results from the CORRECT randomised study [61] showed that, as compared with placebo, regorafenib prolonged overall survival in patients previously treated with all approved standard therapies. Lonsurf is comprised of an antineoplastic thymidine-based nucleoside analogue, trifluridine, and the thymidine phosphorylase (TPase) inhibitor, tipiracil hydrochloride. Trifluridine is cytotoxic antimetabolite, tipiracil is a thymidine phosphorylase inhibitor, it inhibits trifluridine metabolism and has antiangiogenic properties as well [62]. RECOURSE study confirmed clinically meaningful and statistically significant survival benefit of Lonsurf plus best supportive care compared to placebo plus best supportive care improving overall survival to 7.2 months from 5.2 months [63]. It is commonly used third line treatment for metastatic colon cancer. It is generally well tolerated by patients without any significant side effects.

Conclusion

Older patients with colorectal cancer are widely under-represented within clinical trials despite their prevalence within cancer services. Consequently, there is an insufficiency in the evidence that is available. This can create difficulties for the treating oncologist seeking guidance in managing this particular patient group. Historically, age alone was a factor which may have determined a patient's treatment plan. More recently there has been a rise in focus on our older populations and geriatric assessment tools have been increasingly implemented in clinical practice. In early-stage disease, clinical discussions are based around the ability of older patients to undergo successful curative surgical procedures. Where adjuvant therapy may be contemplated a risk versus benefit approach should be used considering other concomitant conditions and life expectancy. In patients with metastatic disease, the focus is often surrounding a patient's suitability to proceed with systemic treatments such as chemotherapy with a primary focus on low toxicity regimens. Careful considerations are to be made with regard to comorbidities, baseline organ function and the toxicity profile of the treatment. Chronological age should not be considered in insolation. Furthermore, increased risks can be reduced with simple adjustments to regimens and dosage, allowing one to minimise toxicity without comprising benefit and negatively impacting on the patient's quality of life. Individual case discussions are encouraged to reach the best outcomes for patients. Clear, concise discussions need to take place between the oncologist, the patient and their families to ensure a fully informed decision can be reached. Multidisciplinary discussions are pivotal to ensuring the patient is offered the most suitable treatment and to avoid under or over treating. Using a frailty score can aid the accurate assessment of an individual, thus aiding the creation of a truly personalised care plan.

References

1. Noone AM, Howlader N, Krapcho M, Miller D, Brest A, Yu M, Ruhl J, Tatalovich Z, Mariotto A, Lewis DR, Chen HS, Feuer EJ, Cronin KA. SEER Cancer Statistics Review, 1975–2015. https://seer.cancer.gov/csr/1975_2015/, based on November 2017 SEER data submission, posted to the SEER web site, April 2018.: National Cancer Institute; 2018.
2. Handforth C, Clegg A, Young C, Simpkins S, Seymour MT, Selby PJ, et al. The prevalence and outcomes of frailty in older cancer patients: a systematic review. Ann Oncol. 2015;26(6):1091–101.

3. Soler G, Ruffinelli Rodriguez JC, Legido R, Martinez Villacampa M, Perez FJ, Pardo-Burdalo B, et al. Detection of frailty in elderly colorectal càncer patients: Is G8 a good screening tool? Ann Oncol. 2018;29:viii191.
4. Boakye D, Rillmann B, Walter V, Jansen L, Hoffmeister M, Brenner H. Impact of comorbidity and frailty on prognosis in colorectal cancer patients: a systematic review and meta-analysis. Cancer Treat Rev. 2018;64:30–9.
5. Extermann M, Aapro M, Bernabei R, Cohen HJ, Droz JP, Lichtman S, et al. Use of comprehensive geriatric assessment in older cancer patients: recommendations from the task force on CGA of the International Society of Geriatric Oncology (SIOG). Crit Rev Oncol Hematol. 2005;55(3):241–52.
6. Wildiers H, Kenis C. Comprehensive geriatric assessment (CGA) in older oncological patients: Why and how? J Geriatr Oncol. 2012;3(2):174–6.
7. Shaukat A, Kahi CJ, Burke CA, Rabeneck L, Sauer BG, Rex DK. ACG clinical guidelines: colorectal cancer screening 2021. Am J Gastroenterol. 2021;116(3):458–79.
8. Ma W, Wang K, Nguyen LH, Joshi A, Cao Y, Nishihara R, et al. Association of screening lower endoscopy with colorectal cancer incidence and mortality in adults older than 75 years. JAMA Oncol. 2021;7(7):985–92.
9. Gooiker GA, Dekker JWT, Bastiaannet E, van der Geest LGM, Merkus JWS, van de Velde CJH, et al. Risk factors for excess mortality in the first year after curative surgery for colorectal cancer. Ann Surg Oncol. 2012;19(8):2428–34.
10. Dekker JW, Gooiker GA, Bastiaannet E, van den Broek CB, van der Geest LG, van de Velde CJ, et al. Cause of death the first year after curative colorectal cancer surgery; a prolonged impact of the surgery in elderly colorectal cancer patients. Eur J Surg Oncol. 2014;40(11):1481–7.
11. Hines RB, Chatla C, Bumpers HL, Waterbor JW, McGwin G Jr, Funkhouser E, et al. Predictive capacity of three comorbidity indices in estimating mortality after surgery for colon cancer. J Clin Oncol. 2009;27(26):4339–45.
12. Gröne J, Kreis ME. Personalized treatment of colorectal cancer in old age. Der Chirurg; Zeitschrift fur alle Gebiete der operativen Medizen. 2013;84(4):305–9.
13. Jafari MD, Jafari F, Halabi WJ, Nguyen VQ, Pigazzi A, Carmichael JC, et al. Colorectal cancer resections in the aging US population: a trend toward decreasing rates and improved outcomes. JAMA Surg. 2014;149(6):557–64.
14. Fagard K, Leonard S, Deschodt M, Devriendt E, Wolthuis A, Prenen H, et al. The impact of frailty on postoperative outcomes in individuals aged 65 and over undergoing elective surgery for colorectal cancer: a systematic review. J Geriatr Oncol. 2016;7(6):479–91.
15. Souwer ETD, Bastiaannet E, Steyerberg EW, Dekker J-WT, van den Bos F, Portielje JEA. Risk prediction models for postoperative outcomes of colorectal cancer surgery in the older population - a systematic review. J Geriatr Oncol. 2020;11(8):1217–28.
16. Kristjansson SR, Rønning B, Hurria A, Skovlund E, Jordhøy MS, Nesbakken A, et al. A comparison of two pre-operative frailty measures in older surgical cancer patients. J Geriatr Oncol. 2012;3(1):1–7.
17. Snowden CP, Prentis J, Jacques B, Anderson H, Manas D, Jones D, et al. Cardiorespiratory fitness predicts mortality and hospital length of stay after major elective surgery in older people. Ann Surg. 2013;257(6):999–1004.
18. Chan KE, Pathak S, Smart NJ, Batchelor N, Daniels IR. The impact of cardiopulmonary exercise testing on patients over the age of 80 undergoing elective colorectal cancer surgery. Colorectal Dis. 2016;18(6):578–85.
19. Swart M, Carlisle JB. Case-controlled study of critical care or surgical ward care after elective open colorectal surgery. Br J Surg. 2012;99(2):295–9.
20. Kim YJ. Colorectal cancer surgery in elderly patients. Ann Coloproctol. 2017;33(4):121–2.
21. Antoniou SA, Antoniou GA, Koch OO, Pointner R, Granderath FA. Laparoscopic colorectal surgery confers lower mortality in the elderly: a systematic review and meta-analysis of 66,483 patients. Surg Endosc. 2015;29(2):322–33.

22. Hamaker ME, Prins MC, Schiphorst AH, van Tuyl SA, Pronk A, van den Bos F. Long-term changes in physical capacity after colorectal cancer treatment. J Geriatr Oncol. 2015;6(2):153–64.
23. Bagnall NM, Malietzis G, Kennedy RH, Athanasiou T, Faiz O, Darzi A. A systematic review of enhanced recovery care after colorectal surgery in elderly patients. Colorectal Dis. 2014;16(12):947–56.
24. Snijders HS, van den Broek CB, Wouters MW, Meershoek-Klein Kranenbarg E, Wiggers T, Rutten H, et al. An increasing use of defunctioning stomas after low anterior resection for rectal cancer. Is this the way to go? Eur J Surg Oncol. 2013;39(7):715–20.
25. Papamichael D, Audisio RA, Glimelius B, de Gramont A, Glynne-Jones R, Haller D, et al. Treatment of colorectal cancer in older patients: International Society of Geriatric Oncology (SIOG) consensus recommendations 2013. Ann Oncol. 2015;26(3):463–76.
26. Erlandsson J, Holm T, Pettersson D, Berglund Å, Cedermark B, Radu C, et al. Optimal fractionation of preoperative radiotherapy and timing to surgery for rectal cancer (Stockholm III): a multicentre, randomised, non-blinded, phase 3, non-inferiority trial. Lancet Oncol. 2017;18(3):336–46.
27. Martijn H, Vulto JC. Should radiotherapy be avoided or delivered differently in elderly patients with rectal cancer? Eur J Cancer (Oxford, England: 1990). 2007;43(15):2301–6.
28. Kennedy ED, Schmocker S, Victor C, Baxter NN, Kim J, Brierley J, et al. Do patients consider preoperative chemoradiation for primary rectal cancer worthwhile? Cancer. 2011;117(13):2853–62.
29. Argilés G, Tabernero J, Labianca R, Hochhauser D, Salazar R, Iveson T, et al. Localised colon cancer: ESMO Clinical Practice Guidelines for diagnosis, treatment and follow-up. Ann Oncol. 2020;31(10):1291–305.
30. Haller DG, O'Connell MJ, Cartwright TH, Twelves CJ, McKenna EF, Sun W, et al. Impact of age and medical comorbidity on adjuvant treatment outcomes for stage III colon cancer: a pooled analysis of individual patient data from four randomized, controlled trials. Ann Oncol. 2015;26(4):715–24.
31. Rosati G, Galli F, Lonardi S, Dotti KF, Ronzoni M, Zampino MG, et al. Oxaliplatin plus fluoropyrimidines as adjuvant therapy for colon cancer in elderly patients: a subgroup analysis from TOSCA trial. Ann Oncol. 2020;31:S410–S1.
32. Labianca R, Lonardi S, Rosati G, Di Bartolomeo M, Ronzoni M, Pella N, et al. FOLFOX4/XELOX in stage II–III colon cancer: efficacy and safety results of the Italian Three Or Six Colon Adjuvant (TOSCA) trial. Ann Oncol. 2017;28:v614.
33. André T, Meyerhardt J, Iveson T, Sobrero A, Yoshino T, Souglakos I, et al. Effect of duration of adjuvant chemotherapy for patients with stage III colon cancer (IDEA collaboration): final results from a prospective, pooled analysis of six randomised, phase 3 trials. Lancet Oncol. 2020;21(12):1620–9.
34. Iveson TJ, Sobrero AF, Yoshino T, Souglakos I, Ou F-S, Meyers JP, et al. Duration of adjuvant doublet chemotherapy (3 or 6 months) in patients with high-risk stage II colorectal cancer. J Clin Oncol. 2021;39(6):631–41.
35. Twelves C, Scheithauer W, McKendrick J, Seitz JF, Van Hazel G, Wong A, et al. Capecitabine versus 5-fluorouracil/folinic acid as adjuvant therapy for stage III colon cancer: final results from the X-ACT trial with analysis by age and preliminary evidence of a pharmacodynamic marker of efficacy. Ann Oncol. 2012;23(5):1190–7.
36. Chintala L, Vaka S, Baranda J, Williamson SK. Capecitabine versus 5-fluorouracil in colorectal cancer: where are we now? Oncol Rev. 2011;5(2):129–40.
37. Lund CM, Vistisen KK, Olsen AP, Bardal P, Schultz M, Dolin TG, et al. The effect of geriatric intervention in frail older patients receiving chemotherapy for colorectal cancer: a randomised trial (GERICO). Br J Cancer. 2021;124(12):1949–58.
38. Schmoll HJ, Van Cutsem E, Stein A, Valentini V, Glimelius B, Haustermans K, et al. ESMO Consensus Guidelines for management of patients with colon and rectal cancer. a personalized approach to clinical decision making. Ann Oncol. 2012;23(10):2479–516.

39. Van Cutsem E, Cervantes A, Nordlinger B, Arnold D. Metastatic colorectal cancer: ESMO Clinical Practice Guidelines for diagnosis, treatment and follow-up. Ann Oncol. 2014;25(Suppl 3):iii1–9.
40. Hamaker ME, van Rixtel B, Thunnissen P, Oberndorff AH, Smakman N, ten Bokkel HD. Multidisciplinary decision-making on chemotherapy for colorectal cancer: an age-based comparison. J Geriatr Oncol. 2015;6(3):225–32.
41. Seymour MT, Maughan TS, Ledermann JA, Topham C, James R, Gwyther SJ, et al. Different strategies of sequential and combination chemotherapy for patients with poor prognosis advanced colorectal cancer (MRC FOCUS): a randomised controlled trial. Lancet (London, England). 2007;370(9582):143–52.
42. Koopman M, Antonini NF, Douma J, Wals J, Honkoop AH, Erdkamp FL, et al. Sequential versus combination chemotherapy with capecitabine, irinotecan, and oxaliplatin in advanced colorectal cancer (CAIRO): a phase III randomised controlled trial. Lancet (London, England). 2007;370(9582):135–42.
43. Figer A, Perez-Staub N, Carola E, Tournigand C, Lledo G, Flesch M, et al. FOLFOX in patients aged between 76 and 80 years with metastatic colorectal cancer: an exploratory cohort of the OPTIMOX1 study. Cancer. 2007;110(12):2666–71.
44. Maindrault-Goebel F, Lledo G, Chibaudel B, Mineur L, Andre T, Bennamoun M, et al. Final results of OPTIMOX2, a large randomized phase II study of maintenance therapy or chemotherapy-free intervals (CFI) after FOLFOX in patients with metastatic colorectal cancer (MRC): a GERCOR study. J Clin Oncol. 2007;25(18_suppl):4013.
45. Seymour MT, Thompson LC, Wasan HS, Middleton G, Brewster AE, Shepherd SF, et al. Chemotherapy options in elderly and frail patients with metastatic colorectal cancer (MRC FOCUS2): an open-label, randomised factorial trial. Lancet (London, England). 2011;377(9779):1749–59.
46. Liposits G, Eshøj HR, Möller S, Winther SB, Skuladottir H, Ryg J, et al. Quality of life in vulnerable older patients with metastatic colorectal cancer receiving palliative chemotherapy—the randomized NORDIC9-study. Cancers. 2021;13(11):2604.
47. Rousseau F, Bugat R, Ducreux M, Cvitkovic F, Carola E, Gisselbrecht M, et al. Effect of XELOX on functional ability among elderly patients with metastatic colorectal cancer: results from the FNCLCC/GERICO 02 phase II study. J Geriatr Oncol. 2011;2(2):105–11.
48. Aaldriks AA, van der Geest LGM, Giltay EJ, le Cessie S, Portielje JEA, Tanis BC, et al. Frailty and malnutrition predictive of mortality risk in older patients with advanced colorectal cancer receiving chemotherapy. J Geriatr Oncol. 2013;4(3):218–26.
49. Sorbye H, Cvancarova M, Qvortrup C, Pfeiffer P, Glimelius B. Age-dependent improvement in median and long-term survival in unselected population-based Nordic registries of patients with synchronous metastatic colorectal cancer. Ann Oncol. 2013;24(9):2354–60.
50. Cunningham D, Lang I, Marcuello E, Lorusso V, Ocvirk J, Shin DB, et al. Bevacizumab plus capecitabine versus capecitabine alone in elderly patients with previously untreated metastatic colorectal cancer (AVEX): an open-label, randomised phase 3 trial. Lancet Oncol. 2013;14(11):1077–85.
51. Cassidy J, Saltz LB, Giantonio BJ, Kabbinavar FF, Hurwitz HI, Rohr UP. Effect of bevacizumab in older patients with metastatic colorectal cancer: pooled analysis of four randomized studies. J Cancer Res Clin Oncol. 2010;136(5):737–43.
52. Gilabert M, Ries P, Chanez B, Triby S, Francois E, Lièvre A, et al. Place of anti-EGFR therapy in older patients with metastatic colorectal cancer in 2020. J Geriatr Oncol. 2020;11(8):1229–36.
53. Swierkowski M, Ptak-Chmielewska A, Sliwczynski A, Czeleko T, Teter Z, Szczylik C. Efficacy of panitumumab and cetuximab in elderly patients (aged ≥75) with chemotherapy-refractory wild-type KRAS exon 2 metastatic colorectal cancer (mCRC): retrospective analysis of data from nationwide drug-reimbursement-access program. Ann Oncol 2017;28:v178.
54. Gouverneur A, Salvo F, Berdaï D, Moore N, Fourrier-Réglat A, Noize P. Inclusion of elderly or frail patients in randomized controlled trials of targeted therapies for the treatment of metastatic colorectal cancer: a systematic review. J Geriatr Oncol. 2018;9(1):15–23.

55. Jehn CF, Böning L, Kröning H, Possinger K, Lüftner D. Cetuximab-based therapy in elderly comorbid patients with metastatic colorectal cancer. Br J Cancer. 2012;106(2):274–8.
56. Mineur L, François E, Phelip JM, Guimbaud R, Plassot C, Smith DM, et al. Cetuximab (CTX) in first-line treatment of elderly patients with metastatic colorectal cancer (mCRC), KRAS wild type: French multicentre prospective community-based registry and results. J Clin Oncol. 2017;35(4_suppl):760.
57. Lonardi S, Schirripa M, Buggin F, Antonuzzo L, Merelli B, Boscolo G, et al. First-line FOLFOX plus panitumumab versus 5FU plus panitumumab in RAS-BRAF wild-type metastatic colorectal cancer elderly patients: The PANDA study. J Clin Oncol. 2020;38(15_suppl):4002.
58. Pietrantonio F, Cremolini C, Aprile G, Lonardi S, Orlandi A, Mennitto A, et al. Single-Agent panitumumab in frail elderly patients with advanced RAS and BRAF wild-type colorectal cancer: challenging drug label to light up new hope. Oncologist. 2015;20(11):1261–5.
59. Van Cutsem E, Tabernero J, Lakomy R, Prenen H, Prausová J, Macarulla T, et al. Addition of aflibercept to fluorouracil, leucovorin, and irinotecan improves survival in a phase III randomized trial in patients with metastatic colorectal cancer previously treated with an oxaliplatin-based regimen. J Clin Oncol. 2012;30(28):3499–506.
60. Tabernero J, Van Cutsem E, Lakomý R, Prausová J, Ruff P, van Hazel GA, et al. Aflibercept versus placebo in combination with fluorouracil, leucovorin and irinotecan in the treatment of previously treated metastatic colorectal cancer: prespecified subgroup analyses from the VELOUR trial. Eur J Cancer (Oxford, England: 1990). 2014;50(2):320–31.
61. Grothey A, Van Cutsem E, Sobrero A, Siena S, Falcone A, Ychou M, et al. Regorafenib monotherapy for previously treated metastatic colorectal cancer (CORRECT): an international, multicentre, randomised, placebo-controlled, phase 3 trial. Lancet (London, England). 2013;381(9863):303–12.
62. Lenz HJ, Stintzing S, Loupakis F. TAS-102, a novel antitumor agent: a review of the mechanism of action. Cancer Treat Rev. 2015;41(9):777–83.
63. Mayer RJ, Van Cutsem E, Falcone A, Yoshino T, Garcia-Carbonero R, Mizunuma N, et al. Randomized trial of TAS-102 for refractory metastatic colorectal cancer. N Engl J Med. 2015;372(20):1909–19.

Chapter 20
Prostate Cancer in Older Adults with Frailty

Andrea Luciani, Cristina Falci, Fausto Petrelli, and Giuseppe Colloca

Introduction

Prostate cancer represents the second most common malignancy among males, after lung cancer, with above 1.2 million new cases registered worldwide according to GLOBOCAN 2020 estimates [1]. Aging is a key risk factor and in the population of the United States of America, it is estimated that 1 in 12 adults above 70 years will develop prostate cancer [2, 3]. While the median age at diagnosis of prostate cancer is 66 years, the proportion of older adults is expected to continue increasing due to the fast aging of western populations [4]. In fact, it is projected that by 2040 patients aged 65 years and older will represent 70% of new cases [5]. While the median age of patients who die because of prostate cancer is 80 years, many older adults with prostate cancer will die from competing causes, particularly if comorbid and with frailty [6, 7].

In 2010, Bechis et al. studied the impact of age on prostate cancer treatment delivery and mortality by using data from the Cancer of the Prostate Strategic Urologic Research Endeavor (CaPSURE), a longitudinal, observational disease registry of men with biopsy-proven prostate cancer [8]. In total, 11,790 patients with localized disease (clinical stage up to T3aN0M0) were considered for analysis, of which 1706 were aged ≥75 years. Regarding this older cohort, 26% presented with high-risk disease, compared to 10–18% in the younger cohorts. Moreover, the older cohort had a significantly higher risk of cancer-specific

A. Luciani (✉) · F. Petrelli
Medical Oncology Department, ASST-Bergamo Ovest, Treviglio, Italy
e-mail: andrea_luciani@asst-bgovest.it

C. Falci
Medical Oncology Department, Istituti Oncologico Veneto, Padova, Italy
e-mail: cristina.falci@ioveneto.it

G. Colloca
Geriatric Unit, Policlinico Gemelli, Rome, Italy

F. Gomes (ed.), *Frailty in Older Adults with Cancer*,
https://doi.org/10.1007/978-3-030-89162-6_20

mortality (HR = 1.86, 95% CI 1.17–2.97, $p = 0.009$) compared to those younger than 55 years of age. Older men were also more likely to receive just hormone therapy and after controlling for possible confounders like comorbidity burden, older men with high-risk tumors receiving local therapy had a 46% reduction in mortality compared with those treated conservatively. The author concluded that treatment decisions in older adults with prostate cancer should be driven by disease prognostic factors and tumor-independent life expectancy rather than chronological age alone.

If we consider that older adults may present with more high-risk disease and higher cancer-specific mortality, as above-described, that raises the question about the value of prostate cancer screening in the older population. In 2018, the United States of America preventive services task force updated the 2012 recommendations and classified as "low value" any prostate-specific antigen (PSA)-based screening performed in men aged 70 years or older [9]. Controversially, some authors strongly support PSA screening of prostate cancer for high-risk men, including African Americans, men with family history of prostate cancer and men aged 70–80 (provided they are healthy since they have a higher chance of high-risk tumors) [10, 11]. But if the rationale of prolonging PSA screening beyond the cut-off of 70 years may be discussed for patients who enjoy relatively good health (that means an estimated ≥10-years life expectancy), patients with frailty should be excluded from prostate cancer screening strategies. In fact, people aged ≥70 years who are in the lowest health condition quartile, have an estimated life expectancy shorter than 10 years, ranging from 6.7 years at 70 years, to 4.9 years at 75 years, 3.3 years at 80 years, until 2.2 years at 85 years [12].

Ultimately, the optimal management of older men with prostate cancer and frailty, both in the early and in the metastatic setting is challenging and represents a public health worry that is expected to further increase in the next decades [13]. This chapter will review the current evidence regarding the treatment of prostate cancer in older patients with frailty, from an early stage to a metastatic setting.

Frailty in Patients with Prostate Cancer

Frailty is defined as a state of increased vulnerability toward stressors due to a multisystem reduction in reserve capacity [2]. Frailty is more prevalent with increasing age, but high chronological age does not necessarily lead to frailty. In the scenario of older adults with cancer, a systematic review in 2015 by Handforth et al. assessed the prevalence of frailty [14]. A total of 20 studies were included with 2916 cancer patients aged ≥70 years, which identified a median prevalence of frailty of 42%. These patients have an increased risk of toxicity from medical treatment, radiation therapy, and postoperative complications after cancer surgery [14]. Moreover, frailty is associated with other negative outcomes such as institutionalization, functional decline, and mortality [15].

In the setting of prostate cancer, few studies described the geriatric features of this population, such as frailty. A study from the Surveillance, Epidemiology and

End Results-Medicare (SEER-Medicare), explored the life expectancy in a population-based cohort of 96,032 men aged >65 years with early-stage prostate cancer with Gleason scores ≤7 [16]. The proportion of patients with a Charlson comorbidity index score of 0 (low burden of comorbidity) at diagnosis was between 75 and 81% in patients aged 66–79 but this proportion dropped to 33% in patients aged 80+. The life expectancy was shorter than 10 years for men aged 66–69 with Charlson scores ≥2, men aged 70–74 with Charlson scores ≥1 and men aged 75+ regardless of comorbidity status. Another study using the SEER database focused on the relationships between age, comorbidity, and the natural history of prostate cancer [17]. The cumulative, not cancer-specific mortality rates were 24%, 33%, 46%, and 57% for men with 0, 1, 2, and ≥3 comorbidities, respectively. In contrast, the rates of cancer-specific mortality (at the same time point) were much lower at 3%, 7%, and 18% for men with low-, intermediate-, and high-risk prostate cancer. Lastly, a prospective cohort study recruited 181 men aged ≥70 years with histologically proven prostate cancer, early stage, with any primary tumor size and Gleason score, who were deemed candidates to receive radiotherapy and endocrine treatment [18]. Patients completed a comprehensive geriatric assessment (CGA) and 31% were defined as having "CGA needs," i.e., they had at least one component of the geriatric assessments impaired. This is notable if one considers that this study population was favorably selected and included only patients deemed eligible for cancer treatment.

The International Society of Geriatric Oncology (SIOG) has published guidelines for the management of the older adult with prostate cancer and three treatment-oriented categories of older adults with cancer, which could be identified from geriatric assessment—fit, vulnerable, and frail were outlined [13]. Whilst the "fit" older adults should receive full treatment similar to a fit younger patient, the "frail" older person should be offered mainly palliative care. The intermediate category, the older "vulnerable" person, would need an individualized approach [13]. The most recent recommendations by SIOG on prostate cancer further emphasize the use of geriatric assessments to guide these treatment decisions rather than age alone [19]. Ultimately, treatment decisions should take into account the risk of dying from prostate cancer (e.g., tumor grade and stage) vs other causes (e.g., comorbidities burden and frailty), and also the patient individual risk with a treatment and their preferences and goals of care [19, 20].

Management of Early-Stage and locally Advanced Prostate Cancer

Localized prostate cancer is divided into risk groups, high, medium and low, which help guide treatments decisions depending on how likely it is that cancer will grow quickly or spread. The risk group depends on the size of the tumor, the grade of the tumor (Gleason score), and the PSA level. For example, a high-risk disease means the patient has a large tumor or a high-grade tumor or a high PSA level

High Risk Localized Disease and Locally Advanced Disease

There are several treatment options that may be considered in this setting. Nonetheless, Vernooij et al. performed a population-based study in the Netherlands where the survival rates of older patients with localized high-risk disease remained lower compared with younger patients due to the suboptimal treatment received [21].

An analysis of SEER-Medicare database revealed that among men aged ≥75 years and diagnosed with locally advanced or high-risk screen-detected cancers, only 40% received androgen deprivation therapy (ADT) alone [22]. This real-world non-randomized study was performed to verify the advantage of ADT plus radiotherapy versus ADT alone (previously reported in two randomized trials [23, 24]) in older patients with high-risk locally advanced prostate cancer. ADT plus radiotherapy was associated with survival benefits of similar magnitude in older men aged 76–85 years with locally advanced prostate cancer and older men aged 65–85 years with screen-detected high-risk prostate cancer [22].

Regarding surgery with radical prostatectomy, a retrospective study included 1008 patients with high-risk prostate cancer who underwent this treatment across 14 centers between 1988 and 2014.

Age and Charlson Comorbidity Index were the major determinants of other-cause mortality, but their impact on cancer-specific mortality was minimal. Therefore, patients aged 60 years or above died primarily from other causes and when patients had Charlson score ≥2, no deaths were related to prostate cancer. Focusing on this, Sivaraman et al. performed a retrospective analysis on 7651 older patients (aged 70+) with high-risk disease to identify the appropriate level of Charlson Comorbidity Index in order to achieve survival benefit from radical prostatectomy. When patients had Charlson ≥2, all the recorded deaths in the study (40.7%) were related to other causes (not cancer), highlighting the importance of the competing causes of death. Another similar analysis of a multi-institutional cohort of 3828 men treated with radical prostatectomy for high-risk prostate cancer also showed that the cancer-specific mortality rate for these patients was 5.9%, while the mortality from other causes was 14.3%. Age and Charlson Comorbidity Index were again the major determinants of other-cause mortality [25–27].

Therefore, older patients with frailty and high-risk or locally advanced prostate cancer should be considered for upfront active anti-cancer treatment. However, it is key to understand the severity of frailty and the competing comorbid conditions, in order to assess if the prognosis is more likely to be determined by cancer or their overall health status.

Low-Risk Disease

In the context of clinically localized mainly low-risk prostate cancer, the ProtecT study compared the outcomes for watchful waiting, radical prostatectomy, and external-beam radiotherapy in men aged 50–69 years between 1999 and 2009 [28]. A total of 2664 patients received a diagnosis of localized prostate cancer and 1643 were randomized (1:1:1) to observation, radical prostatectomy, or radiotherapy. At a median of 10 years follow-up, cancer-specific survival was at least 98.8% in all treatment groups, with no significant difference between them. This study highlighted the potential harm of overtreatment in this low-risk group of patients, in terms of costs and morbidity [28].

The Scandinavian Prostate Cancer Group Study Number 4 (SPCG-4) was a randomized trial of radical prostatectomy versus watchful waiting in men with localized prostate cancer (any age) diagnosed between 1989 and 1999 (before the era of PSA testing). After 23 years of follow-up, this trial found a significant absolute reduction in the rate of death from prostate cancer and in the risk of metastases in the radical-prostatectomy group. However, this benefit was more prominent in those with intermediate-risk disease and younger patients. Patients diagnosed with low-risk disease or aged 65 and above, had no reduction in the risk of death from prostate cancer and had a small yet significant reduction in the risk of metastasis of about 10% [29, 30]. Similar findings were reported by the PIVOT trial [29, 31].

Lu Yao et al. published a SEER database analysis of 31,137 men aged ≥65 years (median age at diagnosis of 75 years) diagnosed with stage T1–T2 prostate cancer during 1992–2009 and managed initially conservatively (i.e., no active treatment at diagnosis). For men with Gleason 5–7 disease, the 15-year cancer-specific mortality was 5.7% for men aged 65–74 years and 10% for men aged ≥75 years. However, for men with Gleason 8–10, the cancer-specific mortality rates were 22% and 27%, respectively. Analysis by comorbidity status showed that patients with a comorbidity score of 0 had mortality rates similar to the entire group, whereas patients with a higher comorbidity score had lower cancer-specific mortality rates because of deaths from competing risks [32].

Therefore, the available evidence suggests that for older patients with frailty and low-risk disease, a conservative approach, such as watchful waiting is the most appropriate option.

Intermediate Risk Disease

As described in the above sub-sections, in this context there is a stronger rationale to offer upfront anti-cancer treatment. Yet these older patients are still less likely to be offered active treatment compared to their younger counterparts. In a hospital-based database, 40–45% of patients over 80 years old did not receive radical treatment [33]. But data from the SEER database showed how an active treatment could produce a survival benefit in this setting, even in older patients [34, 35]. The problematic however is the presence of frailty and often significant comorbidities, which may deem upfront active treatment inappropriate, favoring instead a conservative approach for the majority of these older patients with frailty and intermediate-risk disease. Ultimately, this should always be an individualized decision and geriatric assessment will support this decision-making.

Management of Advanced Metastatic Prostate Cancer

As is the case in localized/locally advanced disease, treatment of advanced prostate cancer is dictated by a preliminary evaluation of risk factors. The initial management will depend on a pretreatment assessment of the patients' life expectancy and overall medical condition (including comorbidities and frailty). Moreover, there is a wide range of cancer-specific considerations, such as the presence or absence of symptoms, the clinical TNM staging, the burden/volume of the disease (e.g., the number of metastatic sites), the pretreatment PSA level, the Gleason score in the pretreatment biopsy and the results of pretreatment imaging studies (showing, for example, the site of bone fractures, nodal compression or visceral disease) [19].

Hormone-Sensitive Disease

The mainstay of treatment for hormone-sensitive prostate cancer is ADT with luteinizing hormone-releasing hormone (LHRH) analogs (e.g., goserelin, leuprorelin) or antiandrogens (e.g., bicalutamide). Despite the obvious implications in sexual activity and satisfaction, a large prospective observational study conducted on a large cohort of more than 1000 patients (25% of those had metastatic prostate cancer) showed that the other domains of health-related quality of life (HRQoL) are improved or unchanged with the LHRH agonist therapy [36]. However, it is important to note that the use of ADT in the medium-long term is associated with a wide range of issues, such as the increased risk of osteopenic bone fracture and metabolic syndrome with cardiovascular disease [37–40]. This is described in more detail in a subsequent section, as these are of particular concern for those older patients with frailty.

The addition of other systemic agents (antiandrogens or chemotherapy) is a common strategy in metastatic hormone-sensitive prostate cancer. The LATITUDE (Long-Acting Therapy to Improve Treatment Success in Daily Life) study of abiraterone added to ADT showed that the magnitude of benefit in older patients was reduced compared to younger men [41]. In patients older than 75 years (20% of total), the difference in overall survival (OS) was not statistically significant (HR 0.82, 95% CI 0.53–1.27), whereas radiographic progression-free survival (PFS) remained statistically significant. Similarly, in the STAMPEDE study of abiraterone, PFS for men over the age of 70 improved in those receiving abiraterone in addition to ADT. However, differences in prostate cancer-specific mortality (HR 0.80, 95% CI 0.54–1.17) and OS (HR 0.94, 95% CI 0.69–1.29) were not statistically significant [42]. The use of docetaxel in addition to ADT in older patients with metastatic hormone-sensitive prostate cancer was also explored in several studies. In the CHAARTED study, a benefit in OS was confirmed with the addition of docetaxel and this benefit persisted in those over 70 years (HR 0.43, 95% CI 0.23–0.78) [43], but this was not significant in the STAMPEDE study (HR 0.90, 95% CI 0.64–1.26)

[44]. In a pooled analysis of STAMPEDE, CHAARTED, and LATITUDE trials, PFS was significantly better with the addition of docetaxel (HR 0.51, 95% CI 0.42–0.61) or abiraterone (HR 0.48, 95% CI 0.36–0.64) in patients older than 70 years with metastatic hormone-sensitive prostate cancer. However, OS did not improve with either docetaxel (HR 0.86, 95% CI 0.69–1.07) or abiraterone (HR 0.85, 95% CI 0.67–1.08) in this setting.

Therefore, whilst combination strategies are the recommended first-line treatment in healthy older men, for those with more comorbid conditions and frailty, ADT alone may be the most appropriate treatment option. In this context, and despite not being supported by robust data, intermittent ADT may be an appropriate strategy rather than continuous ADT to decrease the medium-long term side effect profile [19].

Hormone-Resistant Disease

Once prostate cancer becomes hormone-resistant, ADT should be continued but associated with further systemic therapies despite the ideal sequence of treatment being unclear. A study investigated the discontinuation of scheduled treatment in older patients with the hormone-resistant disease and documented a high discontinuation rate of 58%. Whilst the leading cause was progressive disease/death, 22% of these cases were due to adverse events/toxicity. Patients aged 80 and above, those with poor performance status as well as those with compromised functional or nutritional status were at a higher risk in bivariate analyses, but an impairment in ADL was the only independent factor for older patients in the multivariate analysis [45]. This highlights the importance of an appropriate decision-making regarding treatment for older patients, particularly with frailty in this setting.

Until recently, docetaxel was the only treatment available to improve OS in this setting, but several other agents have become available such as abiraterone, enzalutamide, radium-223, and cabazitaxel, providing further options to consider before and after docetaxel treatment.

Docetaxel (75 mg/m^2 every 3 weeks) is a chemotherapy option for hormone-resistant prostate cancer, which resulted in similar outcomes in older men, including those ≥75 years [46]. In a pooled analysis of three prospective trials assessing docetaxel/prednisone, an analysis stratified by age (≥vs < 75 years) was performed. Despite no difference in OS between the age groups, older patients were more likely to have adverse events ($p < 0.001$), any fatal adverse events ($p = 0.007$), anemia ($p < 0.001$), and neutropenia ($p < 0.001$) [47]. Older age may affect docetaxel renal clearance and it is well-established that these patients have a higher risk of treatment-induced toxicity [48, 49]. Due to the limited tolerance of chemotherapy in those with frailty, particularly due to myelosuppression-related issues, a lower dose of docetaxel or modified schedules, such as biweekly, should be considered [19, 50, 51]. The use of primary prophylaxis with G-CSF should also be considered. Cabazitaxel is a newer chemotherapy tubulin-binding taxane that was shown to prolong OS in patients with hormone-resistant prostate cancer progressing after docetaxel therapy [52]. In older patients, the toxicity is manageable provided that for patients with more than 75 years old the prophylactic use of G-CSF is guarantee [53]. Ultimately, data on the role of chemotherapy agents in the sub-group of older patients with prostate cancer and frailty is scarce, hence that a decision should be supported by geriatric assessments. But in this setting, chemotherapy options may not be appropriate over best supportive care alone, due to its tolerability, depending on the severity of frailty.

Before treatment with chemotherapy (docetaxel), a newer generation of hormone therapies, either abiraterone or enzalutamide provide significant benefits in men younger and older than 75 years in the setting of minimally symptomatic or asymptomatic hormone-resistant prostate cancer [54, 55]. Even in the real world, the effectiveness and safety of these treatments were relatively similar between older and younger patients; however, treatment discontinuation due to adverse events was more frequent in the older age group [56]. A real-world study focusing on abiraterone also documented that patients with poor performance status were less likely to achieve a 50% reduction on PSA levels and had a shorter time to PSA progression, with shorter time on treatment and shorter overall survival [57]. Enzalutamide showed a better survival outcome when given pre-docetaxel compared to an earlier generation of hormonotherapy, bicalutamide [58]. It significantly reduced the risk of disease progression or death in patients aged 75+ (HR 0.59, 95% CI 0.37–0.92, $p = 0.018$). The time to PSA progression was also significantly prolonged with enzalutamide vs bicalutamide in these older patients. There were some differences in terms of adverse events between older (75+) and younger patients. For example, atrial fibrillation, urinary tract infections, falls, decreased appetite were more common in the older sub-group on enzalutamide. In the randomized PREVAIL study, comparing enzalutamide to placebo in hormone-resistant prostate cancer before chemotherapy with docetaxel, it was demonstrated that older patients on enzalutamide had a similar benefit to younger patients in terms of PFS, OS and safety, yet a higher number of reported falls [59]. Another option to mitigate the risk of toxicity with enzalutamide is reducing the dose of (≤80 mg/day) [60]. This reduced dose still demonstrated a high tumor response rate and survival benefit and it could be an option for those older patients more vulnerable or with frailty.

Even in the post-docetaxel setting, the response rates for abiraterone or enzalutamide are similar in older and younger men, with a mostly similar pattern of adverse events. However, and similarly to above, some toxicities were more common in older men on abiraterone (atrial fibrillation and tachycardia) and on enzalutamide (peripheral edema, fatigue, and diarrhea) studies [61, 62]. In this setting, a cohort of patients aged 80 and above enrolled in the Italian abiraterone patient program, had a PSA response rate of 48.9%, the median PFS and OS of 8 and 18 months, respectively [63]. Moreover, the differences in toxicities between the older and younger age groups were not relevant. Despite the retrospective nature of this study, abiraterone was active and safe in this older population and lead to clinical outcomes similar to those observed in younger patients.

Lastly, for patients with bone metastases and no visceral or bulky lymph node metastases, after the failure of docetaxel, a course of radium-223 may be attempted. Despite myelosuppression and renal clearance being a cause of concern in older patients treated with radium-223, radiopharmaceuticals are generally less toxic than chemotherapy and so may be used in the treatment of older patients. The subgroup analyses from the ALSYMPCA trial of radium-223 and the early access program confirmed its positive effect on bone-related complications with decreased hospitalizations and a favorable toxicity profile in older patients [64–67].

Therefore, the management of these older patients with frailty and hormone-resistant prostate cancer is complex. Chemotherapy options may be adjusted in terms of dose, schedule, and supportive measures, but even then, these will not be appropriate for the majority of older patients with frailty. Abiraterone and enzalutamide may be suitable for a larger proportion of these patients, but their selection should also take into consideration their toxicity profile. Best supportive care instead of any active anti-cancer treatment should also be considered and discussed in this setting.

Medium to Long-Term Consequences of Prostate Cancer Treatments

A *metabolic syndrome* can develop with the long-term use of ADT [68]. This consists of abdominal obesity, high cholesterol levels, high blood pressure, and high glucose levels, which in turn significantly increases the cardiovascular risk of a patient with prostate cancer. For this reason, it is important to monitor these patients and actively control these risk factors.

Sarcopenia and *bone mass density* can also result from treatment with ADT due to both factors implicit in the treatment and reduced patient activity [69, 70]. These can impact patient outcomes but are also potentially reversible, for this reason, it is key to diagnose or prevent it. Testosterone deficiency is a known risk factor for osteopenia and osteoporosis in older men [71]. Estradiol, which is primarily obtained through testosterone aromatization, is also needed for normal bone development and the maintenance of healthy bone density in men [72]. The negative effect of testosterone and estradiol suppression due to the use of ADT may result in a decrease in bone density of 13% each year [73]. Since there is a physiological reduction of lean/muscle mass and bone mass with aging, it is particularly relevant to monitor older men on ADT. Apart from physical activity, the use of antiresorptive therapy with denosumab plus or minus the addition of calcium and vitamin D represents a companion treatment to preserve mineral bone density.

Urinary incontinence (UI) has been highlighted as a possible consequence particularly after radical prostatectomy but also possible, to a lesser extent, after brachytherapy [74]. After 2 years, urinary incontinence was reported by 15% of surgically treated patients [75]. For patients treated with brachytherapy and transurethral resection, UI can occur until 25% of individuals [76, 77]. Risk factors for urinary incontinence include those with large tumors, patients with previous transurethral resection of prostate (TURP) and those who experienced acute grade 2 or above urinary toxicity during brachytherapy [78].

Sexual dysfunction is an important consideration when discussing treatment options, as it ultimately influences the patient HRQoL and that of his partner, compromising all aspects of sexual health both in terms of erectile function but also self-image, mental health and the relationship with one's partner [79]. Erectile dysfunction and loss of sexual desire, are commonly experienced by patients on ADT [80]. In a recent study, 82% of patients on ADT reported erectile problems and 64% experienced loss of sexual desire [81]. This loss of sexual desire is often linked with iatrogenic deficiency of testosterone.

After prostate radiotherapy, patients also often report impaired sexual function; including erectile dysfunction, increased time until orgasm, decreased intensity of orgasm, and/or dry ejaculation [82]. Radiation-induced sexual dysfunction results from a concert of neurological, vascular, and endocrine perturbations [83]. The etiology of impotence after radical prostatectomy is unclear although a variety of potential factors have been cited: neurogenic, psychogenic, and possibly vascular [84]. A study has found variation between open and robotic surgery, with fewer complications, improved sexual function, and increased use of high volume surgeons in the robotic group, possibly reflecting differences in quality between approaches, differences in practice patterns, and/or biases in patient selection [85]. Preservation of neurovascular bundles at the time of radical prostatectomy influences the recovery of sexual function after radical prostatectomy for localized prostate cancer. Recovery of sexual function after radical prostatectomy is an important component of HRQoL after surgery [84, 85]. In men with poor pre-operative erectile function, recovery of function is unlikely even with nerve-sparing, and efforts to spare the nerves may increase the risk for positive margins, particularly for men with higher-risk cancers.

Conclusion

Older patients with prostate cancer represent one of the largest cancer sub-groups. These patients can benefit from standard anti-cancer treatments similarly to their younger counterparts, provided that they have a good overall health status. Frailty plays a key role in this and older patients with frailty and comorbidity are at an increased risk of adverse events during cancer treatments. Moreover, these patients often have poorer prognoses which may be led by competing conditions and not primarily by cancer. In order to appropriately support and manage these patients, geriatric assessments should be included to better understand the potential risks and benefits, which in turn informs the shared decision-making. These may be used to determine if a patient is fit, vulnerable, or frail and therefore guide if they should be considered for optimal treatment, modified treatment, or no anti-cancer treatment. Lastly, more research is required in this field and the design of clinical trials should reflect the populations and their goals of care.

References

1. Globocan 2020: estimated cancer incidence, mortality and prevalence worldwide in 2020. International Agency for Reseach on Cancer (IARC). 2020.
2. 2020. Atlanta: American Cancer Society, American Cancer Society. Cancer Facts & Figures 2020.
3. Siegel RL, Miller KD, Jemal A. Cancer statistics. CA Cancer J Clin. 2020;70:7–30.
4. Globocan 2018: estimated cancer incidence mapwi: International Agency for Reseach on Cancer (IARC). 2018.
5. Wong MC, Goggins WB, Wang HH, et al. Global incidence and mortality for prostate cancer: analysis of temporal patterns and trends in 36 countries. Eur Urol. 2016;70:862–74.
6. Institute. NC: SEERCancer Stat Facts: prostate cancer. 2018.
7. Smith BDSG, Hurria A, et al. Future of cancer incidence in the United States: burdens upon an aging, changing nation. J Clin Oncol. 2009;27:2758–65.
8. Bechis SKCP, Cooperberg MR. Impact of age at diagnosis on prostate cancer treatment and survival. J Clin Oncol. 2011;29(2):235–41.
9. US Preventive Services Task Force GD, Curry SJ, et al. Screening for prostate cancer: US preventive services task force recommendation statement [published correction appears in JAMA]. JAMA 2018;319(18):1901–13.
10. Shah N IV. Frequency of Gleason score 7 to 10 in 5100 elderly prostate canceer patients. Rev Urol. 2016;18(4):181–7.
11. Shah N IV. Comment on low-value prostate cancer screening among older men within the veterans health administration. J Am Geriatr Soc. 2020;68(1):219–20.
12. Walter LCCK. Cancer screening in elderly patients: a framework for individualized decision making. JAMA. 2001;285:2750–6.
13. Droz J-PAG, Gillessen S, et al. Management of prostate cancer in elderly patients: recommendations of a task force of the International Society of Geriatric Oncology. Eur Urol. 2017;72:521–31.
14. Handforth CCA, Young C, et al. The prevalence and outcomes of frailty in older cancer patients: a systematic review. Ann Oncol. 2015;26(6):1091–101.
15. Morley JEVB, van Kan GA, et al. Frailty consensus: a call to action. J Am Med Dir Assoc. 2013;14(6):392–7.
16. Daskivich TJLJ, Dick AW, et al. Variation in treatment associated with life expectancy in a population-based cohort of men with early-stage prostate cancer. Cancer. 2014;120(23):3642–50.
17. Daskivich TJ, Fan KH, Koyama T, et al. Effect of age, tumor risk, and comorbidity on competing risks for survival in a U.S. population-based cohort of men with prostate cancer. Ann Intern Med. 2013;158(10):709–17.
18. Osborne GEC, Appleyard SA, Gilbert DC, et al. Comprehensive geriatric assessment in men aged 70 years or older with localised prostate cancer undergoing radical radiotherapy. Clin Oncol (R Coll Radiol). 2017;29:609–16.
19. Boyle HJ, Alibhai S, Decoster L, et al. Updated recommendations of the International Society of Geriatric Oncology on prostate cancer management in older patients. Eur J Cancer. 2019;116:116–36.
20. D'Amico AV, Moul JW, Carroll PR, et al. Surrogate end point for prostate cancer-specific mortality after radical prostatectomy or radiation therapy. J Natl Cancer Inst. 2003;95:1376–83.
21. Vernooij RWM, van Oort I, de Reijke TM, et al. Nationwide treatment patterns and survival of older patients with prostate cancer. J Geriatr Oncol. 2019;10:252–8.
22. Bekelman JE, Mitra N, Handorf EA, et al. Effectiveness of androgen-deprivation therapy and radiotherapy for older men with locally advanced prostate cancer. J Clin Oncol. 2015;33:716–22.
23. Warde P, Mason M, Ding K, et al. Combined androgen deprivation therapy and radiation therapy for locally advanced prostate cancer: a randomised, phase 3 trial. Lancet. 2011;378:2104–11.

24. Widmark A, Klepp O, Solberg A, et al. Endocrine treatment, with or without radiotherapy, in locally advanced prostate cancer (SPCG-7/SFUO-3): an open randomised phase III trial. Lancet. 2009;373:301–8.
25. Briganti A, Joniau S, Gontero P, et al. Identifying the best candidate for radical prostatectomy among patients with high-risk prostate cancer. Eur Urol. 2012;61:584–92.
26. Briganti A, Spahn M, Joniau S, et al. Impact of age and comorbidities on long-term survival of patients with high-risk prostate cancer treated with radical prostatectomy: a multi-institutional competing-risks analysis. Eur Urol. 2013;63:693–701.
27. Sivaraman A, Ordaz Jurado G, Cathelineau X, et al. Older patients with low Charlson score and high-risk prostate cancer benefit from radical prostatectomy. World J Urol. 2016;34:1367–72.
28. Hamdy FC, Donovan JL, Lane JA, et al. 10-year outcomes after monitoring, surgery, or radiotherapy for localized prostate cancer. N Engl J Med. 2016;375:1415–24.
29. Bill-Axelson A, Holmberg L, Garmo H, et al. Radical prostatectomy or watchful waiting in early prostate cancer. N Engl J Med. 2014;370:932–42.
30. Bill-Axelson A, Holmberg L, Ruutu M, et al. Radical prostatectomy versus watchful waiting in early prostate cancer. N Engl J Med. 2011;364:1708–17.
31. Wilt TJ, Jones KM, Barry MJ, et al. Follow-up of prostatectomy versus observation for early prostate cancer. N Engl J Med. 2017;377:132–42.
32. Lu-Yao GL, Albertsen PC, Moore DF, et al. Fifteen-year outcomes following conservative management among men aged 65 years or older with localized prostate cancer. Eur Urol. 2015;68:805–11.
33. Yang DD, Mahal BA, Muralidhar V, et al. Receipt of definitive therapy in elderly patients with unfavorable-risk prostate cancer. Cancer. 2017;123:4832–40.
34. Nanda A, Chen M-H, Moran BJ, et al. Predictors of prostate cancer-specific mortality in elderly men with intermediate-risk prostate cancer treated with brachytherapy with or without external beam radiation therapy. Int J Radiat Oncol Biol Phys. 2010;77:147–52.
35. Wong YN, Mitra N, Hudes G, et al. Survival associated with treatment vs observation of localized prostate cancer in elderly men. JAMA. 2006;296:2683–93.
36. Lebret T, Culine S, Davin JL, Hennequin C, Mignard JP, Moreau JL, et al. Quality of life of 1276 elderly patients with prostate cancer, starting treatment with a gonadotropin-releasing hormone agonist: results of a French observational study. Aging Male; 2014.
37. Bakhireva LN, Barrett-Connor E, Kritz-Silverstein D, Morton DJ. Modifiable predictors of bone loss in older men: a prospective study. Am J Prev Med. 2004.
38. Shahinian VB, Yong-Fang K, Freeman JL, Goodwin JS. Risk of fracture after androgen deprivation for prostate cancer. N Engl J Med. 2005.
39. Braga-Basaria M, Dobs A, Muller DC, Carducci MA, John M, Egan J, et al. Metabolic syndrome in men with prostate cancer undergoing long-term androgen-deprivation therapy. J Clin Oncol. 2006.
40. Ford ES, Giles W, Dietz WH. Prevalence of the metabolic syndrome among US adults: findings from the Third National Health and Nutrition Examination Survey. J Am Med Assoc. 2002.
41. Fizazi K, Tran N, Fein L, Matsubara N, Rodriguez-Antolin A, Alekseev BY, et al. Abiraterone plus prednisone in metastatic, castration-sensitive prostate cancer. N Engl J Med. 2017.
42. James ND, de Bono J, Spears MR, Clarke NW, Mason MD, Dearnaley DP, et al. Abiraterone for prostate cancer not previously treated with hormone therapy. N Engl J Med. 2017.
43. Kyriakopoulos CE, Chen Y, Carducci MA, Liu G, Jarrard DF, Hahn NM, et al. Chemohormonal therapy in metastatic hormone-sensitive prostate cancer: long-term survival analysis of the randomized phase III E3805 chaarted trial. J Clin Oncol. 2018.
44. James ND, Sydes M, Clarke NW, Mason MD, Dearnaley DP, Spears MR, et al. Addition of docetaxel, zoledronic acid, or both to first-line long-term hormone therapy in prostate cancer (STAMPEDE): Survival results from an adaptive, multiarm, multistage, platform randomised controlled trial. Lancet. 2016.
45. Honecker F, Wedding U, Kallischnigg G, Schroeder A, Klier J, Frangenheim T, et al. Risk factors for unplanned discontinuation of scheduled treatment in elderly patients with castration-resistant prostate cancer: results of the IBuTu study. J Cancer Res Clin Oncol. 2018.

46. Berthold DR, Pond G, Soban F, De Wit R, Eisenberger M, Tannock IF. Docetaxel plus prednisone or mitoxantrone plus prednisone for advanced prostate cancer: updated survival in the TAX 327 study. J Clin Oncol. 2008.
47. Abdel-Rahman O. Efficacy and toxicity outcomes of elderly castrate-resistant prostate cancer patients treated with docetaxel—a pooled analysis of 3 randomized studies. Urol Oncol Semin Orig Investig. 2020.
48. Crombag MRBS, Dorlo T, van der Pan E, van Straten A, Bergman AM, van Erp NP, et al. Exposure to docetaxel in the elderly patient population: a population pharmacokinetic study. Pharm Res 2019.
49. Kongsted P, Svane I, Lindberg H, Sengeløv L. Predictors of chemotherapy-induced toxicity and treatment outcomes in elderly versus younger patients with metastatic castration-resistant prostate cancer. Clin Genitourin Cancer. 2016.
50. Italiano A, Ortholan C, Oudard S, Pouessel D, Gravis G, Beuzeboc P, et al. Docetaxel-based chemotherapy in elderly patients (age 75 and older) with castration-resistant prostate cancer. Eur Urol. 2009.
51. Hervonen P, Joensuu H, Joensuu T, et al. Biweekly docetaxel is better tolerated than conventional three-weekly dosing for advanced hormone-refractory prostate cancer. Anticancer Res. 2012;32:953–6.
52. de Bono JS, Oudard S, Ozguroglu M, et al. Prednisone plus cabazitaxel or mitoxantrone for metastatic castration-resistant prostate cancer progressing after docetaxel treatment: a randomised open-label trial. Lancet. 2010;376:1147–54.
53. Heidenreich A, Bracarda S, Mason M, et al. Safety of cabazitaxel in senior adults with metastatic castration-resistant prostate cancer: results of the European compassionate-use programme. Eur J Cancer. 2014;50:1090–9.
54. Beer TM, Armstrong A, Rathkopf DE, Loriot Y, Sternberg CN, Higano CS, et al. Enzalutamide in metastatic prostate cancer before chemotherapy. N Engl J Med. 2014.
55. Ryan CJ, Smith M, De Bono JS, Molina A, Logothetis CJ, De Souza P, et al. Abiraterone in metastatic prostate cancer without previous chemotherapy. N Engl J Med. 2013.
56. Beardo P, Osman I, San José B, Llarena R, Congregado B, Campá J, et al. Safety and outcomes of new generation hormone-therapy in elderly chemotherapy-naive metastatic castration-resistant prostate cancer patients in the real world. Arch Gerontol Geriatr. 2019.
57. Azad AA, Eigl B, Leibowitz-Amit R, Lester R, Kollmannsberger C, Murray N, et al. Outcomes with abiraterone acetate in metastatic castration-resistant prostate cancer patients who have poor performance status. Eur Urol. 2015.
58. Shore ND, Chowdhury S, Villers A, Klotz L, Robert Siemens D, Phung D, et al. Efficacy and safety of enzalutamide versus bicalutamide for patients with metastatic prostate cancer (TERRAIN): a randomised, double-blind, phase 2 study. Lancet Oncol. 2016.
59. Graff JN, Baciarello G, Armstrong AJ, Higano CS, Iversen P, Flaig TW, et al. Efficacy and safety of enzalutamide in patients 75 years or older with chemotherapy-naive metastatic castrationresistant prostate cancer: Results from PREVAIL. Ann Oncol. 2016;
60. Vinh-Hung V, Natchagande G, Joachim C, Gorobets O, Drame M, Bougas S, et al. Low-dose enzalutamide in late-elderly patients (≥ 75 years old) presenting with metastatic castration-resistant prostate cancer. Clin Genitourin Cancer. 2020.
61. Mulders PFA, Molina A, Marberger M, Saad F, Higano CS, Chi KN, et al. Efficacy and safety of abiraterone acetate in an elderly patient subgroup (aged 75 and older) with metastatic castration-resistant prostate cancer after docetaxel-based chemotherapy. Eur Urol. 2014.
62. Sternberg CN, de Bono J, Chi KN, Fizazi K, Mulders P, Cerbone L, et al.. Improved outcomes in elderly patients with metastatic castration-resistant prostate cancer treated with the androgen receptor inhibitor enzalutamide: results from the phase III AFFIRM trial. Ann Oncol. 2014.
63. Maines F, Caffo O, De Giorgi U, Fratino L, Lo Re G, Zagonel V, et al. Safety and clinical outcomes of abiraterone acetate after docetaxel in octogenarians with metastatic castration-resistant prostate cancer: results of the Italian compassionate use named patient programme. Clin Genitourin Cancer. 2016.

64. Sartor O, Coleman R, Nilsson S, Heinrich D, Staudacher K, Garcia-Vargas J, Vogelzang N et al. Radium-223(R a-223) safety and efficacy in prostate cancer with bone metastases: phase 3 ALSYMPCA study findings stratified by age. BJU Int. 2013.
65. O'Sullivan J JD, Widmark A, Syndikus I, James N, Dall'Oglio M, et al. Hematologic safety of radium-223 dichloride (Ra-223) in the phase 3 ALSYMPCA trial in castration-resistant prostate cancer (CRPC) patients with bone metastases: baseline prognostic factor subgroup analysis. Eur J Cancer. 2013.
66. Parker C, Zhan L, Cislo P, Reuning-Scherer J, Vogelzang NJ, Nilsson S, et al. Effect of radium-223 dichloride (Ra-223) on hospitalisation: an analysis from the phase 3 randomised Alpharadin in Symptomatic Prostate Cancer Patients (ALSYMPCA) trial. Eur J Cancer. 2017.
67. Vogelzang NJ, Coleman R, Michalski JM, Nilsson S, O'Sullivan JM, Parker C, et al. Hematologic safety of radium-223 dichloride: baseline prognostic factors associated with myelosuppression in the ALSYMPCA Trial. Clin Genitourin Cancer. 2017.
68. Braga-Basaria M, Dobs AS, Muller DC, et al. Metabolic syndrome in men with prostate cancer undergoing long-term androgen-deprivation therapy. J Clin Oncol. 2006;24:3979–83.
69. Smith MR, Saad F, Egerdie B, et al. Sarcopenia during androgen-deprivation therapy for prostate cancer. J Clin Oncol. 2012;30:3271–6.
70. Kacker R, Conners W, Zade J, Morgentaler A. Bone mineral density and response to treatment in men younger than 50 years with testosterone deficiency and sexual dysfunction or infertility. J Urol. 2014.
71. Golds G, Houdek D, Arnason T. Male hypogonadism and osteoporosis: the effects, clinical consequences, and treatment of testosterone deficiency in bone health. Int J Endocrinol. 2017.
72. Russell N, Grossmann M. Estradiol as a male hormone. Eur J Endocrinol. 2019;181(1):R23–43.
73. Guise TA, Oefelein M, Eastham JA, Cookson MS, Higano CS, Smith MR. Estrogenic side effects of androgen deprivation therapy. Rev Urol. 2007;9(4):163–80.
74. Liu M, Pickles T, Berthelet E, et al. Urinary incontinence in prostate cancer patients treated with external beam radiotherapy. Radiother Oncol. 2005;74(2):197–201.
75. Vernooij RWM, Cremers R, Jansen H, et al. Urinary incontinence and erectile dysfunction in patients with localized or locally advanced prostate cancer: a nationwide observational study. Urol Oncol Semin Orig Investig. 2020;38(9):735.e17–25.
76. Leapman MS, Stone NN, Mock S, et al. Urinary incontinence following prostate brachytherapy. Urology. 2016;95:151–7.
77. Mock S, Leapman M, Stock RG, et al. Risk of urinary incontinence following post-brachytherapy transurethral resection of the prostate and correlation with clinical and treatment parameters. J Urol. 2013;190:1805–10.
78. Doiron RC, Witten J, Rourke KF. The scope, presentation, and management of genitourinary complications in patients presenting with high-grade urethral complications after radiotherapy for prostate cancer. Can Urol Assoc J. 2020;15(1):E6–E10.
79. Mauro M, Di MG, Giorgio RI. Problems in defining sexual dysfunction in prostate cancer patients. IJIR Your Sex Med J. 2020.
80. Duthie CJ, Calich H, Rapsey CM, Wibowo E. Maintenance of sexual activity following androgen deprivation in males. Crit Rev Oncol Hematol. 2020;153:103064.
81. Wibowo E, Wassersug R, Robinson JW, Matthew A, McLeod D, Walker LM. How are patients with prostate cancer managing androgen deprivation therapy side effects? Clin Genitourin Cancer. 2019;17(3):e408–19.
82. Telöken T. Management of erectile dysfunction secondary to treatment for localized prostate cancer. Cancer Control. 2001;8(6):540–5.
83. Feldman HA, Goldstein I, Hatzichristou DG, Krane RJ, McKinlay JB. Impotence and its medical and psychosocial correlates: results of the Massachusetts male aging study. J Urol. 1994;151(1):54–61.
84. Walsh PC, Donker P. Impotence following radical prostatectomy: insight into etiology and prevention. J Urol. 2017;197:S165–70.
85. Alemozaffar M, Regan M, Cooperberg MR, et al. Prediction of erectile function following treatment for prostate cancer. J Am Med Assoc. 2011;306(11):1205–14.

Chapter 21
Renal Cell Carcinoma in Older Adults with Frailty

Tanujaa Rajasekaran, Anupama Roy Chowdhury, and Ravindran Kanesvaran

Introduction

Renal cell carcinoma (RCC) is a disease entity whereby malignant cells are found in the lining of the tubules within the kidney. It is the 16th most common cancer and 17th most lethal cancer in the world [1]. Worldwide in 2018, there were more than 400,000 newly diagnosed RCC cases and nearly 180,000 RCC-related deaths, which is projected to significantly increase by 2030 [1]. RCC accounts for 3% of adult malignancies and can exist in both sporadic and hereditary forms. It is a clinically and pathologically heterogenous disease, with clear cell renal cell carcinoma (CCRCC) being the dominant subtype accounting for over 75% of all RCCs [2]. Other subtypes include papillary RCC (type I and type II), chromophobe RCC, hereditary cancer syndromes, multilocular cystic RCC, collecting duct carcinoma, medullary carcinoma, mucinous tubular and spindle cell carcinoma, neuroblastoma-associated RCC, Xp11.2 translocation-*TFE3* carcinoma and a few more rare types, which are collectively known as non-clear cell RCC [2]. At diagnosis, about one third of all RCC patients are metastatic, and recurrence rates for those treated for localized disease are as high as 50% [3].

RCC predominantly affects a significant proportion of older adults with a median age at diagnosis of 64 years [3]. Whilst the pivotal phase III trials in metastatic RCC

T. Rajasekaran · R. Kanesvaran (✉)
Division of Medical Oncology, National Cancer Centre, Singapore, Singapore

Duke-NUS Medical School, Singapore, Singapore
e-mail: tanujaa.rajasekaran@singhealth.com.sg; ravindran.kanesvaran@singhealth.com.sg

A. R. Chowdhury
Duke-NUS Medical School, Singapore, Singapore

Department of General Medicine, Sengkang General Hospital, Singapore, Singapore
e-mail: anupama.roy.chowdhury@singhealth.com.sg

F. Gomes (ed.), *Frailty in Older Adults with Cancer*,
https://doi.org/10.1007/978-3-030-89162-6_21

have shown no differences in efficacy and toxicity in older patients (65+ years) compared to younger patients [3, 4]; older patients are usually underrepresented in clinical trials, and the majority of data for those with either metastatic RCC or localized disease come from unpowered sub-group analyses. Although new drugs approved for the treatment of RCC were assessed in trials without an upper age limitation and included patients over 65 years, older adults with frailty were mainly excluded indirectly due to the strict inclusion criteria. In fact, clinical trials tend to select those patients in better health and with fewer co-morbidities, rather than the unselected older patients who are vulnerable or with significant frailty who are commonly seen in real-world clinical practice.

Frailty is a physiological syndrome characterized by decreased reserve and diminished resistance to stressors resulting from cumulative decline across multiple physiological systems and causing vulnerability to adverse outcomes [5]. The utility of identifying someone with frailty allows for provision of care commensurate with the patient's needs, circumstances and perceived benefit from proposed treatment. This is particularly relevant in the oncology clinic where treatments come with significant risk of adverse events, morbidity and even mortality. It avoids undertreatment and particularly overtreatment in patients in whom the burden of treatment and its adverse effects would outweigh its benefits.

Overall there is limited guidance in the current literature on how best to treat older adults with frailty who were diagnosed with RCC. This chapter will review the latest evidence regarding the treatment of RCC and apply this into best practice approaches for the treatment of the older adults with frailty and RCC, from an early stage to the metastatic setting.

Frailty in Patients with RCC

Normal ageing does cause a gradual decline in physiological reserve; however, this decline is accelerated in frailty resulting in failure of homeostatic mechanisms. A small insult such as a minor infection, surgery or new drug may result in a disproportionate change in health state including physical and cognitive functioning [6]. These physiologic changes that occur with ageing can affect the pharmacokinetics and pharmacodynamics of various therapies used in the treatment of RCC. A decrease in liver mass and blood flow may lead to a decline in liver function. The cytochrome P450 microsomal enzyme system has been reported to decline with increasing age and may have a significant impact on drug metabolism, given that most of the targeted agents for metastatic RCC are metabolized via this system [7]. In the ageing kidney, there is a decrease in blood flow, a proportion of glomeruli are lost and these are replaced by fat and fibrotic tissue. This, coupled with the presence of RCC leads to impairment of the glomerular filtration rate which affects the pharmacokinetics of targeted cancer therapies. However some studies have shown that some targeted therapies, like sunitinib, are efficacious with an acceptable toxicity profile in patients with impaired kidney function as well [8]. With the recent emergence of immune checkpoint inhibitors in the setting of metastatic RCC, it can be assumed that age-related changes of the immune system (immunosenescence) might also affect the efficacy and toxicity of immunotherapy in older patients with frailty. It is known that the expression of immune checkpoints on T-cells increases with age, hence making this potentially an important target with immune-oncology drugs, which now form one of the standards of care in RCC [9].

It is estimated that 17% of newly diagnosed older patients with metastatic RCC have frailty at diagnosis [10]. The most evidence-based method to detect and stratify frailty would be by means of a geriatric assessment, although screening tools are also a good strategy to identify those at higher risk who may benefit the most from a geriatric assessment. A geriatric assessment is a multidimensional, multidisciplinary diagnostic instrument designed to collect data on the medical, psychosocial and functional capabilities and limitations of the older individual. Therefore, it is a very useful method to identify those with frailty and it is the most appropriate tool to predict functional age of older RCC patients [11]. In the setting of RCC, polypharmacy and drug interactions can be problematic when, for example, a patient is offered treatment with a vascular endothelial growth factor (VEGF) tyrosine kinase inhibitor, as the concurrent use of proton pump inhibitors can inhibit the absorption of this targeted treatment, leading to lower serum concentration levels and lower efficacy [12]. In another example, a prospective study performed nutritional assessments in 300 patients with metastatic RCC planned to be treated with targeted therapies. Depending on the tool used, between 21 and 32% of patients were at risk of malnutrition and this was an independent predictor of survival [13]. Hence it is important for the treating oncologist to work together with a multidisciplinary team to ensure that older patients with RCC who are found to have deficits in one of more geriatric assessment are optimized and adequate support provided throughout the continuum of cancer care.

In general, older patients with frailty differ from their younger counterparts when it comes to decision-making processes related to their cancer therapy. Older patients, particularly those with frailty, differ in that they are less likely to trade quality of life for an improvement in overall survival compared to younger more fit patients [14, 15]. In addition, one other aspect that needs to be taken into consideration is cognitive frailty even before embarking on treatment. Depending on the degree of cognitive compromise a patient has, he may not have the mental capacity to make an informed decision on his treatment. Compliance to prescribed treatment is another factor to consider when treating older patients with frailty. For example, the treatment for metastatic RCC involves oral therapies which have several advantages including not requiring intravenous access, hence avoiding its associated complications and reducing travelling to hospital. However oral administration comes with its own disadvantages, specifically with the problem of drug compliance. Older patients with frailty may be less compliant to oral medication compared to their younger counterparts, due to reasons such as polypharmacy, memory related cognitive impairment and general physical decline [16]. Poor compliance can lead to both decreased drug efficacy and increased toxicities if the patient persists in taking medication during rest periods (with sunitinib, for example, which has a 2-week rest period after 4 weeks of treatment). In order to improve compliance and ensure that patients, particularly those with frailty, are able to seek help for treatment related toxicities, it is key to ascertain the social support the patient has. For patients with poor social support and lack of adequate supervision for monitoring of compliance and adverse events, prescription of these oral targeted therapies may not be appropriate. In these circumstances, intravenous options with the use of immunotherapy should be considered as a reasonable alternative option.

Management of Localized RCC

The increasing use of imaging in the investigation of various symptoms, particularly in older patients, has resulted in an increased detection of small renal masses (<4 cm), of which a substantial number are RCC [17]. For the management of localized RCC there are a number of treatment options available, which vary depending on the size and site of the tumour. However, for older adults with frailty, depending on its severity not all options are appropriate.

A radical nephrectomy may not be an appropriate option for many of these older adults with frailty; therefore, nephron-sparing surgeries or partial nephrectomy is the treatment of choice for localized small RCC based on their location [18, 19]. However, for those deemed unsuitable for surgery, there is a need to consider alternative options to control symptoms and maintain quality of life. Ablative therapies, such as cryotherapy or radiofrequency, have been developed for the treatment of small renal tumours as an alternative to nephron-sparing surgery, with the goal of reducing operative morbidity. A systematic review comparing cryoablation versus partial nephrectomy reported higher rates of tumour progression with cryoablation but both had similar low rates of distant metastases of less than 2% [20], hence making it a suitable option for many of these older adults with frailty. Another alternative to control symptoms is by renal artery embolization if the tumour is causing symptoms like bleeding [21].

Importantly, after the initial treatment of a localized RCC, there is currently no clear data to support the role of adjuvant therapy even in the fittest older adults [22–24].

Another important consideration in the decision-making for these older adults with frailty and RCC is the possibility of active surveillance for their small renal masses [25]. Some of these small renal masses can be slow-growing and may not impact on the long-term either the quality of life or the survival of this sub-group of patients with a reduced life expectancy. Therefore, active surveillance is an appropriate alternative to surgical or medical interventions for small renal masses, particularly for this sub-group of patients.

Management of Metastatic RCC

Clear Cell Metastatic RCC

Role of Cytoreductive Nephrectomy

The role of cytoreductive nephrectomy had been studied specifically in older patients with metastatic RCC and there was no significant difference between the older and younger group of patients in terms of overall survival (OS) [26]. This study also showed that the perioperative mortality of patients older than 75 years of age was significantly higher than that seen in younger patients. In older adults with frailty, one can extrapolate the data from this study to imply that they are likely to suffer from higher perioperative mortality if they were to undergo such procedure in the setting of metastatic RCC, and as such, the vast majority of these patients should not be offered cytoreductive nephrectomy.

Systemic Therapies

Patients with metastatic RCC should first be stratified into the appropriate prognostic risk group as defined by either the Memorial Sloan Kettering Cancer Center (MSKCC) or the International Metastatic Renal Cell Carcinoma Database (IMDC) criteria [27]. The choice of treatment for patients with advanced disease has been based on prognostic risk factors. For example, The International Metastatic Renal Cell Carcinoma Database Consortium (IMDC) prognostic model integrates six adverse factors and stratifies patients into favourable-, intermediate- or poor-risk groups. These six factors are Karnofsky performance status, time from diagnosis to systemic therapy, haemoglobin below upper limit of normal, serum calcium, neutrophil and platelets above upper limit of normal. Older patients with metastatic RCC and frailty are more likely to have one or more of the above criteria, rendering the majority of them as either IMDC intermediate- or poor- risk [28].

The systemic therapy landscape for metastatic RCC is rapidly evolving (Table 21.1). Immunotherapy has become a standard of care across all the IMDC risk groups. This is because of substantial benefit shown in the CheckMate-214 and Keynote-426 trials [29–31]. In CheckMate-214, nivolumab and ipilimumab were compared against sunitinib in treatment-naïve advanced RCC patients. The nivolumab and ipilimumab combination showed an improvement in both OS and progression free survival (PFS) benefit in patients who were IMDC intermediate and poor risk [29]. Similarly in Keynote-426, a combination of pembrolizumab and axitinib was compared against sunitinib in previously untreated advanced RCC patients. Pembrolizumab and axitinib improved OS and PFS in all IMDC patient sub-groups [30]. Both these immunotherapy combinations also showed an improvement in quality of life and objective response rate (ORR) compared to sunitinib.

Table 21.1 Summary of systemic therapies from pivotal trials in the setting of metastatic RCC

Treatment line	Phase 3 trial	Tumour type	Median age (years)	Age of oldest patient (years)	Median PFS (months)	Median OS (months)	Recommendations for older adults with frailty
1st	Pembrolizumab/ Axitinib [30]	Clear cell	62	89	15.2	NR	Use single agent Pembrolizumab
1st	Nivolumab/ Ipilimumab [29]	Clear cell	62	85	11.6	NR	Use single agent Nivolumab
1st	Sunitinib [36]	Clear cell	62	87	11	26.4	To consider dose reduction to 37.5 mg [40]
1st	Pazopanib [35]	Clear cell	59	85	9.2	22.9	Consider dose reduction to 600 mg daily if not well tolerated
2nd (after 1–2 antiangiogenic therapy)	Nivolumab [37]	Clear cell	62	88	4.6	25.0	Use as prescribed if progression on TKI in the first line
2nd (after at least 1 VEGFR TKI)	Cabozantinib [38]	Clear cell	63	86	7.4	–	Consider starting dose of 40 mg daily and escalating to full dose if tolerating well
2nd (after VEGFR TKI, cytokine-based systemic therapy)	Axitinib [39]	Clear cell	61	82	8.3	20.1	Consider starting at 5 mg daily and titrating to twice daily dose if tolerating

NR not reported, *OS* overall survival, *PFS* progression free survival, *TKI* tyrosine kinase inhibitor, *VEGFR* vascular endothelial growth factor receptor

While both these trials included older adults, they excluded patients with frailty as previously described.

However if the frailty of these older patients is mainly attributable to their extensive cancer burden, the above mentioned immunotherapy combinations may potentially be considered, since the treatment will target its leading factor. However, older patients more often have multifactorial frailty which makes such decisions particularly challenging. Therefore, a safer and usually more appropriate option for older adults with frailty is single agent immunotherapy. Single agent pembrolizumab was assessed in cohort A of Keynote-427 [32]. This was a phase 2 single arm trial in previously untreated patients with advanced clear cell RCC. The study demonstrated a ORR of 33.6% and a median PFS of 6.9 months. Also 86% of patient with a positive response to treatment, had their response lasting at least 3 months [32]. While patients with poor performance status were excluded from this study, the clinical benefits and manageable toxicity profile of single agent pembrolizumab makes it a viable treatment option in this sub-group of patients.

The use of antiangiogenic therapy with VEGF tyrosine kinase inhibitor (e.g. sunitinib and pazopanib) for older adults with frailty can be considered, despite these patients having mainly a IMDC of intermediate and poor risk, as previously described [33]. Prior to the advent of immune checkpoint inhibitors, sunitinib and pazopanib were considered standard of care for patients with newly diagnosed metastatic RCC [34–36]. A study comparing patient preference between sunitinib and pazopanib reported that a majority of metastatic RCC patients prefer pazopanib due to its better toxicity profile and quality of life [34]. Although this was not an older adult specific study, the lower toxicities and better quality of life assessment make pazopanib a possible better choice for older adults with frailty.

For patients with cancer progression on initial systemic therapy, who have frailty and further deteriorated, best supportive care may be the most appropriate option. But some patients may still continue suitable to consider second line therapy. The choice of second line therapy will be dependent not just on the patient performance status and overall fitness but also on the prior treatment received. For patients with frailty who progressed after initial treatment with a VEGF tyrosine kinase inhibitor, single agent immunotherapy with nivolumab can be considered [37]. In Checkmate 025 trial, patients with metastatic RCC who had progressed on VEGF tyrosine kinase inhibitor were randomized to nivolumab or everolimus. The patients on the nivolumab arm had an improved survival [37]. And for patients progressing on initial single agent pembrolizumab, they can be switched to a VEGF tyrosine kinase inhibitor. Studies in the second line indicate that treatment with nivolumab or cabozantinib (a multikinase inhibitor) may be suitable options for older patients with metastatic RCC after these were found to have superior efficacy and better tolerability when compared with everolimus [37, 38]. Based on the safety data, nivolumab may be the preferred option for metastatic RCC patients with frailty as evidenced by the lower rate of dose discontinuations and dose reductions compared to cabozantinib [37, 38]. Axitinib, a second generation VEGF tyrosine kinase inhibitor, is also approved as the second line treatment of metastatic RCC patients and is another suitable option for selected metastatic RCC patients with frailty [3, 39].

Regarding the use of the above-described targeted therapies with tyrosine kinase inhibitors, in the context of older adults with frailty, a possible strategy to better tailor these treatments is to consider starting with a reduced dose and to consider a dose escalation to full dose, once adequate tolerability has been established [40]. For example, starting sunitinib at 37.5 mg instead of 50 mg has shown to be better tolerated and still maintained its efficacy [40].

There are several treatment options for the management of patients with metastatic RCC; therefore, the potential toxicity with systemic therapy is of particular concern in older adults with frailty. Awareness of the key toxicities of concern for these patients (Table 21.2), alongside appropriate prophylactic measures, patient education and close monitoring of toxicity and quality of life, are all key to provide good quality care. But it is equally important to know when not to treat might be the best option, considering the balance of risk-benefit. In fact, for those older patients with frailty and a limited disease burden, upfront active surveillance may be an appropriate option based on a recent multi-centre phase 2 study [41].

Non-clear Cell RCC

The major subtypes of non-clear cell RCC are papillary, chromophobe, collecting duct, translocation and unclassified carcinomas. Ideally, a specific treatment should be instituted based on the histological subtype. However, there is a lack of good quality data for this sub-group of patients due to the rarity of these tumours. Much of the data for non-clear cell RCC patients have been derived from subset analyses from large clinical trials that had both clear cell RCC and non-clear cell RCC patients or small retrospective analyses.

The ASPEN phase 2 study looked at the various types of metastatic non-clear cell RCC and their responses to targeted therapies [42]. The study outcome showed that sunitinib significantly increased PFS compared with everolimus in metastatic non-clear cell RCC. However, the OS was not different between the two treatment

Table 21.2 Systemic therapies and special considerations in older patients with frailty

Line of treatment	Drug	Specific considerations in older adults with frailty
1st	Pembrolizumab [32]	Monitor for fatigue, diarrhoea, rash, HTN, hypothyroidism
1st	Pazopanib [35]	Monitor for GI toxicity, HTN, anorexia
2nd	Nivolumab [37]	Monitor for fatigue, nausea, pruritis, diarrhoea and rare endocrinopathies such as hypothyroidism, hypophysitis, and adrenal insufficiency
2nd	Cabozantinib [38]	Monitor for HTN, diarrhoea, fatigue
2nd	Axitinib [39]	Monitor for HTN, diarrhoea, fatigue

HTN hypertension

groups, although there were differences in treatment effect between the various histologic subtypes and prognostic risk groups. The role of checkpoint inhibitors in non-clear cell RCC was studied in cohort B of the Keynote-427 trial [32]. This was a single arm phase 2 study with pembrolizumab in treatment-naïve non-clear cell RCC patients. Single agent pembrolizumab had an ORR of 24.8% and the majority of responders had durable responses of 6 months or more. Although older patients with frailty were not recruited in both the ASPEN and Keynote-427 trials, one can extrapolate the use of these drugs in this population based on the predictable toxicity profile of sunitinib and pembrolizumab, and by applying the same selection principles used in the setting of clear cell RCC.

Conclusion

There is limited data specific to older adults from prospective clinical trials in the treatment of RCC, and there is virtually no data for those living with frailty and RCC. However, there are some retrospective and subset analyses of trial data to assist clinical teams in selecting the most appropriate treatment for this sub-group of patients. A very important determinant of treatment choice should be a thorough assessment with a geriatric assessment. All older adults with RCC should undergo such assessments, including a discussion of their goals of care. Lastly, these patients should also have their case discussed within a multidisciplinary tumour board, before being advised on the most appropriate management plan.

References

1. Bray F, Ferlay J, Soerjomataram I, Siegel RL, Torre LA, Jemal A, et al. Global cancer statistics 2018: GLOBOCAN estimates of incidence and mortality worldwide for 36 cancers in 185 countries. CA Cancer J Clin. 2018;68:394–424.
2. Moch H, Cubilla AL, Humphrey PA, Reuter VE, Ulbright TM. The 2016 WHO classification of tumours of the urinary system and male genital organs-part a: renal, penile, and testicular tumours. Eur Urol. 2016;70(1):93–105.
3. Kanesvaran R, Le Saux O, Motzer R, et al. Elderly patients with metastatic renal cell carcinoma: position paper from International Society of Geriatric Oncology. Lancet Oncol. 2018;19:e317–26.
4. Hahn AW, Esther J, Haaland B, et al. Patterns of treatment in metastatic renal cell carcinoma for older versus younger patients. J Geriatr Oncol. 2020;11(4):724–6.
5. Fried LP, et al. Frailty in older adults: evidence for a phenotype. J Gerontol A Biol Sci Med Sci. 2001;56(3):M146–56.
6. Clegg A, et al. Frailty in elderly people. Lancet. 2013;381:752–62.
7. Wauthier V, Verbeeck RK, Calderon PB. The effect of ageing on cytochrome p450 enzymes: consequences for drug biotransformation in the elderly. Curr Med Chem. 2007;14(7):745–57.
8. Kim KH, Kim HY, Kim HR, Sun JM, Lim HY, Lee HJ, et al. Efficacy and toxicity of sunitinib in patients with metastatic renal cell carcinoma with renal insufficiency. Eur J Cancer. 2014;50(4):746–52.

9. Hurez V, Padron AS, Svatek RS, Curiel TJ. Considerations for successful cancer immunotherapy in aged hosts. Clin Exp Immunol. 2017;187(1):53–63.
10. Pierantoni F, Basso U, Maruzzo M, et al. Comprehensive geriatric assessment is an independent prognostic factor in older patients with metastatic renal cell cancer treated with first-line Sunitinib or Pazopanib: a single center experience. J Geriatr Oncol. 2021;12(2):290–7.
11. Kanesvaran R, Li H, Koo KN, Poon D. Analysis of prognostic factors of comprehensive geriatric assessment and development of a clinical scoring system in elderly Asian patients with cancer. J Clin Oncol Off J Am Soc Clin Oncol. 2011;29(27):3620–7.
12. Lalani AA, McKay RR, Lin X, Simantov R, Kaymakcalan MD, Choueiri TK. Proton pump inhibitors and survival outcomes in patients with metastatic renal cell carcinoma. Clin Genitourin Cancer. 2017;15:724–32.
13. Gu W, Zhang G, Sun L, Ma Q, Cheng Y, Zhang H, et al. Nutritional screening is strongly associated with overall survival in patients treated with targeted agents for metastatic renal cell carcinoma. J Cachexia Sarcopenia Muscle. 2015;6(3):222–30.
14. Yellen SB, Cella DF, Leslie WT. Age and clinical decision making in oncology patients. J Natl Cancer Inst. 1994;86(23):1766–70.
15. Puts MT, Tapscott B, Fitch M, Howell D, Monette J, Wan-Chow-Wah D, et al. A systematic review of factors influencing older adults' decision to accept or decline cancer treatment. Cancer Treat Rev. 2015;41(2):197–215.
16. Biganzoli L, Lichtman S, Michel JP, Papamichael D, Quoix E, Walko C, et al. Oral single-agent chemotherapy in older patients with solid tumours: a position paper from the International Society of Geriatric Oncology (SIOG). Eur J Cancer. 2015;51(17):2491–500.
17. Sun M, Thuret R, Abdollah F, Lughezzani G, Schmitges J, Tian Z, et al. Age-adjusted incidence, mortality, and survival rates of stage-specific renal cell carcinoma in North America: a trend analysis. Eur Urol. 2011;59(1):135–41.
18. Chow WB, Rosenthal RA, Merkow RP, Ko CY, Esnaola NF, American College of Surgeons National Surgical Quality Improvement P, et al. Optimal preoperative assessment of the geriatric surgical patient: a best practices guideline from the American College of Surgeons National Surgical Quality Improvement Program and the American Geriatrics Society. J Am Coll Surg 2012;215(4):453–466.
19. Miller C, Raza SJ, Davaro F, et al. Trends in the treatment of clinical T1 renal cell carcinoma for octogenarians: analysis of the National Cancer Database. J Geriatr Oncol. 2019;10(2):285–91.
20. Klatte T, Grubmuller B, Waldert M, Weibl P, Remzi M. Laparoscopic cryoablation versus partial nephrectomy for the treatment of small renal masses: systematic review and cumulative analysis of observational studies. Eur Urol. 2011;60(3):435–43.
21. Imgard LE, Fernstrom I, Haverling M, Ljungqvist A, et al. Treatment of renal adenocarcinoma by embolic occlusion of the renal circulation. Br J Urol. 1973;45:474–9.
22. Ravaud A, Motzer RJ, Pandha HS, George DJ, Pantuck AJ, Patel A, et al. Adjuvant sunitinib in high-risk renal-cell carcinoma after nephrectomy. N Engl J Med. 2016;375(23):2246–54.
23. Haas NB, Manola J, Uzzo RG, Flaherty KT, Wood CG, Kane C, et al. Adjuvant sunitinib or sorafenib for high-risk, non-metastatic renal-cell carcinoma (ECOG-ACRIN E2805): a double-blind, placebo-controlled, randomised, phase 3 trial. Lancet. 2016;
24. Gyawali B, Ando Y. Adjuvant Sunitinib for high-risk resected renal cell carcinoma: a meta-analysis of ASSURE and S-TRAC trials. Ann Oncol. 2016;
25. Borghesi M, Brunocilla E, Volpe A, Dababneh H, Pultrone CV, Vagnoni V, et al. Active surveillance for clinically localized renal tumors: an updated review of current indications and clinical outcomes. Int J Urol. 2015;22(5):432–8.
26. Kader AK, Tamboli P, Luongo T, Matin SF, Bell K, Jonasch E, et al. Cytoreductive nephrectomy in the elderly patient: the M. D. Anderson Cancer Center experience. J Urol. 2007;177(3):855–60. discussion 60–1
27. Heng DY, Xie W, Regan MM, Warren MA, Golshayan AR, Sahi C, et al. Prognostic factors for overall survival in patients with metastatic renal cell carcinoma treated with vascular

endothelial growth factor-targeted agents: results from a large, multicenter study. J Clin Oncol Off J Am Soc Clin Oncol.
28. Hale P, Hahn AW, Rathi N, et al. Treatment of metastatic renal cell carcinoma in older patients: a network meta-analysis. J Geriatr Oncol. 2019;10(1):149–54.
29. Motzer RJ, Tannir NM, McDermott DF, et al. Nivolumab plus ipilimumab versus sunitinib in advanced renal-cell carcinoma. N Engl J Med. 2018;378:1277.
30. Rini BI, Plimack ER, Stus V, et al. Pembrolizumab plus axitinib versus sunitinib for advanced renal-cell carcinoma. N Engl J Med. 2019;380:1116.
31. Araujo DV, Wells JC, Hansen AR, Dizman N, et al. Efficacy of immune-checkpoint inhibitors (ICI) in the treatment of older adults with metastatic renal cell carcinoma (mRCC) – an International mRCC Database Consortium (IMDC) analysis. J Geriatr Oncol. 2021;12(5):820–6.
32. Lee JL, Ziobro M, Gafanov R, et al. KEYNOTE-427 cohort B: first-line pembrolizumab (pembro) monotherapy for advanced non–clear cell renal cell carcinoma (NCC-RCC). J Clin Oncol. 2019;15S
33. Schmidinger M, Porta C, Oudard S, Dénéchère G, et al. Real-world experience with sunitinib treatment in patients with metastatic renal cell carcinoma: Clinical outcome according to risk score. J Clin Oncol. 2019;37(7_suppl):606.
34. Escudier B, Porta C, Bono P, Powles T, Eisen T, Sternberg CN, et al. Randomized, controlled, double-blind, cross-over trial assessing treatment preference for pazopanib versus sunitinib in patients with metastatic renal cell carcinoma: PISCES Study. J Clin Oncol Off J Am Soc Clin Oncol. 2014;32(14):1412–8.
35. Motzer RJ, Hutson TE, Cella D, Reeves J, Hawkins R, Guo J, et al. Pazopanib versus sunitinib in metastatic renal-cell carcinoma. N Engl J Med. 2013;369(8):722–31.
36. Motzer RJ, Hutson TE, Tomczak P, Michaelson MD, Bukowski RM, Rixe O, et al. Sunitinib versus interferon alfa in metastatic renal-cell carcinoma. N Engl J Med. 2007;356(2):115–24.
37. Motzer RJ, Escudier B, McDermott DF, George S, Hammers HJ, Srinivas S, et al. Nivolumab versus everolimus in advanced renal-cell carcinoma. N Engl J Med. 2015;373(19):1803–13.
38. Choueiri TK, Escudier B, Powles T, Mainwaring PN, Rini BI, Donskov F, et al. Cabozantinib versus everolimus in advanced renal-cell carcinoma. N Engl J Med. 2015;373(19):1814–23.
39. Rini BI, Escudier B, Tomczak P, Kaprin A, Szczylik C, Hutson TE, et al. Comparative effectiveness of axitinib versus sorafenib in advanced renal cell carcinoma (AXIS): a randomised phase 3 trial. Lancet. 2011;378(9807):1931–9.
40. Kanesvaran R, Tan HS, Tan MH. An attenuated dose of sunitinib shows equal efficacy and with higher dose discontinuations in elderly patients compared with younger patients with metastatic renal cell carcinoma (mRCC). J Geriatr Oncol. Prostate, Bladder, Kidney Cancer in Elderly Patients SP019. 2014;5(Suppl 2).
41. Rini BI, Dorff TB, Elson P, Rodriguez CS, Shepard D, Wood L, et al. Active surveillance in metastatic renal-cell carcinoma: a prospective, phase 2 trial. Lancet Oncol. 2016;17(9):1317–24.
42. Armstrong AJ, Halabi S, Eisen T, Broderick S, Stadler WM, Jones RJ, et al. Everolimus versus sunitinib for patients with metastatic non-clear cell renal cell carcinoma (ASPEN): a multicentre, open-label, randomised phase 2 trial. Lancet Oncol. 2016;17(3):378–88.

Chapter 22
Cutaneous Melanoma in Older Adults with Frailty

Sophia Callaghan, Caroline Donovan, Paul Lorigan, and Avinash Gupta

Introduction

Older age is associated with a higher incidence of melanoma and a higher disease-related mortality [1, 2]. In the United Kingdom (UK), between 2015 and 2017, 28% of all new cutaneous melanoma cases were diagnosed in people aged 75 years and over and 45% of disease-related deaths occurred in this age group [2]. From 1991 to 2011, the UK incidence rate rose by 4.5% per annum and although the incidence for people aged <65 years is expected to plateau, for those >65 years, and particularly >80 years, incidence is predicted to continue rising [3].

Older age has been identified as an independent negative prognostic factor for melanoma and the explanation for this is likely to be multifactorial [4]. Adverse disease-related prognostic factors for melanoma include greater Breslow thickness, tumour ulceration and mitotic count, which are all found more commonly at diagnosis in older patients [4–6]. Factors relating to ageing host biology may include lymphatic dysfunction causing more distant metastasis via haematogenous spread; immunosenescence, organ dysfunction, comorbidities, declining physiological reserve and frailty syndrome [7]. The risk of Vitamin D deficiency is higher in older patients and is associated with poorer survival outcomes for melanoma patients [8, 9]. Whilst its supplementation is recommended for melanoma patients with a deficiency [10], studies are currently investigating the potential protective effect of supplementation on melanoma outcomes, such as recurrence [11, 12].

S. Callaghan · C. Donovan · A. Gupta (✉)
Medical Oncology Department, The Christie NHS Foundation Trust, Manchester, UK
e-mail: sophia.callaghan1@nhs.net; caroline.donovan3@nhs.net; avinash.gupta@nhs.net

P. Lorigan
Medical Oncology Department, The Christie NHS Foundation Trust, Manchester, UK

Division of Medical Sciences, The University of Manchester, Manchester, UK
e-mail: paul.lorigan@nhs.net

F. Gomes (ed.), *Frailty in Older Adults with Cancer*,
https://doi.org/10.1007/978-3-030-89162-6_22

Evidence shows that older patients with melanoma are less likely to receive management in line with national guidance and there may be a number of reasons for this [5, 6, 13, 14]. Whilst some of the differences in the management may be due to appropriate treatment selection, it is key to explore the risk of under-treatment, as well as over-treatment in this subgroup of patients.

In recent years, the introduction of BRAF targeted therapy and immunotherapy, specifically the immune system checkpoint inhibitors (CPI) pembrolizumab, nivolumab and ipilimumab, has drastically changed the management and prognosis for patients with melanoma, with a significant improvement in patient outcomes. Immunotherapy is potentially effective in all patients, however, a 2011–2015 review of the US National Cancer Database identified 11,944 patients with melanoma, of whom 25% received immunotherapy [15]. Patients aged >60 years were 31% less likely to receive immunotherapy compared to younger patients [15]. Contrary to immunotherapy, BRAF targeted therapy is only potentially effective in the 40–60% of patients, those whose melanomas contain a BRAF mutation [16]. However, the frequency of BRAF mutation decreases with increasing age, which limits the use of this treatment in older patients, and it may have contributed to their underrepresentation in these clinical trials [1, 17].

Despite the differences between older and younger patients with melanoma and the potential impact on treatment outcomes, age subgroup analyses from clinical trials and retrospective reviews of real-world data have shown comparable efficacy and tolerability across all age groups. However, the efficacy and safety of these treatments has not been evaluated as extensively in the older patient group with frailty, as the selection criteria for clinical trials usually exclude these patients indirectly via a strict set of criteria, such as performance status and comorbidities [1, 4]. Therefore, this chapter outlines the management of an older patient with frailty through the different stages of cutaneous melanoma, summarises the available evidence in this patient group and discusses the challenges and limitations treating teams face in this setting.

Frailty in Patients with Cutaneous Melanoma

Frailty and pre-frailty affect over half of older patients with cancer and there is a higher incidence of melanoma in older patients [18]. Such patients with both cancer and frailty are more likely to experience postoperative complications, systemic therapy intolerance, disease progression and death [18].

An adequate assessment of older patients is paramount, and as part of the standard functional assessment of patients, oncologists assess Performance Status (PS) using tools such as the Eastern Cooperative Oncology Group (ECOG) scale; however, these do not accurately identify functional impairment in older patients with cancer [19, 20]. The use of formal geriatric assessments (GA) in oncology is widely recommended as standard practice and this should evaluate domains including functional status, comorbidity, cognition, mental health status, nutrition, social support, polypharmacy and the presence of geriatric syndromes [21]. A GA can aid decision-making in a number of ways as it can identify issues missed during routine assessment, guide intervention to improve a patient's functional capacity and fitness pre-treatment and estimate treatment outcomes and severe treatment-related toxicity for some diseases and treatments [21]. The use of screening tools such as the 'Geriatric 8' (G8) to identify patients who require a more comprehensive assessment should also be considered [22]. Geriatric assessment tools are not disease- or treatment-specific and there are sparse data on the use of a GA in predicting immunotherapy-related outcomes and toxicity risk [23].

One study looked at sarcopenia, an objective measure of frailty, as a prognostic indicator in patients with Stage III melanoma undergoing Completion Lymph Node Dissection (CLND) [24]. The total cross-sectional area of the psoas muscles and the density in Hounsfield Units on CT imaging was used as a measure of sarcopenia. There were significant associations between psoas muscle density and both disease-free survival and distant disease-free survival, after adjusting for known prognostic factors including age [24].

The presence of comorbidities is another important consideration in this patient group. Older patients with advanced melanoma are highly likely to have pre-existing comorbidities which can impact on their eligibility for treatment and require treating teams to work closely with other specialties to optimise patient care and outcomes [25]. Whilst CPI are safe to use in patients with mild to moderate renal impairment and mild hepatic impairment, there should be caution with CPI use in patients with severe renal impairment and moderate to severe hepatic impairment as there are few data for these groups [26–28]. Similar recommendations should be followed in patients with BRAF mutations treated with BRAF and MEK inhibitors. For those patients with pre-existing cardiovascular disease, caution is advised for the use of BRAF and MEK inhibition as trials reported treatment-related adverse events (AEs), including prolonged-QT interval, hypertension and a reduction in ejection fraction (EF) [29, 30]. For those with a history of significant retinopathy, caution is advised due to the risk of serous neuroretinal detachment due to retinal oedema during treatment with combination BRAF and MEK inhibitors [31]. This can be asymptomatic or present with blurred vision, reduced visual acuity and photophobia [31]. Lastly, some subgroups of patients, including those with active autoimmune disease, previous organ transplant and chronic immunosuppression, will require more individualised management considerations, as use of immunotherapy will be more challenging and possibly contraindicated.

Linked with the comorbidity burden, particularly in older patients with frailty, are polypharmacy and drug interactions. However, of particular importance is the use of corticosteroids. These are often used for the management of immune-related AEs, and they can exacerbate pre-existing medical conditions such as hypertension, diabetes, congestive cardiac failure and mood disorders [31–33].

Apart from the above-mentioned considerations, which are of paramount importance for older patients with frailty, the patient's symptoms, burden of disease, tumour BRAF status and the potential treatment impact on their functional capacity and quality of life should all play a role in the decision-making. This is a particularly challenging group of patients and currently most management decisions for older patients with frailty are based on extrapolation from pivotal trials not designed for this population, combined with pockets of published real-world data and clinician experience.

Management of Early-Stage (Stage 0–II) Cutaneous Melanoma

The optimum management of primary invasive cutaneous melanoma is surgical excision with recommended wide local excision margins based on the tumour thickness [34, 35]. Older patients with frailty may present a challenge to surgical teams due to the anatomical site of the lesion, comorbidities and anaesthetic risk. In fact, older patients often experience a longer time to definitive excision and 16.8%, compared to 5% of younger patients, have insufficient excision margins ($p < 0.001$) [6]. Narrow margin excision may be acceptable in certain circumstances to maintain function, cosmesis or reduce morbidity. This is particularly relevant for cases of head and neck melanoma, which are diagnosed more frequently in older patients [6]. Alternative treatment approaches should also be considered particularly in this group of patients and there is an increasing body of evidence supporting the use of Mohs Micrographic Surgery. This can spare tissue as the surgical margins (both peripheral and deep) are tailored by the surgeon to the histological findings in real time [34, 36].

A sentinel lymph node biopsy (SLNB) identifies the presence of micro-metastatic nodal disease, which determines staging, predicts prognosis and guides further management. This is a standard of care staging procedure for the majority of patients [37–39]. However, studies have observed that older patients are less likely to undergo an SLNB due to physician recommendation, patient choice and significant comorbidities [13, 14]. As an example, a retrospective study in France observed that SLNB was performed in 23.3% of older patients, compared to 41.4% of younger patients ($p < 0.001$) [6]. Whilst there may be a lower incidence of SLN positivity in older patients [40], studies have reported that around a quarter of SLNB undertaken in older patients were positive, highlighting the value of this staging procedure, especially as there are now adjuvant treatments to reduce the risk of recurrence in patients with nodal involvement [13, 14, 41]. However, SLNB may be unsuitable depending on the severity of frailty as it also requires a general anaesthetic. Therefore, some alternatives may be considered, such as the use of focused ultrasound monitoring following lymphoscintigraphy to identify sentinel nodes [42]. High-definition ultrasound is a specialised technique that is highly operator dependent, hence that where appropriate other cross-sectional imaging techniques can also be used [37, 42].

Considerations Regarding Lentigo Maligna and Lentigo Maligna Melanoma

Lentigo Maligna (LM), a form of in situ melanoma more frequently diagnosed in older patients, is characterised by larger lesions which develop on chronically sun exposed areas such as the head and neck, but do not invade below the epidermis [34, 43]. LM requires extensive surgical margins, beyond the obvious lesion, for adequate clearance due to its tendency for subclinical extension [43]. In some cases, radiotherapy can provide an alternative to surgery for the primary treatment of LM when patients are not suitable for surgery or when adequate margins are not obtainable [34, 43]. Another alternative is imiquimod 5% cream, which has been investigated as an alternative treatment when either surgery or radiotherapy is not feasible [43, 44]. Studies have shown clearance rates of at least 75% when topical imiquimod is used first line, however a phase II study reported conflicting evidence with only a 37% rate of pathological clearance [43–45]. There is a higher risk of recurrence with imiquimod compared to surgery and radiotherapy but after clear discussion of the evidence, risks and benefits, this may be a reasonable option for patients with LM and significant frailty [34, 43, 46]. Importantly, if the malignant melanocytes in an LM lesion invade below the epidermis, this is no longer an in situ melanoma but instead an invasive melanoma, the Lentigo Maligna Melanoma (LMM), and it should be treated as such.

Management of Resectable Locally Advanced and Metastatic (Stage III–IV) Cutaneous Melanoma

Regional lymph node involvement, or in-transit metastases (ITM), upstage a melanoma to Stage III. Further staging classification is based on the number of metastatic nodes and whether the nodes were clinically detected or occult (i.e. detected only by SLNB) [39]. There is no benefit of completing lymph node dissection (CLND) for patients only with SLN positive disease [47, 48]. But for patients with clinically or radiologically detected nodal disease, CLND remains part of the initial surgical management [49]. However, given the significant risk of surgical complications with CLND, including wound infection, lymphoedema and neurological damage, it is important to consider this option on a case by case basis, especially in older patients with frailty [7]. Whilst the preferred initial approach for the management of ITM is a narrow margin excision, if this is not possible (due to the number of lesions, their location, patient fitness and risk of morbidity) other options may be considered including isolated limb infusion, electrochemotherapy, intralesional talimogene laherparepvec (T-VEC), palliative systemic therapies or radiotherapy [35]. These will be described in more detail in the next section.

Regarding the use of adjuvant treatments, three pivotal trials have shown that adjuvant treatment with BRAF directed targeted therapy (dabrafenib plus trametinib) or anti-PD-1 immunotherapy (pembrolizumab or nivolumab) is associated with a significant improvement in relapse-free survival and distant metastasis free survival. Based on these studies, these treatments are now approved for the management of resected Stage III and resected Stage IV melanoma [50–54]. The age subgroup analyses in these studies suggest similar efficacy in older and younger patients (Table 22.1). Adjuvant therapies are administered for up to 1 year, unless there is disease recurrence, unacceptable toxicity or withdrawal of patient consent. Other than the requirement of a BRAF V600 mutation for targeted therapy, there is yet no evidence to support the use of 1 treatment over the other in the adjuvant setting [49]. However, given the heterogeneity of the older and frail population, adjuvant treatment needs to be considered on a case-by-case basis. Despite their frailty, some

Table 22.1 Summary of the key clinical trials for BRAF targeted therapy and immunotherapy in the adjuvant setting

Clinical trial	Key outcomes	Treatment-related Grade 3/4 adverse events	Age subgroup analysis
CheckMate 238 [50] Nivo Vs. Ipi in patients with resected IIIB, IIIC or IV melanoma (AJCC v7 staging).	3-year RFS: 58% with Nivo 45% with Ipi 32% improvement in RFS with Nivo compared to Ipi	Nivo 14.4% Ipi 45.9%	35% and 34% improvement in RFS with Nivo compared with Ipi for patients <65 years and >65 years, respectively.
KEYNOTE-054 [51, 52] Pembro Vs. Placebo in patients with resected stage IIIA (>1 mm deposit) to IIIC melanoma (AJCC v7 staging).	3-year RFS: 64% with Pembro 44% with Placebo 44% improvement in RFS with Pembro compared to placebo	Pembro 14.7%	43% and 45% improvement in RFS with Pembro compared to placebo for patients <65 years and >65 years, respectively.
COMBI-AD [53, 54] Dab + Tram Vs. Placebo in patients with BRAF-mutant resected stage IIIA (>1 mm deposit) to IIIC melanoma (AJCC v7 staging).	3-year RFS: 59% with Dab + Tram 40% with placebo 5-year RFS: 52% with Dab + Tram 36% with placebo	Dab + Tram 41%	49% and 62% improvement in RFS with Dab and Tram compared to placebo for patients <65 years and >65 years, respectively.

Nivo Nivolumab, *Ipi* Ipilimumab, *Pembro* Pembrolizumab, *Dab* Dabrafenib, *Tram* Trametinib, *RFS* relapse-free survival patients will have a sufficient life expectancy to benefit from adjuvant therapy. A discussion with the patient, carefully considering the potential benefit weighed against the risk of toxicity is required. When the life expectancy is likely to be more limited by frailty and comorbid conditions than a possible recurrence of melanoma, the use of adjuvant treatment (with risk of toxicity and impact on quality of life) may be inappropriate. Therefore, patients with low-risk stage III melanoma or those not fit enough for adjuvant treatment should undergo observation with regular clinical examination and imaging follow-up according to established clinical guidelines [35, 38, 49].

Management of Unresectable Locally Advanced and Metastatic (Stage III–IV) Cutaneous Melanoma

The introduction of targeted therapy and immunotherapy has revolutionised the management of advanced melanoma and the prognosis for patients. The outcomes for efficacy, safety and age subgroup analysis from the most relevant clinical trials and pooled analyses are summarised in Table 22.2 [29, 30, 55–61].

Targeted Therapy

Patients with sensitising BRAF mutations may be offered oral targeted therapy with BRAF inhibitors, such as dabrafenib, encorafenib and vemurafenib, combined with MEK inhibitors, such as trametinib, binimetinib and cobimetinib. BRAF targeted therapy is only potentially effective in the 40–60% of patients whose melanomas contain a BRAF mutation [16]. However, as previously described, the frequency of BRAF mutation decreases with increasing age [1, 17].

Targeted therapy is usually continued until there is evidence of disease progression, or unacceptable toxicity. BRAF targeted treatment involves one of three different combination regimens: oral dabrafenib 150 mg BD plus trametinib 2 mg OD, binimetinib 45 mg BD plus encorafenib 450 mg OD or vemurafenib 960 mg BD plus cobimetinib 60 mg OD.

There are several factors which may influence treatment selection, including tablet load, dose timing and toxicity profiles. Treatment with dabrafenib and trametinib requires a patient to store trametinib in a fridge and take a total of five capsules/tablets daily on an empty stomach, with strict timing of doses which could be difficult for some older patients with frailty to comply with. Encorafenib plus binimetinib and vemurafenib plus cobimetinib combinations can be taken independently of food but involve taking significantly more capsules/tablets, 12 and 11 daily, respectively. Fever and rigours are more common with dabrafenib plus trametinib

Table 22.2 Summary of the key clinical trials for BRAF targeted therapy and immunotherapy for advanced melanoma

Clinical trial	Stages of melanoma (AJCC v7)	ECOG PS	Treatment arms	Key outcomes	Treatment-related Grade 3/4 AE	Age subgroup analysis
Pooled analysis of COMBI-d & COMBI- v [29, 30, 55]	Unresectable stage IIIC or IV, BRAF-mutant melanoma	0 or 1	COMBI-d [29] • Dab + Tram • Dab + Placebo COMBI-v [30] • Dab + Tram • Vem	Five-year outcomes with Dab +Tram: Median PFS of 11.1 months and median OS of 25.9 months. 5 year OS rate 34% and PFS rate 19%. DCR of 91% and ORR of 68% with 19% achieving CR.	Dab +Tram: 35–52% 18% discontinued due to AEs	Multivariate analysis of baseline factors for patients who remained progression free at 5 years suggested that older age (in 10 year increments) was significantly associated with prolonged duration of PFS ($p = 0.02$) and OS ($p = 0.04$).
COLUMBUS [56, 57]	Unresectable stage IIIB, IIIC or IV BRAF-mutant melanoma	0 or 1	• Enco • Vem • Enco + Bini	Three year outcomes with Enco +Bini: Median PFS of 14.9 months and median OS of 33.6 months. 2 year OS rate 57.6%.	Enco +Bini: 58%. 6% discontinued treatment due to AEs.	Enco + Bini compared to Vem: 45% improvement in PFS in patients <65 years and 34% improvement in PFS for patients >65 years (median follow-up of 16.6 months). At 3 years, 29% improvement in OS for patients <65 years and 37% improvement in OS for patients >65 years.
Keynote-006 [58, 59]	Unresectable stage III or IV	0 or 1	• Pembro 2 weekly • Pembro 3 weekly • Ipi 2 weekly	Five-year outcomes for the combined Pembro arms: Median PFS of 8.4 months and median OS of 32.7 months. 5 year OS rate of 38.7% and PFS rate of 23%. DCR of 63% and ORR of 42% with 14% achieving CR.	Pembro 17% Ipi 20%	Improvement in PFS with Pembro compared to Ipi was similar in patients younger than 65 years (41%) and older than 65 years (43%). Improvement in OS with Pembro compared to Ipi was observed in patients younger and older than 65 years, however it did not reach statistical significance in either group.

CheckMate-067 [60]	Unresectable stage III or IV	0 or 1	• Nivo + Ipi • Nivo • Ipi	Five-year outcomes: Nivo + Ipi PFS rate 36%, median PFS of 11.5 months. OS rate 52%, median OS >60 months. ORR of 58% with 22% achieving CR. Nivo alone PFS rate 29%, median PFS of 6.9 months. OS rate 44%, median OS of 36.9 months. ORR of 45% with 19% achieving CR.	Nivo + Ipi 59% Nivo alone 23%	Improvement in PFS with Nivo, compared to Ipi, was similar in patients younger (44%) and older than 65 years (51%). Improvement in OS with Nivo, compared to Ipi, was similar in patients <65 years (40%) and >65 years (31%). 27% improvement in PFS with Ipi + Nivo compared to Nivo in patients younger than 65 years and 11% improvement in patients over 65 years although it did not reach statistical significance. Improvement in OS with Ipi + Nivo compared to Nivo was similar in patients younger and older than 65 years, however it did not reach statistical significance.
Pooled analysis from phase II and phase III trials with Ipilimumab & secondary analysis included data from expanded access programme [61]	Previously treated and untreated advanced melanoma	0 or 1 in clinical trial 0–2 in EAP	Ipi 3 mg/kg or 10 mg/kg every 3 weeks for 4 doses	OS of 21% with a plateau in the survival curve around 3 years and extending up to 10 years for some patients.	Not analysed in this pooled analysis, but grade 3/4 AEs affected 28% in the Checkmate 067 trial.	Not reviewed in this pooled analysis. Similar improvement in OS with Ipi compared to gp100 vaccine in older patients (39%) and younger patients (35%).

ECOG PS Eastern Cooperative Oncology Group performance status, *AE* adverse event, *PFS* progression-free survival, *OS* overall survival, *DCR* disease control rate, *ORR* objective response rate, *CR* complete response, *Dab* Dabrafenib, *Tram* Trametinib, *Enco* Encorafenib, *Bini* Binimetinib, *Vem* Vemurafenib, *Nivo* Nivolumab, *Pembro* Pembrolizumab, *Ipi* Ipilimumab and gastrointestinal toxicity occurs more frequently with encorafenib plus binimetinib and vemurafenib plus cobimetinib, which should be considered during patient assessment and treatment selection [31]. Overall, health related quality of life measures are similar or improved compared with baseline whilst on combination targeted therapy and actually better for combination targeted therapy vs monotherapy [62, 63].

The age subgroup analyses of the pivotal trials of targeted therapy suggest the overall efficacy is similar in older and younger patient groups (Table 22.2). Meanwhile, an on-going retrospective study, using patient data from the French database MELBASE, aims to analyse the tolerance of targeted therapy in older patients with melanoma (NCT03155217).

Based on the safety data from the clinical trials, there are a few key considerations for patients with comorbidities and frailty. Risks and benefits of BRAF and MEK inhibition should be carefully considered in patients with cardiovascular risk factors, as these drugs can cause QT-prolongation, impaired myocardial function and hypertension. For frailer patients who experience fever and GI toxicity, closer monitoring and prompt management with fluid and electrolyte replacement is required to avoid hypovolaemia, hypotension and acute renal failure [31]. The management of toxicity generally involves interrupting dosing, until the toxicity resolves, and then resuming treatment, either at the same dose or a lower dose, depending on the severity of the toxicity [31]. Older patients with frailty may not be able to tolerate full doses of these drugs due to the associated side effects, however they are often able to tolerate lower doses quite well.

Ultimately, whilst patients with BRAF-mutant melanoma have the option of either treatment with immunotherapy or targeted therapy with a combination of BRAF and MEK inhibitors, targeted therapy is generally the preferred first line treatment for symptomatic patients requiring early response, as this can induce rapid disease regression and symptomatic relief, and these are a good option for older patients with frailty [35, 64].

Immunotherapy with CPI

The introduction of immunotherapy with CPI revolutionised the treatment of melanoma patients, but it is challenging to predict benefit and tolerability with CPI. The age subgroup analyses suggest there is no significant difference in efficacy between patients older and younger than 65 years (Table 22.2). However older patients recruited to clinical trials are not representative of older patients particularly as those with frailty are mostly excluded. However, several retrospective reviews have analysed real-world data and reported no significant difference in efficacy and tolerability between age groups [65–72]. Retrospective studies have assessed the impact of ECOG PS, comorbidities and indirect frailty markers on immunotherapy outcomes in older patients [67, 68, 73]. Data of 318 patients with advanced melanoma, treated with anti-CTLA-4 or/and anti-PD-1 between

2011 and 2017 were analysed [68]. Eighty-two patients were aged >70 years and 84% had comorbidities including hypertension, cardiovascular disease and diabetes. Overall survival and toxicity were similar for patients all age groups, and the presence of comorbidities was not associated with increased risk of toxicity [68]. A review of 40 patients with advanced melanoma who received first line anti-PD1 monotherapy found overall response rate and rate of severe toxicity were similar between patients <70 years and >70 years [67]. This study also considered indirect frailty markers in patients >70 years which included ECOG PS ≥ 2, a fall in the previous 6 months and a Charlson comorbidity score ≥11, and found there were similar rates of response and toxicity in patients identified as 'frail' [67]. The recently published ELDERS study was a prospective cohort study of patients starting single-agent CPI for the management of melanoma or lung cancer which was designed to primarily assess the incidence of severe toxicity (immune-related) between 2 age cohorts (<70 vs ≥70 years) [74]. The study was negative for its primary aim with no significant difference in severe toxicity between younger and older patients. Moreover, this study was amongst the first to incorporate frailty and geriatric assessments in the context of CPI treatment, for patient characterisation. Frailty (assessed by G8 screening tool) was identified in half of the older patients on CPI but it was not associated with a higher risk of severe toxicity. It was however a predictor of hospital admission (mainly due to the cancer and comorbidity instead of treatment-related), as well as a predictor of risk of death. The authors concluded that although frailty did not increase the risk of immune-related toxicity, it impacted the patients' ability to cope with adverse events (treatment-related or not) [74].

Whilst combination CPI with nivolumab plus ipilimumab is more effective than monotherapy, this is not appropriate for older patients with frailty given the high incidence of high-grade toxicity (over 50%) [4, 60]. Therefore, treatment with PD-1 inhibitor monotherapy, either nivolumab or pembrolizumab, is usually more appropriate given the positive survival outcomes and significantly lower rates of high-grade toxicity (about 10%) [4, 35, 64]. Current regimens are nivolumab 480 mg 4 weekly and pembrolizumab 200 mg 3 weekly or 400 mg 6 weekly. Pembrolizumab dosing every 6 weeks has demonstrated comparable safety and efficacy to 3 weekly dosing and so can be considered particularly for patients who will benefit from fewer hospital visits [75].

For PD-1 inhibitors, the most commonly reported toxicity is fatigue, rash, pruritus, diarrhoea, nausea and arthralgia [76]. One retrospective study found a higher incidence of arthritis (10.8%, $p = 0.02$) in patients aged 65–74 years and a trend towards more immune-related endocrinopathy in patients over 75 years, who received anti-PD-1 and or PD-L1 [69]. Another study which included patients with PS 2–3 (26%) found no statistically significant difference in toxicity between groups with low and high ECOG PS [73]. The ELDERS study reported a relatively similar toxicity profile between older and younger patients, however the duration of systemic steroid used to manage severe toxicity seemed to be potentially longer in older patients which could have significant consequences particularly for those patients with frailty and a high comorbidity burden [74].

There are a number of published guidelines for management of immunotherapy-related toxicity, including by the European Society of Medical Oncology [77]. Underpinning all of them are direct symptom reporting, prompt investigation and usually early management with steroid immunosuppression. Immune-related endocrinopathies often require lifelong hormone replacement and monitoring. Closer monitoring is required for older patients with frailty as symptoms and signs can be subtle and non-specific, such as memory loss or cognitive decline secondary to immune-related hypothyroidism [78]. The use of corticosteroids is a key part of the management for more severe toxicity related to both targeted therapy and especially immunotherapy, with the potential need for high doses of steroids to manage such toxicity. Patients with frailty and those with comorbidities are more at risk of iatrogenic events related to corticosteroid use, such as worsening diabetes, hypertension, congestive cardiac failure and delirium [32, 76, 78]. In addition, the impact of a hospital admission for treatment and recovery could be more significant for this subgroup of patients [4].

Overall treatment with single-agent CPI is a good and appropriate option for older patients with melanoma and frailty, however the higher toxicity risk of CPI combinations precludes their use for the vast majority of these patients. Lastly, for older patients with frailty and progressive disease with CPI treatment (and, where appropriate, BRAF targeted therapy), further options are very limited and best supportive care is often the most appropriate option.

Other Treatments

Prior to 2011, chemotherapy with single-agent dacarbazine was the standard of care systemic treatment for advanced melanoma. However, it had poor response rates of around 15% as a first line therapy and very few patients achieved a durable response [79]. Combination chemotherapy has demonstrated no improved survival benefit compared to dacarbazine alone [80]. The use of chemotherapy is now generally a last resort for the treatment of melanoma and would not be recommended for an older patient with frailty, given the high risk of toxicity and low chance of any benefit.

Radiotherapy can also be considered for the palliative treatment of symptomatic skin, subcutaneous, lymph node and bone metastases. Denosumab can also be used to help manage symptomatic bone metastases [81]. Both are appropriate and may play a role in the management of older patients with frailty.

The management of localised, unresectable disease depends on the volume and location of the disease, history of previous recurrence, the fitness of the patient and the risk of treatment-related toxicity weighed against potential benefit. Generally, if the patient is well enough, systemic therapies are considered first due to the significant progression-free survival and overall survival benefit. If there are concerns regarding patient fitness for systemic treatment, other options may include isolated limb infusion, electrochemotherapy or T-VEC [35, 82]. Isolated limb infusion of high dose chemotherapy has shown an ORR around 70% with complete responses in up to 30% of patients, and low rates of severe toxicity [82]. Retrospective data has shown comparable efficacy and tolerability in younger and older patients, with an age cut-off at 75 years [83]. Electrochemotherapy can be considered for disease on the trunk, head and neck as well as limbs and has demonstrated an ORR of 80–90% with complete responses in up to 60% with minimal toxicity [84]. The intralesional injection of T-VEC, a modified oncolytic herpes simplex virus, may also be considered for patients who are unable to have regional therapies or for small volume disease on the trunk, head and neck. It is well tolerated with minor side effects including fatigue, fever, flu-like symptoms and injection site pain [85]. All these options are potentially appropriate for older patients with frailty.

Considerations Regarding Brain Metastases

The incidence of melanoma brain metastases (MBM) is reported as 43% in clinical studies and 75% in autopsy series [86]. Prognosis is usually poor with a median overall survival of 4–6 months [86]. If picked up early, management can include neurosurgical resection or stereotactic radiosurgery (SRS) [35]. Both BRAF targeted therapy and combination immunotherapy have been shown to be effective against brain metastases [87–89]. The COMBI-MB study evaluated the efficacy and safety of dabrafenib plus trametinib in patients with MBM. Results showed high intracranial response rates of about 56%, but limited survival benefit, with a median progression-free survival of about 6 months and median overall survival of about 11 months in patients with both asymptomatic and symptomatic MBM [89]. For patients with asymptomatic MBM, combination immunotherapy is associated with a similar intracranial response rates (56%) and longer overall survival, based on two small studies, and this has become standard of care for patients fit enough to receive this, considering its toxicity [87, 88]. Whole brain radiotherapy has demonstrated improvement in some neurological symptoms but no improvement in overall survival, and a high incidence of associated neurocognitive decline [86, 90]. Data from other types of cancer suggest patients with a poor PS and short life expectancy do not benefit from this more than steroids and best supportive care [91].

For older patients with significant frailty, best supportive is the most appropriate management for the vast majority of such patients since the treatment modalities available pose significant risk of toxicity and debility [35]. The potential exception is for patients with BRAF-mutant melanoma, where treatment with targeted therapy may still be appropriate, based on the results of the COMBI-MB study, which included patients with symptomatic MBM, with or without previous local brain therapy and an ECOG PS of 0–2 [89]. Of note, for those with mild frailty or pre-frailty, treating clinicians may discuss the risks and benefits of the other treatment options available, ideally after liaising with their local neuro-oncology multidisciplinary team.

Conclusion

The management of older patients with frailty and melanoma is fundamentally based on the guidelines and recommendations for all patients with melanoma. But the suitability of the available treatments and the balance of risk-benefit are often significantly different in the older sub-population with frailty. This needs to be carefully considered throughout the continuum of cancer care so that the management plan can be adequately tailored to this challenging group of patients. The development of specific biomarkers to accurately predict individual patient benefit and toxicity risk from melanoma treatments is an active area of research [92, 93]. In the future this will hopefully help identify older patients with frailty who are most likely to benefit from and tolerate treatment for their melanoma.

References

1. Iglesias-Pena N, Paradela S, Tejera-Vaquerizo A, Boada A, Fonseca E. Cutaneous melanoma in the elderly: review of a growing problem. Actas Dermosifiliogr. 2019;110(6):434–47. https://doi.org/10.1016/j.ad.2018.11.009.
2. Cancer Research UK: Melanoma skin cancer statistics. https://www.cancerresearchuk.org/health-professional/cancerstatistics/statistics-by-cancer-type/melanoma-skin-cancer#heading-Five. Accessed 22 August 2020; 2020.
3. Whiteman DC, Green AC, Olsen CM. The growing burden of invasive melanoma: projections of incidence rates and numbers of new cases in six susceptible populations through 2031. J Invest Dermatol. 2016;136(6):1161–71. https://doi.org/10.1016/j.jid.2016.01.035.
4. Bastiaannet E, Battisti N, Loh KP, de Glas N, Soto-Perez-de-Celis E, Baldini C, et al. Immunotherapy and targeted therapies in older patients with advanced melanoma; Young International Society of Geriatric Oncology review paper. J Geriatr Oncol. 2019;10(3):389–97. https://doi.org/10.1016/j.jgo.2018.06.009.
5. Rees MJ, Liao H, Spillane J, Speakman D, McCormack C, Donahoe S, et al. Melanoma in the very elderly, management in patients 85years of age and over. J Geriatr Oncol. 2018;9(5):488–93. https://doi.org/10.1016/j.jgo.2018.01.001.
6. Ciocan D, Barbe C, Aubin F, Granel-Brocard F, Lipsker D, Velten M, et al. Distinctive features of melanoma and its management in elderly patients: a population-based study in France. JAMA Dermatol. 2013;149(10):1150–7. https://doi.org/10.1001/jamadermatol.2013.706.
7. Garcovich S, Colloca G, Sollena P, Andrea B, Balducci L, Cho WC, et al. Skin cancer epidemics in the elderly as an emerging issue in geriatric oncology. Aging Dis. 2017;8(5):643–61. https://doi.org/10.14336/ad.2017.0503.
8. Fang S, Sui D, Wang Y, Liu H, Chiang YJ, Ross MI, et al. Association of vitamin D levels with outcome in patients with melanoma after adjustment for C-reactive protein. J Clin Oncol. 2016;34(15):1741–7. https://doi.org/10.1200/jco.2015.64.1357.
9. Timerman D, McEnery-Stonelake M, Joyce CJ, Nambudiri VE, Hodi FS, Claus EB, et al. Vitamin D deficiency is associated with a worse prognosis in metastatic melanoma. Oncotarget. 2017;8(4):6873–82. https://doi.org/10.18632/oncotarget.14316.
10. National Institute for Health and Care Excellence. Melanoma: assessment and management. NICE guideline [NG14]. https://www.nice.org.uk/guidance/ng14/chapter/1-recommendations (2015). Accessed 31 August 2020; 2020.
11. De Smedt J, Van Kelst S, Boecxstaens V, Stas M, Bogaerts K, Vanderschueren D, et al. Vitamin D supplementation in cutaneous malignant melanoma outcome (ViDMe): a randomized controlled trial. BMC Cancer. 2017;17(1):562. https://doi.org/10.1186/s12885-017-3538-4.

12. Saw RP, Armstrong BK, Mason RS, Morton RL, Shannon KF, Spillane AJ, et al. Adjuvant therapy with high dose vitamin D following primary treatment of melanoma at high risk of recurrence: a placebo controlled randomised phase II trial (ANZMTG 02.09 Mel-D). BMC Cancer. 2014;14:780. https://doi.org/10.1186/1471-2407-14-780.
13. Grotz TE, Puig CA, Perkins S, Ballman K, Hieken TJ. Management of regional lymph nodes in the elderly melanoma patient: patient selection, accuracy and prognostic implications. Eur J Surg Oncol. 2015;41(1):157–64. https://doi.org/10.1016/j.ejso.2014.10.051.
14. Sabel MS, Kozminski D, Griffith K, Chang AE, Johnson TM, Wong S. Sentinel lymph node biopsy use among melanoma patients 75 years of age and older. Ann Surg Oncol. 2015;22(7):2112–9. https://doi.org/10.1245/s10434-015-4539-7.
15. Jain V, Hwang WT, Venigalla S, Nead KT, Lukens JN, Mitchell TC, et al. Association of age with efficacy of immunotherapy in metastatic melanoma. Oncologist. 2020;25(2):e381–e5. https://doi.org/10.1634/theoncologist.2019-0377.
16. Cheng L, Lopez-Beltran A, Massari F, MacLennan GT, Montironi R. Molecular testing for BRAF mutations to inform melanoma treatment decisions: a move toward precision medicine. Mod Pathol. 2018;31(1):24–38. https://doi.org/10.1038/modpathol.2017.104.
17. Menzies AM, Haydu LE, Visintin L, Carlino MS, Howle JR, Thompson JF, et al. Distinguishing clinicopathologic features of patients with V600E and V600K BRAF-mutant metastatic melanoma. Clin Cancer Res. 2012;18(12):3242–9. https://doi.org/10.1158/1078-0432.Ccr-12-0052.
18. Ethun CG, Bilen MA, Jani AB, Maithel SK, Ogan K, Master VA. Frailty and cancer: implications for oncology surgery, medical oncology, and radiation oncology. CA Cancer J Clin. 2017;67(5):362–77. https://doi.org/10.3322/caac.21406.
19. Repetto L, Fratino L, Audisio RA, Venturino A, Gianni W, Vercelli M, et al. Comprehensive geriatric assessment adds information to Eastern Cooperative Oncology Group performance status in elderly cancer patients: an Italian Group for Geriatric Oncology Study. J Clin Oncol. 2002;20(2):494–502. https://doi.org/10.1200/jco.2002.20.2.494.
20. Jolly TA, Deal AM, Nyrop KA, Williams GR, Pergolotti M, Wood WA, et al. Geriatric assessment-identified deficits in older cancer patients with normal performance status. Oncologist. 2015;20(4):379–85. https://doi.org/10.1634/theoncologist.2014-0247.
21. Wildiers H, Heeren P, Puts M, Topinkova E, Janssen-Heijnen ML, Extermann M, et al. International Society of Geriatric Oncology consensus on geriatric assessment in older patients with cancer. J Clin Oncol. 2014;32(24):2595–603. https://doi.org/10.1200/jco.2013.54.8347.
22. Kenis C, Decoster L, Van Puyvelde K, De Grève J, Conings G, Milisen K, et al. Performance of two geriatric screening tools in older patients with cancer. J Clin Oncol. 2014;32(1):19–26. https://doi.org/10.1200/jco.2013.51.1345.
23. Welaya K, Loh KP, Messing S, Szuba E, Magnuson A, Mohile SG, et al. Geriatric assessment and treatment outcomes in older adults with cancer receiving immune checkpoint inhibitors. J Geriatr Oncol. 2020;11(3):523–8. https://doi.org/10.1016/j.jgo.2019.05.021.
24. Sabel MS, Lee J, Cai S, Englesbe MJ, Holcombe S, Wang S. Sarcopenia as a prognostic factor among patients with stage III melanoma. Ann Surg Oncol. 2011;18(13):3579–85. https://doi.org/10.1245/s10434-011-1976-9.
25. Rai P, Shen C, Kolodney J, Kelly KM, Scott VG, Sambamoorthi U. Prevalence and risk factors for multimorbidity in older US patients with late-stage melanoma. J Geriatr Oncol. 2021;12(3):388–93. https://doi.org/10.1016/j.jgo.2020.09.019.
26. FDA: KEYTRUDA. Highlights of prescribing information. https://www.accessdata.fda.gov/drugsatfda_docs/label/2019/125514Orig1s054lbl.pdf. Accessed 22 August 2020; 2020.
27. FDA: OPDIVO Highlights of prescribing information. https://www.accessdata.fda.gov/drugsatfda_docs/label/2018/125554s058lbl.pdf. Accessed 22 August 2020; 2020.
28. FDA: YERVOY. Highlights of prescribing information. https://www.accessdata.fda.gov/drugsatfda_docs/label/2018/125377s094lbl.pdf. Accessed 22 August 2020; 2020.
29. Long GV, Stroyakovskiy D, Gogas H, Levchenko E, De Braud F, Larkin J, et al. Dabrafenib and trametinib versus dabrafenib and placebo for Val600 BRAF-mutant melanoma: a multicentre, double-blind, phase 3 randomised controlled trial. Lancet. 2015;386(9992):444–51.
30. Robert C, Karaszewska B, Schachter J, Rutkowski P, Mackiewicz A, Stroiakovski D, et al. Improved overall survival in melanoma with combined dabrafenib and trametinib. N Engl J Med. 2015;372(1):30–9. https://doi.org/10.1056/NEJMoa1412690.

31. Heinzerling L, Eigentler TK, Fluck M, Hassel JC, Heller-Schenck D, Leipe J, et al. Tolerability of BRAF/MEK inhibitor combinations: adverse event evaluation and management. ESMO Open. 2019;4(3):e000491. https://doi.org/10.1136/esmoopen-2019-000491.
32. Alkharabsheh O, Kannarkatt P, Kannarkatt J, Karapetyan L, Laird-Fick HS, Al-Janadi A. An overview of the toxicities of checkpoint inhibitors in older patients with cancer. J Geriatr Oncol. 2018;9(5):451–8. https://doi.org/10.1016/j.jgo.2018.02.002.
33. Daste A, Chakiba C, Domblides C, Gross-Goupil M, Quivy A, Ravaud A, et al. Targeted therapy and elderly people: a review. Eur J Cancer. 2016;69:199–215. https://doi.org/10.1016/j.ejca.2016.10.005.
34. Dowling J, McGregor SP, Williford P. Update on current treatment recommendations for primary cutaneous melanoma. Dermatol Clin. 2019;37(4):397–407. https://doi.org/10.1016/j.det.2019.06.001.
35. National Comprehensive Cancer Network: NCCN Clinical Practice Guidelines in Oncology - Cutaneous Melanoma. Version 3.2020. https://www.nccn.org/professionals/physician_gls/pdf/cutaneous_melanoma.pdf (2020). Accessed 22 August 2020; 2020.
36. Beaulieu D, Fathi R, Srivastava D, Nijhawan RI. Current perspectives on Mohs micrographic surgery for melanoma. Clin Cosmet Investig Dermatol. 2018;11:309–20. https://doi.org/10.2147/ccid.S137513.
37. Peach H, Board R, Cook M, Corrie P, Ellis S, Geh J, et al. Current role of sentinel lymph node biopsy in the management of cutaneous melanoma: a UK consensus statement. J Plast Reconstr Aesthet Surg. 2020;73(1):36–42. https://doi.org/10.1016/j.bjps.2019.06.020.
38. Wong SL, Faries MB, Kennedy EB, Agarwala SS, Akhurst TJ, Ariyan C, et al. Sentinel lymph node biopsy and management of regional lymph nodes in melanoma: American Society of Clinical Oncology and Society of Surgical Oncology Clinical Practice guideline update. Ann Surg Oncol. 2018;25(2):356–77. https://doi.org/10.1245/s10434-017-6267-7.
39. Gershenwald JE, Scolyer RA, Hess KR, Sondak VK, Long GV, Ross MI, et al. Melanoma staging: evidence-based changes in the American Joint Committee on Cancer eighth edition cancer staging manual. CA Cancer J Clin. 2017;67(6):472–92. https://doi.org/10.3322/caac.21409.
40. Balch CM, Thompson JF, Gershenwald JE, Soong SJ, Ding S, McMasters KM, et al. Age as a predictor of sentinel node metastasis among patients with localized melanoma: an inverse correlation of melanoma mortality and incidence of sentinel node metastasis among young and old patients. Ann Surg Oncol. 2014;21(4):1075–81. https://doi.org/10.1245/s10434-013-3464-x.
41. Koskivuo I, Hernberg M, Vihinen P, Virolainen S, Talve L, Seppänen M, et al. Sentinel lymph node biopsy and survival in elderly patients with cutaneous melanoma. Br J Surg. 2011;98(10):1400–7. https://doi.org/10.1002/bjs.7565.
42. Ipenburg NA, Thompson JF, Uren RF, Chung D, Nieweg OE. Focused ultrasound surveillance of lymph nodes following lymphoscintigraphy without sentinel node biopsy: a useful and safe strategy in elderly or frail melanoma patients. Ann Surg Oncol. 2019;26(9):2855–63. https://doi.org/10.1245/s10434-019-07505-6.
43. Swetter SM, Tsao H, Bichakjian CK, Curiel-Lewandrowski C, Elder DE, Gershenwald JE, et al. Guidelines of care for the management of primary cutaneous melanoma. J Am Acad Dermatol. 2019;80(1):208–50. https://doi.org/10.1016/j.jaad.2018.08.055.
44. Tio D, van Montfrans C, Ruijter CGH, Hoekzema R, Bekkenk MW. Effectiveness of 5% topical imiquimod for lentigo maligna treatment. Acta Derm Venereol. 2019;99(10):884–8. https://doi.org/10.2340/00015555-3241.
45. Marsden JR, Fox R, Boota NM, Cook M, Wheatley K, Billingham LJ, et al. Effect of topical imiquimod as primary treatment for lentigo maligna: the LIMIT-1 study. Br J Dermatol. 2017;176(5):1148–54. https://doi.org/10.1111/bjd.15112.
46. Forschner A, Heinrich V, Pflugfelder A, Meier F, Garbe C. The role of radiotherapy in the overall treatment of melanoma. Clin Dermatol. 2013;31(3):282–9. https://doi.org/10.1016/j.clindermatol.2012.08.009.
47. Leiter U, Stadler R, Mauch C, Hohenberger W, Brockmeyer N, Berking C, et al. Complete lymph node dissection versus no dissection in patients with sentinel lymph node biopsy positive melanoma (DeCOG-SLT): a multicentre, randomised, phase 3 trial. Lancet Oncol. 2016;17(6):757–67. https://doi.org/10.1016/s1470-2045(16)00141-8.

48. Faries MB, Thompson JF, Cochran AJ, Andtbacka RH, Mozzillo N, Zager JS, et al. Completion dissection or observation for sentinel-node metastasis in melanoma. N Engl J Med. 2017;376(23):2211–22. https://doi.org/10.1056/NEJMoa1613210.
49. Ascierto PA, Borgognoni L, Botti G, Guida M, Marchetti P, Mocellin S, et al. New paradigm for stage III melanoma: from surgery to adjuvant treatment. J Transl Med. 2019;17(1):266. https://doi.org/10.1186/s12967-019-2012-2.
50. Weber J, Mandala M, Del Vecchio M, Gogas HJ, Arance AM, Cowey CL, et al. Adjuvant nivolumab versus ipilimumab in resected stage III or IV melanoma. N Engl J Med. 2017;377(19):1824–35. https://doi.org/10.1056/NEJMoa1709030.
51. Eggermont AM, Blank CU, Mandalà M, Long GV, Atkinson V, Dalle S, et al. Pembrolizumab versus placebo after complete resection of high-risk stage III melanoma: New recurrence-free survival results from the EORTC 1325-MG/Keynote 054 double-blinded phase III trial at three-year median follow-up. J Clin Oncol. 2020;38(15_suppl):10000. https://doi.org/10.1200/JCO.2020.38.15_suppl.10000.
52. Eggermont AMM, Blank CU, Mandala M, Long GV, Atkinson V, Dalle S, et al. Adjuvant pembrolizumab versus placebo in resected stage III melanoma. N Engl J Med. 2018;378(19):1789–801. https://doi.org/10.1056/NEJMoa1802357.
53. Long GV, Hauschild A, Santinami M, Atkinson V, Mandalà M, Chiarion-Sileni V, et al. Adjuvant dabrafenib plus trametinib in stage III BRAF-mutated melanoma. N Engl J Med. 2017;377(19):1813–23. https://doi.org/10.1056/NEJMoa1708539.
54. Hauschild A, Dummer R, Santinami M, Atkinson V, Mandalà M, Kirkwood JM, et al. Long-term benefit of adjuvant dabrafenib + trametinib (D+T) in patients (pts) with resected stage III BRAF V600–mutant melanoma: Five-year analysis of COMBI-AD. J Clin Oncol. 2020;38(15_suppl):10001. https://doi.org/10.1200/JCO.2020.38.15_suppl.10001.
55. Robert C, Grob JJ, Stroyakovskiy D, Karaszewska B, Hauschild A, Levchenko E, et al. Five-year outcomes with dabrafenib plus trametinib in metastatic melanoma. N Engl J Med. 2019;381(7):626–36. https://doi.org/10.1056/NEJMoa1904059.
56. Dummer R, Ascierto PA, Gogas HJ, Arance A, Mandala M, Liszkay G, et al. Overall survival in patients with BRAF-mutant melanoma receiving encorafenib plus binimetinib versus vemurafenib or encorafenib (COLUMBUS): a multicentre, open-label, randomised, phase 3 trial. Lancet Oncol. 2018;19(10):1315–27. https://doi.org/10.1016/s1470-2045(18)30497-2.
57. Dummer R, Ascierto PA, Gogas HJ, Arance A, Mandala M, Liszkay G, et al. Encorafenib plus binimetinib versus vemurafenib or encorafenib in patients with BRAF-mutant melanoma (COLUMBUS): a multicentre, open-label, randomised phase 3 trial. Lancet Oncol. 2018;19(5):603–15. https://doi.org/10.1016/s1470-2045(18)30142-6.
58. Robert C, Schachter J, Long GV, Arance A, Grob JJ, Mortier L, et al. Pembrolizumab versus ipilimumab in advanced melanoma. N Engl J Med. 2015;372(26):2521–32. https://doi.org/10.1056/NEJMoa1503093.
59. Robert C, Ribas A, Schachter J, Arance A, Grob JJ, Mortier L, et al. Pembrolizumab versus ipilimumab in advanced melanoma (KEYNOTE-006): post-hoc 5-year results from an open-label, multicentre, randomised, controlled, phase 3 study. Lancet Oncol. 2019;20(9):1239–51. https://doi.org/10.1016/s1470-2045(19)30388-2.
60. Larkin J, Chiarion-Sileni V, Gonzalez R, Grob JJ, Rutkowski P, Lao CD, et al. Five-year survival with combined nivolumab and ipilimumab in advanced melanoma. N Engl J Med. 2019;381(16):1535–46. https://doi.org/10.1056/NEJMoa1910836.
61. Schadendorf D, Hodi FS, Robert C, Weber JS, Margolin K, Hamid O, et al. Pooled analysis of long-term survival data from phase II and phase III trials of ipilimumab in unresectable or metastatic melanoma. J Clin Oncol. 2015;33(17):1889–94. https://doi.org/10.1200/jco.2014.56.2736.
62. Grob JJ, Amonkar MM, Karaszewska B, Schachter J, Dummer R, Mackiewicz A, et al. Comparison of dabrafenib and trametinib combination therapy with vemurafenib monotherapy on health-related quality of life in patients with unresectable or metastatic cutaneous BRAF

Val600-mutation-positive melanoma (COMBI-v): results of a phase 3, open-label, randomised trial. Lancet Oncol. 2015;16(13):1389–98. https://doi.org/10.1016/s1470-2045(15)00087-x.
63. Gogas H, Dummer R, Ascierto P, Arance A, Mandala M, Liszkay G, et al. 1245PQuality-of-life (QoL) in COLUMBUS part 1: a phase 3 trial of encorafenib (ENCO) plus binimetinib (BINI) versus vemurafenib (VEM) or ENCO in braf-mutant melanoma. Ann Oncol. 2017;28 https://doi.org/10.1093/annonc/mdx377.031.
64. Keilholz U, Ascierto PA, Dummer R, Robert C, Lorigan P, van Akkooi A, et al. ESMO consensus conference recommendations on the management of metastatic melanoma: under the auspices of the ESMO Guidelines Committee. Ann Oncol. 2020; https://doi.org/10.1016/j.annonc.2020.07.004.
65. Friedman CF, Horvat TZ, Minehart J, Panageas K, Callahan MK, Chapman PB, et al. Efficacy and safety of checkpoint blockade for treatment of advanced melanoma (mel) in patients (pts) age 80 and older (80+). Am Soc Clin Oncol.2016.
66. Chiarion Sileni V, Pigozzo J, Ascierto PA, Grimaldi AM, Maio M, Di Guardo L, et al. Efficacy and safety of ipilimumab in elderly patients with pretreated advanced melanoma treated at Italian centres through the expanded access programme. J Exp Clin Cancer Res. 2014;33(1):30. https://doi.org/10.1186/1756-9966-33-30.
67. Archibald WJ, Victor AI, Strawderman MS, Maggiore RJ. Immune checkpoint inhibitors in older adults with melanoma or cutaneous malignancies: The Wilmot Cancer Institute experience. J Geriatr Oncol. 2020;11(3):496–502. https://doi.org/10.1016/j.jgo.2019.07.005.
68. Cybulska-Stopa B, Ługowska I, Jagodzińska-Mucha P, Koseła-Paterczyk H, Kozak K, Klimczak A, et al. Immune checkpoint inhibitors therapy in older patients ($\geq$ 70 years) with metastatic melanoma: a multicentre study. Postepy Dermatol Alergol. 2019;36(5):566–71. https://doi.org/10.5114/ada.2018.79940.
69. Betof AS, Nipp RD, Giobbie-Hurder A, Johnpulle RAN, Rubin K, Rubinstein SM, et al. Impact of age on outcomes with immunotherapy for patients with melanoma. Oncologist. 2017;22(8):963–71. https://doi.org/10.1634/theoncologist.2016-0450.
70. Barailler H, Salomon G, Dutriaux C, Prey S, Gérard E, Dousset L, et al. Adverse events, need for hospitalization and systemic immunosuppression in very older patients (over 80 years) treated with anti-PD-1 for metastatic melanoma. J Geriatr Oncol. 2020. doi:https://doi.org/10.1016/j.jgo.2020.03.003.
71. van Holstein Y, Kapiteijn E, Bastiaannet E, van den Bos F, Portielje J, de Glas NA. Efficacy and adverse events of immunotherapy with checkpoint inhibitors in older patients with cancer. Drugs Aging. 2019;36(10):927–38. https://doi.org/10.1007/s40266-019-00697-2.
72. Howell AV, Gebregziabher M, Thiers BH, Paulos CM, Wrangle JM, Hunt KJ, et al. Immune checkpoint inhibitors retain effectiveness in older patients with cutaneous metastatic melanoma. J Geriatr Oncol. 2021;12(3):394–401. https://doi.org/10.1016/j.jgo.2020.09.023.
73. Wong A, Williams M, Milne D, Morris K, Lau P, Spruyt O, et al. Clinical and palliative care outcomes for patients of poor performance status treated with antiprogrammed death-1 monoclonal antibodies for advanced melanoma. Asia Pac J Clin Oncol. 2017;13(6):385–90. https://doi.org/10.1111/ajco.12702.
74. Gomes F, Lorigan P, Woolley S, Foden P, Burns K, Yorke J, et al. A prospective cohort study on the safety of checkpoint inhibitors in older cancer patients - the ELDERS study. ESMO Open. 2021;6(1):100042. https://doi.org/10.1016/j.esmoop.2020.100042.
75. Mallika Lala OA, Chartash E, Kalabis M, Su S-C, De Alwis D, Sinha V, Jain L. Pembrolizumab 400mg Q6W dosing: first clinical outcomes data from Keynote-555 cohort B in metastatic melanoma patients. 2020 AACR Virtual Meeting Abstract CT042.2020.
76. Helissey C, Vicier C, Champiat S. The development of immunotherapy in older adults: New treatments, new toxicities? J Geriatr Oncol. 2016;7(5):325–33. https://doi.org/10.1016/j.jgo.2016.05.007.
77. Haanen J, Carbonnel F, Robert C, Kerr KM, Peters S, Larkin J, et al. Management of toxicities from immunotherapy: ESMO Clinical Practice Guidelines for diagnosis, treatment and follow-up. Ann Oncol. 2017;28(suppl_4):iv119–iv42. https://doi.org/10.1093/annonc/mdx225.

78. Friedman CF, Wolchok JD. Checkpoint inhibition and melanoma: considerations in treating the older adult. J Geriatr Oncol. 2017;8(4):237–41. https://doi.org/10.1016/j.jgo.2017.04.003.
79. Gupta A, Gomes F, Lorigan P. The role for chemotherapy in the modern management of melanoma. Melanoma Manag. 2017;4(2):125–36. https://doi.org/10.2217/mmt-2017-0003.
80. Nashan D, Müller ML, Grabbe S, Wustlich S, Enk A. Systemic therapy of disseminated malignant melanoma: an evidence-based overview of the state-of-the-art in daily routine. J Eur Acad Dermatol Venereol. 2007;21(10):1305–18. https://doi.org/10.1111/j.1468-3083.2007.02475.x.
81. Coleman R, Body JJ, Aapro M, Hadji P, Herrstedt J. Bone health in cancer patients: ESMO Clinical Practice Guidelines. Ann Oncol. 2014;25(Suppl 3):iii124–37. https://doi.org/10.1093/annonc/mdu103.
82. Perone JA, Farrow N, Tyler DS, Beasley GM. Contemporary approaches to in-transit melanoma. J Oncol Pract. 2018;14(5):292–300. https://doi.org/10.1200/jop.18.00063.
83. Kroon HM, Coventry BJ, Giles MH, Henderson MA, Speakman D, Wall M, et al. Safety and efficacy of isolated limb infusion chemotherapy for advanced locoregional melanoma in elderly patients: an Australian Multicenter Study. Ann Surg Oncol. 2017;24(11):3245–51. https://doi.org/10.1245/s10434-017-6046-5.
84. Testori A, Ribero S, Bataille V. Diagnosis and treatment of in-transit melanoma metastases. Eur J Surg Oncol. 2017;43(3):544–60. https://doi.org/10.1016/j.ejso.2016.10.005.
85. Andtbacka RHI, Collichio F, Harrington KJ, Middleton MR, Downey G, Öhrling K, et al. Final analyses of OPTiM: a randomized phase III trial of talimogene laherparepvec versus granulocyte-macrophage colony-stimulating factor in unresectable stage III-IV melanoma. J Immunother Cancer. 2019;7(1):145. https://doi.org/10.1186/s40425-019-0623-z.
86. Glitza Oliva I, Tawbi H, Davies MA. Melanoma brain metastases: current areas of investigation and future directions. Cancer J. 2017;23(1):68–74. https://doi.org/10.1097/ppo.0000000000000237.
87. Long GV, Atkinson V, Lo S, Sandhu S, Guminski AD, Brown MP, et al. Combination nivolumab and ipilimumab or nivolumab alone in melanoma brain metastases: a multicentre randomised phase 2 study. Lancet Oncol. 2018;19(5):672–81. https://doi.org/10.1016/s1470-2045(18)30139-6.
88. Tawbi HA, Forsyth PA, Algazi A, Hamid O, Hodi FS, Moschos SJ, et al. Combined nivolumab and ipilimumab in melanoma metastatic to the brain. N Engl J Med. 2018;379(8):722–30. https://doi.org/10.1056/NEJMoa1805453.
89. Davies MA, Saiag P, Robert C, Grob JJ, Flaherty KT, Arance A, et al. Dabrafenib plus trametinib in patients with BRAF(V600)-mutant melanoma brain metastases (COMBI-MB): a multicentre, multicohort, open-label, phase 2 trial. Lancet Oncol. 2017;18(7):863–73. https://doi.org/10.1016/s1470-2045(17)30429-1.
90. Cohen JV, Tawbi H, Margolin KA, Amravadi R, Bosenberg M, Brastianos PK, et al. Melanoma central nervous system metastases: current approaches, challenges, and opportunities. Pigment Cell Melanoma Res. 2016;29(6):627–42. https://doi.org/10.1111/pcmr.12538.
91. Mulvenna P, Nankivell M, Barton R, Faivre-Finn C, Wilson P, McColl E, et al. Dexamethasone and supportive care with or without whole brain radiotherapy in treating patients with non-small cell lung cancer with brain metastases unsuitable for resection or stereotactic radiotherapy (QUARTZ): results from a phase 3, non-inferiority, randomised trial. Lancet. 2016;388(10055):2004–14. https://doi.org/10.1016/s0140-6736(16)30825-x.
92. Gibney GT, Weiner LM, Atkins MB. Predictive biomarkers for checkpoint inhibitor-based immunotherapy. Lancet Oncol. 2016;17(12):e542–e51. https://doi.org/10.1016/s1470-2045(16)30406-5.
93. Teng F, Meng X, Kong L, Yu J. Progress and challenges of predictive biomarkers of anti PD-1/PD-L1 immunotherapy: a systematic review. Cancer Lett. 2018;414:166–73. https://doi.org/10.1016/j.canlet.2017.11.014.

Chapter 23
Gastroesophageal Cancer in Older Adults with Frailty

Daniel Swinson, Noor Mohammed, Andy Cockbain, Simon J. Howell, and Mohan Hingorani

Introduction

Gastric and oesophageal cancers combined, account for 8% of cancer related deaths, which is the the 5th highest in the United Kingdom (UK). The 10-year survival for either is poor, at less than 20% and 15%, respectively. Whilst the incidence of gastric cancer has fallen, the incidence of oesophageal cancer has climbed modestly over the last 2 decades [1, 2]

The incidence of gastro-oesophageal (GO) cancer is strongly related to age, with most new cases diagnosed in people aged 65 years and over, and 41% in people aged

D. Swinson (✉)
Medical Oncology Department, St James's University Hospital, Leeds Teaching Hospitals Trust, Leeds, UK
e-mail: daniel.swinson@nhs.net

N. Mohammed
Gastroenterology Department, St James's University Hospital, Leeds Teaching Hospitals Trust, Leeds, UK
e-mail: noor.mohammed@nhs.net

A. Cockbain
Upper Gastrointestinal Surgery Department, St James's University Hospital, Leeds Teaching Hospitals Trust, Leeds, UK
e-mail: andy.cockbain@nhs.net

S. J. Howell
Anaesthesiology Department, St. James's University Hospital, Leeds, UK

Leeds Institute of Medical Research at St James's, University of Leeds, Leeds, UK
e-mail: simon.howell@nhs.net

M. Hingorani
Clinical Oncology Department, Hull University Teaching Hospitals NHS Trust, Hull, UK
e-mail: mohan.hingorani@nhs.net

F. Gomes (ed.), *Frailty in Older Adults with Cancer*,
https://doi.org/10.1007/978-3-030-89162-6_23

75 and over. Obesity, alcohol and smoking are important risk factors, meaning that many of these patients will be challenged by other health conditions [1, 2]. Therefore, frailty and geriatric conditions are prevalent in the population with GO cancer, with some studies reporting that up to 67% of patients with oesophageal cancer are functionally impaired. Moreover, several of these studies found that functional impairment or frailty was significantly associated with adverse health outcomes [3]

This chapter reviews the current evidence regarding the management of GO cancer in older patients, the individual contributions of the multidisciplinary team and how frailty may influence the management of cancer

Management of Early-Stage and Locally Advanced GO Cancer

Endoscopic Management

Early cancers in the upper GI tract are increasingly diagnosed in older people. Contributing factors are an ageing population, continued surveillance of Barrett's in older patients, and both technological improvements in the optics of newer endoscopes and dye-based assessments aiding endoscopic diagnosis [4]. Different techniques are available for endoscopic removal of pre-neoplastic and early cancers, which are usually performed safely in patients with frailty.

Endoscopic mucosal resection (EMR) is commonly used to resect many types of GO lesions. EMR has shown to be effective in resecting Barrett's dysplasia. It is a simple, quick, and safe method of resection that is usually performed as a day-case procedure. However, as the name suggests, EMR is beneficial in only mucosal disease. Hence, one has to be careful in selecting lesions that are limited to mucosal layer only. A disadvantage of this technique is that larger lesions can only be resected in piecemeal fashion making histological confirmation of a clear margin difficult.

Endoscopic submucosal dissection (ESD) is increasingly available. It has the advantage of resecting larger lesions en-bloc and can also be used to resect cancers with early submucosal involvement (defined as SM1). Deeper submucosal involvement (defined as SM2 or SM3) precludes this technique due to the increased risk of nodal involvement. Nevertheless, ESD is seen as organ-preserving endoscopic surgery in suitable cases [5, 6].

Full-thickness resection (FTR) can tackle deeper lesions smaller than 2.5 cm in length involving the muscularis propria layer and provides the pathologist with a full-thickness specimen. Evidence for use of this technique for upper GI cancers is limited and it remains unclear where it fits into the treatment algorithm.

Endoscopic ablative therapies such as photodynamic therapy (PDT), radiofrequency ablation (RFA), cryoablation, and argon plasma coagulation (APC) are employed to destroy the field of change within Barrett's mucosa and to control disease progression. These techniques are used as adjuncts to the resection techniques described above.

Ultimately, selecting patients for appropriate endoscopic resection technique requires a multidisciplinary approach. In the West endoscopic findings are combined with radiological assessments including endoscopic ultrasound (EUS) to characterize lesions. The Japanese favour use of advanced endoscopic techniques alone. Table 23.1 outlines our institution's approach, which techniques are used for different lesions, and when surgery may be routinely considered and how these decisions are influenced by patient frailty status.

Surgical Management

Surgery remains the mainstay of treatment for fit older patients with a locally advanced gastric cancer or a distal oesophageal adenocarcinoma. For oesophageal squamous cell carcinoma, surgery alone is uncommon (unless small tumours, up to T2 and N0) and definitive chemo-radiotherapy is more likely to be considered.

For the majority of patients on a surgical pathway, optimal treatment will involve pre-operative chemo(radio)therapy [7]. However, this multi-modality approach is often not appropriate for the older patient with frailty. The decision-making process depends on not just the severity of frailty but also on tumour factors (e.g. stage and lymph node burden) and clinical factors (e.g. bleeding or obstruction).

Assessment of Surgical Fitness

The assessment of peri-operative risk rests on three pillars: the magnitude of the planned surgery, burden of comorbidity, and the functional status of the patient. Assessment begins in the outpatient clinic with a detailed medical history, including a discussion of a patient's exercise tolerance. Whilst there is a growing body of evidence across different types of cancer surgery supporting an association between

Table 23.1 Types of resection based on patient frailty, histology and local extent of GO cancer

Pathology	Frailty	Mucosal				Submucosal	
		Ulcer (−)		Ulcer (+)		<500 μm	>500 μm
Size of cancer		≤2 cm	>2 cm	≤3 cm	>3 cm	≤3 cm	Any size
Differentiated type histology	No	EMR/ESD	ESD	ESD	ESD	ESD	Surgery
	Yes	EMR	EMR/ESD	ESD	ESD	ESD	Chemo-radiotherapy
Undifferentiated type histology	No	ESD	Surgery	Surgery	Surgery	Surgery	Surgery
	Yes	ESD	ESD	ESD	Chemo-radiotherapy	ESD	Chemo-radiotherapy

EMR endoscopic mucosal resection, *ESD* endoscopic submucosal dissection poorer functional capacity and an increased risk of adverse outcomes, there is no universally accepted objective measurement of a patient's fitness. Cardiopulmonary exercise testing (CPET) is widely used for assessment of functional capacity prior to upper gastrointestinal surgery [8]. The six-minute walk and hand grip tests have also been described [9, 10]. Fitness for surgery should be considered as a continuum of risk, and CPETs should not be applied with binary cut-offs but be considered as part of the holistic assessment of the patient. That said, an anaerobic threshold of less than 9 ml/kg/minute would be considered high risk, and less than 8 would almost universally preclude oesophagectomy. Lower anaerobic thresholds may sometimes be acceptable for patients undergoing gastrectomy. In the UK, older surgical patients are increasingly reviewed by POPS clinics (proactive care of the older patient undergoing surgery) [11]. These bring together a multidisciplinary team that includes an anaesthetist, an elderly care physician, and other healthcare professionals.

An issue of particular concern in both patients with frailty and those with GO cancer is the prevalence of malnutrition and sarcopenia. The phenotypic definition of frailty includes unintentional weight loss as a criterion [12]. Where the obstructive and systemic effects of GO cancer are added to this the patient may rapidly become very malnourished. Such malnutrition is associated with poorer short- and long-term outcomes [13, 14]. There is an association between sarcopenia as identified by indexed measurements of the psoas muscle on CT scan and adverse post-operative outcomes, although this remains more of a research parameter than a clinical tool to guide decision-making [15–18]. It is important to assess dysphagia symptoms and nutritional intake at all stages of the treatment pathway and to consider interventions such as enteral tube feeding, particularly for patients taking less than 50% of their prescribed calorie intake [19]. In some patients, self-expanding metal stents may be indicated to help relieve obstructive symptoms and improve nutritional intake. They are more commonly used in patients on a palliative pathway and the decision to stent a patient on a curative treatment pathway should only be taken after consultation with the multidisciplinary team.

A number of studies have demonstrated an association between frailty and adverse outcome following upper gastrointestinal cancer surgery, albeit these are often relatively small single-centre case-series [17, 20–27]. The European Society of Medical Oncology suggests performing a geriatric assessment may aid determination of a patient's functional age prior to commencing treatment of older patients with gastric cancer [28], recognizing that performance status is not a good predictor of tolerance of chemotherapy. A full Comprehensive Geriatric Assessment (CGA) can be resource intensive, and studies have shown that an abbreviated assessment can still identify patients at increased risk of functional decline of death in the next 2 years and that comorbidity, polypharmacy, and activities of daily living components of the CGA predict post-operative complications after gastrointestinal cancer surgery [29, 30]. Pre-operative identification of issues such as social isolation, depressive symptoms, and impairment of activities of daily living would be particularly beneficial for major cancer surgery, such as gastrectomy and oesophagectomy, as these operations have a significant impact on patient's post-operative quality of life.

Surgical Considerations and Outcomes

There are important differences between surgery for gastric cancer and that for oesophageal cancers. For gastric cancer, a subtotal or total gastrectomy will be performed supine, either laparoscopically or through an open midline or rooftop incision. The operation is confined to the abdominal cavity, and may take in the order of 2–4 h. By contrast, an oesophagectomy is a longer, more complex operation involving 2 or 3 stages. It may take in the order of 4–6 h. In the 2-stage Ivor Lewis operation, the patient first undergoes an abdominal stage (open or laparoscopic) to mobilize the stomach and distal oesophagus and form a stomach tube (conduit) which will ultimately replace the resected oesophagus. The patient is then turned into a lateral position, and a thoracic stage performed (right fifth thoracotomy, or thoracoscopic). The right lung is deflated to facilitate access to resect the oesophagus and a thoracic stage performed (right fifth thoracotomy, or thoracoscopic) to allow resection of the oesophagus. The gastric conduit is then pulled up into the mediastinum and an anastomosis formed to restore the continuity of the GI tract. In the 3-stage McKeown operation, a third incision is made over the left neck and the gastric conduit brought up to the neck to anastomose onto the cervical oesophagus. Other surgical approaches exist, including the trans-hiatal and left thoracoabdominal approach for oesophageal cancers, and robotic surgery for both gastric and oesophageal surgery is also available in some centres. The approach depends on either local expertise and facilities, or specific technical factors, and is broadly speaking independent of the assessment of a patient's fitness for surgery.

It is more complex to quantify the risks of gastrectomy or oesophagectomy in older patients with frailty. Published surgical outcomes come predominantly from retrospective case-series reporting outcomes in older patients (using difference age cut-offs) and without any assessment of frailty. This heterogeneity, together with the inherent selection bias of patients put forward for surgery in each study, and inconsistent definitions of post-operative complications make it difficult to generalize the results [31–33]. Table 23.2 summarizes surgical outcomes following oesophagectomy from two retrospective series and a large systematic review.

Table 23.2 Outcomes following oesophagectomy for different age-groups

Study	Treatment	Number	Age cut	Mortality	Pulmonary Complications	Cardiac Complications
Pultrum 2010	Oesophagectomy	64 170	≥70 <70	Peri-operative 11 vs 5% (n/s)	56 vs 42% OR = 1.75 (0.98–3.12)	38 vs 16% OR = 3.18 (1.66–6.10)
Lester 2017	CRT & Surgery	202 369	≥65 <65	90 day 5.4 vs 2.2%	37.6 vs. 23% OR = 2.02 (1.39–2.93)	24.8 vs. 13% OR = 2.20 (1.42–3.42)
Markar 2013	Oesophagectomy	2573 9531	≥70 <70	In-hospital 7.8 vs. 4.2% OR = 1.87 (1.54–2.26)	21.8 vs. 19.5% OR = 1.49 (1.29–1.71)	18.7 vs. 13.2% OR 2.06 (1.75–2.41)

When counselling older patients for surgery, the estimate of operative risks quoted often pertain to fit younger patients with an acknnowledgement that they will be higher for frail and older patients. It is, therefore, key that surgical teams consider how to best incoporate the limited information available into their consultations, to better inform the older patient with frailty in the decision-making and consent process. Ultimately, older patients with moderate to severe frailty are unlikely to be appropriate candidates for surgery, but the main challenge in decision-making is for those with mild to moderate frailty.

The final consideration in all patients is what treatment outcomes are important to the patient. Both gastrectomy and oesophagectomy can result in a prolonged functional recovery and significantly impact the patients' quality of life. Factors such as post-operative dysphagia, stricturing, dumping syndrome, reduced gastric capacity, fatigue and chronic pain, especially from a thoracotomy, can all be important factors for a patient to consider before deciding whether to undergo surgical or non-surgical treatment. These outcomes are poorly studied, rarely reported, and can be difficult to discuss in the outpatient clinic but are of crucial importance for the decision-making.

Peri-operative Systemic Therapy

Patients with localized disease amenable to surgery are routinely considered for peri-operative chemotherapy resulting in a modest survival benefit [34–37]. Real-world data exploring trends in treatment show older patients with localized oesophageal cancer are more frequently offered definitive chemo-radiotherapy but the rates of peri-operative chemotherapy or neoadjuvant chemo-radiotherapy and surgery are increasing [38, 39]. These real-world data also suggest there is a survival advantage for the combination treatment strategies. Since there is less morbidity associated with gastric surgery, it is reasonable to assume that older patients with gastric cancer also have a survival advantage with combination strategies.

Data from clinical trials is more limited regarding older patients as these have not specifically addressed the use of systemic therapy in older surgical patients and some trials even included an upper age limit at 75 years [34, 40]. Extrapolating results from the GO2 trial which was designed for older and frail patients with advanced GO cancer, suggests combination chemotherapy can be delivered safely and whilst disease control rates were not influenced by dose, response rate was and this may be more important in the curative than palliative-intent setting [41].

A pooled analysis of four pivotal studies of chemotherapy in the pre or peri-operative setting (MAGIC, ST03, OEO2, OEO5) comprising of 3265 patients (20% aged over 70) investigated the impact of age on outcomes. Both operative rates and survival were similar for patients aged above and below 70, but older patients experienced more neutropenia [42, 43]. Of note tumour regression was observed more frequently in older patients and this may reflect pharmacokinetic differences resulting in higher drug exposure. Whilst an argument could be made here for reducing the dose of chemotherapy on this inference, the above-described GO2 trial data argues otherwise.

More recently the FLOT4 trial has made the case for the use of taxane- fluoropyrimidine platinum triplet chemotherapy, but <25% of patients were aged above 70 years [35]. A small randomized phase II trial recruiting patients over 65 concluded this regimen was deliverable in older patients albeit with markedly increased toxicity impacting patient quality of life [44]. Importantly, the proportion of patients with this triplet regimen who underwent resection was lower than comparative patients in the pooled analysis (74.5% vs 81%).

Age alone should not be considered a barrier to systemic therapy for older surgical patients. However, older patients are significantly under-represented in the available datasets, particularly those with some degree of frailty. Therefore, although peri-operative chemotherapy should be considered for these patients, alternative approaches such as surgery alone, definitive chemo-radiotherapy, or radical radiotherapy can be utilised where there are significant concerns regarding patient fitness.

Definitive Chemo-Radiotherapy

Definitive chemo-radiotherapy has a role for those patients not suitable or eligible to a surgical approach. Table 23.3 summarizes the non-surgical options and outcomes for patients in this setting according to their level of frailty.

The role of definitive chemo-radiotherapy in the management of locally advanced oesophageal cancer was established by the RTOG_8501 study; 25% of patients were aged over 70; mostly with squamous cell carcinoma. Patients were randomized between radical radiotherapy alone (in 64 Gy) or chemo-radiotherapy (in 50 Gy over 25 fractions along with cisplatin/5 Fluorouracil 2 cycles induction before radiotherapy and 2 cycles concurrently). The overall survival at 5 years for the combination was 26% [95% CI (15%–37%)] compared with 0% following only radiotherapy, the combined regimen was associated with increased risk of significant toxicity (44% vs 25%, being life-threatening in 20% vs 3%, respectively) [45, 46]. Several other studies have consistently demonstrated the benefits of definitive chemo-radiotherapy in terms of objective complete response rates and long-term survival [47–49]. In addition, at least 2 randomized studies have compared definitive chemo-radiotherapy with neoadjuvant chemo-radiotherapy followed by planned oesophagectomy and showed no difference in overall survival [50, 51]. Therefore, definitive chemo-radiotherapy is an accepted standard of care in patients with squamous cell carcinoma of oesophagus and it can be considered in patients with adenocarcinoma sub-type who are not fit for an esophagectomy.

However, focusing on older patients with frailty, this regimen warrants optimal renal function with glomerular filtration rate of at least 50 ml/minute and Eastern Cooperative Oncology Group (ECOG) PS 0–1. Therefore, depending on the severity of frailty, many older patients may not be suitable for a cisplatin-based definitive

Table 23.3 Non-surgical therapeutic options and outcomes in patients with localized cancer of oesophagus based on frailty scores

Rockwood clinical frailty score	Treatment options	Survival outcomes	Expected toxicities
• 1–2 (very fit/ well) • 3 (managing well).	• d-CRT with cisplatin/ fluoropyrimidine, • Alternative to surgery in SqCC of oesophagus OR in patients with AC who refuse surgery.	• 5-year OS: 20–30% (higher in SqCC).	• Grade 3 toxicity: Non-haematological (40%), haematological (20%).
• 4 (vulnerable) • 5 (mildly frail).	• d-CRT with carboplatin/ paclitaxel.	• 1-year OS: 82% 2-year OS: 50% • Median OS 24 months.	• Grade 3 toxicity: Non-haematological (20–30%) haematological (5–10%).
• 4 (vulnerable) • 5 (mildly frail).	• Radical RT 50 Gy in 16 fractions 50–55 Gy in 20 fractions.	• 3-year OS: 30–50% • 5-year OS: 10–20%.	• Grade 3 toxicity: 15%.
• 6 (moderately frail).	• Palliative RT (30 Gy in 10 fractions) + brachytherapy (12–14 Gy in 2 fractions).	• 1-year OS: 18–20%.	• Grade 3 toxicity: 30%.
• 6 (moderately frail).	• Palliative RT 20 Gy in 5 fractions 30 Gy in 10 fractions.	• Median OS: 6 months.	• Grade 3 toxicity: <10%.
• 7 (severely frail).	Stent if appropriate		
• 8–9 (very severely frail/terminally ill).	Best supportive care		

AD adenocarcinoma, *d-CRT* definitive chemo-radiotherapy, *OS* overall survival, *RT* palliative radiotherapy, *SqCC* squamous cell carcinoma, *yr* year

chemo-radiotherapy and alternatives, such as with a different chemotherapy backbone or even radical radiotherapy alone, should be considered.

Carboplatin/paclitaxel may be considered as an alternative chemotherapy regimen to combine with radiotherapy, following results from the CROSS study, which investigated neoadjuvant chemo-radiotherapy followed by surgery for OG cancer [40]. Whilst there are no randomized studies comparing carboplatin/ paclitaxel to cisplatin/ fluoropyrimidine, the use of this alternative regimen for patients with frailty is supported by 2 retrospective studies. The first, from the Netherlands, observed similar survival outcomes with higher completion rates (82% vs 57%, $P = 0.010$) and less toxicity for the carboplatin/ paclitaxel combination with radiotherapy [52]. The second study, from the UK, reviewed 214 patients with a median age of 73 years (39.7% of patients aged 75 or over and 18.7% aged 80 or over). The median progression-free survival and OS were 16.33 months and 24.28 months, respectively. The incidence of grade 3 or higher toxicity was 33% and there were no treatment-related deaths [53]. Therefore, the use of definitive chemo-radiotherapy with carboplatin/ paclitaxel has steadily increased driven by its safety profile.

Radical Radiotherapy

For older patients with oesophageal cancer considered unfit for the previous treatment modalities, radical radiotherapy represents the last radical treatment option available. The RTOG-8501 study showed no long-term survivors with radical radiotherapy and therefore many oncologists do not consider it to be a curative-intent option [46]. There is a paucity of research exploring radical radiotherapy as a single treatment modality for oesophageal cancer, but four prospective studies have compared radical radiotherapy with definitive chemo-radiotherapy. The fractionation schedules varied but the majority of these studies found that the 5-year survival of radical radiotherapy was higher than reported by the RTOG-8501 study, yet still less than 10% [54–57].

Two retrospective single-centre series of radical radiotherapy using hypo-fractionated protocols have been published. The long-term survival figures for both exceed those reported by the prospective studies of definitive chemo-radiotherapy described. The Manchester series consisted mainly of squamous cell carcinoma and used dose ranges between 45 and 52.5 Gy in 15 or 16 fractions over 3 weeks, reporting 3- and 5-year overall survival rates of 27% and 21%, respectively. The Leeds series included a more balanced cohort of squamous and adenocarcinoma and used mostly 50 Gy in 16 fractions (80% of cases) or 50–52.5 Gy in 20 fractions. The 3-year overall survival was 56.9%, which was similar to their own cohort of patients with definitive chemo-radiotherapy. The hypo-fractionated protocols were well tolerated in both centre series. The Manchester series reported oesophageal stricturing in a quarter of patients with long-term survival, managed by dilation. The Leeds series reported a 2.5-fold reduction in grade 3 toxicity compared to chemo-radiotherapy [58, 59]. Ultimately, radical radiotherapy potentially with hypo-fractionated protocols has a role in the management of patients with oesophageal cancer not suitable for definitive chemo-radiotherapy, particularly for those older patients with significant frailty.

Palliative Radiotherapy

A significant proportion of older patients with frailty and oesophageal cancer are not appropriate for radical/curative-intent treatment and are usually managed with a palliative-intent, with either palliative radiotherapy or insertion of an oesophageal stent to achieve rapid palliation of symptoms.

Palliative radiotherapy consists of either fractionated external beam radiotherapy (EBRT) or intraluminal brachytherapy (ILBT). These techniques may be used alone or combined. Radiotherapy has been shown to be extremely effective in palliation of dysphagia with more durable and sustained improvement in swallowing function compared to an oesophageal stent. In a retrospective single-centre analysis palliative radiotherapy, where 90% received 20 Gy in 5 fractions, there was an improvement in dysphagia in more than 75% of patients. Subsequent intervention with stent was needed in 25% of patients and 5 patients received a repeat schedule of palliative radiotherapy with median overall survival of 6 months [60]. A series from Leeds with a median age of 74 years treated patients with either 20 Gy over 5 fractions or 30 Gy over 10 fractions and improvements in dysphagia were observed in 52% and 60% of patients, respectively. Both the median time to deterioration of swallowing (4.5 and 3.9 months) and the median overall survival times (6.2 and 6.9 months) were similar. The incidence of grade 3 toxicity was less than 10% in both groups [61].

The insertion of self-expanding oesophageal stents can achieve rapid palliation of dysphagia and is the preferred option in patients with significant obstruction and high dysphagia scores [Mellow-Pinkas ≥ 3 (swallowing limited to liquids)] [62]. At least 2 randomized studies have assessed the effects of palliative radiotherapy after stent insertion with the aim of maintaining swallowing function and preventing tumour-related complications (e.g., stent blockage from tumour ingrowth, bleeding, etc.). The first, an older and smaller study reported improved duration of symptom control; the second, reported in 2020, was larger and found no benefit other than reduced bleeding, numbers need to treat = 12 [63, 64].

ILBT involves intraluminal placement of an applicator (6–10 mm in diameter) under endoscopic or fluoroscopic guidance followed by after-loading with a high-dose rate stepped Iridium (Ir^{192}) or cobalt (Co^{60}) radioactive source. The dose is usually prescribed 5 mm from the surface of the applicator and is delivered in single or multiple (typically 2–3) fractions [65]. Two randomized trials studies comparing ILBT with stent insertion showed more lasting effects on health-related quality of life, and dysphagia scores and a significantly lower overall complication rate in the brachytherapy arm in comparison to the stent arm [66, 67]. Another study of 219 patients randomized to ILBT alone or ILBT followed by EBRT. Patients received ILBT in 2 fractions of 8 Gy and EBRT was delivered using 30 Gy in 10 fractions. The dysphagia-relief experience was significantly improved with combined therapy, for an absolute benefit of +18% at 200 days from randomization ($p = 0.019$). The study reported median overall survival of 188 days and 1-year survival of 18% although there was no survival difference between the two arms [68]. Therefore, combining ILBT and EBRT is feasible and can be considered in patients who are not appropriate for radical radiotherapy. This is a particular advantage in the presence of cardiopulmonary morbidity since the dose to the heart and lungs is significantly reduced compared to conventional radical radiotherapy protocols.

Management of Advanced GO Cancer

Advanced GO cancer is often a morbid disease, and its impact will vary for patients at different stages of life. Older patients will frequently be challenged by multimorbidity, frailty and often have carer responsibilities [69, 70]. Decision-making in this setting is challenging and clear guidance on the benefits of specific treatments for this group, whose circumstances are highly variable, is key.

Up until recently, pivotal trials guiding the use of systemic therapy have included patients with a median age in the low 60s and even late 50s [35, 71–74]. A UK national audit suggested up to half of older patients may not be considered fit for standard treatment. A national survey in 2011 reported a wide variation in the treatment of older patients with use of standard regimens at reduced doses, non-standard combinations or single agent treatments. A separate region wide study with a specific focus on treating older patients reported higher treatment rates suggesting such a focus may provide better outcomes [75, 76].

Evidence from pivotal trials describes a disease initially chemo-sensitive with symptom improvement recorded in over 70% of patients and an improvement in median overall survival times from 3–5 to 8–12 months [77–81]. Single-agent fluoropyrimidines likely provide some survival benefit but the addition of a platinum agent or irinotecan is considered optimal [28, 36, 81–83]. Evidence for adding a third cytotoxic agent is controversial. The REAL2 trial established epirubicin, oxaliplatin, and capecitabine (EOCap) as a standard of care in the UK and remains a recognized regimen although the evidence for the addition of an anthracycline is limited [28, 36, 73, 74, 81]. The addition of docetaxel may improve survival but at the expense of significant toxicity [84]. Better tolerated taxane containing schedules have been explored but are not in routine use [28].

There has been limited success with targeted therapies. A notable exception is Trastuzumab which improves survival with minimal additional toxicity for patients with HER2 positive disease [71]. Two phase III trials of checkpoint inhibitors have been presented in abstract form. Pembrolizumab, as a single agent, afforded similar outcomes to chemotherapy but achieved no additive benefit with chemotherapy [85]. Nivolumab in contrast improved survival and may represent a new standard of care [86].

In 2011, fifty UK oncologists were surveyed, 49 reported regularly altering treatment for older patients by reducing dose and/or numbers of drugs. There was significant variation in clinical practice, and none reported using a geriatric assessment to aid decisions [87]. The survey exemplified a clear unmet need; in response the 321GO and GO2 trials were conducted. The 321GO trial was a 3-arm phase II pick the winner trial comparing 3 treatments: capecitabine alone, oxaliplatin and capecitabine (OCap), and epirubicin, oxaliplatin, capecitabine (EOCap), all delivered at 80% of standard dose. Eligible patients were considered unsuitable for full dose EOCap on the basis of age or frailty. The median age of patients recruited was 75. The 2-drug combination (OCap) produced the best balance of efficacy and toxicity [87].

The GO2 study was a phase III trial recruiting from a similar population and compared 3 doses levels of OCap with the aim to establish the minimally effective dose [41]. All patients underwent a comprehensive health assessment from which a 9-domain frailty score was calculated. The study was powered to demonstrate equivalence in terms of progression-free survival. Overall treatment utility (OTU), a novel composite endpoint of clinical and patient reported outcomes was measured at 9 weeks. A good OTU was achieved if there was disease control, no significant toxicity, or drop in quality of life and a positive patient valuation of treatment. An intermediate OTU was obtained if there was progression and no other negative factor or vice versa. A poor OTU was obtained if there were both progression and another negative factor or the patient had died. The primary endpoint was met establishing the lowest dose level, oxaliplatin 78 mg/m^2 q3 weekly and capecitabine 375 mg/m^2 bd daily, as a new standard of care for older-and-or-frail patients. This dose level produced the highest rate of good OTU. No patient group benefited from higher dosing. A multivariate model identified frailty, neutrophil to lymphocyte ratio (NLR), and patient reported quality of life using the EQ-5D visual analogue score as independent predictors of OTU outcomes. For example, a mildly frail patient with baseline EQ-5D = 55 and NLR = 3.0 (predictive score = 1) had a 44% probability of good OTU and 27% probability of poor OTU. Conversely, a severely frail patient with baseline EQ-5D = 45 and NLR = 5.0 (score = 0) had only 18% probability of good OTU and 57% probability of poor OTU [41].

The GO2 trial represents a landmark moment for this population of patients. Clinicians can now base treatment discussions on a firm evidence base without the need to extrapolate from data based on younger fitter patients. Description of differing OTU outcomes during patient consultations may aid patient understanding on the likelihood of differing treatment experiences and aid delicate decision-making. The multivariate analysis may permit further tailoring of these discussions allowing for the impact of disease and patient factors. Further work is needed to validate the predictive factors identified, better understand how we can incorporate these tools in busy oncology clinics, and how effectively such data meets patients' information needs when considering the use of chemotherapy.

Conclusion

A new evidence base is now emerging on how to manage the older cancer patient which includes a more granular assessment of patient fitness, minimally effective dosing and the incorporation of a geriatric multidisciplinary team. The GO2 model provides a framework for informed decision-making for a diverse patient group based on both traditional oncology outcomes and patient reported assessment of treatment value. Moreover, the American Society of Clinical Oncology recommends the use of geriatric assessments, such as the CARG and CRASH tools, which incorporate patient, frailty, and treatment parameters to provide an estimate of the risk of toxicity [88]. In 2020, 3 randomized controlled trials explored the benefit of adding CGA to the standard care of cancer patients in terms of improving high grade toxicity and health-related quality of life, all these studies met their primary endpoint [89–92].

There is a growing body of evidence providing better treatment options for older patients and those with frailty at all stages of GO cancer, which are delivered by different members of the multidisciplinary team. Careful consideration of an older patient's fitness including both their comorbid state and presence of frailty should be undertaken during the clinical decision-making, and future research should aim to clarify who is best served with less intense treatments.

References

1. CRUK. https://www.cancerresearchuk.org/health-professional/cancer-statistics/statistics-by-cancer-type/oesophageal-cancer#heading-Six. 2021, January.
2. CRUK. https://www.cancerresearchuk.org/health-professional/cancer-statistics/statistics-by-cancer-type/stomach-cancer. 2021, January.
3. van Deudekom FJ, Klop HG, Hartgrink HH, et al. Functional and cognitive impairment, social functioning, frailty and adverse health outcomes in older patients with esophageal cancer, a systematic review. J Geriatric Oncol. 2018;9:560–8.
4. Luo H, Xu G, Li C, et al. Real-time artificial intelligence for detection of upper gastrointestinal cancer by endoscopy: a multicentre, case-control, diagnostic study. Lancet Oncol. 2019;20:1645–54.
5. Curvers WL, Bansal A, Sharma P, Bergman JJ. Endoscopic work-up of early Barrett's neoplasia. Endoscopy. 2008;40:1000–7.
6. Allum WH, Blazeby JM, Griffin SM, et al. Guidelines for the management of oesophageal and gastric cancer. Gut. 2011;60:1449.
7. (NICE). Oesophago-gastric cancer: assessment and management in adults NICE guideline [NG83] Published date: 24 January 2018. https://www.nice.org.uk/guidance/ng83. 2018.
8. Carney A, Dickinson M. Anesthesia for esophagectomy. Anesthesiol Clin. 2015;33:143–63.
9. Inoue T, Ito S, Kanda M, et al. Preoperative six-minute walk distance as a predictor of postoperative complication in patients with esophageal cancer. Dis Esophagus. 2020;33
10. Sato S, Nagai E, Taki Y, et al. Hand grip strength as a predictor of postoperative complications in esophageal cancer patients undergoing esophagectomy. Esophagus. 2018;15:10–8.
11. Harari D, Hopper A, Dhesi J, et al. Proactive care of older people undergoing surgery ('POPS'): designing, embedding, evaluating and funding a comprehensive geriatric assessment service for older elective surgical patients. Age Ageing. 2007;36:190–6. Epub 2007 Jan 2027
12. Fried LP, Tangen CM, Walston J, et al. Frailty in older adults: evidence for a phenotype. J Gerontol A Biol Sci Med Sci. 2001;56:M146–56.
13. Chen FF, Zhang FY, Zhou XY, et al. Role of frailty and nutritional status in predicting complications following total gastrectomy with D2 lymphadenectomy in patients with gastric cancer: a prospective study. Langenbeck's Arch Surg. 2016;401:813–22.
14. Tegels JJ, de Maat MF, Hulsewé KW, et al. Value of geriatric frailty and nutritional status assessment in predicting postoperative mortality in gastric cancer surgery. J Gastrointest Surg. 2014;18:439–45. discussion 445-436
15. Makiura D, Ono R, Inoue J, et al. Preoperative sarcopenia is a predictor of postoperative pulmonary complications in esophageal cancer following esophagectomy: a retrospective cohort study. J Geriatr Oncol. 2016;7:430–6.
16. Sheetz KH, Zhao L, Holcombe SA, et al. Decreased core muscle size is associated with worse patient survival following esophagectomy for cancer. Dis Esophagus. 2013;26:716–22.
17. Shen Y, Hao Q, Zhou J, Dong B. The impact of frailty and sarcopenia on postoperative outcomes in older patients undergoing gastrectomy surgery: a systematic review and meta-analysis. BMC Geriatr. 2017;17:188.
18. Wagner D, DeMarco MM, Amini N, et al. Role of frailty and sarcopenia in predicting outcomes among patients undergoing gastrointestinal surgery. World J Gastrointest Surg. 2016;8:27–40.
19. Miller KR, Bozeman MC. Nutrition therapy issues in esophageal cancer. Curr Gastroenterol Rep. 2012;14:356–66.
20. Al-Batran SE, Homann N, Pauligk C, et al. Effect of neoadjuvant chemotherapy followed by surgical resection on survival in patients with limited metastatic gastric or gastroesophageal junction cancer: the AIO-FLOT3 trial. JAMA Oncol. 2017;3:1237–44.
21. Lu J, Zheng HL, Li P, et al. High preoperative modified frailty index has a negative impact on short- and long-term outcomes of octogenarians with gastric cancer after laparoscopic gastrectomy. Surg Endosc. 2018;32:2193–200.
22. Hirpara DH, Kidane B, Rogalla P, et al. Frailty assessment prior to thoracic surgery for lung or esophageal cancer: a feasibility study. Support Care Cancer. 2019;27:1535–40.

23. Giannotti C, Sambuceti S, Signori A, et al. Frailty assessment in elective gastrointestinal oncogeriatric surgery: predictors of one-year mortality and functional status. J Geriatr Oncol. 2019;10:716–23.
24. Tanaka T, Suda K, Inaba K, et al. Impact of frailty on postoperative outcomes for laparoscopic gastrectomy in patients older than 80 years. Ann Surg Oncol. 2019;26:4016–26.
25. Misawa N, Higurashi T, Tachikawa J, et al. Clinical impact of evaluation of frailty in endoscopic submucosal dissection for early gastric cancer in elderly patients. Geriatr Gerontol Int. 2020;20:461–6.
26. Osaki T, Saito H, Shimizu S, et al. Modified frailty index is useful in predicting non-home discharge in elderly patients with gastric cancer who undergo gastrectomy. World J Surg. 2020;44:3837–44.
27. Partnership TAaPCPS. Anaesthesia and perioperative care PSP 2014-15. In National Institute of Academic Anaesthesia. 2015.
28. Smyth EC, Verheij M, Allum W, et al. Gastric cancer: ESMO clinical practice guidelines for diagnosis, treatment and follow-up. Ann Oncol. 2016;27:v38–49.
29. Joharatnam-Hogan N, Shiu KK, Khan K. Challenges in the treatment of gastric cancer in the older patient. Cancer Treat Rev. 2020;85:101980.
30. Xue DD, Cheng Y, Wu M, Zhang Y. Comprehensive geriatric assessment prediction of postoperative complications in gastrointestinal cancer patients: a meta-analysis. Clin Interv Aging. 2018;13:723–36.
31. Lester SC, Lin SH, Chuong M, et al. A multi-institutional analysis of Trimodality therapy for esophageal cancer in elderly patients. Int J Radiat Oncol Biol Phys. 2017;98:820–8.
32. Markar SR, Karthikesalingam A, Thrumurthy S, et al. Systematic review and pooled analysis assessing the association between elderly age and outcome following surgical resection of esophageal malignancy. Dis Esophagus. 2013;26:250–62.
33. Pultrum BB, Bosch DJ, Nijsten MW, et al. Extended esophagectomy in elderly patients with esophageal cancer: minor effect of age alone in determining the postoperative course and survival. Ann Surg Oncol. 2010;17:1572–80.
34. Medical Research Council Oesophageal Cancer Working Group. Surgical resection with or without preoperative chemotherapy in oesophageal cancer: a randomised controlled trial. Lancet. 2002;359:1727–33.
35. Al-Batran S-E, Homann N, Pauligk C, et al. Perioperative chemotherapy with fluorouracil plus leucovorin, oxaliplatin, and docetaxel versus fluorouracil or capecitabine plus cisplatin and epirubicin for locally advanced, resectable gastric or gastro-oesophageal junction adenocarcinoma (FLOT4): a randomised, phase 2/3 trial. Lancet. 2019;393:1948–57.
36. Alderson D, Cunningham D, Nankivell M, et al. Neoadjuvant cisplatin and fluorouracil versus epirubicin, cisplatin, and capecitabine followed by resection in patients with oesophageal adenocarcinoma (UK MRC OE05): an open-label, randomised phase 3 trial. Lancet Oncol. 2017;18:1249–60.
37. Cunningham D, Stenning SP, Smyth EC, et al. Peri-operative chemotherapy with or without bevacizumab in operable oesophagogastric adenocarcinoma (UK medical research council ST03): primary analysis results of a multicentre, open-label, randomised phase 2-3 trial. Lancet Oncol. 2017;18:357–70.
38. Koëter M, van Putten M, Verhoeven RHA, et al. Definitive chemoradiation or surgery in elderly patients with potentially curable esophageal cancer in the Netherlands: a nationwide population-based study on patterns of care and survival. Acta Oncol. 2018;57:1192–200.
39. Verma V, Haque W, Zheng D, et al. Patterns of care and outcomes of elderly esophageal cancer patients not meeting age-based criteria of the CROSS trial. Am J Clin Oncol. 2019;42:67–74.
40. van Hagen P, Hulshof MC, van Lanschot JJ, et al. Preoperative chemoradiotherapy for esophageal or junctional cancer. N Engl J Med. 2012;366:2074–84.
41. Hall PS, Swinson D, Cairns DA, et al. Efficacy of reduced-intensity chemotherapy with Oxaliplatin and Capecitabine on quality of life and cancer control among older and frail patients with advanced gastroesophageal cancer: the GO2 phase 3 randomized clinical trial. JAMA Oncol. 2021;7:869–77.

42. Trumper M, Ross PJ, Cunningham D, et al. Efficacy and tolerability of chemotherapy in elderly patients with advanced oesophago-gastric cancer: a pooled analysis of three clinical trials. Eur J Cancer. 2006;42:827–34.
43. Athauda A, Nankivell M, Langley RE, et al. Impact of sex and age on chemotherapy efficacy, toxicity and survival in localised oesophagogastric cancer: a pooled analysis of 3265 individual patient data from four large randomised trials (OE02, OE05, MAGIC and ST03). Eur J Cancer. 2020;137:45–56.
44. Lorenzen S, Pauligk C, Homann N, et al. Feasibility of perioperative chemotherapy with infusional 5-FU, leucovorin, and oxaliplatin with (FLOT) or without (FLO) docetaxel in elderly patients with locally advanced esophagogastric cancer. Br J Cancer. 2013;108:519–26.
45. Cooper JS, Guo MD, Herskovic A, et al. Chemoradiotherapy of locally advanced esophageal cancer: long-term follow-up of a prospective randomized trial (RTOG 85-01). Radiation Therapy Oncology Group. JAMA. 1999;281:1623–7.
46. Herskovic A, Martz K, Al-Sarraf M, et al. Combined chemotherapy and radiotherapy compared with radiotherapy alone in patients with cancer of the esophagus. N Engl J Med. 1992;326:1593–8.
47. Kato K, Muro K, Minashi K, et al. Phase II study of chemoradiotherapy with 5-fluorouracil and cisplatin for stage II-III esophageal squamous cell carcinoma: JCOG trial (JCOG 9906). Int J Radiat Oncol Biol Phys. 2011;81:684–90.
48. Kato K, Nakajima TE, Ito Y, et al. Phase II study of concurrent chemoradiotherapy at the dose of 50.4 Gy with elective nodal irradiation for stage II-III esophageal carcinoma. Jpn J Clin Oncol. 2013;43:608–15.
49. Tahara M, Fuse N, Mizusawa J, et al. Phase I/II trial of chemoradiotherapy with concurrent S-1 and cisplatin for clinical stage II/III esophageal carcinoma (JCOG 0604). Cancer Sci. 2015;106:1414–20.
50. Bedenne L, Michel P, Bouché O, et al. Chemoradiation followed by surgery compared with chemoradiation alone in squamous cancer of the esophagus: FFCD 9102. J Clin Oncol. 2007;25:1160–8.
51. Stahl M, Stuschke M, Lehmann N, et al. Chemoradiation with and without surgery in patients with locally advanced squamous cell carcinoma of the esophagus. J Clin Oncol. 2005;23:2310–7.
52. Honing J, Smit JK, Muijs CT, et al. A comparison of carboplatin and paclitaxel with cisplatinum and 5-fluorouracil in definitive chemoradiation in esophageal cancer patients. Ann Oncol. 2014;25:638–43.
53. Owens R, Cox C, Gomberg S, et al. Outcome of weekly carboplatin-paclitaxel-based definitive Chemoradiation in Oesophageal cancer in patients not considered to be suitable for platinum-Fluoropyrimidine-based treatment: a multicentre, retrospective review. Clin Oncol (R Coll Radiol). 2020;32:121–30.
54. Slabber CF, Nel JS, Schoeman L, et al. A randomized study of radiotherapy alone versus radiotherapy plus 5-fluorouracil and platinum in patients with inoperable, locally advanced squamous cancer of the esophagus. Am J Clin Oncol. 1998;21:462–5.
55. Araújo CM, Souhami L, Gil RA, et al. A randomized trial comparing radiation therapy versus concomitant radiation therapy and chemotherapy in carcinoma of the thoracic esophagus. Cancer. 1991;67:2258–61.
56. Smith TJ, Ryan LM, Douglass HO, et al. Combined chemoradiotherapy vs. radiotherapy alone for early stage squamous cell carcinoma of the esophagus: a study of the eastern cooperative oncology group 11Other participating institutions: Albany Medical College, Albany, NY (CA 06594); Albert Einstein College of Medicine, Bronx, NY (CA 14958); University of California-Irvine, Orange, CA; Case Western Reserve University, Cleveland, OH (CA 14548); Chicago Medical School, Chicago, IL (CA 14144); Colorado Cancer Research Program, Denver, CO; Downstate Medical Center, Brooklyn, NY; University of Florida-Gainesville, Gainesville, FL; Fox Chase Cancer Center, Philadelphia, PA (CA 18281); Indiana University Medical Center, Indianapolis, IN (CA 49883); Medical College of Ohio, Toledo, OH; University of Medicine

and Dentistry of New Jersey, Newark, NJ; University of Minnesota, Minneapolis, MN (CA 20365); New York University Medical Center, New York, NY (CA 16395); Newark Beth Israel Medical Center, Newark, NJ; Rush-Presbyterian-St. Luke's Medical Center, Chicago, IL (CA 25988); University of Pretoria, Pretoria, South Africa (CA 21692); Natalie Warren Bryant Cancer Center, Tulsa, OK; Vermont Regional Cancer Center, Burlington, VT. Int J Radiat Oncol Biol Phys. 1998;42:269–76.

57. Wobbes T, Baron B, Paillot B, et al. Prospective randomised study of split-course radiotherapy versus cisplatin plus split-course radiotherapy in inoperable squamous cell carcinoma of the oesophagus. Eur J Cancer. 2001;37:470–7.
58. Sykes AJ, Burt PA, Slevin NJ, et al. Radical radiotherapy for carcinoma of the oesophagus: an effective alternative to surgery. Radiother Oncol. 1998 Jul;48(1):15–21. https://doi.org/10.1016/s0167-8140(98)00037-1.
59. Jones CM, Spencer K, Hitchen C, et al. Hypofractionated radiotherapy in Oesophageal cancer for patients unfit for systemic therapy: a retrospective single-Centre analysis. Clin Oncol (R Coll Radiol). 2019;31:356–64.
60. Murray LJ, Din OS, Kumar VS, et al. Palliative radiotherapy in patients with esophageal carcinoma: a retrospective review. Pract Radiat Oncol. 2012;2:257–64.
61. Parikh SP, Goody R, Coen O, et al. Palliative radiotherapy to the oesophagus: less is just as good. Clin Oncol. 2019;31:e9.
62. Martin EJ, Bruggeman AR, Nalawade VV, et al. Palliative radiotherapy versus esophageal stent placement in the management of patients with metastatic esophageal cancer. J Natl Compr Canc Netw. 2020;18:569–74.
63. Javed A, Pal S, Dash NR, et al. Palliative stenting with or without radiotherapy for inoperable esophageal carcinoma: a randomized trial. J Gastrointest Cancer. 2012;43:63–9.
64. Byrne AT, Adamson D, Porter C, et al. Radiotherapy after esophageal cancer stenting (ROCS): a pragmatic randomized controlled trial evaluating the role of palliative radiotherapy in maintaining swallow. J Clin Oncol. 2020;38:4569.
65. Lettmaier S, Strnad V. Intraluminal brachytherapy in oesophageal cancer: defining its role and introducing the technique. J Contemp Brachytherapy. 2014;6:236–41.
66. Homs MY, Steyerberg EW, Eijkenboom WM, et al. Single-dose brachytherapy versus metal stent placement for the palliation of dysphagia from oesophageal cancer: multicentre randomised trial. Lancet. 2004;364:1497–504.
67. Bergquist H, Wenger U, Johnsson E, et al. Stent insertion or endoluminal brachytherapy as palliation of patients with advanced cancer of the esophagus and gastroesophageal junction. Results of a randomized, controlled clinical trial. Dis Esophagus. 2005;18:131–9.
68. Rosenblatt E, Jones G, Sur RK, et al. Adding external beam to intra-luminal brachytherapy improves palliation in obstructive squamous cell oesophageal cancer: a prospective multi-Centre randomized trial of the International Atomic Energy Agency. Radiother Oncol. 2010;97:488–94.
69. Extermann M. Measuring comorbidity in older cancer patients. Eur J Cancer. 2000;36:453–71.
70. Lees J, Chan A. Polypharmacy in elderly patients with cancer: clinical implications and management. Lancet Oncol. 2011;12:1249–57.
71. Bang YJ, Van Cutsem E, Feyereislova A, et al. Trastuzumab in combination with chemotherapy versus chemotherapy alone for treatment of HER2-positive advanced gastric or gastro-oesophageal junction cancer (ToGA): a phase 3, open-label, randomised controlled trial. Lancet. 2010;376:687–97.
72. Cunningham D, Allum WH, Stenning SP, et al. Perioperative chemotherapy versus surgery alone for resectable gastroesophageal cancer. N Engl J Med. 2006;355:11–20.
73. Cunningham D, Starling N, Rao S, et al. Capecitabine and Oxaliplatin for advanced Esophagogastric cancer. N Engl J Med. 2008;358:36–46.
74. Ross P, Nicolson M, Cunningham D, et al. Prospective randomized trial comparing mitomycin, cisplatin, and protracted venous-infusion fluorouracil (PVI 5-FU) with epirubicin, cisplatin, and PVI 5-FU in advanced esophagogastric cancer. J Clin Oncol. 2002;20:1996–2004.

75. Hall PS, Lord SR, Collinson M, et al. A randomised phase II trial and feasibility study of palliative chemotherapy in frail or elderly patients with advanced gastroesophageal cancer (321GO). Br J Cancer. 2017;116:472–8.
76. Audit NE-G. https://www.augis.org/outcomes-data-2019/. 2019.
77. Findlay M, Cunningham D, Norman A, et al. A phase II study in advanced gastro-esophageal cancer using epirubicin and cisplatin in combination with continuous infusion 5-fluorouracil (ECF). Ann Oncol. 1994;5:609–16.
78. Murad AM, Santiago FF, Petroianu A, et al. Modified therapy with 5-fluorouracil, doxorubicin, and methotrexate in advanced gastric cancer. Cancer. 1993;72:37–41.
79. Glimelius B, Ekström K, Hoffman K, et al. Randomized comparison between chemotherapy plus best supportive care with best supportive care in advanced gastric cancer. Ann Oncol. 1997;8:163–8.
80. Pyrhönen S, Kuitunen T, Nyandoto P, Kouri M. Randomised comparison of fluorouracil, epidoxorubicin and methotrexate (FEMTX) plus supportive care with supportive care alone in patients with non-resectable gastric cancer. Br J Cancer. 1995;71:587–91.
81. Wagner AD, Syn NL, Moehler M, et al. Chemotherapy for advanced gastric cancer. Cochrane Database Syst Rev. 2017;8:Cd004064.
82. Koizumi W, Narahara H, Hara T, et al. S-1 plus cisplatin versus S-1 alone for first-line treatment of advanced gastric cancer (SPIRITS trial): a phase III trial. Lancet Oncol. 2008;9:215–21.
83. Guimbaud R, Louvet C, Ries P, et al. Prospective, randomized, multicenter, phase III study of fluorouracil, leucovorin, and irinotecan versus epirubicin, cisplatin, and capecitabine in advanced gastric adenocarcinoma: a French intergroup (Fédération francophone de Cancérologie digestive, Fédération Nationale des Centres de Lutte Contre le cancer, and Groupe Coopérateur Multidisciplinaire en Oncologie) study. J Clin Oncol. 2014;32:3520–6.
84. Van Cutsem E, Moiseyenko VM, Tjulandin S, et al. Phase III study of docetaxel and cisplatin plus fluorouracil compared with cisplatin and fluorouracil as first-line therapy for advanced gastric cancer: a report of the V325 study group. J Clin Oncol. 2006;24:4991–7.
85. Tabernero J, Van Cutsem E, Bang Y-J, et al. Pembrolizumab with or without chemotherapy versus chemotherapy for advanced gastric or gastroesophageal junction (G/GEJ) adenocarcinoma: the phase III KEYNOTE-062 study. J Clin Oncol. 2019;37:LBA4007-LBA4007.
86. Moehler M, et al. LBA6_PR - Nivolumab (nivo) plus chemotherapy (chemo) versus chemo as first-line (1L) treatment for advanced gastric cancer/gastroesophageal junction cancer (GC/GEJC)/esophageal adenocarcinoma (EAC): first results of the CheckMate 649 study. Ann Oncol. 2020, September;31(Suppl_4):S1142–215. https://doi.org/10.1016/annonc/annonc325.
87. Hall PS. A randomised phase II trial and feasibility study of palliative chemotherapy in frail or elderly patients with advanced gastroesophageal cancer (321GO). Br J Cancer. 2017;116(114):472–8.
88. Mohile SG, Dale W, Somerfield MR, Hurria A. Practical assessment and Management of Vulnerabilities in older patients receiving chemotherapy: ASCO guideline for geriatric oncology summary. J Oncol Pract. 2018;14:442–6.
89. Wee-Kheng Soo MK, Alun Pope, Phillip Parente, Peteris Darzins, Ian D. Davis. Integrated geriatric assessment and treatment (INTEGERATE) in older people with cancer planned for systemic anticancer therapy. https://meetinglibrary.asco.org/record/186699/abstract 2020.
90. Mohile SG, Mohamed MR, Culakova E, et al. A geriatric assessment (GA) intervention to reduce treatment toxicity in older patients with advanced cancer: a University of Rochester Cancer Center NCI community oncology research program cluster randomized clinical trial (CRCT). J Clin Oncol. 2020;38:12009.
91. Soto-Perez-de-Celis E, Aapro M, Muss H. ASCO 2020: the geriatric assessment comes of age. Oncologist. 2020;25:909–12.
92. Li D, Sun C-L, Kim H, et al. Geriatric assessment-driven intervention (GAIN) on chemotherapy toxicity in older adults with cancer: a randomized controlled trial. J Clin Oncol. 2020;38:12010.

Chapter 24
Hepatopancreaticobiliary Cancer in Older Adults with Frailty

Zainul Abedin Kapacee, Nicola de Liguori Carino, Angela Lamarca, Richard A. Hubner, Juan W. Valle, and Mairéad G. McNamara

Introduction

Malignancies of the hepatopancreaticobiliary (HPB) tract encompass cancers of the liver, pancreas and biliary tract. Primary liver cancer or hepatocellular carcinoma (HCC) is a cancer of the hepatocytes and tends to occur in the context of chronic liver disease and liver cirrhosis [1]. Cancers of the biliary tract (BTC) can be further subdivided into gallbladder, ampulla of Vater and cholangiocarcinoma (cancers of the intrahepatic bile ducts, perihilar region and distal bile duct). The most common histological subtype for pancreatic and biliary cancers are adenocarcinomas [2, 3].

Hepatopancreaticobiliary cancers are more common in older people and the prognosis, particularly in the advanced setting, remains poor, with median overall survival (OS) ranging from 8-12 months or less. The relative 5-year survival in European countries for HPB malignancies, grouped collectively, ranges from 7-18% [4]. In the United Kingdom (UK), between 2015 and 2017, 43%, 47% and 52% of all new cases of HCC, pancreatic ductal adenocarcinomas (PDAC) and BTC, respectively, were in patients aged over 75 years [5–7]. The peak incidence for all these cancers was in patients aged 80-85 years. In the United States (US), data from

Z. A. Kapacee
Department of Medical Oncology, The Christie NHS Foundation Trust, Manchester, UK
e-mail: Zainul.Kapacee@nhs.net

N. de Liguori Carino
Regional Hepato-Pancreato-Biliary Unit, Manchester Royal Infirmary, Manchester, UK
e-mail: Nicola.DeLiguoriCarino@mft.nhs.uk

A. Lamarca · R. A. Hubner · J. W. Valle · M. G. McNamara (✉)
Department of Medical Oncology, The Christie NHS Foundation Trust, Manchester, UK

Division of Cancer Sciences, University of Manchester, Manchester, UK
e-mail: Angela.Lamarca@nhs.net; Richard.Hubner@nhs.net; Juan.Valle@nhs.net; Mairead.McNamara@nhs.net

F. Gomes (ed.), *Frailty in Older Adults with Cancer*,
https://doi.org/10.1007/978-3-030-89162-6_24

the surveillance, epidemiology and end results (SEER) programme (between 2013 and 2017) reported that the median age of patients diagnosed with PDAC was 70 years and 38% of all new cases were in patients aged over 75 [8]. The median age of patients with HCC and intrahepatic cholangiocarcinomas was 65 years and 23% of cases were in patients aged over 75 [9].

Frailty is more common in older patients. Whilst there is no universal age cut-off for 'older', 70 years is often chosen as the older age cut-off [10, 11]. Frailty becomes more prevalent with advancing age, but it is not exclusive to the ageing process. Frailty can be directly lead or worsen by many of the signs, symptoms and complications attributed to the disease process in HPB malignancies, which subsequently impacts on the treatment options available to these patients.

A number of tools have been devised to assess frailty, one example is the Rockwood clinical frailty scale (CFS) which categorises patients using a 9-point descriptive scale [12, 13]. Broadly categorised, patients who score 1-3 are typically non-frail patients, those who score 4 are pre-frail, 5-6 are mild to moderately frail, 7-8 are severely frail and 9 are terminally ill [13]. In the context of advanced HPB malignancies, in the absence of anticancer treatment, the prognosis can be less than 6 months and so a score of 9 is therefore unhelpful in grading frailty in these patients. Patients with severe frailty (CFS scores 7-8) are unlikely to be fit for anticancer treatment, with best supportive care and symptom control favoured. Therefore, this chapter will focus on the management of older patients with mild to moderate frailty and HPB cancers, where cancer treatment may still be of benefit, from early to advanced cancer stages.

Signs and Symptoms of HPB Malignancies and Relation to Frailty

Some problems arising from HPB malignancies are likely to impact on frailty, which include pancreatic exocrine insufficiency, biliary obstruction, diabetes mellitus, liver dysfunction, duodenal obstruction, anorexia, disease-related pain and depression (Fig. 24.1).

Pancreatic Exocrine Insufficiency

Pancreatic exocrine insufficiency (PEI) is common in patients with ampullary carcinomas, PDAC and extrahepatic cholangiocarcinoma (hilar and distal bile duct cholangiocarcinoma) situated close to the head of the pancreas; these cause PEI due to obstructed flow of pancreatic secretions secondary to tumour. Other causes include impaired production of the digestive enzymes due to inflammation, fibrosis and infiltration of pancreatic acinar cells by cancer cells, altered enteric pH, due to reduced bicarbonate production and altered anatomy after pancreatic surgery [14].

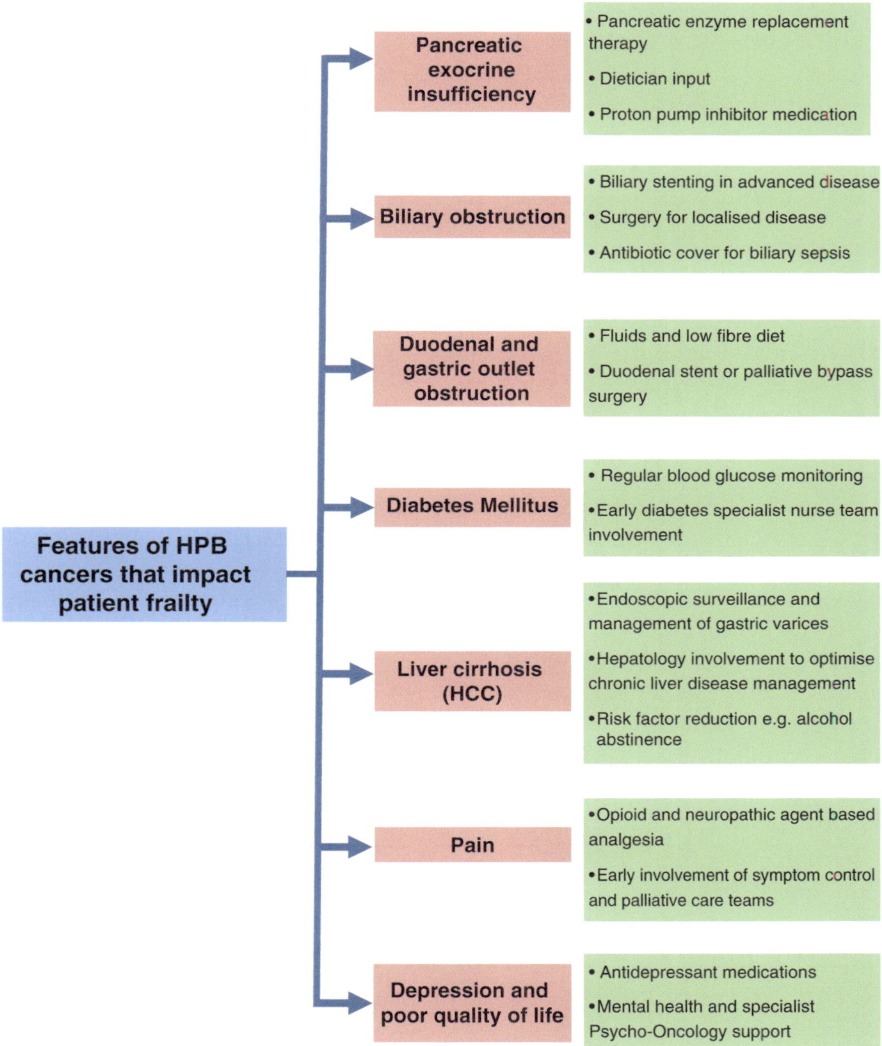

Fig. 24.1 Signs and symptoms associated with hepatopancreaticobiliary cancers in the context of frailty and recommended interventions

The common symptoms associated with PEI include abdominal pain, anorexia, nausea and vomiting, steatorrhoea, flatus and weight loss. Pancreatic exocrine insufficiency is predominantly determined from the clinical history and whilst a number of investigations for diagnosis of PEI exist such as faecal elastase testing, confirming PEI can often be a diagnostic challenge [15]. Pancreatic enzyme replacement therapy (PERT) forms the mainstay of treatment, but challenges with titration according to meal portions/components, issues with poor tolerance and compliance are common [14]. Polypharmacy and compliance with medications are additional factors to consider in older patients who may take inadequate PERT, due to the number of tablets often required for sufficient replacement. Nutritional deficiencies due to impaired digestion and absorption can accelerate weight loss and sarcopenia, which can also lead to or exacerbate existing frailty in patients

Disruption of Enterohepatic Circulation of Bile Acids

Cancers of the pancreaticobiliary tract can cause obstruction of the normal enterohepatic circulation of bile acids. Bile duct strictures due to extrinsic tumour compression or local invasion impede the normal flow of bile into the duodenum. A common presenting symptom of these cancers is painless obstructive jaundice which can be alleviated by stenting, either by endoscopic retrograde cholangiopancreatography (ERCP) and/or radiological percutaneous transhepatic cholangiography (PTC), depending on the site of obstruction [16]. Until such intervention takes place, patients often become systemically unwell with jaundice and frequently report symptoms including anorexia, nausea and vomiting, intractable itching and severe fatigue [16]. Patients are also at profound risk of infection due to biliary stasis and jaundice and can require intravenous antibiotics and fluids for concomitant biliary sepsis. Pre-operative biliary drainage for resectable disease remains controversial; most studies report a greater rate of complications and no improvement in survival outcome with peri-operative biliary drainage and direct 'fast-track' surgery is recommended [17, 18]. In the majority of patients who present with advanced disease, however, biliary drainage is a time critical 'life-saving' intervention and should be performed urgently to limit the detrimental effects of jaundice, which can trigger or exacerbate patient frailty.

Impaired Blood Glucose Control in Pancreatic Ductal Adenocarcinoma

The relationship between cancers involving the pancreas and diabetes is complex. Longstanding Type 2 Diabetes Mellitus (DM) is a known risk factor for developing PDAC, but it's also understood that pancreatogenic diabetes mellitus, or Type 3c DM (cancer-related DM), is a separate entity: the pathophysiology of which is proposed to involve pancreatic glandular inflammation and subsequent irreversible fibrotic damage, leading to islet cell loss [19]. Anorexia, weight loss, infection and concomitant steroid use are common factors that can cause significant disruption to blood glucose control in patients with PDAC. Prolonged periods of hyperglycaemia and erratic blood glucose control can lead to symptoms of polyuria, polydipsia, dehydration and fatigue. These patients also have increased susceptibility to infections, diabetic emergencies and long-term sequelae of end-organ macrovascular and microvascular complications, which can all exacerbate patient frailty [20, 21].

Liver Cirrhosis in HCC

Patients typically develop HCC in the context of underlying liver cirrhosis. The underlying aetiology of HCC is the same as those that lead to chronic liver disease and liver cirrhosis, namely: alcohol, viral hepatitis B and C and non-alcoholic fatty liver disease. Chronic liver disease and liver cirrhosis lead to a catabolic physiological state due to impaired liver synthetic function of proteins, such as albumin, and increased muscle breakdown, and the scarring from cirrhosis increases vascular resistance within the liver, causing portal hypertension. Ageing is associated with decline in hepatic function and reserve, over time, and in patients with existing chronic liver disease the risk of decompensation and mortality increases with age [22]. Furthermore patients with liver cirrhosis often have co-existing frailty with less physiological reserve to overcome environmental stressors such as an acute illness, surgery or anticancer therapy [23]. This can lead to decompensated liver disease with complications such as ascites, gastrointestinal variceal bleeding, jaundice and encephalopathy, which carry a high mortality risk [24]. It is therefore vital that patients with HCC and liver cirrhosis are optimised prior to any anticancer treatments, which may include abstinence from alcohol (if applicable), appropriate surveillance and management of varices, control of portal hypertension and regular laxatives to reduce the risk of hepatic encephalopathy [25, 26].

Management of Patients with Pancreatic Ductal Adenocarcinoma

Surgery for Localised Disease

Surgery is the only potentially curative treatment for patients with PDAC, but only 15–20% present with disease that is amenable to surgical resection. For tumours of the head and uncinate process of the pancreas, the cancer is excised via a pancreaticoduodenectomy (Whipple's procedure), which involves complex reconstruction of the remnant pancreas, common bile duct and small bowel. Cancers of the body and tail of the pancreas are usually excised by partial pancreatectomy ± splenectomy. Pancreatic resection surgeries are associated with significant post-operative morbidity and potential complications. Retrospective studies suggest that older patients are less likely to be offered surgery. Retrospective studies comparing older patients (age cut-off range of 70–80 years) vs younger patients who have undergone pancreatic surgery highlight that there is no consensus view on whether increasing age is associated with poorer outcomes [27–30]. Careful patient selection and high-volume experienced centres performing surgeries are factors that can reduce morbidity and mortality in older patients. Patients of any age are required to have adequate cardiovascular and respiratory fitness and an Eastern Cooperative Oncology Group (ECOG) performance score (PS) of 0-1, at least, to be considered for surgery. There is a paucity of data exploring PDAC resection surgery in patients with frailty, with the geriatric oncology surgical assessment and functional recovery after surgery (GOSAFE) trial currently underway [31], but at present given the required fitness parameters, it is often unlikely that patients with frailty would be eligible for curative surgery.

Adjuvant Chemotherapy for Localised Disease

There are different chemotherapy regimens available in the adjuvant setting with triplet, doublet and monotherapy options, the choice of which depends on patient fitness, post-operative recovery, existing co-morbidities and patient preference (Fig. 24.2) [32, 33]. The recurrence rate after PDAC resection is in excess of 80% and previous clinical trials, notably ESPAC-1 [34] and CONKO-001 [35], have demonstrated survival benefit with adjuvant chemotherapy compared to surveillance alone.

Modified FOLFIRINOX is a three-drug combination of 5-flurouracil (5-FU)/folinic acid, irinotecan and oxaliplatin given in 2-weekly cycles over 6 months. To date, this adjuvant regimen has demonstrated the greatest median OS of 54.4 months and 36% reduction in risk of death compared to single agent adjuvant therapy with gemcitabine in patients with resected PDAC [32]. The oldest patient recruited to the triple-drug arm in this trial was 79 years and only 19% of patients were aged 70 years or above. Whilst older age was not a limiting factor to recruitment, given the associated toxicities, all patients required an ECOG PS of 0-1, and thus most patients with frailty would not be suitable for chemotherapy combination [32].

Gemcitabine-based chemotherapy regimens are the mainstay of treatment for patients who are not fit enough for modified FOLFIRINOX. The ESPAC-4 clinical trial, published in 2017, established the gemcitabine and capecitabine combination as a standard of care adjuvant option for patients with resected PDAC [33], resulting in a median OS of 28.0 months (95% CI 23.5–31.5 months). This study included patients of ECOG PS of 2 and the oldest patient treated was 81 years, with 48% of patients being over 65 years. Furthermore, there was no difference in risk of death on comparison of age subgroups of <65 and ≥65 years [33]. The trial reported that gemcitabine/capecitabine was well tolerated, with similar toxicity profiles to gemcitabine monotherapy except for grade 3–4 neutropenia and plantar-palmar erythema (PPE), which was more frequent in all patients given combination therapy ($p<0.0001$). Gemcitabine and capecitabine combination may be a suitable treatment option for carefully selected patients, even in patients with frailty, provided there is close monitoring of patient functioning and treatment toxicities.

Single-agent adjuvant gemcitabine is usually well tolerated and more often used for patients with significant co-morbidities or who have had a delayed post-operative recovery. One study reported that patients over 70 years with PDAC are less likely to be offered adjuvant chemotherapy, and the most common reason for this was underlying frailty [36]. In most centres, patients with mild to moderate frailty are most likely to be offered monotherapy with gemcitabine [3]. Where there is clinical uncertainty regarding opting for combination chemotherapy using gemcitabine and

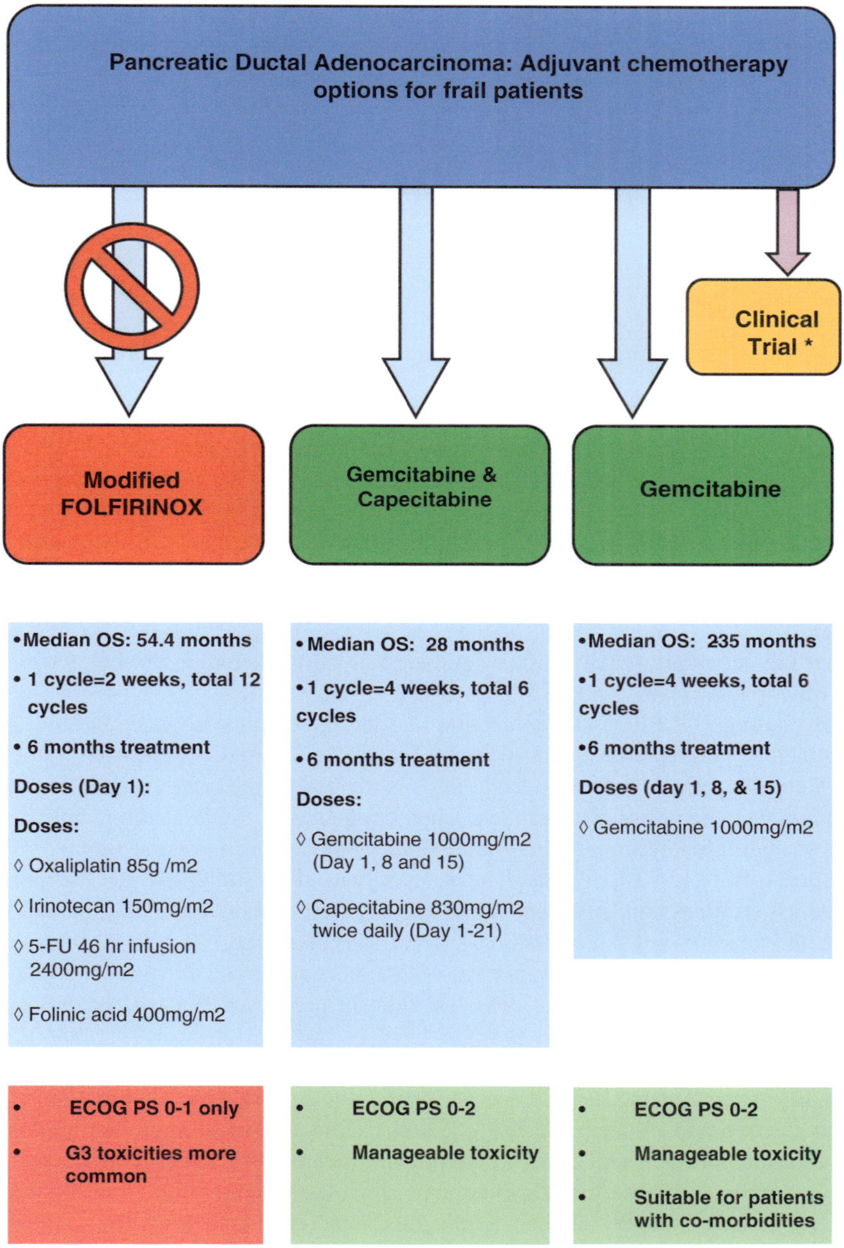

Fig. 24.2 Summary of adjuvant chemotherapy regimens and their suitability for older patients with mild to moderate frailty following pancreatic ductal adenocarcinoma resection. (*red = unsuitable; amber = may be suitable in carefully selected patients; green = suitable for the majority; Abbreviations: OS, overall survival; ECOG PS, Eastern Cooperative Oncology Group performance score)*

capecitabine or single agent gemcitabine, patients may be commenced on doublet therapy with the option to dose reduce both agents or omit capecitabine from subsequent cycles if unacceptable toxicities are encountered [3].

Palliative Chemotherapy for Advanced Disease

Despite advances in treatment management, the 5-year OS in patients with advanced PDAC remains fixed at less than 3% and median OS ranges from 6-8 months with systemic treatment. Given the poor survival outcomes in advanced disease, decisions regarding treatment for older patients with frailty need careful consideration (Fig. 24.3).

The chemotherapy regimen availability in advanced disease is similar to those employed in the adjuvant setting. Palliative FOLFIRINOX has the best OS outcome, to date, with a median OS of 11.1 [37]. However, the inclusion criteria for this study mandated that all patients had an ECOG PS 0-1 and the maximum age limit of patients randomised to this treatment was 76 years. This three-drug combination was associated with a higher incidence of grade 3–4 toxicities, such as neutropenia, thrombocytopenia and diarrhoea, compared to gemcitabine. Age >65 years was also found to be an independent adverse prognostic factor for OS, and given the anticipated toxicity, this regimen may be challenging and inappropriate for older patients with frailty [37].

Excluding FOLFIRINOX, other first line regimens in the advanced PDAC setting include gemcitabine as a core agent. The MPACT trial demonstrated a survival advantage in patients with advanced PDAC in the first-line setting with combination gemcitabine and nab-paclitaxel [38], when compared to single agent gemcitabine. The median age of patients recruited to this combination treatment was 62 years (range 27–86) and 42% of patients were ≥65 years. This study used the Karnofsky PS to assess fitness for treatment (scale 10-100, greater score indicating greater fitness and functioning). All patients required a Karnofsky score of ≥70 for inclusion. Furthermore, in patients ≥65 years, the reduction in risk of death with combination gemcitabine and nab-paclitaxel was less than in patients <65 years, hazard ratio (HR) 0.81 [95% CI 0.63–1.03] and 0.65 [95% confidence interval (CI) 0.53–0.79], respectively. There were also more frequent grade 3 toxicities of neutropenia, anaemia, thrombocytopenia, fatigue and peripheral neuropathy with combination gemcitabine and nab-paclitaxel, and 41% of patients in this cohort required chemotherapy dose reductions. So, whilst older patients and those with borderline performance status are not ineligible for this treatment, given the observed toxicity profile and unclear benefit in those ≥65 years, gemcitabine/nab-paclitaxel may not be suitable for older and/or frail patients.

Combination gemcitabine/capecitabine may be a treatment option for patients with advanced PDAC >70 years and those with frailty. This clinical trial included older patients, with a median age of 62 years (range 37–82) and also those of ECOG PS 2 [39]. Treatment was well tolerated, with comparable toxicity profiles for

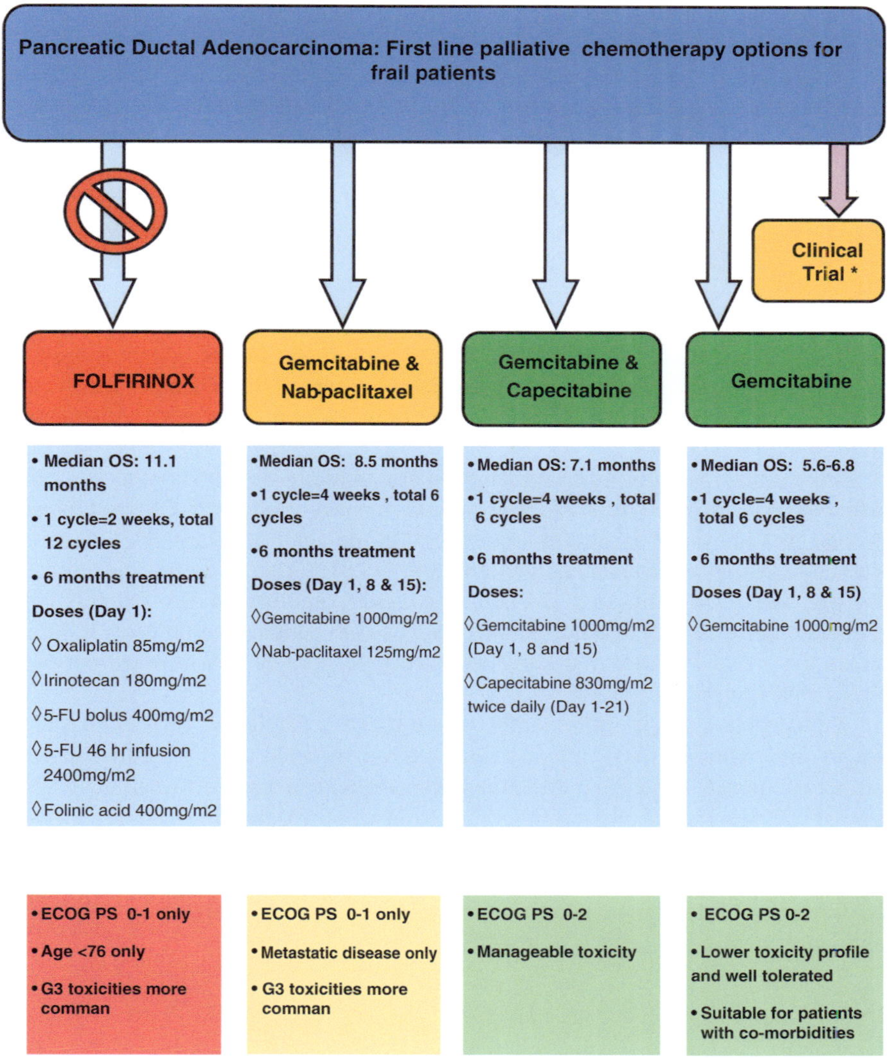

Fig. 24.3 Summary of palliative chemotherapy regimens and their suitability for older patients with mild to moderate frailty and advanced pancreatic ductal adenocarcinoma. (*red = unsuitable; amber = may be suitable in carefully selected patients; green = suitable for the majority; Abbreviations: OS, overall survival; ECOG PS, Eastern Cooperative Oncology Group performance score)*

gemcitabine/capecitabine and gemcitabine monotherapy. Grade 3-4 PPE and neutropenia were more common with combination chemotherapy (4% and 35% respectively) compared to gemcitabine monotherapy (0% and 22%, respectively). However, the survival advantage with doublet treatment was modest with a median

OS of 7.1 months compared to 6.2 months for patients receiving gemcitabine monotherapy HR 0.86 ($p = 0.08$) [39].

Gemcitabine monotherapy was established as standard of care first-line treatment in patients with advanced PDAC in 1997 [40] and has been the comparator arm in most subsequent pivotal trials [37–39]. The original study reported a median OS of 5.65 months with gemcitabine monotherapy and this has remained similar in subsequent literature ranging from 5-7 months [37–40]. In current clinical practice, gemcitabine monotherapy is the treatment choice for patients with existing co-morbidities, ECOG PS 2, who may gain symptomatic clinical benefit from chemotherapy. In the original study, the primary endpoint was clinical benefit response rate for symptoms of pain, functionality (assessed by Karnofsky PS) and weight loss; 23.8% of patients were found to have symptomatic benefit in one or more of these domains with gemcitabine treatment [40]. Given the satisfactory safety profile, gemcitabine monotherapy is often the preferred option for older patients with mild to moderate frailty.

Second-line palliative chemotherapies are unlikely to be suitable for older patients with frailty. The NAPOLI-1 phase 3 study confirmed OS benefit with second-line liposomal irinotecan with 5-FU/folinic acid, but Karnofsky PS scores <90 and age >65 were associated with poorer OS [41]. Other second-line regimens include the oxaliplatin and 5-FU/folinic acid combination for patients with gemcitabine-refractory disease, but has been used in patients with preserved fitness (Karnofsky PS >70) after first-line chemotherapy, and thus benefit in patients with frailty is less clear [42].

A prospective single centre study, where patients diagnosed with PDAC of all stages were assessed for frailty on diagnosis, were defined as frail if they had three or more abnormalities in grip strength, gait speed, weight loss, self-reported exhaustion or self-reported physical activity. This study reported that 25% of patients were identified as frail and had a significantly increased risk of death ($p<0.001$) compared with non-frail patients [43]. It is clear that for patients with severe frailty, best supportive care with management of disease-related symptoms is preferred to systemic anticancer treatment.

Management of Patients with Biliary Tract Cancers

Surgery for Localised Disease

Surgical resection for BTC can entail liver resection, cholecystectomy, pancreaticoduodenectomy (Whipple's procedure) and biliary reconstruction depending on the location of the cancer within the biliary tract [3]. Metastatic disease, multifocal liver disease and involvement of porta hepatis structures preclude curative surgery [44]. In retrospective studies, older age has not prevented patients being offered curative surgery and similar survival outcomes have been observed comparing older (>70 years) and younger patients [45, 46]. Patients with an ECOG PS ≥2 are less likely to be offered surgical intervention [46]; it may be inferred that a significant proportion of these patients are also likely to have frailty, and thus curative surgery may only be feasible for some of these patients. The previously mentioned GOSAFE trial is underway and includes comprehensive frailty assessments in patients >70 years undergoing cancer surgery and it recruits those for elective BTC resection, which may help address some of these unknowns [31].

Adjuvant Chemotherapy for Localised Disease

Since the BILCAP study, published in 2019, the recommended standard of care adjuvant chemotherapy is oral capecitabine commenced within 16 weeks of BTC resection [47]. A clear survival advantage was demonstrated in the pre-specified per-protocol analysis with median OS of 53 months compared to 36 months in the capecitabine and observation cohorts, respectively, p=0.028. In this study, the median age of patients receiving capecitabine was 62 years (55–68) and included patients of ECOG PS 0-2. Treatment was well tolerated with the most common toxicities being plantar-palmar erythrodysesthesia, fatigue and diarrhoea. Although patients older than 60 years were under-represented in this study, accounting for only 35% of trial recruitment with 18% receiving capecitabine, capecitabine was relatively well tolerated and thus in wider clinical practice, age >70 years and frailty may not be a prohibitive factor for adjuvant treatment (Fig. 24.4).

Palliative Chemotherapy for Advanced Disease

The cisplatin/gemcitabine combination is well established as the standard of care for patients with recurrent, locally advanced or metastatic BTC [48]. The Advanced Biliary tract Cancer (ABC)-02 study recruited patients with a median age of 63.9 years (range 32.8–81.9) and an ECOG PS 0-2, with 13% patients having an ECOG PS of 2. The median OS was 11.7 months in patients receiving combination chemotherapy compared to 8.1 months with gemcitabine monotherapy, with manageable toxicity profiles in both cohorts. An evaluation of patients from this study and 12 other prospective BTC studies reported no significant difference in progression-free survival or OS between the older cohort (≥70 years) and those <70 years [49]. Furthermore, all age subgroups demonstrated a favourable outcome with combination treatment. A meta-analyses of two randomised trials, including the ABC-02 data, reported that patients with ECOG PS 2 may derive the least benefit from combination cisplatin/gemcitabine treatment and thus gemcitabine monotherapy may be more suitable for less fit patients [50].

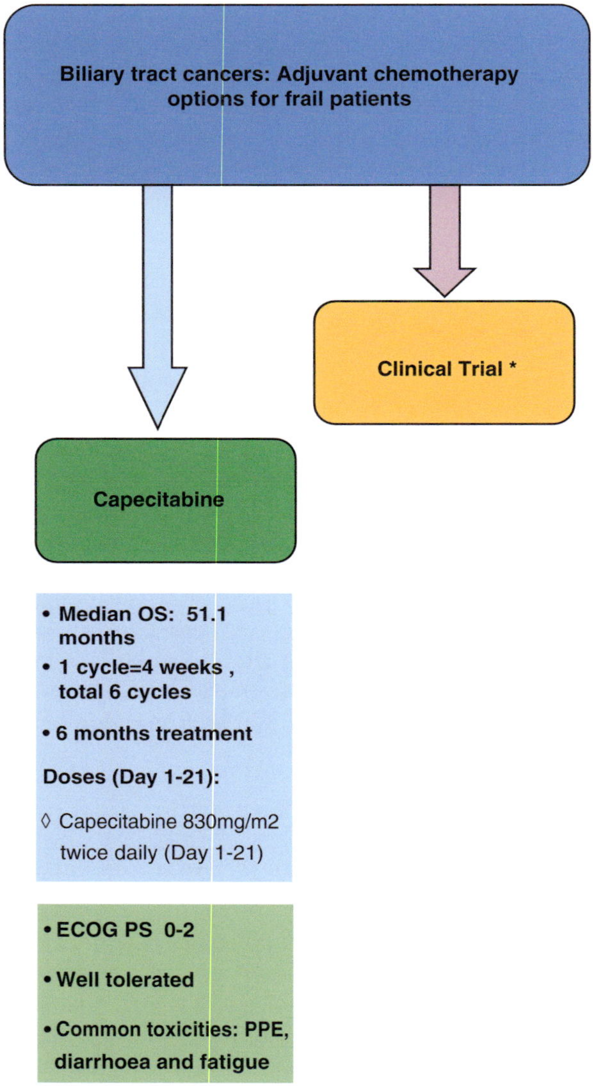

Fig. 24.4 Summary of adjuvant chemotherapy regimens and their suitability for older patients with mild to moderate frailty following biliary tract cancer resection. (*amber = may be suitable in carefully selected patients; green = suitable for the majority*; *Abbreviations: OS, overall survival; ECOG PS, Eastern Cooperative Oncology Group performance score)*

Combination 5FU and oxaliplatin is recommended as second-line palliative treatment for advanced BTC [51]. A retrospective study (n=378) found that only a quarter of the patients received second-line therapy with the majority (95%) having an ECOG PS 0-1. Patients >60 years were also less likely to receive second-line chemotherapy (p=0.001) [52]. From the available data patients >70 years and those with frailty may lack the fitness for second-line chemotherapy. Interestingly abstract data from the ABC-06 study has shown that active symptom control after first line cisplatin gemcitabine offered a median 5.3 month survival and thus may be an option for older patients with frailty (Fig. 24.5) [51].

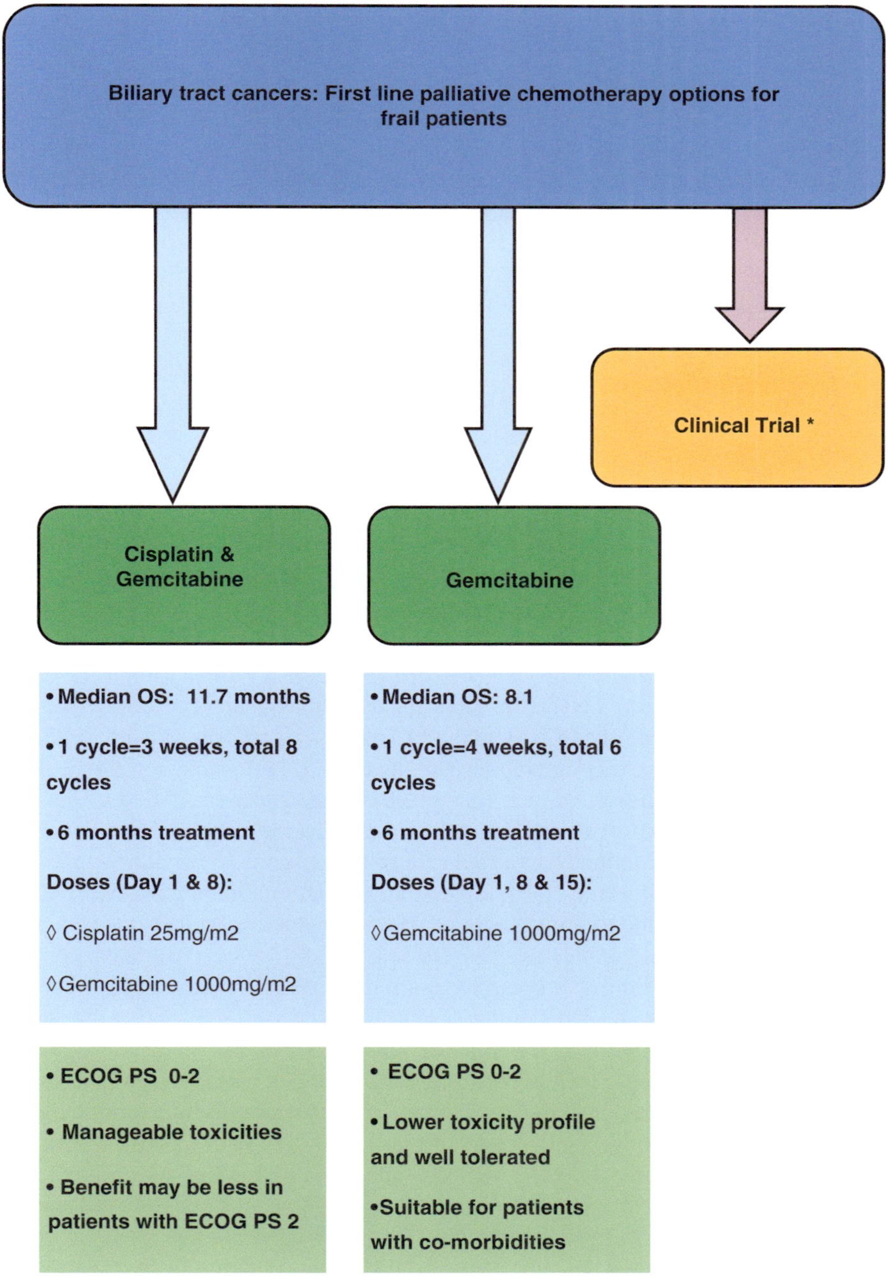

Fig. 24.5 Summary of palliative chemotherapy regimens and their suitability for older patients with mild to moderate frailty and advanced biliary tract cancer. (*amber = may be suitable in carefully selected patients; green = suitable for the majority*; *Abbreviations: OS, overall survival; ECOG PS, Eastern Cooperative Oncology Group performance score)*

Management of Patients with Hepatocellular Carcinoma

Patients tend to develop HCC in the context of existing liver cirrhosis and may have existing frailty and other co-morbidities. The Barcelona Clinic Liver Cancer (BCLC) algorithm is the most widely used staging system to determine localised or advanced disease and subsequently guide management for patients with HCC (Table 24.1) [53]. The choice of treatment is based upon the degree of tumour burden, current liver function measured (using the Child Pugh score) and the patient's ECOG PS. Where disease remains confined to the liver, with lower tumour burden, localised liver-directed therapies such as surgical resection, radiofrequency ablation and transarterial chemoembolisation can be employed. For advanced HCC, where there is multifocal disease with macrovascular invasion and/or extrahepatic spread, systemic treatments are required [54].

Liver-Directed Treatments for Localised Disease

Patients with a solitary HCC can potentially be treated curatively with surgical resection, and for patients with lesions <5 cm or up to 3 lesions (each <3 cm), they can be considered for liver transplantation as per the Milan criteria [55]. Data from the US and European liver transplant registries indicate a growing trend for older patients ≥ 65 years being deemed eligible for liver transplantation [56]. However, increasing age, particularly in patients ≥70 years, was associated with a higher waiting list mortality rate compared to patients aged 18–49 years, and the proportion of patients who underwent liver transplantation also decreased with increasing age (≥70 years). One study of 294 patients awaiting liver transplant found that 17% of patients were frail (defined as a Fried Frailty Index score >3) and these patients had greater waitlist mortality [57]. Liver transplantation for patients with HCC remains challenging due to a multitude of factors, including limited donor supply and disease progression whilst awaiting transplant [58]. Liver transplantation carries the risk of significant post-operative complications and with a need for long-term immunosuppressive medications, and is unlikely to be an option for older patients with frailty [59].

Liver resection is more widely performed for localised disease and many retrospective studies have demonstrated similar treatment and survival outcomes in older and younger patient subgroups undergoing resection, although these independent single centre studies have used different age cut-offs to define the older patient and the cut-off point ranges from 70-80 years [60]. Age >70 years alone does not appear to be a contraindication to liver resection for localised HCC and individualised assessment of older patients is advocated [61]. However, suitability for liver resection, as recommended by the BCLC algorithm, requires normal liver function and a good functional baseline of ECOG PS 0-1. A recent study explored survival outcomes in patients over 75 years after surgical resection for HCC and found that

Table 24.1 Adapted summary of the Barcelona Clinic Liver Cancer (BCLC) algorithm for staging and management options for hepatocellular cancers [53, 54]

BCLC stage		Tumour burden	Liver function (CP score)	ECOG PS	Treatment options
0	Very early	Solitary nodule <2 cm	A	0-1	Resection or ablation
A	Early	Solitary nodule >2 cm or 2-3 nodules ≤3 cm	A	0-1	Transplant, resection or ablation
B	Intermediate	Multinodular: >3 nodules or ≥2 nodules > 3 cm	A, B (caution)	0-1	Embolisation: TACE or SIRT
C	Advanced	Macrovascular invasion or extrahepatic spread	A, B (caution)	0-2	Systemic therapies
D	Terminal	Macrovascular invasion or extrahepatic spread	B, C	>2	Best supportive care

Abbreviations: *CP* Child Pugh, *ECOG PS* Eastern cooperative oncology group performance status, *TACE* Trans-arterial chemoembolisation, *SIRT* selective internal radiation treatment

patients with frailty (CFS score >4) were less likely to be offered surgical resection, and that those with frailty had greater post-operative complications and worse survival outcomes ($p<0.05$) [62]. Patients with frailty may not have sufficient cardiorespiratory fitness, and the presence of other co-morbidities may preclude resection, hence data on surgery and outcomes in this patient group with resectable HCC is limited [61].

Radiofrequency ablation (RFA) is a potentially curative treatment which is suitable for small HCCs that fulfil the Milan criteria [55]. This treatment has advantages over surgery, being less invasive, associated with less morbidity and usually requires a shorter duration of hospitalisation. These factors mean RFA may be considered for older patients with frailty unfit for surgical resection. However, RFA may be an inferior treatment to surgical resection, as a number of studies report poorer survival outcomes for patients undergoing RFA, when compared to surgical resection [63, 64]. There is a lack of consensus, as other studies have reported comparable survival outcomes [65, 66]. Furthermore, in one meta-analysis of over 11,000 patients undergoing RFA, age ≥65 years and declining liver function (Child Pugh B vs Child Pugh A function and albumin-bilirubin score 1 vs 0) were predictive of worse OS (both $p<0.0001$) [67]. Older patients with HCC and frailty are more likely to have lower serum albumin and abnormal liver function [23]. Ultimately, RFA may be an appropriate option for older patients with mild to moderate frailty due to fewer associated toxicities, but the OS benefit may be limited.

For intermediate stage HCC (Barcelona Class B), non-curative loco-regional treatments such as transarterial chemoembolisation (TACE) or selective internal radiation therapy (SIRT) can be considered [54]. TACE is the standard of care treatment for patients with intermediate stage HCC [68], and a number of retrospective studies have shown similar survival outcomes in older (>70 years) and younger patients [60, 69]. The American Association for the Study of Liver Diseases guidance recommends consideration of TACE for patients with Child Pugh A and highly selected Child Pugh B liver dysfunction, ECOG PS 0 and tumours without macrovascular invasion [70]. There is a paucity of data for outcomes in patients using frailty scoring tools. SIRT involves transarterial infusion of yttrium-90 microspheres which delivers localised radiotherapy to the targeted tumour, and a meta-analysis reports similar survival outcomes comparing TACE and SIRT in appropriate patients with HCC [71]. Small single centre studies have not shown age to be a prognostic factor in patients treated with SIRT, but similar to TACE, outcomes for patients with frailty are not known [72].

The management of localised HCC is complex and in clinical practice, patients may receive different therapeutic approaches over time. Some studies have also explored patient outcomes with combination treatments such as combined RFA and TACE [73]. Outcomes in older patients ≥70 years appear similar to younger patients <70 years for localised disease, but most available data is from retrospective single centre studies and predominantly from the Asia-Pacific region, where HCC is most prevalent (hepatitis B-related). These small studies may not reflect the outcomes in older patients with frailty of Europe and the Americas, due to differences in HCC aetiology, ethnicity, socio-economic factors and healthcare systems.

Systemic Therapy for Advanced Disease

Advanced HCC is defined as multifocal disease within the liver not amenable to localised therapies or where there is extrahepatic spread of disease. In this setting the backbone treatment for patients consists of targeted therapies (Fig. 24.6). For a number of years, the first-line treatment for advanced HCC has been sorafenib, which offers patients a median OS of 8–12 months [74, 75]. Sorafenib is a small molecule multikinase inhibitor targeting Raf-1, B-Raf, Vascular Endothelial Growth Factor Receptor (VEGFR) 1, 2 and 3 and Platelet Derived Growth Factor Receptor (PDGFR) and had been the first-line standard of care for these patients for the past decade. A meta-analysis of 30 studies reporting use of sorafenib in patients with advanced HCC (n=8000) found that risk factors which had a negative influence on OS on multivariable analysis were ECOG PS ≥2 and Child Pugh B liver dysfunction [76]. However, older age was neither prognostic nor predictive of treatment-related death. The most commonly-reported toxicities of all grades were plantar-palmar erythrodysesthesia, diarrhoea, fatigue and hypertension. Older patients are much more likely to have pre-existing hypertension with up to 90% of patients aged over 55 years likely to develop hypertension in their remaining lifespan [77]. Use of targeted therapies in older patients can worsen blood pressure control and increase the risk of cardiovascular complications. Patients with frailty may be less likely to gain benefit from targeted therapy, but one large retrospective study has shown that sorafenib can be given in carefully selected patients, including those with poorer liver function, at a lower dose such as 200 mg twice a day or 200 mg once day, depending on the patients' degree of frailty [78].

Lenvatinib is another targeted therapy which demonstrated similar survival outcomes to sorafenib but with a more favourable toxicity profile, and is often used for

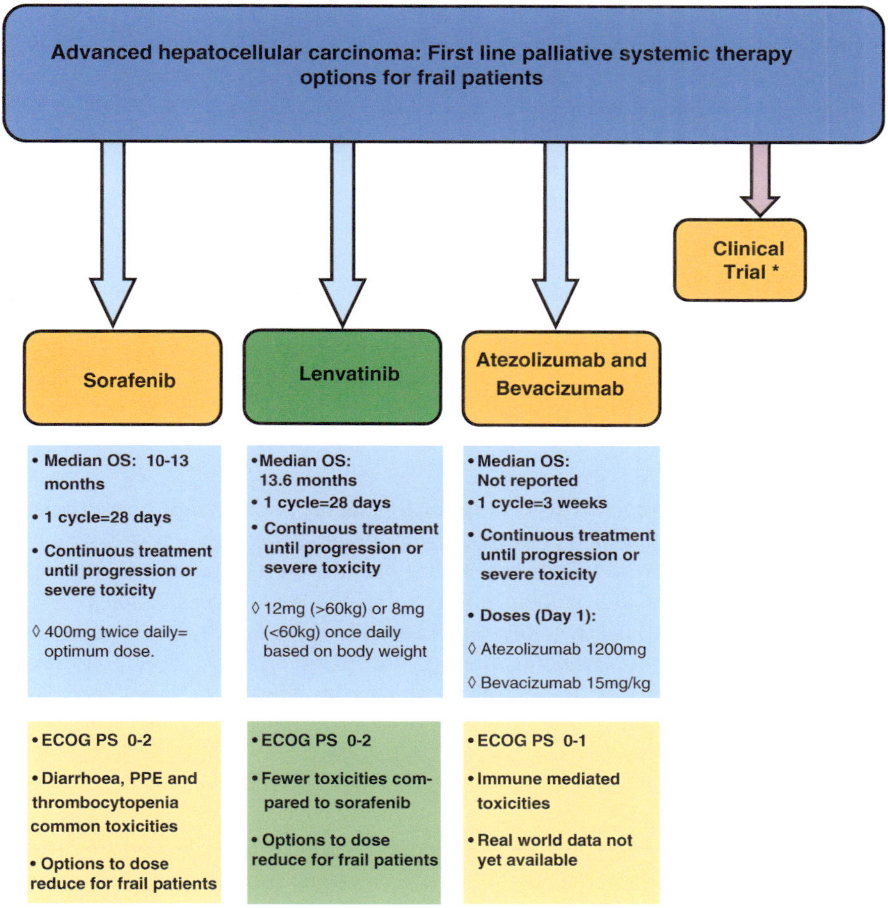

Fig. 24.6 Summary of palliative targeted treatments and their suitability for older patients with mild to moderate frailty and advanced hepatocellular carcinoma. *(amber = may be suitable in carefully selected patients; green = suitable for the majority; Abbreviations: OS, overall survival; ECOG PS, Eastern Cooperative Oncology Group performance score)*

patients intolerant of sorafenib, and so may be prescribed for carefully selected older patients with frailty [79]. There are now a number of second-line targeted therapies potentially available, namely regorafenib [80], ramucirumab [81] and cabozantinib [82], but most trial designs for these agents required patients to have ECOG PS scores of 0-1, normal liver function, and importantly to have progressed following treatment with sorafenib and previously tolerated this in the first-line setting. These trials have recruited patients >70 years and found no differences in survival outcomes, but the benefit of second-line therapies in patients with frailty is less clear [83].

Recently, in early 2020, combination immunotherapy and anti-angiogenic treatment with atezolizumab and bevacizumab has superseded survival outcomes achieved with sorafenib and is set to become the new standard of care in the first-line advanced setting [84]. All patients recruited to this landmark trial had an ECOG PS 0-1, Child Pugh A liver function and a median age of 64 years (56–71) in patients receiving atezolizumab/bevacizumab and 66 years (59–71) in those receiving sorafenib. Serious adverse events occurred more frequently in patients receiving atezolizumab/bevacizumab compared to those receiving sorafenib, but a longer time to deterioration of patient-reported quality of life and functioning was observed in the combination arm. Real-world data from prospective studies, once this treatment has been more widely used, will shed light as to its suitability for older patients with frailty.

Conclusion

The management of patients with HPB malignancies is challenging and patients with advanced disease have a poor prognostic outlook. It is key to address cancer-related symptoms early in the patients' management to limit deterioration in patients functioning and to enhance patients ability to receive anticancer therapies. Whilst older patients are significantly under-represented in clinical trials, most studies suggest they have similar survival outcomes to younger cohorts [83, 85, 86]. However, data on older patients with frailty and its impact on patient outcomes with HPB malignancies is particularly limited, and most outcome data is inferred from performance status scores which place emphasis on patient activity. Whilst this is relevant to frailty, other aspects such as cognition, nutrition, sarcopenia, mobility and balance may be overlooked.

For patients with localised disease, surgical resection offers the only potentially curative option, but there is a high risk of recurrence and patient with frailty are less likely to be offered curative surgery due to having reduced physiological reserve and a higher risk of significant post-operative complications and long-term morbidity. Therefore, peri-operative rehabilitation and optimising potentially reversible factors such as nutrition, muscle strength and mobility may improve outcomes and treatment options for these patients [87]. Robotic and minimal access surgery may reduce morbidity of HPB resection compared to open techniques, but the survival advantage and suitability older patients with frailty is unclear [88, 89]. The previously mentioned GOSAFE trial is a prospective multicentre study that aims to obtain real-world data on long-term post-operative outcomes in patients >70 years undergoing elective cancer surgery [31]. Patients are assessed for frailty using a comprehensive multimodality approach using the ECOG PS, adapted 3-min 'Mini-Cog' test for cognition, geriatric 8 (G8) scoring tool, timed up and go (TUG) test, aged adjusted Charlson co-morbidity index and nutritional risk screening, amongst others [31]. This study will report on the 30-day morbidity and mortality, 3- and 6-month post-operative functional outcomes. A considerable proportion of these patients have HPB malignancies, therefore the survival and functional outcomes of these patients will be insightful.

In the setting of advanced HPB malignancies, the focus of care is on quality of life and symptom control, given the shorter survival durations anticipated. Opting for anticancer treatments with fewer toxicities and better tolerability are preferred, to preserve functioning and overall quality of life. Clinicians should have a lower threshold to dose reduce, provide treatment breaks or discontinue palliative anticancer therapies if severe toxicities or unacceptable symptoms are encountered.

To improve the management of older patients with HPB malignancies and frailty, dedicated frailty assessments and the gold standard comprehensive geriatric assessment (CGA) should be conducted for older patients and for those in whom frailty is suspected. One interventional Phase IV trial is exploring the use of gemcitabine ± nab-paclitaxel in patients >70 years with advanced PDAC, with the aim to determine whether treatment individualisation by CGA improves functional outcome for these patients (NCT02812992) [90]. Similar trials utilising the CGA or other tailored frailty assessments are needed [91, 92] along with improvements in future therapeutic strategies. Molecular profiling of tumours to identify targetable mutations may improve treatment options for frail patients in the future. Examples of these treatments include olaparib in patients with breast cancer gene 1/2 (BRCA1/2) mutations in PDAC [93], ivosidenib in patients with isocitrate dehydrogenase mutations [94] and fibroblast growth factor receptor related aberrations [95] in cholangiocarcinomas. Immunotherapies are also another modality of treatment, but so far have not shown survival benefit in patients with PDAC. Studies are on-going to investigate the potential additional benefit of immunotherapy, for example, with durvalumab in combination with cisplatin/gemcitabine (NCT03875235) in patients with advanced BTCs [96]. For patients with advanced HCC, first-line combination therapy using programmed cell death ligand-1 (PDL-1) inhibition with atezolizumab and anti-VEGF treatment with bevacizumab has shown improved survival outcomes compared to the standard of care sorafenib [84]. These emerging treatment strategies may be associated with fewer toxicities compared to current cytotoxic regimens, and with increasing use and clinician experience may be suitable for frail patients.

References

1. Vogel A, Cervantes A, Chau I, Daniele B, Llovet JM, Meyer T, et al. Hepatocellular carcinoma: ESMO Clinical Practice Guidelines for diagnosis, treatment and follow-up † Incidence and epidemiology. ESMO Guidel Comm. 2018;29:iv238–55. https://doi.org/10.1093/annonc/mdy308.
2. Valle JW, Borbath I, Khan SA, Huguet F, Gruenberger T, Arnold D. Biliary cancer: ESMO Clinical Practice Guidelines for diagnosis, treatment and follow-up † On behalf of the ESMO Guidelines Committee 2016. Ann Oncol. 2016;27(Suppl 5):v28–37. https://doi.org/10.1093/annonc/mdw324.
3. Ducreux M, Sa Cuhna A, Caramella C, Hollebecque A, Burtin P, Goéré D, et al. Cancer of the pancreas: ESMO Clinical Practice Guidelines for diagnosis, treatment and follow-up †. ESMO Updat Clin Pract Guidel. 2015;26:v56–68. https://doi.org/10.1093/annonc/mdv295.
4. Lepage C, Capocaccia R, Hackl M, Lemmens V, Molina E, Pierannunzio D, et al. Survival in patients with primary liver cancer, gallbladder and extrahepatic biliary tract cancer and pancre-

atic cancer in Europe 1999-2007: results of EUROCARE-5. Eur J Cancer. 2015;51:2169–78. https://doi.org/10.1016/j.ejca.2015.07.034.

5. Pancreatic cancer statistics | Cancer Research UK n.d. https://www.cancerresearchuk.org/health-professional/cancer-statistics/statistics-by-cancer-type/pancreatic-cancer#heading-Two. Accessed July 6, 2020.
6. Liver cancer statistics | Cancer Research UK n.d. https://www.cancerresearchuk.org/health-professional/cancer-statistics/statistics-by-cancer-type/liver-cancer. Accessed July 6, 2020.
7. Gallbladder cancer statistics | Cancer Research UK n.d. https://www.cancerresearchuk.org/health-professional/cancer-statistics/statistics-by-cancer-type/gallbladder-cancer. Accessed July 6, 2020.
8. Pancreatic Cancer — Cancer Stat Facts n.d. https://seer.cancer.gov/statfacts/html/pancreas.html. Accessed July 6, 2020.
9. Liver and Intrahepatic Bile Duct Cancer — Cancer Stat Facts n.d. https://seer.cancer.gov/statfacts/html/livibd.html. Accessed July 6, 2020.
10. Hurria A, Togawa K, Mohile SG, Owusu C, Klepin HD, Gross CP, et al. Predicting chemotherapy toxicity in older adults with cancer: a prospective multicenter study. J Clin Oncol. 2011;29:3457–65. https://doi.org/10.1200/JCO.2011.34.7625. American Society of Clinical Oncology
11. Balducci L, Extermann M. Management of cancer in the older person: a practical approach. Oncologist. 2000;5:224–37. https://doi.org/10.1634/theoncologist.5-3-224.
12. Rockwood K, Song X, MacKnight C, Bergman H, Hogan DB, McDowell I, et al. A global clinical measure of fitness and frailty in elderly people. CMAJ. 2005;173:489–95. https://doi.org/10.1503/cmaj.050051.
13. Juma S, Taabazuing MM, Montero-Odasso M. Clinical frailty scale in an acute medicine unit: a simple tool that predicts length of stay. Can Geriatr J. 2016;19:34–9. https://doi.org/10.5770/cgj.19.196.
14. Powell-Brett S, de Liguori CN, Roberts K. Understanding pancreatic exocrine insufficiency and replacement therapy in pancreatic cancer. Eur J Surg Oncol. 2021;47(3 Pt A):539–44. https://doi.org/10.1016/j.ejso.2020.03.006.
15. Carnie LE, Lamarca A, McNamara MG, Bibby N, O'Reilly DA, Valle JW. The assessment of pancreatic exocrine function in patients with inoperable pancreatic cancer: in need of a new gold-standard. Pancreatology. 2020;20:668–75. https://doi.org/10.1016/j.pan.2020.03.020.
16. Viesca MFY, Arvanitakis M. Early diagnosis and management of malignant distal biliary obstruction: a review on current recommendations and guidelines. Clin Exp Gastroenterol. 2019;12:415–32. https://doi.org/10.2147/CEG.S195714.
17. Sewnath ME, Karsten TM, Prins MH, Rauws EJA, Obertop H, Gouma DJ. A meta-analysis on the efficacy of preoperative biliary drainage for tumors causing obstructive jaundice. Ann Surg. 2002;236:17–27. https://doi.org/10.1097/00000658-200207000-00005.
18. van der Gaag NA, Rauws EAJ, van Eijck CHJ, Bruno MJ, van der Harst E, Kubben FJGM, et al. Preoperative biliary drainage for cancer of the head of the pancreas. N Engl J Med. 2010;362:129–37. https://doi.org/10.1056/NEJMoa0903230.
19. Andersen DK, Korc M, Petersen GM, Eibl G, Li D, Rickels MR, et al. Diabetes, pancreatogenic diabetes, and pancreatic cancer. Diabetes. 2017;66:1103–10. https://doi.org/10.2337/db16-1477.
20. Perkisas S, Vandewoude M. Where frailty meets diabetes. Diabetes Metab Res Rev. 2016;32:261–7. https://doi.org/10.1002/dmrr.2743.
21. Liuu E, Saulnier PJ, Gand E, Ragot S, Valero S, Jamet A, et al. Frailty and diabetes status in older patients with cancer: impact on mortality in the ANCRAGE cohort. Aging Clin Exp Res. 2020;32(9):1809–19. https://doi.org/10.1007/s40520-019-01362-9.
22. Kim IH, Kisseleva T, Brenner DA. Aging and liver disease. Curr Opin Gastroenterol. 2015;31:184–91. https://doi.org/10.1097/MOG.0000000000000176.
23. Laube R, Wang H, Park L, Heyman JK, Vidot H, Majumdar A, et al. Frailty in advanced liver disease. Liver Int. 2018;38:2117–28. https://doi.org/10.1111/liv.13917.

24. Nusrat S, Khan MS, Fazili J, Madhoun MF. Cirrhosis and its complications: Evidence based treatment. World J Gastroenterol. 2014;20:5442–60. https://doi.org/10.3748/wjg.v20.i18.5442.
25. Pinter M, Trauner M, Peck-Radosavljevic M, Sieghart W. Cancer and liver cirrhosis: implications on prognosis and management. ESMO Open. 2016;1(2):e000042. https://doi.org/10.1136/esmoopen-2016-000042.
26. Ismail BES, Cabrera R. Management of liver cirrhosis in patients with hepatocellular carcinoma. Chinese Clin Oncol. 2013;2:4. https://doi.org/10.21037/CCO.V2I4.3026.
27. Makary MA, Winter JM, Cameron JL, Campbell KA, Chang D, Cunningham SC, et al. Pancreaticoduodenectomy in the very elderly. J Gastrointest Surg. 2006;10:347–56. https://doi.org/10.1016/j.gassur.2005.12.014.
28. He W, Zhao H, Chan W, Lopez D, Shroff RT, Giordano SH. Underuse of surgical resection among elderly patients with early-stage pancreatic cancer. Surg (United States). 2015;158:1226–34. https://doi.org/10.1016/j.surg.2015.04.031.
29. Riall TS, Sheffield KM, Kuo YF, Townsend CM, Goodwin JS. Resection benefits older adults with locoregional pancreatic cancer despite greater short-term morbidity and mortality. J Am Geriatr Soc. 2011;59:647–54. https://doi.org/10.1111/j.1532-5415.2011.03353.x.
30. Van Der Geest LGM, Besselink MGH, Van Gestel YRBM, Busch ORC, De Hingh IHJT, De Jong KP, et al. Pancreatic cancer surgery in elderly patients: balancing between short-term harm and long-term benefit. A population-based study in the Netherlands. Acta Oncol (Madr). 2016;55:278–85. https://doi.org/10.3109/0284186X.2015.1105381.
31. Montroni I, Rostoft S, Spinelli A, Van Leeuwen BL, Ercolani G, Saur NM, et al. GOSAFE – geriatric oncology surgical assessment and functional recovery after surgery: early analysis on 977 patients. J Geriatr Oncol. 2020;11:244–55. https://doi.org/10.1016/j.jgo.2019.06.017.
32. Conroy T, Hammel P, Hebbar M, Ben Abdelghani M, Wei AC, Raoul J-L, et al. FOLFIRINOX or gemcitabine as adjuvant therapy for pancreatic cancer. N Engl J Med. 2018;379:2395–406. https://doi.org/10.1056/NEJMoa1809775.
33. Neoptolemos JP, Palmer DH, Ghaneh P, Psarelli EE, Valle JW, Halloran CM, et al. Comparison of adjuvant gemcitabine and capecitabine with gemcitabine monotherapy in patients with resected pancreatic cancer (ESPAC-4): a multicentre, open-label, randomised, phase 3 trial. Lancet. 2017;389:1011–24. https://doi.org/10.1016/S0140-6736(16)32409-6.
34. Neoptolemos JP, Stocken DD, Friess H, Bassi C, Dunn JA, Hickey H, et al. A randomized trial of chemoradiotherapy and chemotherapy after resection of pancreatic cancer. N Engl J Med. 2004;350:1200–10. https://doi.org/10.1056/NEJMoa032295.
35. Oettle H, Neuhaus P, Hochhaus A, Hartmann JT, Gellert K, Ridwelski K, et al. Adjuvant chemotherapy with gemcitabine and long-term outcomes among patients with resected pancreatic cancer: the CONKO-001 randomized trial. JAMA – J Am Med Assoc. 2013;310:1473–81. https://doi.org/10.1001/jama.2013.279201.
36. Malik AK, Lamarca A, Siriwardena AK, O'Reilly D, Deshpande R, Satyadas T, et al. The influence of patients' age on the outcome of treatment for pancreatic ductal adenocarcinoma. Pancreas. 2020;49:201–7. https://doi.org/10.1097/MPA.0000000000001486.
37. Conroy T, Desseigne F, Ychou M, Bouché O, Guimbaud R, Bécouarn Y, et al. FOLFIRINOX versus gemcitabine for metastatic pancreatic cancer. N Engl J Med. 2011;364:1817–25. https://doi.org/10.1056/NEJMoa1011923.
38. Von Hoff DD, Ervin T, Arena FP, Chiorean EG, Infante J, Moore M, et al. Increased survival in pancreatic cancer with nab-paclitaxel plus gemcitabine. N Engl J Med. 2013;369:1691–703. https://doi.org/10.1056/NEJMoa1304369.
39. Cunningham D, Chau I, Stocken DD, Valle JW, Smith D, Steward W, et al. Phase III randomized comparison of gemcitabine versus gemcitabine plus capecitabine in patients with advanced pancreatic cancer. J Clin Oncol. 2009;27:5513–8. https://doi.org/10.1200/JCO.2009.24.2446.
40. Burris HA, Moore MJ, Andersen J, Green MR, Rothenberg ML, Modiano MR, et al. Improvements in survival and clinical benefit with gemcitabine as first- line therapy for

patients with advanced pancreas cancer: a randomized trial. J Clin Oncol. 1997;15:2403–13. https://doi.org/10.1200/JCO.1997.15.6.2403.
41. Wang-Gillam A, Hubner RA, Siveke JT, Von Hoff DD, Belanger B, de Jong FA, et al. NAPOLI-1 phase 3 study of liposomal irinotecan in metastatic pancreatic cancer: final overall survival analysis and characteristics of long-term survivors. Eur J Cancer. 2019;108:78–87. https://doi.org/10.1016/j.ejca.2018.12.007.
42. Oettle H, Riess H, Stieler JM, Heil G, Schwaner I, Seraphin J, et al. Second-line oxaliplatin, folinic acid, and fluorouracil versus folinic acid and fluorouracil alone for gemcitabine-refractory pancreatic cancer: Outcomes from the CONKO-003 Trial. J Clin Oncol. 2014;32:2423–9. https://doi.org/10.1200/JCO.2013.53.6995.
43. Ngo-Huang A, Holmes HM, des Bordes JKA, Parker NH, Fogelman D, Petzel MQB, et al. Association between frailty syndrome and survival in patients with pancreatic adenocarcinoma. Cancer Med. 2019;8:2867–76. https://doi.org/10.1002/cam4.2157.
44. Corrigan LR, Bracken-Clarke DM, Horgan AM. The challenge of treating older patients with pancreaticobiliary malignancies. Curr Probl Cancer. 2018;42:59–72. https://doi.org/10.1016/j.currproblcancer.2018.01.015.
45. Bartsch F, Baumgart J, Tripke V, Hoppe-Lotichius M, Heinrich S, Lang H. Resection of intrahepatic cholangiocarcinoma in elderly patients – Is it reasonable? BMC Surg. 2019;19:157. https://doi.org/10.1186/s12893-019-0620-7.
46. Horgan AM, Knox JJ, Aneja P, Le LW, McKeever L, McNamara MG. Patterns of care and treatment outcomes in older patients with biliary tract cancer. Oncotarget. 2015;6:44995–5004. https://doi.org/10.18632/oncotarget.5707.
47. Primrose JN, Fox RP, Palmer DH, Malik HZ, Prasad R, Mirza D, et al. Capecitabine compared with observation in resected biliary tract cancer (BILCAP): a randomised, controlled, multicentre, phase 3 study. Lancet Oncol. 2019;20:663–73. https://doi.org/10.1016/S1470-2045(18)30915-X.
48. Valle J, Wasan H, Palmer DH, Cunningham D, Anthoney A, Maraveyas A, et al. Cisplatin plus gemcitabine versus gemcitabine for biliary tract cancer for the ABC-02 trial investigators*. N Engl J Med. 2010;14:1273–81. https://doi.org/10.1056/NEJMoa0908721.
49. Mcnamara MG, Bridgewater J, Lopes A, Wasan H, Malka D, Jensen LH, et al. Systemic therapy in younger and elderly patients with advanced biliary cancer: sub-analysis of ABC-02 and twelve other prospective trials. BMC Cancer. 2017;17:262. https://doi.org/10.1186/s12885-017-3266-9.
50. Valle J, Furuse J, Jitlal M, Beare S, Mizuno N, Wasan H, et al. Cisplatin and gemcitabine for advanced biliary tract cancer: a meta-analysis of two randomised trials. Ann Oncol. 2014;25(2):391–8. https://doi.org/10.1093/annonc/mdt540.
51. Lamarca A, Palmer DH, Wasan HS, Ross PJ, Ma YT, Arora A, et al. ABC-06 | A randomised phase III, multi-centre, open-label study of active symptom control (ASC) alone or ASC with oxaliplatin / 5-FU chemotherapy (ASC+mFOLFOX) for patients (pts) with locally advanced / metastatic biliary tract cancers (ABC) previously-treated with cisplatin/gemcitabine (CisGem) chemotherapy. J Clin Oncol. 2019;37:4003. https://doi.org/10.1200/jco.2019.37.15_suppl.4003.
52. Walter T, Horgan AM, McNamara M, McKeever L, Min T, Hedley D, et al. Feasibility and benefits of second-line chemotherapy in advanced biliary tract cancer: a large retrospective study. Eur J Cancer. 2013;49:329–35. https://doi.org/10.1016/j.ejca.2012.08.003.
53. Llovet JM, Brú C, Bruix J. Prognosis of hepatocellular carcinoma: the BCLC staging classification. Semin Liver Dis. 1999;19:329–37. https://doi.org/10.1055/s-2007-1007122.
54. Villanueva A. Hepatocellular carcinoma. N Engl J Med. 2019;380:1450–62. https://doi.org/10.1056/NEJMra1713263.
55. Mazzaferro V, Regalia E, Doci R, Andreola S, Pulvirenti A, Bozzetti F, et al. Liver transplantation for the treatment of small hepatocellular carcinomas in patients with cirrhosis. N Engl J Med. 1996;334:693–700. https://doi.org/10.1056/NEJM199603143341104.
56. Durand F, Levitsky J, Cauchy F, Gilgenkrantz H, Soubrane O, Francoz C. Age and liver transplantation. J Hepatol. 2019;70:745–58. https://doi.org/10.1016/j.jhep.2018.12.009.

57. Lai JC, Feng S, Terrault NA, Lizaola B, Hayssen H, Covinsky K. Frailty predicts waitlist mortality in liver transplant candidates. Am J Transplant. 2014;14:1870–9. https://doi.org/10.1111/ajt.12762.
58. Su F, Yu L, Berry K, Liou IW, Landis CS, Rayhill SC, et al. Aging of liver transplant registrants and recipients: trends and impact on waitlist outcomes, post-transplantation outcomes, and transplant-related survival benefit. Gastroenterology. 2016;150:441–453.e6. https://doi.org/10.1053/j.gastro.2015.10.043.
59. Dolnikov S, Adam R, Cherqui D, Allard MA. Liver transplantation in elderly patients: what do we know at the beginning of 2020? Surg Today. 2020;50:533–9. https://doi.org/10.1007/s00595-020-01996-7.
60. Brunot A, Le Sourd S, Pracht M, Edeline J. Hepatocellular carcinoma in elderly patients: challenges and solutions. J Hepatocell Carcinoma. 2016;3:9. https://doi.org/10.2147/jhc.s101448.
61. Shapey IM, Malik HZ, de Liguori CN. Data driven decision-making for older patients with hepatocellular carcinoma. Eur J Surg Oncol. 2020;47(3 Pt A):576–82. https://doi.org/10.1016/j.ejso.2020.05.023.
62. Yamada S, Shimada M, Morine Y, Imura S, Ikemoto T, Arakawa Y, et al. Significance of frailty in prognosis after hepatectomy for elderly patients with hepatocellular carcinoma. Ann Surg Oncol. 2020;28(1):439–46. https://doi.org/10.1245/s10434-020-08742-w.
63. Huang J, Yan L, Cheng Z, Wu H, Du L, Wang J, et al. A randomized trial comparing radiofrequency ablation and surgical resection for HCC conforming to the Milan criteria. Ann Surg. 2010;252:903–12. https://doi.org/10.1097/SLA.0b013e3181efc656.
64. Li L, Zhang J, Liu X, Li X, Jiao B, Kang T. Clinical outcomes of radiofrequency ablation and surgical resection for small hepatocellular carcinoma: a meta-analysis. J Gastroenterol Hepatol. 2012;27:51–8. https://doi.org/10.1111/j.1440-1746.2011.06947.x.
65. Takahashi H, Mizuta T, Kawazoe S, Eguchi Y, Kawaguchi Y, Otuka T, et al. Efficacy and safety of radiofrequency ablation for elderly hepatocellular carcinoma patients. Hepatol Res. 2010;40:997–1005. https://doi.org/10.1111/j.1872-034X.2010.00713.x.
66. Mirici-Cappa F, Gramenzi A, Santi V, Zambruni A, Di MA, Frigerio M, et al. Treatments for hepatocellular carcinoma in elderly patients are as effective as in younger patients: a 20-year multicentre experience. Gut. 2010;59:387–96. https://doi.org/10.1136/gut.2009.194217.
67. Gardini AC, Marisi G, Canale M, Foschi FG, Donati G, Ercolani G, et al. Radiofrequency ablation of hepatocellular carcinoma: a meta-analysis of overall survival and recurrence-free survival. Onco Targets Ther. 2018;11:6555–67. https://doi.org/10.2147/OTT.S170836.
68. Llovet JM, Bruix J. Systematic review of randomized trials for unresectable hepatocellular carcinoma: Chemoembolization improves survival. Hepatology. 2003;37:429–42. https://doi.org/10.1053/jhep.2003.50047.
69. Hilgard P, Hamami M, El FA, Scherag A, MüLler S, Ertle J, et al. Radioembolization with yttrium-90 glass microspheres in hepatocellular carcinoma: European experience on safety and long-term survival. Hepatology. 2010;52:1741–9. https://doi.org/10.1002/hep.23944.
70. Heimbach JK, Kulik LM, Finn RS, Sirlin CB, Abecassis MM, Roberts LR, et al. AASLD guidelines for the treatment of hepatocellular carcinoma. Hepatology. 2018;67:358–80. https://doi.org/10.1002/hep.29086.
71. Casadei Gardini A, Tamburini E, Iñarrairaegui M, Frassineti GL, Sangro B. Radioembolization versus chemoembolization for unresectable hepatocellular carcinoma: a meta-analysis of randomized trials. Onco Targets Ther. 2018;11:7315–21. https://doi.org/10.2147/OTT.S175715.
72. Meyer C, Christian Pieper C, Matuschek ME, Adrian Maschke T, Enkirch J, Essler M, et al. Yttrium-90 radioembolization of unresectable hepatocellular carcinoma-a single center experience. Onco Targets Ther. 2017;10:4773–85. https://doi.org/10.2147/OTT.S137519.
73. Ni JY, Liu SS, Xu LF, Sun HL, Chen YT. Meta-analysis of radiofrequency ablation in combination with transarterial chemoembolization for hepatocellular carcinoma. World J Gastroenterol. 2013;19:3872–82. https://doi.org/10.3748/wjg.v19.i24.3872.
74. Llovet JM, Ricci S, Mazzaferro V, Hilgard P, Gane E, Blanc J-F, et al. Sorafenib in advanced hepatocellular carcinoma. N Engl J Med. 2008;359:378–90. https://doi.org/10.1056/NEJMoa0708857.

75. Cheng AL, Kang YK, Chen Z, Tsao CJ, Qin S, Kim JS, et al. Efficacy and safety of sorafenib in patients in the Asia-Pacific region with advanced hepatocellular carcinoma: a phase III randomised, double-blind, placebo-controlled trial. Lancet Oncol. 2009;10:25–34. https://doi.org/10.1016/S1470-2045(08)70285-7.
76. McNamara MG, Slagter AE, Nuttall C, Frizziero M, Pihlak R, Lamarca A, et al. Sorafenib as first-line therapy in patients with advanced Child-Pugh B hepatocellular carcinomada meta-analysis. Eur J Cancer. 2018;105:1–9. https://doi.org/10.1016/j.ejca.2018.09.031.
77. Lionakis N, Mendrinos D, Sanidas E, Favatas G, Georgopoulou M, Figueroa X. Hypertension in the elderly. World J Cardiol. 2012;4:135–47. https://doi.org/10.4330/wjc.v4.i5.135.
78. Reiss KA, Yu S, Mamtani R, Mehta R, D'Addeo K, Wileyto EP, et al. Starting dose of sorafenib for the treatment of hepatocellular carcinoma: a retrospective, multi-institutional study. J Clin Oncol. 2017;35:3575–81. https://doi.org/10.1200/JCO.2017.73.8245.
79. Kudo M, Finn RS, Qin S, Han KH, Ikeda K, Piscaglia F, et al. Lenvatinib versus sorafenib in first-line treatment of patients with unresectable hepatocellular carcinoma: a randomised phase 3 non-inferiority trial. Lancet. 2018;391:1163–73. https://doi.org/10.1016/S0140-6736(18)30207-1.
80. Facciorusso A, Abd El Aziz MA, Sacco R. Efficacy of regorafenib in hepatocellular carcinoma patients: a systematic review and meta-analysis. Cancers (Basel). 2019;12:36. https://doi.org/10.3390/cancers12010036.
81. Zhu AX, Kang YK, Yen CJ, Finn RS, Galle PR, Llovet JM, et al. Ramucirumab after sorafenib in patients with advanced hepatocellular carcinoma and increased α-fetoprotein concentrations (REACH-2): a randomised, double-blind, placebo-controlled, phase 3 trial. Lancet Oncol. 2019;20:282–96. https://doi.org/10.1016/S1470-2045(18)30937-9.
82. Abou-Alfa GK, Meyer T, Cheng A-L, El-Khoueiry AB, Rimassa L, Ryoo B-Y, et al. Cabozantinib in patients with advanced and progressing hepatocellular carcinoma. N Engl J Med. 2018;379:54–63. https://doi.org/10.1056/NEJMoa1717002.
83. Kapacee ZA, McNamara MG, de Liguori CN, Lamarca A, Valle JW, Hubner RA. Systemic therapies in advanced hepatocellular carcinoma: how do older patients fare? Eur J Surg Oncol. 2020; https://doi.org/10.1016/j.ejso.2020.03.210.
84. Finn RS, Qin S, Ikeda M, Galle PR, Ducreux M, Kim TY, et al. Atezolizumab plus Bevacizumab in Unresectable Hepatocellular Carcinoma. N Engl J Med. 2020;382:1894–905. https://doi.org/10.1056/NEJMoa1915745.
85. Garcia G, Odaimi M. Systemic combination chemotherapy in elderly pancreatic cancer: a review. J Gastrointest Cancer. 2017;48:121–8. https://doi.org/10.1007/s12029-017-9930-0.
86. McNamara MG, de Liguori CN, Kapacee ZA, Lamarca A, Valle JW. Outcomes in older patients with biliary tract cancer. Eur J Surg Oncol. 2020;47(3 Pt A):569–75. https://doi.org/10.1016/j.ejso.2020.03.202.
87. Carli F, Baldini G. From preoperative assessment to preoperative optimisation of frail older patients. Eur J Surg Oncol. 2020;47(3 Pt A):519–23. https://doi.org/10.1016/j.ejso.2020.06.011.
88. Zhao W, Liu C, Li S, Geng D, Feng Y, Sun M. Safety and efficacy for robot-assisted versus open pancreaticoduodenectomy and distal pancreatectomy: a systematic review and meta-analysis. Surg Oncol. 2018;27:468–78. https://doi.org/10.1016/j.suronc.2018.06.001.
89. Lim C, Salloum C, Tudisco A, Ricci C, Osseis M, Napoli N, et al. Short- and long-term outcomes after robotic and laparoscopic liver resection for malignancies: a propensity score-matched study. World J Surg. 2019;43:1594–603. https://doi.org/10.1007/s00268-019-04927-x.
90. Betge J, Chi-Kern J, Schulte N, Belle S, Gutting T, Burgermeister E, et al. A multicenter phase 4 geriatric assessment directed trial to evaluate gemcitabine +/− nab-paclitaxel in elderly pancreatic cancer patients (GrantPax). BMC Cancer. 2018;18:747. https://doi.org/10.1186/s12885-018-4665-2.
91. Hurria A, Levit LA, Dale W, Mohile SG, Muss HB, Fehrenbacher L, et al. Improving the evidence base for treating older adults with cancer: American Society of Clinical Oncology statement. J Clin Oncol. 2015;33:3826–33. https://doi.org/10.1200/JCO.2015.63.0319.
92. Hurria A. Clinical trials in older adults with cancer: Past and future. Oncology. 2007;21:351–8.

93. Golan T, Hammel P, Reni M, Van Cutsem E, Macarulla T, Hall MJ, et al. Maintenance Olaparib for Germline BRCA-Mutated Metastatic Pancreatic Cancer. N Engl J Med. 2019;381:317–27. https://doi.org/10.1056/NEJMoa1903387.
94. Abou-Alfa GK, Macarulla T, Javle MM, Kelley RK, Lubner SJ, Adeva J, et al. Ivosidenib in IDH1-mutant, chemotherapy-refractory cholangiocarcinoma (ClarIDHy): a multicentre, randomised, double-blind, placebo-controlled, phase 3 study. Lancet Oncol. 2020;21:796–807. https://doi.org/10.1016/S1470-2045(20)30157-1.
95. Lamarca A, Barriuso J, McNamara MG, Valle JW. Molecular targeted therapies: Ready for "prime time" in biliary tract cancer. J Hepatol. 2020;73:170–85. https://doi.org/10.1016/j.jhep.2020.03.007.
96. Oh D-Y, Lee K-H, Lee D-W, Kim TY, Bang J-H, Nam A-R, et al. Phase II study assessing tolerability, efficacy, and biomarkers for durvalumab (D) ± tremelimumab (T) and gemcitabine/cisplatin (GemCis) in chemo-naïve advanced biliary tract cancer (aBTC). J Clin Oncol. 2020;38:4520. https://doi.org/10.1200/jco.2020.38.15_suppl.4520.

Chapter 25
Gynaecological Cancer in Older Adults with Frailty

Christopher Steer, Bridget Josephs, Anthea Cree, and Y. Louise Wan

Introduction

Frailty is best thought of as a syndrome with multiple possible components, rather than a single condition [1]. Whether frailty is defined using the phenotypic model [2] (a collection of key characteristics) or the Rockwood cumulative deficit model [3] (an accumulation of deficits) the findings can be used to predict the vulnerability of the patient to the stressors of the cancer and its treatment. It is important to note that frailty can vary in severity, is not static (can change over time) and is not an inevitable part of ageing [3]. The adequate assessment of older adults with cancer involves the use of multiple geriatric assessment domains. When a comprehensive geriatric assessment (CGA) is combined with a tailored management plan it remains the gold standard for the diagnosis and treatment of frailty [1].

The prevalence and impact of frailty on patients with gynaecological malignancies varies depending upon the definition used and the population of patients studied. In a population-based-study of women undergoing surgery for ovarian

C. Steer (✉)
Border Medical Oncology, Albury Wodonga Regional Cancer Centre, Albury, Australia

University of NSW, Rural Clinical School, Albury Campus, Albury, NSW, Australia
e-mail: csteer@bordermedonc.com.au

B. Josephs
Border Medical Oncology, Albury Wodonga Regional Cancer Centre, Albury, Australia

A. Cree
Clinical Oncology Department, Clatterbridge Cancer Centre, Liverpool, UK
e-mail: anthea.cree@nhs.net

Y. L. Wan
Division of Cancer Sciences, Faculty of Biology, Medicine and Health, University of Manchester, Manchester, UK
e-mail: Yee-loi.Wan@manchester.ac.uk

F. Gomes (ed.), *Frailty in Older Adults with Cancer*,
https://doi.org/10.1007/978-3-030-89162-6_25

cancer (that used the definition of frailty as a collection of attributes including homelessness and poverty) it was suggested that 30% of the patients aged under 60 years and only 11% of patients aged over 80 years met the frailty criteria [4]. Despite this, the available literature in multiple series of patients with gynaecological cancer suggests that a phenotypic frailty score can predict inability to complete chemotherapy and guide clinician choice of less aggressive treatment [5], that frailty can be measured and predicts outcomes in women with ovarian cancer undergoing surgery [6, 7] and chemotherapy [8].

Whilst multiple retrospective studies of women with gynaecological cancer have outlined the prevalence and impact of frailty, the role of geriatric assessment and guided intervention is being defined in prospective studies of a general population of older adults with cancer [9]. We can infer from these prospective studies that CGA will lead to improvement in discussion about age-related concerns [10], decreased treatment toxicity and improved quality of life [9, 11] without an impact on survival.

This chapter will cover all subsites of gynaecological cancer and provide a review of the evidence available for their management from early to advanced stages. Whilst it is often clear in the clinical setting that patients with severe frailty are best served with supportive and palliative care only, those with mild to moderate frailty may benefit from active anti-cancer treatment.

Ovarian Cancer

Ovarian cancer is the fifth most common cause of cancer death in women and the leading cause of gynaecologic cancer-related deaths in developed countries. Median age at diagnosis in both the United States of America (USA) and United Kingdom (UK) is 63 years, and the majority of cases occur in women in their seventh and eighth decades of life [12, 13]. Despite predominately being a cancer of older women, epidemiological studies show that increasing age in patients with ovarian cancer is associated with delayed diagnoses, potentially adverse tumour biology, less treatment, higher rates of treatment toxicity and poorer survival [14, 15]. In addition, older women are under-represented in clinical trials and there is a paucity of data related to the management of older patients with ovarian cancer, including considerations to frailty, which can make the application of standard treatment challenging.

Investigation of Suspected Ovarian Cancer

Epithelial ovarian cancer accounts for the majority of cases of ovarian cancer (~90%) [16]. For most patients, the diagnosis of ovarian cancer is typically not made until the presence of advanced disease, with the cancer having spread throughout the peritoneal cavity and/or involving lymph nodes. Older patients with frailty may be more likely to present with stage IV disease [14]. In general, patients may present with subacute symptomatology including pelvic or abdominal pain, bloating, early satiety, fatigue, constipation and urinary symptoms. Other patients may present acutely with a malignant bowel obstruction, pleural effusion or venous thromboembolism. Another situation may include the incidental discovery of an adnexal mass on imaging performed for another reason.

Routine work-up of a patient with suspected ovarian cancer should include basic laboratory tests and a baseline CA-125 tumour marker. Imaging studies may include an ultrasound of the abdomen and pelvis to evaluate an adnexal or pelvic mass. Computed tomography of the chest, abdomen and pelvis is performed to assess stage and extent of disease. Tissue is required to obtain a histological diagnosis prior to starting systemic treatment. In the surgically fit patient with disease considered likely to be completely resectable on imaging, this may be acquired at the time of surgical debulking. In those deemed either too frail or to have too extensive disease to benefit from upfront surgery, tissue may be obtained radiologically via a biopsy of an omental cake, nodal mass or occasionally an ovarian mass. Where possible a sample of tissue should also be sent for somatic BRCA testing and blood for germline BRCA testing. Positive cytology from ascitic or peritoneal fluid may be sufficient grounds to start systemic anti-cancer treatment in patients in whom a tissue biopsy has failed to give a definitive result and in whom surgery is not possible [16–18].

In an older patient with severe frailty and with clinical, biochemical and radiological findings suspicious for ovarian cancer, patients and clinicians may opt for best supportive care over invasive investigations.

Management of Ovarian Cancer

Treatment decisions should not be made on the basis of chronological age alone. Treatment should be tailored to the individual taking into account their symptoms, extent of disease, comorbidities, cognition, support system, preferences and life goals. The impact of potential loss of independence and institutionalisation as a consequence of treatment is also an important consideration. Overall, older women with ovarian cancer receive less chemotherapy, are less likely to have surgery with curative intent and are more likely not to be offered treatment altogether [14]. Regardless of age, patients with ovarian cancer who fulfil frailty criteria have a shorter progression free and overall survival [19].

The CGA, the Pre-operative Assessment of Cancer in the Elderly (PACE) and the CARG score for pre-chemotherapy assessment, have all been suggested as useful tools to assess the ovarian cancer patient with respect to frailty and prediction of adverse treatment outcomes [20, 21]. At present, there is only one tool in the literature tailored specifically to ovarian cancer patients. Known as the Geriatric Vulnerability Score (GVS), this score was developed to identify those women with the highest risk of death based on geriatric covariates. It is the sum of five prognostic factors indicative of poorer survival: low serum albumin level (<35 g/L), low activities of daily living (ADL) score (<6), low instrumental ADL score (<25), lymphopenia (<1 g/L) and a high score on the Hospitalised Anxiety and Depression Scale (>14). In their initial prospective study, the authors showed that patients with a GVS of ≥3 had significantly decreased overall survival (11.5 vs 21.7 months; hazard ratio [HR] 2.94), lower rates of chemotherapy completion (62 vs 82%; odds ratio [OR] 2.8, $p = 0.04$), higher incidence of severe adverse events (53 vs 29%; OR 2.8, $p = 0.009$) and higher rates of unplanned hospital admissions (53 vs 30%; 2.6, $p = 0.002$) [22]. This score has been used to select patients considered as vulnerable for inclusion on a randomised trial of chemotherapy and subsequently prospectively validated in this population [23].

Surgery

Standard treatment for advanced epithelial ovarian cancer involves a combination of cytoreductive surgery (CRS) and chemotherapy. Residual tumour remaining after surgery is an important prognostic factor for survival [17, 18].

The aim of surgery performed with curative intent is to resect all visible disease. This will usually entail a salpingo-oophorectomy with hysterectomy and omentectomy as a minimum. Extensive peritonectomies, diaphragmatic stripping, bowel resections and resection of other affected organs, e.g., spleen, liver, bulky lymph nodes, may be required to achieve complete cytoreduction. The latter have the potential to cause significant morbidity [17, 18, 24].

Multiple studies show that older women with advanced ovarian cancer are less likely to undergo surgery, and for those who do have surgery, suboptimal cytoreduction is more common due to receiving less aggressive surgeries [19, 24, 25]. Increasing chronological age is associated with higher incidence of surgical morbidity and mortality as well as higher rates of comorbidities impacting on surgical fitness [6, 24]. However, there is evidence to suggest that, if adequately selected, aggressive optimal cytoreduction is safe and feasible in older patients depending on their degree of frailty [26–28].

For patients deemed unsuitable for primary CRS, an alternative may be neoadjuvant chemotherapy followed by interval CRS. This may be a preferable approach, particularly in patients with frailty and high risk of surgical complications. Compared with primary CRS, neoadjuvant chemotherapy has been shown to be associated with higher rates of optimal cytoreduction, lower perioperative morbidity including less blood transfusions, intensive care unit admissions, reduced length of hospital stay and non-discharge home, e.g. to a rehabilitation centre. Additionally, randomised trials have shown survival outcomes of primary versus interval CRS to be similar [29, 30], although different subgroups may benefit from different approaches [31]. However, in the event of severe frailty, surgery is not an appropriate treatment option.

Chemotherapy

Standard first-line chemotherapy for advanced ovarian cancer involves the combination of 3-weekly carboplatin (AUC 5 or 6) and paclitaxel (175 mg/m^2). It is usually given for 6 cycles following primary cytoreductive surgery, or in the case of neoadjuvant chemotherapy, 3 cycles are given pre-surgery and 3 cycles post [17, 18]. In older patients with frailty in whom risk of falls is of particular concern, single-agent carboplatin may be preferred as this regimen is better tolerated and reduces the risk of peripheral neuropathy, alopecia and fever associated with the addition of paclitaxel. Additionally, the ICON3 study in 2002 concluded that the combination of carboplatin and paclitaxel was not superior to single-agent carboplatin and CAP (cyclophosphamide, doxorubicin, cisplatin) as first-line chemotherapy for ovarian cancer [32]. However, this finding is at odds with multiple other studies demonstrating better outcomes with combination treatment. The recent evidence from the EWOC-1 trial suggest that combination chemotherapy is in fact feasible in patients with frailty.

In this trial, women with a geriatric vulnerability score (GVS) ≥3 aged over 70 years were randomised to either 3-weekly carboplatin and paclitaxel, 3-weekly carboplatin alone or weekly combination therapy. In their preliminary report, the investigators found that the median progression free survival was significantly increased in those receiving 3-weekly combination of carboplatin and paclitaxel compared to single-agent carboplatin (12.5 months versus 4.8 months) [33]. It was, however, underpowered to determine whether weekly or three weekly dosing of carboplatin was superior in terms of tolerability and efficacy.

Whilst not specific to older women, MITO-7 did compare weekly versus 3-weekly carboplatin and paclitaxel in women with stage IC-IV ovarian cancer. No difference in median progression free survival was identified between the two trial arms (18.3 months vs 17.3 months respectively, HR 0.96, $p = 0.06$). The weekly regime however, was associated with better quality of life scores and fewer toxic effects, including reduced incidence of neuropathy and serious haematologic toxicity [34], but did not account for the potential increased burden of attending for weekly chemotherapy. Given this lack of clear evidence, shared decision-making between the clinician and patient may be recommended to consider the merits of one regimen over the other.

In the setting of ovarian cancer recurrence and considering the utility of palliative chemotherapy, it is key to weigh up the quality of life over the risk of treatment toxicity. Treatment for recurrent ovarian cancer is divided into platinum-sensitive and platinum-resistant disease as defined by the platinum free interval; i.e. less than 6 months for platinum-resistant disease and greater than 6 months for platinum-sensitive disease [18].

For patients with platinum-sensitive disease, platinum-based doublet therapy is a standard treatment [17, 18]. However, in older patients with recurrent platinum-sensitive disease, increasing age is associated with poorer survival and reduced response to chemotherapy [35]. If considering further treatment, carboplatin and pegylated liposomal doxorubicin may be an option as demonstrated in the CALYPSO trial in patients aged ≥70, with this combination having lower rates of toxicity including peripheral neuropathy compared with carboplatin + paclitaxel with similar overall survival [36].

For older patients with platinum-resistant disease, chemotherapy is given as a single agent with options including pegylated liposomal doxorubicin, topotecan, gemcitabine, vinorelbine and paclitaxel [17, 18]. However, in the setting of platinum-resistant disease where chemotherapy response rates are low in the order of 10–25% [37], discussion with the patient and their caregivers to explore their preferences, highlighting risks of toxicity and low chance of disease palliation, is very important. Rather than undertaking further chemotherapy, a focus on best supportive care measures may be more appropriate.

Targeted Therapies

Bevacizumab is a monoclonal antibody targeting vascular endothelial growth factor that inhibits tumour angiogenesis. A number of trials have shown the addition of bevacizumab to both first-line chemotherapy followed by bevacizumab maintenance (ION-7, GOG-218) and in recurrent disease (OCEANS, AURELIA) improves progression free survival particularly in patients with poor prognostic features, e.g. stage IV disease and suboptimal debulking [38–41]. Data focusing on the use of bevacizumab in older patients with frailty however is scarce.

The single arm ROSiA study involving 121 patients aged ≥70 years evaluated extended duration bevacizumab for up to 24 months in first-line ovarian cancer treatment. Whilst median progression free survival was similar, compared with younger patients, patients ≥70 years had higher incidences of anaemia, diarrhoea, asthenia, grade ≥ 3 hypertension and thromboembolic events [42]. Another single arm trial, OTILIA, involving 284 patients aged ≥70 years, showed age was not associated with worse outcomes [43]. Authors of both ROSiA and OTILA trials both concluded that bevacizumab is a tolerable first-line treatment that should be considered in patients irrespective of age. Whilst there is limited evidence to guide decisions about the use of bevacizumab in older patients with frailty, the limited additional benefit of this agent should be balanced against the likelihood of toxicity such as hypertension and thromboembolic events.

Poly-ADP-ribose polymerase (PARP) inhibitors are oral agents approved for use as maintenance therapy after platinum-based chemotherapy in the first line and relapsed setting in patients with recurrent ovarian cancer and evidence of a homologous recombination defect, e.g. BRCA mutation [44, 45]. Whilst PARP inhibitors demonstrate improved progression free survival, there is limited evidence of the utility and safety of these agents in older patients with frailty. The SOLO1 trial did include patients up to 84 years of age, however in SOLO2, there were no patients above 63 years of age. Additionally, despite being oral agents, PARP inhibitors are associated with significant toxicity such as nausea and anaemia and should be used with caution in this sub-group of patients.

Radiotherapy

Radiotherapy no longer has a role in adjuvant treatment for patients with ovarian cancer and its use in disseminated disease is limited. However, for patients with symptomatic localised disease, palliative radiotherapy can be helpful [46].

Best Supportive Care and Surveillance

In an older woman with advanced ovarian cancer and significant frailty, following shared decision-making, ideally supported by a CGA, a decision may be done in favour of best supportive care over any anti-cancer treatment. This may happen at any time during the patient cancer journey, including at diagnosis or after a period of treatment. Supportive measures include management of ovarian cancer-related symptoms such as abdominal/pelvic pain, nausea, constipation and breathlessness. For symptomatic ascites or pleural effusions, management can include therapeutic paracentesis or pleurocentesis, respectively. Should a patient be requiring regular drainages, insertion of a pleurX catheter for home based drainages may be considered [16]. Patients may encounter problems with malignant bowel obstructions and in this context measures such as nasogastric tubes may be useful for symptomatic relief. Malignant bowel obstructions are one of the common causes of death in women with relapsed/refractory ovarian cancer.

It is also paramount to link the patient in with the palliative care/hospice team and there is data to suggest that early referral is beneficial [47]. Encouraging end of life discussions and advanced care planning discussion are also important and these are usually associated with less aggressive medical care near death [48].

Lastly, for those patients on surveillance, data from a randomised study showed no survival or quality of life benefit with routine measurement of Ca125 for detecting relapse and starting treatment early based on a rising Ca125 level [49].

Endometrial Cancer

Endometrial cancer is the most common cancer of the female reproductive tract in high income countries. Its incidence increases with age; with the peak incidence in the 65–70 age group. In 2018, the incidence of endometrial cancer was 11.1 per 100,000 women in high income countries; compared to 3.3 per 100,000 in low and middle income countries [50].

Endometrial cancer arises from the endometrial lining of the uterus. The most common form of endometrial cancer, endometrioid endometrial cancer which represents 80% of all endometrial cancers, is hormonally driven. Thus, factors which increase a woman's lifetime exposure to oestrogens are linked to an increased risk of endometrial cancer. Women presenting with endometrial cancer may, therefore, have various other comorbidities and are at higher risk of cardiovascular morbidity [51]. Careful assessment of fitness for treatment is, therefore, needed to guide shared decision-making.

The strongest prognostic factor for survival is stage at diagnosis. Most women will present with early-stage disease that is confined to the uterus. Prognosis for these women is good with five-year survival rates are in the region of 90% in this group [52]. Other prognostic factors include histological type, tumour grade, presence of lymphovascular invasion and molecular subtype.

The role of age as a prognostic factor is controversial. Older women appear to have significantly shorter overall survival, cancer specific survival and recurrence free survival than their younger counterparts [53]. This has been attributed to the higher incidence of unfavourable tumour characteristics in these women, delayed presentation, increasing comorbidities and undertreatment. Treatment of these high-grade cancers will often require a combination of surgery, chemotherapy and radiotherapy to achieve the best chance of cure. Paradoxically, the percentage of older women with high-grade disease receiving these radical treatments is much lower than in their younger counterparts [54]. Frailty has been shown to be predictive of poorer overall and cancer specific survival outcomes, even after accounting for the effect of age, tumour characteristics and comorbidities in endometrial cancer [55].

Investigation of Suspected Endometrial Cancer

Affected women will commonly present with postmenopausal bleeding. Older women tend to be diagnosed at later stages and present as emergencies [53]. This may be because symptoms go unrecognised due to various psychosocial factors associated with increasing frailty or that the prevalence of atypical symptoms in these age groups is higher. Therefore, investigation for endometrial cancer should also be offered to postmenopausal women presenting with new vaginal discharge, vaginal discharge in association with thrombocytosis or haematuria or haematuria in the presence of anaemia, thrombocytosis or diabetes [56].

The first-line investigation for a woman with suspected endometrial cancer is a pelvic ultrasound to determine endometrial thickness. Transvaginal ultrasounds are more informative than transabdominal scans for determining endometrial abnormalities and are well tolerated in postmenopausal women. Transvaginal ultrasound has a positive predictive value of approximately 15% and a negative predictive value of 99.6% when a cut off of 4 mm is used [57]. Symptomatic women with an endometrial thickness of greater than 4 mm should, therefore, be offered further investigations in the form of an endometrial biopsy. However, in an older patient with severe frailty and a suspicion of endometrial cancer, patients and clinicians may opt for best supportive care over invasive investigations.

Management of Endometrial Cancer

Surgical Treatment

The mainstay of treatment of postmenopausal women with endometrial cancer is a hysterectomy and bilateral salpingo-oophorectomy and is often curative in women with early-stage endometrial cancer. Population based studies suggest that there may be an age bias in patient selection; with older women less likely to receive a hysterectomy [58, 59]. Surgical resection, however, is associated with rapid relief of symptomatic bleeding and has been shown to be related to improved survival outcomes in all age groups [59]. It should, therefore, be considered in all women deemed medically fit.

Assessment of lymph nodes is also advocated in women with higher risk disease to determine the need for adjuvant therapies, e.g. non-endometrioid cancers, myoinvasive cancers involving more than half of the myometrium [60]. Meta-analyses have found no evidence that systematic pelvic and para-aortic lymphadenectomy decreases the risk of death or recurrence in women with presumed stage 1 disease [61]. However, lymphadenectomy is associated with a significant increase in surgical morbidity and operative times. Longer operative times have been associated with a higher incidence of post-operative delirium, particularly in patients with cognitive impairment [62]. The increasing use of sentinel node approaches to assess lymph node spread may reduce morbidity and operative times; potentially increasing the proportion of older women considered for nodal assessment.

Minimal access surgery is the standard of care in endometrial cancer and has been shown to have similar oncological outcomes to the open approach [63]. It has the advantage of lower blood loss, shorter inpatient stays, less opioid use and better quality of life postoperatively. However, laparoscopic and robotic approaches require the patient to be positioned in steep Trendelenburg for long periods. This position is associated with an increased risk of blindness in patients with glaucoma [64]. Nonetheless, minimal access surgery is associated with a lower risk of surgical morbidity than the open approach [63]. Both approaches, however, are performed under general anaesthetic which has an inherent associated morbidity in the older patient with frailty. Vaginal hysterectomy may be an alternative for these patients as it can be performed under regional anaesthesia; although it does not routinely allow for salpingo-oophorectomy or nodal resection. Regardless of approach, post-operative morbidity is higher in patients with frailty. Therefore, pre-operative optimisation and individualised post-operative support should be offered to older patients with frailty to optimise outcomes.

Radical surgery is rarely performed in the older patient with frailty and with advanced disease as the risk of morbidity and loss of independent function is exceptionally high when compared to any gain in terms of lifespan. In some centres, neoadjuvant chemotherapy is offered with the aim of reducing the need for bowel, urological or upper-abdominal surgery to achieve clearance; similar to ovarian cancer. The value of surgical cytoreduction in this setting has not been evaluated in this patient group in prospective studies.

Radiotherapy

Radiotherapy has a role in the management of endometrial cancer as adjuvant therapy after hysterectomy, reducing local recurrence in patients with early and more advanced stage disease. However, this has not been shown to translate to an increase in overall survival and comes at the expense of acute and late toxicity [65].

The adoption of three-dimensional radiotherapy planning techniques such as intensity modulated radiotherapy (IMRT) and volumetric modulated arc therapy (VMAT) reduces bladder and bowel toxicity, the incidence of pelvic insufficiency fractures and in some cases the time required to deliver the treatments. These aspects are particularly important in frail patients where there is a higher incidence of incontinence, poor mobility, need for assistance with personal care and in whom longer treatments may be particularly uncomfortable.

In patients with high intermediate risk disease, brachytherapy (internal radiotherapy treatment) plays an important role. It has been shown to be as effective as external beam radiotherapy at reducing vaginal vault recurrence, the most common site of relapse, but with fewer side effects [66]. It is a quick treatment, usually taking around 10 mins on 4 occasions over a fortnight and does not require a general anaesthetic. It is well tolerated even in less fit patients, although may be difficult to administer in patients with cognitive impairment. It could be considered in high-risk patients who do not want to undergo external beam radiotherapy although is likely to be associated with an increased risk of pelvic nodal recurrence.

In patients with local recurrence, who have not received adjuvant external beam radiotherapy, a combination of brachytherapy and external beam radiotherapy can be curative. In patients with vaginal only relapse, treated with salvage radiotherapy, a five-year overall survival of greater than 50% has been reported [67].

Primary radiotherapy may be considered as a palliative treatment in patients considered unfit for surgery and may lead to long-term control, especially in early-stage disease [68].

Systemic Therapy

In endometrial cancer, adjuvant chemotherapy is now offered to those at the highest risk of distant recurrence. Meta-analyses show that post-operative platinum-based chemotherapy is associated with better recurrence free survival and overall survival irrespective of radiation treatment in patients with both locally advanced disease (stage 3) and in select patients with early-stage high-risk endometrial cancer (e.g. serous endometrial cancer) [69]. However, in these trials, there were more pelvic recurrences in patients treated with chemotherapy alone. Multi-modal therapies may, therefore, be associated with the best chance of cure. PORTEC-3 trial demonstrated that women with Stage 3 and serous cancers had better survival outcomes when radiotherapy was combined with chemotherapy compared to radiotherapy alone [70]. However, this was associated with a worse toxicity profile, with increased rates of long-term peripheral neuropathy.

Carboplatin and paclitaxel doublet chemotherapy may be considered in patients with surgically unresectable disease. The majority of these patients will have a high symptom burden and often are also frail. Adequate assessment of frailty to determine suitability for treatment, predict toxicities and to guide treatment decisions is, therefore, crucial as determining the most effective regimen that minimises toxicity is challenging. Previous studies have not studied the tolerability of different chemotherapy regimens in older and/or frail patients with endometrial cancer and therefore data is often extrapolated from women with ovarian cancer. This has its limitations as the typical disease course in these two cancers is inherently different.

Unlike in ovarian cancer, there are limited treatment choices in women presenting with recurrent metastatic endometrial cancer. Rechallenge with platinum and taxane regimens may produce a response in those women who have had an initial complete response to chemotherapy. For women with localised recurrences following radiotherapy, pelvic exenteration may be considered. However, given the high rate of associated morbidity and relatively low 5-year survival rates, this is rarely performed in older patients with frailty.

Best Supportive Care and Surveillance

Patients with severe frailty and unfit for standard surgical, systemic or radiation therapies may be offered hormonal therapies to manage bleeding symptoms. These usually consist of oral or intrauterine progestogens. Modest response rates of between 10–25% have been reported [71]. Ultimately the focus is on best supportive care.

For those on surveillance, a holistic approach should be used when considering the optimum follow-up schedule and an individual's needs. There should also be a focus on modifying risk factors for cardiovascular disease and metabolic syndrome as recurrence and treatment related side effects are less common after surgery. In these women, having patient initiated follow-up, group education sessions and general practitioner led risk factor monitoring is likely to be sufficient [72].

Cervical, Vaginal and Vulvar Cancer

The majority of cervical and vaginal cancers and vulvar cancers are related to high-risk human papilloma virus (HPV) infection, particularly HPV 16 and HPV 18. Squamous cell carcinoma is the most common histology followed by adenocarcinoma, other rarer histologies include melanoma, basal cell carcinoma and sarcoma [73]. 85% of cases of cervical cancer occur in patients from low and middle income countries, with over 500,000 women diagnosed in 2012 [74]. These countries will also see the largest rise in the proportion of the population over the age of 60 years and therefore must be central in any strategies developed to treat older patients.

In high income countries, they are rare cancers, with around 3000 patients diagnosed with cervical cancer, 1400 with vulvar cancer and 250 with vaginal cancer every year in the UK. The highest rates of cervical cancer are in younger patients with only 9% of cases occurring in those over the age of 75 years. However, older patients may present with higher stage disease [75]. Current guidance suggests discontinuing cervical screening at 65 years in patients without abnormal smears but this is somewhat controversial [76]. Inevitably, stopping screening in older patients means that cervical cancers in older women are only diagnosed once they become symptomatic which is typically at later stages [77]. Vulvar cancer is more common in older women with 44% of patients in the UK aged over 75 at diagnosis. In contrast to cervical cancer, rates of disease are increasing [78]. Women with HPV related cervical cancer are at increased risk of other HPV related cancers later in life, e.g. vulvar cancer or vaginal cancer [79]. This can complicate treatment as previous treatments can limit therapeutic options, especially in the case of radiotherapy.

Investigation of Suspected Cervical, Vulvar and Vaginal Cancer

The presentation of cervical, vulvar and vaginal cancers may be delayed in older patients, especially those with cognitive impairment. Patients who present with symptomatic vulval lesions have a relatively high risk of malignancy [80]. Clinical examination is extremely important in diagnosis, with direct visualisation required. Biopsies can generally be taken under local anaesthesia but examination under anaesthetic may be required if there are concerns regarding disease extent or patient tolerance. MRI is recommended to assess local disease extent; however, frail patients may struggle to tolerate this. CT or PET-CT is recommended to exclude metastatic disease [75]. It is important to consider if suitable treatment options are available according to patient's frailty as well as patient preference prior to investigation.

Management of Cervical, Vulvar and Vulvar Cancer

Surgery

There is some evidence that older patients are not offered appropriate surgery management. However, in patients with frailty it may be appropriate to perform less radical surgery, acknowledging a higher risk of relapse. It is also important to consider the potential need for adjuvant treatment, prior to surgery as tri-modality treatment is associated with increased mortality and may be avoided by non-surgical treatment.

In patients with micro invasive cervical cancer, which is usually discovered at screening and less commonly seen in older women, localised excisional techniques such as large loop excisions of the transition zone or cone biopsies can be performed under local or regional anaesthetic. For cervical lesions less than 2 cm (stage 1B1) disease, radical hysterectomy, to excise the uterus, cervix and surrounding parametria with lymph node surgery is recommended but simple hysterectomy can be considered for low risk disease. The decision regarding whether to offer open or minimal access surgery to women with early-stage cervical cancer has been further complicated by the results of the LACC trial [81]. This trial was the first to demonstrate that patients undergoing minimal access radical hysterectomy were more likely to suffer recurrence than those having open procedures and has led to the move away from minimal access surgery in this setting. However, this is likely to come at the cost of increased perioperative morbidity, especially in frail patients. For patients with IB3 to IIA2 disease, the evidence comparing surgery and definitive chemotherapy radiotherapy is weak [82]. A meta-analyses of retrospective data suggested survival outcomes are better in patients who received surgery followed by adjuvant therapy but this is at the expense of worse genitourinary toxicities [83]. Without randomised evidence, the true benefits are unclear and definitive radiotherapy (with concurrent chemotherapy if possible) is often more appropriate for frail patients.

Surgery is the main treatment for patients with vulvar cancer. Surgical practice has evolved to support less radical resections, including wide local excision, which reduces morbidity. In patients with greater than Stage 1b1 (i.e. a lesion greater than 2 cm or invades by greater than 1 mm), inguinofemoral node surgery should be considered. To reduce morbidity, sentinel node biopsy can be performed in women with a lesion less than 4 cm and full groin node dissection or radiotherapy can be safely avoided in those with no evidence of nodal metastasis [84]. In stage 4 disease, which involves the anus or urethra, neoadjuvant chemotherapy or radiotherapy maybe used to avoid exenterative surgery [85].

Surgery can also be used for early vaginal cancer but it can be difficult to obtain clear margins and adjuvant therapy is often required [86].

Palliative surgery is an option in symptomatic older patients with frailty in whom a curative approach is not an option.

Radiotherapy

The standard of care for locally advanced cervical cancer is external beam radiotherapy with concurrent cisplatin chemotherapy followed by image guided brachytherapy [87]. The additional overall survival benefit of chemotherapy is approximately 6% [88], and as it increases the risk of both long- and short-term toxicity, omission may be considered in older patients with frailty. There are a number of case series of selected older patients with cervical cancer, showing excellent compliance with external beam radiotherapy treatment, which is delivered 5 days a week for 5 weeks [89, 90]. Side effects have been discussed in the endometrial cancer section.

Brachytherapy is used to deliver a boost to the tumour whilst minimising doses to organs at risk and is superior to a boost delivered with external beam radiotherapy [91]. It is generally performed under general anaesthetic, but regional anaesthetic can also be used in unfit patients. It is tolerated by the majority of patients but the applicator remains in place for a number of hours and it may not be suitable for patients with severe cognitive impairment.

The evidence from cervical cancer is extrapolated to the treatment of vulval or vaginal cancer, with the use of concurrent chemoradiotherapy. In some cases brachytherapy is possible, if not an external beam boost can be used.

Both external beam radiotherapy and brachytherapy can be used in the palliative setting and are particularly effective in controlling bleeding [92].

Systemic Therapy

There is limited evidence to support neoadjuvant chemotherapy for vulvar or cervical cancer, although sometimes it is considered to downstage disease prior to radiotherapy or surgery.

In patients with cervical cancer, the recommended first-line palliative treatment regimen is a platinum agent, paclitaxel and bevacizumab [93]. There is minimal evidence to guide treatment choice in vulvar cancer or vaginal cancer. In frail patients, a single agent could be used. The risk and benefits of chemotherapy should be considered carefully as side effects are similar to patients treated for ovarian cancer but response rates may be lower. There is no gold standard second line treatment option.

Best Supportive Care and Surveillance

Many older patients, particularly with severe frailty may not be eligible for optimum treatments. Patients with cervical, vulval and vaginal cancer may experience significant pain as well as other problems including discharge, lymphedema, urinary or faecal incontinence and fistulae. Management of fungating vulvar lesions can be particularly difficult. Therefore, the supportive of a multidisciplinary team is key. There is also growing interest in the use of electro chemotherapy to treat inoperable or recurrent vulvar tumours, but it is not widely available.

Most relapses in patients with squamous cell carcinoma happen within the first 2 years, however late relapse or second primary malignancy can occur and close clinical follow-up is recommended. There is no standardised imaging follow-up protocol but MR assessment at 3 months is often performed. In patients with vulvar and vaginal cancer, clinical examination is very important to identify local recurrence.

Late toxicity including bladder, bowel, pelvic and sexual dysfunction is relatively common [94] and if not manageable with simple interventions specialist support should be considered. Low-grade side effects may have a significant impact on frail patient's quality of life, for example, bowel or urinary urgency leading to incontinence in patients with poor mobility. Care must also be taken if pharmacological interventions are used, for example, to treat urinary incontinence as they may not be tolerated [95]. A holistic approach with support from a geriatrician and allied health professionals can maximise quality of life following treatment.

Conclusion

Increasing numbers of older patients are diagnosed with gynaecological malignancies. Although the order and importance of different treatment modalities vary between different subsites, the principles of treatment are the same. The management of the older patient with frailty is challenging and a genuinely patient centred care must be supported by a CGA, considering the wishes of the patient as well as the details of the cancer. Further research is required on the optimal management of these patients, not only focussed on anti-cancer treatment but also on improving supportive care.

References

1. Wyrko Z. Frailty at the front door. Clin Med J R Coll Physicians London. 2015; https //doi.org/10.7861/clinmedicine.15-4-377.
2. Fried LP, Tangen CM, Walston J, et al. Frailty in older adults: evidence for a phenotype. Journals Gerontol - Ser A Biol Sci Med Sci. 2001; https://doi.org/10.1093/gerona/56.3.m146.
3. Rockwood K, Fox RA, Stolee P, Robertson D, Beattie BL. Frailty in elderly people: an evolving concept. CMAJ. 1994;150(4):489–95.
4. Sia TY, Wen T, Cham S, Friedman AM, Wright JD. Effect of frailty on postoperative readmissions and cost of care for ovarian cancer. Gynecol Oncol. 2020; https://doi.org/10.1016/j.ygyno.2020.08.024.
5. Hay CM, Donovan HS, Campbell GB, Taylor SE, Wang L, Courtney-Brooks M. Chemotherapy in older adult gynecologic oncology patients: can a phenotypic frailty score predict tolerance? Gynecol Oncol. 2019; https://doi.org/10.1016/j.ygyno.2018.11.031.
6. Kumar A, Langstraat CL, DeJong SR, McGree ME, Bakkum-Gamez JN, Weaver AL, LeBrasseur NK, Cliby WA. Functional not chronologic age: frailty index predicts outcomes in advanced ovarian cancer. Gynecol Oncol. 2017; https://doi.org/10.1016/j.ygyno.2017.07.126.
7. Yao TT, DeJong SR, McGree ME, Weaver AL, Cliby WA, Kumar A. Frailty in ovarian cancer identified the need for increased postoperative care requirements following cytoreductive surgery. Gynecol Oncol. 2019; https://doi.org/10.1016/j.ygyno.2018.12.025.
8. Narasimhulu DM, McGree ME, Weaver AL, Jatoi A, LeBrasseur NK, Glaser GE, Langstraat CL, Block MS, Kumar A. Frailty is a determinant of suboptimal chemotherapy in women with advanced ovarian cancer. Gynecol Oncol. 2020;158:646–52.

9. Soto-Perez-de-Celis E, Aapro M, Muss H. ASCO 2020: the geriatric assessment comes of age. Oncologist. JAMA 2018;319(18):1901–913. https://doi.org/10.1634/theoncologist.2020-0804.
10. Mohile SG, Epstein RM, Hurria A, et al. Communication with older patients with cancer using geriatric assessment: a cluster-randomized clinical trial from the National Cancer Institute Community oncology research program. JAMA Oncol. 2020; https://doi.org/10.1001/jamaoncol.2019.4728.
11. Soo W-K, King M, Pope A, Parente P, Darzins P, Davis ID. Integrated geriatric assessment and treatment (INTEGERATE) in older people with cancer planned for systemic anticancer therapy. J Clin Oncol. 2020; https://doi.org/10.1200/jco.2020.38.15_suppl.12011.
12. Ovarian Cancer — Cancer Stat Facts.
13. Ovarian cancer incidence statistics | Cancer Research UK.
14. Fourcadier E, Trétarre B, Gras-Aygon C, Ecarnot F, Daurès JP, Bessaoud F. Under-treatment of elderly patients with ovarian cancer: a population based study. BMC Cancer. 2015; https://doi.org/10.1186/s12885-015-1947-9.
15. Tortorella L, Vizzielli G, Fusco D, Cho WC, Bernabei R, Scambia G, Colloca G. Ovarian cancer management in the oldest old: improving outcomes and tailoring treatments. Aging Dis. 2017; https://doi.org/10.14336/AD.2017.0607.
16. Lheureux S, Gourley C, Vergote I, Oza AM. Epithelial ovarian cancer. Lancet. 2019; https://doi.org/10.1016/S0140-6736(18)32552-2.
17. National Comprehensive Cancer Network (2020) NCCN Clinical Practice Guidelines in Oncology: Ovarian cancer including fallopian tube and primary peritoneal cancer.
18. Ledermann JA, Raja FA, Fotopoulou C, Gonzalez-Martin A, Colombo N, Sessa C. Newly diagnosed and relapsed epithelial ovarian carcinoma: ESMO clinical practice guidelines for diagnosis, treatment and follow-up. Ann Oncol. 2013; https://doi.org/10.1093/annonc/mdt333.
19. Narasimhulu DM, McGree ME, Weaver AL, Jatoi A, LeBrasseur NK, Glaser GE, Langstraat CL, Block MS, Kumar A. Frailty is a determinant of suboptimal chemotherapy in women with advanced ovarian cancer. Gynecol Oncol. 2020; https://doi.org/10.1016/j.ygyno.2020.05.046.
20. Walter LC, Chair V, Baumgartner J, et al (2020) Continue NCCN Guidelines version 1.2020 older adult oncology.
21. Wildiers H, Heeren P, Puts M, et al. International society of geriatric oncology consensus on geriatric assessment in older patients with cancer. J Clin Oncol. 2014; https://doi.org/10.1200/JCO.2013.54.8347.
22. Falandry C, Weber B, Savoye AM, et al. Development of a geriatric vulnerability score in elderly patients with advanced ovarian cancer treated with first-line carboplatin: a GINECO prospective trial. Ann Oncol. 2013; https://doi.org/10.1093/annonc/mdt360.
23. Tinquaut F, Freyer G, Pommeret F, et al. Validation of the geriatric vulnerability score (GVS) in older ovarian cancer (oOC) patients: an analysis from the GCIG-ENGOT-GINECO EWOC-1 study. Ann Oncol. 2019; https://doi.org/10.1093/annonc/mdz250.005.
24. Joueidi Y, Dion L, Bendifallah S, et al. Management and survival of elderly and very elderly patients with ovarian cancer: an age-stratified study of 1123 women from the FRANCOGYN group. J Clin Med. 2020;9:1451.
25. Cloven NG, Manetta A, Berman ML, Kohler MF, DiSaia PJ. Management of ovarian cancer in patients older than 80 years of age. Gynecol Oncol. 1999; https://doi.org/10.1006/gyno.1998.5337.
26. Wright JD, Herzog TJ, Powell MA. Morbidity of cytoreductive surgery in the elderly. Am J Obstet Gynecol. 2004; https://doi.org/10.1016/j.ajog.2004.01.078.
27. Fanfani F, Fagotti A, Salerno MG, Margariti PA, Gagliardi ML, Gallotta V, Vizzielli G, Panico G, Monterossi G, Scambia G. Elderly and very elderly advanced ovarian cancer patients: does the age influence the surgical management? Eur J Surg Oncol. 2012; https://doi.org/10.1016/j.ejso.2012.08.003.
28. Filippova OT, Chi DS, Long Roche K, et al. Geriatric co-management leads to safely performed cytoreductive surgery in older women with advanced stage ovarian cancer treated at a tertiary care cancer center. Gynecol Oncol. 2019; https://doi.org/10.1016/j.ygyno.2019.04.683.

29. Vergote I, Tropé CG, Amant F, et al. Neoadjuvant chemotherapy or primary surgery in stage IIIC or IV ovarian cancer. N Engl J Med. 2010; https://doi.org/10.1056/NEJMoa0908806.
30. Kehoe S, Hook J, Nankivell M, et al. Primary chemotherapy versus primary surgery for newly diagnosed advanced ovarian cancer (CHORUS): an open-label, randomised, controlled, non-inferiority trial. Lancet. 2015; https://doi.org/10.1016/S0140-6736(14)62223-6.
31. Onda T, Satoh T, et al. Comparison of survival between upfront primary debulking surgery versus neoadjuvant chemotherapy for stage III/IV ovarian, tubal and peritoneal cancers in phase III randomized trial: JCOG0602. J Clin Oncol. 2018; https://doi.org/10.1200/jco.2018.36.15_suppl.5500.
32. Parmar MKB, Adams M, Balestrino M, et al. Paclitaxel plus carboplatin versus standard chemotherapy with either single-agent carboplatin or cyclophosphamide, doxorubicin, and cisplatin in women with ovarian cancer: the ICON3 randomised trial. Lancet. 2002; https://doi.org/10.1016/S0140-6736(02)09738-6.
33. Falandry C, Savoye AM, Stefani L, et al. EWOC-1: a randomized trial to evaluate the feasibility of three different first-line chemotherapy regimens for vulnerable elderly women with ovarian cancer (OC): a GCIG-ENGOT-GINECO study. J Clin Oncol. 2019;37:5508.
34. Pignata S, Scambia G, Katsaros D, et al. Carboplatin plus paclitaxel once a week versus every 3 weeks in patients with advanced ovarian cancer (MITO-7): a randomised, multicentre, open-label, phase 3 trial. Lancet Oncol. 2014; https://doi.org/10.1016/S1470-2045(14)70049-X.
35. Pignata S, Ferrandina G, Scarfone G, et al. Poor outcome of elderly patients with platinum-sensitive recurrent ovarian cancer: results from the SOCRATES retrospective study. Crit Rev Oncol Hematol. 2009; https://doi.org/10.1016/j.critrevonc.2008.12.010.
36. Wagner U, Marth C, Largillier R, et al. Final overall survival results of phase III GCIG CALYPSO trial of pegylated liposomal doxorubicin and carboplatin vs paclitaxel and carboplatin in platinum-sensitive ovarian cancer patients. Br J Cancer. 2012; https://doi.org/10.1038/bjc.2012.307.
37. Tew WP, Lichtman SM. Ovarian cancer in older women. Semin Oncol. 2008; https://doi.org/10.1053/j.seminoncol.2008.08.007.
38. Burger RA, Brady MF, Bookman MA, et al. Incorporation of bevacizumab in the primary treatment of ovarian cancer. N Engl J Med. 2011; https://doi.org/10.1056/NEJMoa1104390.
39. Perren TJ, Swart AM, Pfisterer J, et al. A phase 3 trial of bevacizumab in ovarian cancer. N Engl J Med. 2011; https://doi.org/10.1056/NEJMoa1103799.
40. Aghajanian C, Blank SV, Goff BA, Judson PL, Teneriello MG, Husain A, Sovak MA, Yi J, Nycum LR. OCEANS: a randomized, double-blind, placebo-controlled phase III trial of chemotherapy with or without bevacizumab in patients with platinum-sensitive recurrent epithelial ovarian, primary peritoneal, or fallopian tube cancer. J Clin Oncol. 2012; https://doi.org/10.1200/JCO.2012.42.0505.
41. Pujade-Lauraine E, Hilpert F, Weber B, et al. Bevacizumab combined with chemotherapy for platinum-resistant recurrent ovarian cancer: the AURELIA open-label randomized phase III trial. J Clin Oncol. 2014; https://doi.org/10.1200/JCO.2013.51.4489.
42. Selle F, Colombo N, Korach J, Mendiola C, Cardona A, Ghazi Y, Oza AM. Safety and efficacy of extended bevacizumab therapy in elderly (≥70 years) versus younger patients treated for newly diagnosed ovarian cancer in the international ROSiA study. Int J Gynecol Cancer. 2018; https://doi.org/10.1097/IGC.0000000000001221.
43. Mustea A, Wimberger P, Oskay-Oezcelik G, et al. Impact of age on the safety and efficacy of bevacizumab (BEV)-containing therapy in patients (pts) with primary ovarian cancer (OC): analyses of the OTILIA German non-interventional study on behalf of the north-eastern German Society of Gynaecological Onc. Ann Oncol. 2016;27:vi299.
44. Ledermann J, Harter P, Gourley C, et al. Olaparib maintenance therapy in platinum-sensitive relapsed ovarian cancer. N Engl J Med. 2012; https://doi.org/10.1056/NEJMoa1105535
45. Pujade-Lauraine E, Ledermann JA, Selle F, et al. Olaparib tablets as maintenance therapy in patients with platinum-sensitive, relapsed ovarian cancer and a BRCA1/2 mutation (SOLO2/

ENGOT-Ov21): a double-blind, randomised, placebo-controlled, phase 3 trial. Lancet Oncol. 2017; https://doi.org/10.1016/S1470-2045(17)30469-2.
46. Fields EC, McGuire WP, Lin L, Temkin SM. Radiation treatment in women with ovarian cancer: past, present, and future. Front Oncol. 2017;7:177.
47. Lewin SN, Buttin BM, Powell MA, Gibb RK, Rader JS, Mutch DG, Herzog TJ. Resource utilization for ovarian cancer patients at the end of life: how much is too much? Gynecol Oncol. 2005; https://doi.org/10.1016/j.ygyno.2005.07.102.
48. Wright AA, Zhang B, Ray A, et al. Associations between end-of-life discussions, patient mental health, medical care near death, and caregiver bereavement adjustment. JAMA - J Am Med Assoc. 2008; https://doi.org/10.1001/jama.300.14.1665.
49. Rustin GJS, Van Der Burg MEL, Griffin CL, et al. Early versus delayed treatment of relapsed ovarian cancer (MRC OV05/EORTC 55955): a randomised trial. Lancet. 2010; https://doi.org/10.1016/S0140-6736(10)61268-8.
50. Bray F, Ferlay J, Soerjomataram I, Siegel RL, Torre LA, Jemal A. Global cancer statistics 2018: GLOBOCAN estimates of incidence and mortality worldwide for 36 cancers in 185 countries. CA Cancer J Clin. 2018; https://doi.org/10.3322/caac.21492.
51. Soisson S, Ganz PA, Gaffney D, et al. Long-term cardiovascular outcomes among endometrial cancer survivors in a large, population-based cohort study. J Natl Cancer Inst. 2018; https://doi.org/10.1093/jnci/djy070.
52. Office for National Statistics (2019) Cancer survival in England: adult, stage at diagnosis and childhood - patients followed up to 2018. Off. Natl. Stat.
53. Lachance JA, Everett EN, Greer B, Mandel L, Swisher E, Tamimi H, Goff B. The effect of age on clinical/pathologic features, surgical morbidity, and outcome in patients with endometrial cancer. Gynecol Oncol. 2006;101:470–5.
54. Clark LH, Jackson AL, Gehrig PA, Bae-Jump V, Van Le L, Ko EM. Adjuvant treatment and clinical trials in elderly patients with endometrial cancer: a time for change? Int J Gynecol Cancer. 2016; https://doi.org/10.1097/IGC.0000000000000605.
55. Driver JA, Viswanathan AN. Frailty measure is more predictive of outcomes after curative therapy for endometrial cancer than traditional risk factors in women 60 and older. Gynecol Oncol. 2017; https://doi.org/10.1016/j.ygyno.2017.03.010.
56. NICE Guidelines (2017) Suspected cancer: recognition and referral | guidance and guidelines | NICE. In: NICE Guid.
57. Ciatto S, Cecchini S, Gervasi G, Landini A, Zappa M, Crocetti E. Association of endometrial thickness assessed at transvaginal ultrasonography to endometrial cancer in postmenopausal women asymptomatic or with abnormal uterine bleeding. Radiol Med. 2002;104(5-6):437–42.
58. Wright JD, Lewin SN, Barrena Medel NI, Sun X, Burke WM, Deutsch I, Herzog TJ. Endometrial cancer in the oldest old: tumor characteristics, patterns of care, and outcome. Gynecol Oncol. 2011; https://doi.org/10.1016/j.ygyno.2011.02.040.
59. Ahmed A, Zamba G, DeGeest K, Lynch CF. The impact of surgery on survival of elderly women with endometrial cancer in the SEER program from 1992-2002. Gynecol Oncol. 2008; https://doi.org/10.1016/j.ygyno.2008.06.026.
60. Colombo N, Creutzberg C, Amant F, et al. ESMO-ESGO-ESTRO consensus conference on endometrial cancer: diagnosis, treatment and follow-up. Ann Oncol. 2016; https://doi.org/10.1093/annonc/mdv484.
61. Frost JA, Webster KE, Bryant A, Morrison J. Lymphadenectomy for the management of endometrial cancer. Cochrane Database Syst Rev. 2017; https://doi.org/10.1002/14651858.CD007585.pub4.
62. Rudolph JL, Marcantonio ER. Postoperative delirium: acute change with long-term implications. Anesth Analg. 2011; https://doi.org/10.1213/ANE.0b013e3182147f6d.
63. Walker JL, Piedmonte MR, Spirtos NM, Eisenkop SM, Schlaerth JB, Mannel RS, Spiegel G, Barakat R, Pearl ML, Sharma SK. Laparoscopy compared with laparotomy for comprehensive surgical staging of uterine cancer: gynecologic oncology group study LAP2. J Clin Oncol. 2009; https://doi.org/10.1200/JCO.2009.22.3248.

64. Rupp-Montpetit K, Moody ML. Visual loss as a complication of non-ophthalmologic surgery: a review of the literature. AANA J. 2004;72:285–92.
65. Kong A, Johnson N, Kitchener HC, Lawrie TA. Adjuvant radiotherapy for stage I endometrial cancer. Cochrane Database Syst Rev. 2012; https://doi.org/10.1002/14651858.CD003916.pub4.
66. Nout RA, Smit VTHBM, Putter H, et al. Vaginal brachytherapy versus pelvic external beam radiotherapy for patients with endometrial cancer of high-intermediate risk (PORTEC-2): an open-label, non-inferiority, randomised trial. Lancet (London, England). 2010;375:816–23.
67. Francis SR, Ager BJ, Do OA, Huang Y-HJ, Soisson AP, Dodson MK, Werner TL, Sause WT, Grant JD, Gaffney DK. Recurrent early stage endometrial cancer: patterns of recurrence and results of salvage therapy. Gynecol Oncol. 2019;154:38–44.
68. van der Steen-Banasik E, Christiaens M, Shash E, Coens C, Casado A, Herrera FG, Ottevanger PB. Systemic review: radiation therapy alone in medical non-operable endometrial carcinoma. Eur J Cancer. 2016;65:172–81.
69. Johnson N, Bryant A, Miles T, Hogberg T, Cornes P. Adjuvant chemotherapy for endometrial cancer after hysterectomy. Cochrane Database Syst Rev. 2011; https://doi.org/10.1002/14651858.CD003175.pub2.
70. de Boer SM, Powell ME, Mileshkin L, et al. Adjuvant chemoradiotherapy versus radiotherapy alone for women with high-risk endometrial cancer (PORTEC-3): final results of an international, open-label, multicentre, randomised, phase 3 trial. Lancet Oncol. 2018;19:295–309.
71. Kokka F, Brockbank E, Oram D, Gallagher C, Bryant A. Hormonal therapy in advanced or recurrent endometrial cancer. Cochrane Database Syst Rev. 2010; https://doi.org/10.1002/14651858.CD007926.pub2.
72. Coleridge S, Morrison J. Patient-initiated follow-up after treatment for low risk endometrial cancer: a prospective audit of outcomes and cost benefits. Int J Gynecol Cancer. 2020;30:1177–82.
73. Seamon LG, Java JJ, Monk BJ, et al. Impact of tumour histology on survival in advanced cervical carcinoma: an NRG oncology/Gynaecologic oncology group study. Br J Cancer. 2018;118:162–70.
74. World Health Organisation (2014) Comprehensive cervical cancer control. WHO Libr Cat Data, p 364.
75. Cohen PA, Jhingran A, Oaknin A, Denny L. Cervical cancer. Lancet. 2019;393:169–82.
76. Kissel M, Rambeau A, Achkar S, Lecuru F, Mathevet P. Challenges and advances in cervix cancer treatment in elder women. Cancer Treat Rev. 2020;84:101976.
77. Darlin L, Borgfeldt C, Widén E, Kannisto P. Elderly women above screening age diagnosed with cervical cancer have a worse prognosis. Anticancer Res. 2014;
78. Kang Y, Smith M, Barlow E, Coffey K, Hacker N, Canfell K. Vulvar cancer in high-income countries: increasing burden of disease. Int J Cancer. 2017;141:2174–86.
79. Gilbert DC, Wakeham K, Langley RE, Vale CL. Increased risk of second cancers at sites associated with HPV after a prior HPV-associated malignancy, a systematic review and meta-analysis. Br J Cancer. 2019;120:256–68.
80. Wiggans A, Coleridge S, Bryant A, Morrison J. Relationship between vulvar symptoms and incidence of vulvar cancer in women referred to a rapid access clinic. Int J Gynecol Obstet. 2019;145:283–6.
81. Ramirez PT, Frumovitz M, Pareja R, et al. Minimally invasive versus abdominal radical hysterectomy for cervical cancer. N Engl J Med. 2018;379:1895–904.
82. Nama V, Angelopoulos G, Twigg J, Murdoch JB, Bailey J, Lawrie TA. Type II or type III radical hysterectomy compared to chemoradiotherapy as a primary intervention for stage IB2 cervical cancer. Cochrane Database Syst Rev. 2018; https://doi.org/10.1002/14651858.CD011478.pub2.
83. Yan R, Zeng Z, Liu F, Zeng Y, He T, Xiang Z, Zhang B, Gong H, Liu L. Primary radical hysterectomy vs chemoradiation for IB2-IIA cervical cancer. Medicine (Baltimore). 2020;99:e18738.

84. Te Grootenhuis NC, Van Der Zee AGJ, Van Doorn HC, et al. Sentinel nodes in vulvar cancer: Long-term follow-up of the GROningen INternational study on sentinel nodes in vulvar cancer (GROINSS-V) i. Gynecol Oncol. 2016; https://doi.org/10.1016/j.ygyno.2015.09.077.
85. Morrison J, Baldwin P, Buckley L, et al. British Gynaecological cancer society (BGCS) vulval cancer guidelines: recommendations for practice. Eur J Obstet Gynecol Reprod Biol. 2020;252:502–25.
86. Zhou W, Yue Y, Pei D. Survival benefit of vaginectomy compared to local tumor excision in women with FIGO stage I and II primary vaginal carcinoma: a SEER study. Arch Gynecol Obstet. 2020; https://doi.org/10.1007/s00404-020-05737-6.
87. Bhatla N, Aoki D, Sharma DN, Sankaranarayanan R. Cancer of the cervix uteri. Int J Gynecol Obstet. 2018;143:22–36.
88. Vale C. Reducing uncertainties about the effects of Chemoradiotherapy for cervical cancer: a systematic review and meta-analysis of individual patient data from 18 randomized trials. J Clin Oncol. 2008;26:5802–12.
89. Hata M, Koike I, Kasuya T, Kaizu H, Matsui T, Inoue T, Miyagi E, Numazaki R, Asai-Sato M, Hirahara F. Radiation therapy for very elderly patients aged 80 years and older with squamous cell carcinoma of the uterine cervix. Am J Clin Oncol Cancer Clin Trials. 2017;40:178–82.
90. Nakamura R, Shimoji Y, Nakasone T, Taira Y, Arakaki Y, Nakamoto T, Ooyama T, Kudaka W, Mekaru K, Aoki Y. Relative dose intensity and overall treatment time in older patients with cervical cancer treated with concurrent chemoradiotherapy. J Geriatr Oncol. 2020;62:20–2.
91. Tanderup K, Eifel PJ, Yashar CM, Pötter R, Grigsby PW. Curative radiation therapy for locally advanced cervical cancer: brachytherapy is NOT optional. Int J Radiat Oncol Biol Phys. 2014;88:537–9.
92. Van Lonkhuijzen L, Thomas G. Palliative radiotherapy for cervical carcinoma, a systematic review. Radiother Oncol. 2011;98:287–91.
93. Tewari KS, DiSaia PJ, Sill MW, et al. Bevacizumab for advanced cervical cancer: final overall survival and adverse event analysis of a randomised, controlled, open-label, phase 3 trial (gynecologic oncology group 240). Lancet. 2017;390:1654–63.
94. Kirchheiner K, Pötter R, Nout RA, Schwartz-Vittrup A, Holzner B, Bentzen SM, Tanderup K. Late, persistent, substantial, treatment-related symptoms after radiation therapy (LAPERS): a new method for longitudinal analysis of late morbidity—applied in the EMBRACE study. Int J Radiat Oncol Biol Phys. 2020; https://doi.org/10.1016/j.ijrobp.2019.10.027.
95. Gibson W, Johnson T, Kirschner-Hermanns R, Kuchel G, Markland A, Orme S, Ostaszkiewicz J, Szonyi G, Wyman J, Wagg A. Incontinence in frail elderly persons: report of the 6th international consultation on incontinence. Neurourol Urodyn. 2020;40(1):38–54.

Chapter 26
Head and Neck Cancer in Older Adults with Frailty

Muhammad Shahid Iqbal, Eleanor Smith, and Charles G. Kelly

Introduction

Head and neck cancer (HNC) is a heterogeneous group of subsites including nasopharynx, oropharynx, hypopharynx, larynx, oral cavity, nasal cavity, paranasal sinuses and salivary glands. The majority of HNC patients present at a locally advanced stage and the management is complex, involving multi-modality treatment including surgery, radiotherapy and/or chemotherapy. These intense treatments are often morbid and are associated with an increased incidence of acute and late treatment-related toxicity.

With a rapidly ageing population, there is an increase in the incidence of HNC in older patients. Approximately 47% of all patients diagnosed with HNC in the United States between 1973 and 2008 were above 65 years of age [1] and this trend continues to increase [2]. In fact, the most recent data showed that around 30% of new HNC patients were aged 70 or older and around 20% were aged 75 or older [3]. Nonetheless, older cancer patients are widely underrepresented in clinical trials [4]. This poses a unique challenge to treat this complex disease in an older population which often suffers from frailty syndrome. Therefore, an appropriate shared decision-making process in this complex group of patients is of paramount importance. A multidisciplinary team approach is required in order to select appropriate patients for the different management options and treatment intensity coupled with the patients' input regarding their goals of care.

A comprehensive geriatric assessment (CGA) is the 'gold standard' tool to identify vulnerable patients and those with frailty. This is defined as 'a multidimensional, interdisciplinary diagnostic process focusing on determining an older

M. S. Iqbal (✉) · E. Smith · C. G. Kelly
Department of Clinical Oncology, Northern Centre for Cancer Care, Freeman Hospital, The Newcastle Upon Tyne Hospitals NHS Foundation Trust, Newcastle upon Tyne, UK
e-mail: Shahid.Iqbal@nhs.net; Eleanor.Smith4@nhs.net; Charles.Kelly1@nhs.net

F. Gomes (ed.), *Frailty in Older Adults with Cancer*,
https://doi.org/10.1007/978-3-030-89162-6_26

person's medical, psychosocial, and functional capabilities to develop a coordinated and integrated plan for treatment and long-term follow-up' [5]. The use of CGA helps in identifying frailty and functional impairments which may not be identified in a routine oncological assessment. This approach can also predict severe treatment-related toxicity and estimate prognosis, which can influence treatment decisions [6]. To optimise the use of available resources, screening tools have been developed to identify those who may benefit the most from CGA. These tools include the FRAIL questionnaire [7], the Rockwood Clinical Frailty Scale [8], the Geriatric-8 (G8) [9], amongst several others. The G8 tool is the most widely used in oncology, including HNC patients, with a sensitivity and specificity to detect frailty on subsequent geriatric assessments of 85% and 64%, respectively. Moreover, 63% of studies found the G8 was associated with survival outcome, whilst 43% studies found an association between the G8 score and the risk of treatment-related complications [10]. Ultimately the incidence of frailty in HNC patients is variable, depending on the tool used and the population assessed. Several studies report different results but in patients undergoing curative treatments the incidence of frailty may reach around 40% [11–13]. Hence that these approaches should be implemented in the management of HNC patients to enhanced personalised care and improve outcomes. This chapter will review the available evidence regarding the management of older patients with HNC and frailty from early to advanced cancer stages.

Management of Early-Stage and Locally Advanced HNC

Surgical Management

Surgery is the mainstay of treatment in early-stage HNC, whilst patients with later stage disease require multi-modality therapy. Goldstein et al. [12] performed a prospective cohort study in the setting of HNC confirming that frailty was an independent predictor for serious postoperative complications and longer length of stay. Moreover, frailty assessment was superior to independent activities of daily living assessment at predicting complications. Bras et al. [13] undertook a small retrospective cohort study to assess postoperative outcomes using the Groningen Frailty Indicator and found that frailty was associated with poor patient experience regarding the postoperative recovery. A study from Adams et al. [14] used a modified frailty index to find that postoperative complications, both serious and any grade, were significantly higher in the population with frailty.

Surgical techniques are evolving. Cocuzza et al. [15] reported that older patients with laryngectomy achieved similar speech outcomes following speech rehabilitation to younger patients. Moreover, supracricoid laryngectomy has been developed for preservation of speech and swallowing function in selected individuals. And several small cases series show this approach is equally valid in selected older patients [16, 17]. Another study from Hassid et al. [18] presented a small case series using transoral robotic surgery in older patients. They used the G8 screening tool and were able to complete all their cases without reverting to open surgery and were also able to reduce operative time.

Ultimately, curative surgical resection in HNC is complex and although a number of studies showed it can be safely applied to selected older adults with similar outcomes to their younger counterparts [18–20], frailty plays a key role in this selection. In fact, if frailty predicts risk of postoperative complications, morbidity and length of stay, patient selection and optimisation for surgery is vital. The severity of frailty is key and as surgical approaches evolve, HNC surgery may potentially be considered for those with mild frailty. Further research is needed to establish how the assessment of the severity of frailty may be used to tailor surgical treatment options and whether pre/rehabilitation strategies can be beneficial in the context of HNC.

Radical Radiotherapy and Chemo-Radiotherapy

Radical radiotherapy involves its use either as definitive primary treatment (i.e. instead of surgery) or adjuvant (i.e. post-surgery). In locally advanced HNC, surgery alone is unlikely to cure the disease by itself and adjuvant radiotherapy is often required to maximise the chance of cure.

The indications of adjuvant radiotherapy are positive or close surgical resection margins where further surgery is not possible, the presence of extranodal extension, stage T3/T4 disease, significant nodal involvement or the presence of neural or vascular involvement. Primary radiotherapy provides an alternative treatment to surgery, as an organ preserving approach, this is particularly useful for early-stage small tumours often with equivalent local cancer control rates and better functional outcomes than surgery [21]. For more locally advanced tumours, surgery is preferred (if resectable), however primary radiotherapy is particularly relevant when an older patient with significant frailty is not eligible for surgery. Nonetheless, indications for their use vary from anatomical subsite to subsite; for example, in primary nasopharyngeal carcinoma, primary radiotherapy is even the treatment of choice, however in the oral cavity or paranasal sinuses, primary radiotherapy is seldom curative.

The use of concomitant chemotherapy (cisplatin-based) with the radiotherapy increases its efficacy but at the expense of more toxicity. A large meta-analysis of 93 trials involving more than 17,000 patients showed that addition of concomitant cisplatin chemotherapy to the radiotherapy resulted in a 19% reduction in the risk of death and an absolute 6.5% increase in 5-year overall survival, compared to radiotherapy alone ($p < 0.0001$) [22]. However, the evidence regarding concomitant chemo-radiotherapy in older patients with HNC and frailty is very limited. There are no phase 3 prospective trials and most data come from retrospective institutional observational studies, with conflicting results [23]. Although the above-mentioned meta-analysis showed patients over 70 years old did not benefit, the actual percentage of patients aged over 70 was only 7.5% [22]. The reason for poorer survival for older patients was a greater number of non-cancer related deaths [24]. Michal et al. [25] compared cisplatin-based chemo-radiotherapy in older versus younger patients and found no difference in outcome, although older patients experienced greater myelosuppression and supportive care requirements. Similarly, Nguyen et al. [26] retrospectively compared chemo-radiotherapy in younger patients versus older patients. There was no difference in 2-year survival rates and the older group tolerated treatment better than the younger group. However, Strom et al. [27] found a statistically significant, higher incidence of acute mortality and a higher rate of hospital admission in an older group as compared to younger patients with HNC.

Lastly, a prospective study by VanderWalde et al. [28] looked at the tolerability of radical radiotherapy in 46 older patients (61% had HNC). This small study found that baseline level of activities of daily living was not associated with poor radiotherapy tolerance in general. However, receiving concomitant chemotherapy increased the likelihood of a poor treatment tolerance. Moreover, impairment of baseline function also increased the likelihood of gastrostomy tube use in patients with HNC. Therefore, whilst this may be an appropriate option for selected older patients with mild frailty, it may not be appropriate for the majority of older patients with frailty. Alternatively, for patients who are ineligible for cisplatin chemotherapy, the use of cetuximab (an immunoglobulin G monoclonal antibody against epidermal growth factor receptor) with radiotherapy has shown benefit [29]. However, its use in less fit patients is not well defined [23]. Carboplatin is another option, commonly used, but again level one evidence for its use is lacking.

Another consideration regarding the delivery of radiotherapy in HNC is the use of different fractionation regimens. A meta-analysis involving 15 trials with 6515 patients, with a median follow-up of 6 years showed an absolute survival benefit of 3.4% at 5 years with the use of hyperfractionated or accelerated radiotherapy (HR 0.92, 95%CI 0.86–0.97; p 0.003). But when assessing the effect in different age groups, this benefit was significantly higher in the younger patients under 50 years (HR 0.78, 95%CI 0.65–0.94). This benefit gradually decreased with increasing age, with no benefit for the patients over 70 years (HR 1.08, 95%CI 0.89–1.30; p 0.007). The possible explanation for this loss of benefit with hyperfractionated radiotherapy in older patients could be due to an excess of non-cancer related deaths, a lower compliance or lower treatment tolerance or a relatively poorer general health status [30]. Other developments have led to the consideration of hypofractionated approaches and an ongoing non-inferiority randomised trial (ELAN-RT) is looking at overall survival and loss of independence in activities of daily living between standard radiotherapy (70 Gy/7 weeks/2 Gy per fraction) versus hypofractionated split-course radiotherapy (55 Gy/7 weeks with 2 weeks interruption/3 Gy per fraction until 30 Gy, after interruption 2.5 Gy per fraction until 55 Gy) in medically inoperable HNC patients [31]. Lastly, there have been significant developments in radiotherapy techniques as well, enhancing the delivery of radiation dosing whilst protecting normal surrounding tissues. Intensity Modulated RadioTherapy (IMRT) is a key example of such developments and Fig. 26.1 shows the practicalities of its delivery.

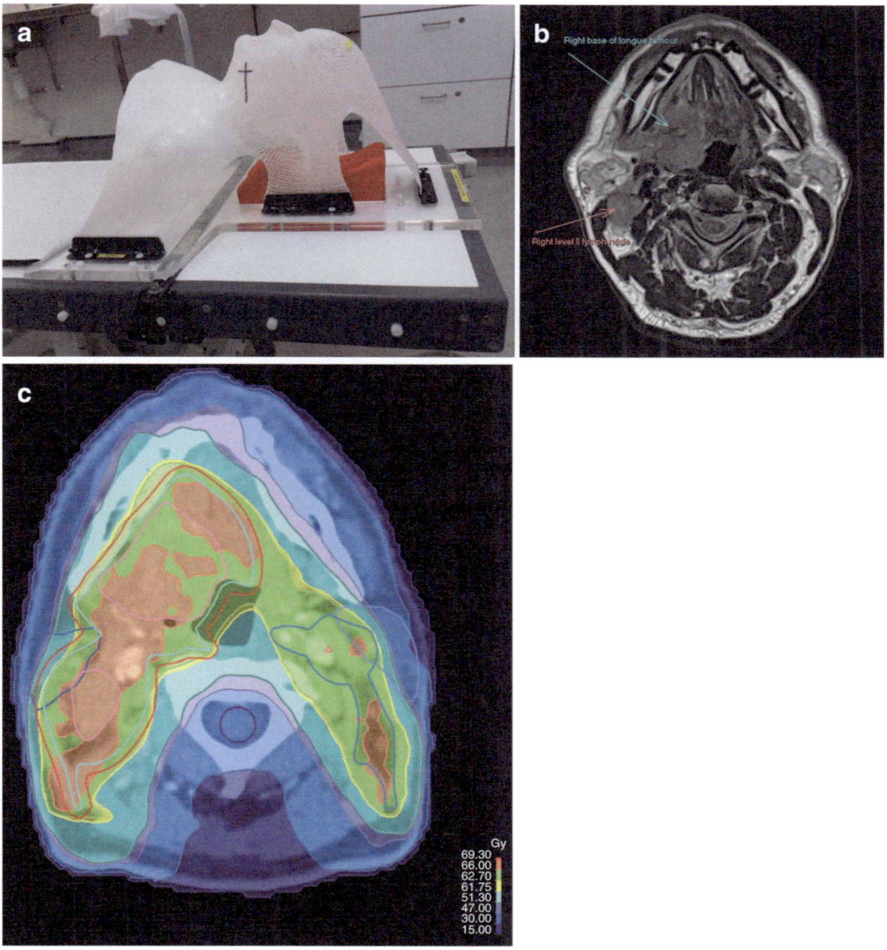

Fig. 26.1 Axial image of diagnostic MRI scan shows right base of tongue tumour and right level II lymph node (**a**). A customised thermoplastic shell for patient immobilisation during the course of radiotherapy (**b**). A volumetric modulated arc therapy plan for T4 N2c right oropharyngeal tumour. Various colour schemes denote different radiotherapy dose levels (**c**)

Managing older patients with frailty and potentially curable HNC poses a significant challenge to finding the optimal balance between treatment intensity and tolerability, in order to achieve the best cancer outcomes. In fact, several studies have reported that older patients with HNC might receive suboptimal treatment when compared to their younger counterparts with the same disease status [32, 33]. As treatment-related toxicities have huge implications on patients' function, especially for speech and swallowing, patient selection is key. This should take into consideration disease status, risk of disease recurrence, patient frailty, comorbidities and preferences, as well as the post-treatment function and quality of life. Only then can a truly shared and informed decision be achieved. In this regard, a comprehensive review by Porceddu and Haddad presented an algorithm of decision for older patients with locoregional HNC, where patient selection for a given treatment modality is based on a systematic approach taking into consideration patients' fitness for treatment. This approach incorporates geriatric assessments, the patients' preference, social support, performance/functional status, life expectancy and comorbidities [34].

Management of Local Recurrence

Despite aggressive management of locoregional HNC, about half of patients still have a recurrence, mainly locally. Management of recurrent locoregional disease and second primary cancers in the previously irradiated field is even more challenging. Although surgery is generally considered first choice for salvage treatment, realistically a significant number of older patients, particularly with frailty, are unfit for surgery. Historically, radical re-irradiation has been considered hazardous; however, with evolving radiotherapy delivery techniques there is increasing interest in re-irradiation. Recently, a multi-institutional re-irradiation collaborative group in the US, entitled MIRI, has published their experience of re-irradiation in the IMRT era. The 2-year overall survival was in the region of 35–45% with overall grade ≥ 3 toxicity of 19%. The same collaborative team also produced criteria for patient selection based on recursive partitioning analysis [35]. Use of stereotactic radiotherapy technique in re-irradiation of HNC is gaining popularity [36]. Similarly, proton therapy has theoretical dosimetric benefit over photon therapy but whether there is a clinical benefit in older HNC patients with frailty is still to be proven.

As salvage surgery or re-irradiation may not be possible, systemic treatment options for advanced disease may then be considered. But best supportive care should also be part of the decision making for older patients with significant frailty.

Palliative Radiotherapy

Approximately 50–70% of patients present with locally advanced HNC. A significant proportion of these patients are not candidates for aggressive curative therapy because of frailty, existing comorbidities, poor performance status or patient choice. These patients with locally advanced HNC disease, not being treated with curative treatment, have only a modest median overall survival of about 6 months [37]. Due to the nature and biology of HNC, patients often suffer from significant symptoms in terms of pain, dysphagia, bleeding or airway compromise. Palliative radiotherapy is often used in order to try to alleviate troublesome symptoms. It also helps in controlling disease progression to some extent and delaying further symptoms. The main aim of using palliative radiotherapy is to achieve effective palliation, ideally with a relatively short treatment duration, without causing significant treatment-related toxicity which may have a detrimental impact on quality of life when there is already a limited life span. A systematic review on the use of palliative radiotherapy in HNC showed that there exists no level one evidence of an optimal dose fractionation [37]. The main evidence has come from retrospective institutional observational case studies. There is a large heterogeneity in clinical practice and the selection of dose fractionation for palliative radiotherapy in HNC ranges from a single fraction to several weeks of radiotherapy [38]. Recently, a phase III randomised control trial comparing 50 Gy in 16 fractions (4 times a week) against 36 Gy in 6 fractions (twice a week) was terminated early because of slow accrual. The total number of patients enrolled was only 34 whilst the planned sample size was 300. There was no significant difference in outcome between treatment regimens, although the acute grade $\geq$ 3 toxicity was less within the short course of radiotherapy [39]. The failure of this properly conducted trial attempted by an experienced multi-centre team highlights the challenges in conducting randomised control trials in this setting. These challenges include finding optimal comparative radiotherapy regimens, patient selection, acceptance of non-curative treatment for non-metastatic disease, suitability of alternatives to radical treatment, estimations of life expectancy and the role of palliative systemic treatments [40]. However, a phase II trial by Fortin et al. [41] used 25 Gy in 5 daily fractions with IMRT which showed a potential advantage of short overall treatment time with adequate symptom control and manageable toxicity.

With evolving techniques of targeted and increasingly precise radiotherapy delivery techniques, there may be the potential to deliver higher dose radiotherapy to those often considered medically unfit for conventional radical treatment, such as many older HNC patients with significant frailty. Gogineni et al. [42] reported treating 66 medically unfit HNC patients with stereotactic radiotherapy. The median age of the patient cohort was 80 years with a median Charlson Comorbidity Index score of 12% and median G8 score 11. The results of these frailty tools indicate a vulnerable group of patients. With 40 Gy delivered in 5 by-weekly fractions, the local control rate was 68% with a median time to local failure of 28.3 months. Twenty-six patients had at least 1-year follow-up and these patients showed a disease free survival of 88%. Treatment toleration was excellent with no grade 4/5 toxicity with only 3% rate of grade 3 toxicity. Whilst stereotactic radiotherapy may provide a 'high grade palliation', the evidence in HNC is still very limited and should not be considered standard of care [36].

Management of Advanced Metastatic HNC

HNC can present at diagnosis with metastatic disease but in other patients the metastatic disease may only develop later in the context of a recurrence after previous radical treatments. In the setting of advanced metastatic disease, often recurrent disease, systemic therapies such as chemotherapy and immunotherapy are the backbone of treatment. However, the primary tumour should ideally also be treated to control the tumour locally and its associated symptoms [21]. The intensity of this management plan should be guided by the burden of disease and the overall patient fitness/frailty.

There is an inverse relationship between comorbidity levels and survival in HNC [43–45] and some evidence of higher recurrence rates in patients with more comorbidities [46, 47]. Moreover, the treatment intent in this setting is palliative, and a significant proportion of patients will not benefit from it. In one study, 175/741 patients had persistent disease after first-line therapy, and 63 of these 175 patients were considered ineligible for further second-line management [48]. Therefore, for patients with severe frailty and a metastatic HNC, it may be that the patient's best interests are served by using best supportive care, rather than reducing quality-of-life and increasing treatment-related morbidity, for what is already a compromised lifespan [49]. Palliative radiotherapy, particularly to the primary tumour, may also play an important role in improving symptoms for some of these patients.

Palliative Chemotherapy and Targeted Therapies

For the non-curative use of chemotherapy, regimen choice depends on performance status, frailty, physiological reserve, renal function and comorbidities present. The commonest regimens used are cisplatin or carboplatin in combination with 5-FU, giving an expected response rate of 30–40% [50]. If impaired renal function, deafness, tinnitus or peripheral neuropathy is present, then carboplatin is preferred to cisplatin as the latter can exacerbate all of these. Alternatively, some older patients with significant frailty may only be suitable for single-agent carboplatin. Methotrexate has a long history of use in HNC but since the introduction of platinum agents its use has been declining and has all but disappeared in palliative clinical practice. The combination of cetuximab with carboplatin or cisplatin and 5-FU can increase response rate and survival as demonstrated in the EXTREME trial [51]. However, the combination of multiple drugs results in more toxicity and this may not be appropriate for older patients with significant frailty. Cetuximab is an anti-EGFR targeted treatment, and it may be an alternatively for patients unfit for platinum-based chemotherapy as a single agent with a response rate of 10–15% [52–54]. Lastly, whilst some patients with advanced disease are offered concomitant chemo-radiotherapy, for older patients with significant frailty systemic therapies alone may be more appropriate [55].

Palliative Immunotherapy (Checkpoint Inhibitors)

The two most common checkpoint inhibitors used in advanced or metastatic HNC are nivolumab and pembrolizumab. Nivolumab was introduced after publication of the Checkmate-141 In the CheckMate-141 trial, nivolumab was compared to a drug of physician's choice (limited to cetuximab, docetaxel or methotrexate) in patients with recurrent HNC within six months of platinum treatment (meaning patients showing early recurrence). Patients on nivolumab showed an improved medial overall survival (7.7 vs 5.1 months) but had a similar progression-free survival time [56]. The CheckMate-714 trial investigated ipilimumab plus nivolumab versus nivolumab alone and this was a negative trial [57]. However, pembrolizumab has been approved in the USA and in Europe for first-line treatment of recurrent HNC in those patients with positive PD-L1 following the positive results from Keynote-048 trial [58, 59]. In this trial, pembrolizumab was investigated as monotherapy or in combination with chemotherapy versus the standard cetuximab with chemotherapy, proving its superiority in terms of overall survival. Although this trial was open to all patients over the age of 18, no one in the trial was over the age of 68, and the median age for patients receiving pembrolizumab and chemotherapy was 61 years. All patients required to be performance status 0 or 1, and even in this relatively young, fit population, 85% of patients showed grade 3+ adverse events in the pembrolizumab and chemotherapy group. This leads to caution in offering combined chemotherapy and immunotherapy to older, more frail patients but further research is needed.

Treatment with checkpoint inhibitors gives a different spectrum of treatment induced morbidity than those experienced with chemotherapy [60]. For the majority of patients who develop toxicity, this tends to be mild which encourages their use in older patients and those with mild frailty who still maintain a good performance status. However, more research is needed to enhance the treatment of advanced metastatic HNC, and there are multiple trials ongoing exploring new therapies and new combinations of therapies. Of particularly interest is the FRAIL IMMUNE (GORTEC 2018–03) study [61] is looking at a combination of durvalumab with carboplatin and paclitaxel in patients over 70 years of age or those with poor renal function or who would be normally excluded from standard chemotherapy or immunotherapy for recurrent HNC.

Conclusion

Patients with HNC often have significant symptoms, in particular swallowing difficulties due to both the tumour and its treatments, which can then lead to malnutrition and poor clinical outcomes. These effects are often more significant in the older patient due to underlying frailty. Therefore, appropriate baseline assessment and a proactive multidisciplinary care are essential, particularly as studies show that health related quality-of-life data can be maintained in older adults [62]. Moreover, when making decisions regarding the management plan, it is crucial to ensure that the patient is likely to complete the treatment, particularly if this has a radical intent. For example, patients should not be placed in a situation where their radical or adjuvant radiotherapy completion is compromised by the addition of chemotherapy. As with radical treatment for HNC some older or more frail patients may benefit from salvage treatment following recurrence and be able to tolerate it, yet identifying which patients can be difficult and using geriatric assessment tools is helpful [63].

The recent implementation of immunotherapy with checkpoint inhibitors for advanced metastatic HNC is expected to continue expanding and this may be a better match for many older patients. However, further research is needed to ensure frailty is not just assessed but supported and managed within a treatment plan for patients with HNC, shaping the decision-making process throughout their cancer journey.

References

1. VanderWalde NA, Fleming M, Weiss J, Chera BS. Treatment of older patients with head and neck cancer: a review. Oncologist. 2013;18(5):568–78. https://doi.org/10.1634/theoncologist.2012-0427.
2. Mourad M, Jetmore T, Jategaonkar AA, Moubayed S, Moshier E, Urken ML. Epidemiological trends of head and neck cancer in the United States: a SEER population study. J Oral Maxillofac Surg. 2017;75(12):2562–72. https://doi.org/10.1016/j.joms.2017.05.008.
3. National Cancer Institute surveillance, epidemiology and end results problem. Available at https://seer.cancer.gov/ (date accessed 19.09.2020).
4. Abbasi J. Older patients (still) left out of cancer clinical trials. JAMA. 2019; https://doi.org/10.1001/jama.2019.17016.
5. Rubenstein LZ, Stuck AE, Siu AL, Wieland D. Impacts of geriatric evaluation and management programs on defined outcomes: overview of the evidence. J Am Geriatr Soc. 1991;39(9 Pt 2):8S–18S. https://doi.org/10.1111/j.1532-5415.1991.tb05927.x.
6. Wildiers H, Heeren P, Puts M, et al. International Society of Geriatric Oncology consensus on geriatric assessment in older patients with cancer. J Clin Oncol. 2014;32(24):2595–603. https://doi.org/10.1200/JCO.2013.54.8347.
7. Morley JE, Malmstrom TK, Miller DK. A simple frailty questionnaire (FRAIL) predicts outcomes in middle aged African Americans. J Nutr Health Aging. 2012;16(7):601–8. https://doi.org/10.1007/s12603-012-0084-2.
8. Rockwood K, Song X, MacKnight C, et al. A global clinical measure of fitness and frailty in elderly people. CMAJ. 2005;173(5):489–95. https://doi.org/10.1503/cmaj.050051.
9. Bellera CA, Rainfray M, Mathoulin-Pelissier S, Mertens C, Delva F, Fonck M, et al. Screening older cancer patients: first evaluation of the G-8 geriatric screening tool. Ann Oncol Off J Eur Soc Med Oncol. 2012;23(8):2166–72. https://doi.org/10.1093/annonc/mdr587.
10. van Walree IC, Scheepers E, van Huis-Tanja L, et al. A systematic review on the association of the G8 with geriatric assessment, prognosis and course of treatment in older patients with cancer. J Geriatr Oncol. 2019;10(6):847–58. https://doi.org/10.1016/j.jgo.2019.04.016.
11. Kwon M, Kim SA, Roh JL, Lee SW, Kim SB, Choi SH, Nam SY, Kim SY. An introduction to a head and neck cancer-specific frailty index and its clinical implications in elderly patients: a prospective observational study focusing on respiratory and swallowing functions. Oncologist. 2016 Sep;21(9):1091–1098. https://doi.org/10.1634/theoncologist.2016-0008. Epub 2016 Jul 1. PMID: 27368883; PMCID: PMC5016072.
12. Goldstein DP, Sklar MC, de Almeida JR, Gilbert R, Gullane P, Irish J, Brown D, Higgins K, Enepekides D, Xu W, Su J, Alibhai SMH. Frailty as a predictor of outcomes in patients undergoing head and neck cancer surgery. Laryngoscope 2020 May;130(5):E340-E345. https://doi.org/10.1002/lary.28222. Epub 2019 Aug 16.
13. Bras L, Peters TT, Wedman J, Plaat BE, Witjes MJ, van Leeuwen BL, van der Laan BF, Halmos GB. Predictive value of the Groningen frailty indicator for treatment outcomes in elderly patients after head and neck, or skin cancer surgery in a retrospective cohort. Clin Otolaryngol. 2015 Oct;40(5):474–82. https://doi.org/10.1111/coa.12409.

14. Adams P, Ghanem T, Stachler R, Hall F, Velanovich V, Rubinfeld I. Frailty as a predictor of morbidity and mortality in inpatient head and neck surgery. JAMA Otolaryngol Head Neck Surg. 2013 Aug 1;139(8):783–9. https://doi.org/10.1001/jamaoto.2013.3969.
15. Cocuzza S, Bonfiglio M, Grillo C, Maiolino L, Malaguarnera M, Martines F, Serra A. Post laryngectomy speech rehabilitation outcome in elderly patients. Eur Arch Otorhinolaryngol 2013 May;270(6):1879–1884. https://doi.org/10.1007/s00405-013-2430-3. Epub 2013 Mar 22.
16. Nam I, Park J, Kim C, Kim S, Cho K, et al. Role of supracricoid partial laryngectomy in the aging era. https://www.redjournal.org/article/S0360-3016(13)03386-5/abstract
17. Allegra E, Franco T, Trapasso S, Domanico R, La Boria A, Garozzo A. Modified supracricoid laryngectomy: oncological and functional outcomes in the elderly. Clin Interv Aging. 2012;7:475–80. https://doi.org/10.2147/CIA.S38410. Epub 2012 Nov 8. PMID: 23152678; PMCID: PMC3496192
18. Hassid SA, Delcour L, Delahaut G, Van Der Vorst S, Lawson G. Transoral robotic surgery and geriatric population: which benefit? B-ENT. 2019;15:63.
19. Otsuki N, Furukawa T, Avinçsal MO, Teshima M, Shinomiya H, Oshikiri T, Nakamura T, Nomura T, Hashikawa K, Nibu KI. Results of free flap reconstruction for patients aged 80 years or older with head and neck cancer. Auris Nasus Larynx 2020 Feb;47(1):123–127. https://doi.org/10.1016/j.anl.2019.04.005. Epub 2019 May 3.
20. Peters TT, Post SF, van Dijk BA, Roodenburg JL, van der Laan BF, Werker PM, Halmos GB. Free flap reconstruction for head and neck cancer can be safely performed in both young and elderly patients after careful patient selection. Eur Arch Otorhinolaryngol 2015 Oct;272(10):2999–3005. https://doi.org/10.1007/s00405-014-3268-z. Epub 2014 Sep 13.
21. Machiels JP, René Leemans C, Golusinski W, Grau C, Licitra L, Gregoire V; EHNS Executive Board. Electronic address: secretariat@ehns.org; ESMO guidelines committee. Electronic address: clinicalguidelines@esmo.org; ESTRO Executive Board. Electronic address: info@estro.org. Squamous cell carcinoma of the oral cavity, larynx, oropharynx and hypopharynx: EHNS-ESMO-ESTRO clinical practice guidelines for diagnosis, treatment and follow-up. Ann Oncol 2020 Nov;31(11):1462–1475. https://doi.org/10.1016/j.annonc.2020.07.011. Epub 2020 Oct 23.
22. Pignon JP, le Maitre A, Maillard E, Bourhis J, MACH-NC Collaborative Group. Metaanalysis of chemotherapy in head and neck cancer (MACH-NC): an update on 93 randomised trials and 17,346 patients. Radiother Oncol. 2009 Jul;92(1):4–14.
23. Iqbal MS, Dua D, Kelly C, Bossi P. Managing older patients with head and neck cancer: the non-surgical curative approach. J Geriatr Oncol. 2018;9(4):411–7. https://doi.org/10.1016/j.jgo.2018.03.016.
24. Kish JA, et al. The effect of age on outcome in prospective, phase III NRG Oncology/RTOG trials of radiotherapy (XRT) +/− chemotherapy in locally advanced (LA) head and neck cancer (HNC). J Clin Oncol 2015;33(Suppl.; abstract 6003).
25. Michal SA, Adelstein DJ, Rybicki LA, et al. Multi-agent concurrent chemoradiotherapy for locally advanced head and neck squamous cell cancer in the elderly. Head Neck. 2012;34(8):1147–52. https://doi.org/10.1002/hed.21891.
26. Nguyen NP, Vock J, Chi A, et al. Impact of intensity-modulated and image-guided radiotherapy on elderly patients undergoing chemoradiation for locally advanced head and neck cancer. Strahlenther Onkol. 2012;188(8):677–83. https://doi.org/10.1007/s00066-012-0125-0.
27. Strom TJ, Naghavi AO, Trotti AM, et al. Increased acute mortality with chemoradiotherapy for locally advanced head and neck cancer in patients ≥70 years. J Geriatr Oncol. 2017;8(1):50–5. https://doi.org/10.1016/j.jgo.2016.09.003.
28. Vanderwalde NA, Deal AM, Comitz E, et al. Functional age and tolerance to radiotherapy: a prospective study of a comprehensive geriatric assessment. J Clin Oncol 2015;33 [Suppl; abstract e20534].
29. Bonner JA, Harari PM, Giralt J, et al. Radiotherapy plus cetuximab for squamous-cell carcinoma of the head and neck. N Engl J Med. 2006;354(6):567–78. https://doi.org/10.1056/NEJMoa053422.

30. Bourhis J, Overgaard J, Audry H, Ang KK, Saunders M, Bernier J, et al. Hyperfractionated or accelerated radiotherapy in head and neck cancer: a meta-analysis. Lancet. 2006;368(9538):843–54.
31. https://clinicaltrials.gov/ct2/show/NCT01864850
32. Juarez JE, Choi J, St John M, Abemayor E, TenNapel M, Chen AM. Patterns of care for elderly patients with locally advanced head and neck cancer. Int J Radiat Oncol Biol Phys. 2017;98(4):767–74. https://doi.org/10.1016/j.ijrobp.2017.01.209.
33. VanderWalde NA, Meyer AM, Liu H, et al. Patterns of care in older patients with squamous cell carcinoma of the head and neck: a surveillance, epidemiology, and end results-medicare analysis. J Geriatr Oncol. 2013;4(3):262–70. https://doi.org/10.1016/j.jgo.2013.03.002.
34. Porceddu SV, Haddad RI. Management of elderly patients with locoregionally confined head and neck cancer. Lancet Oncol. 2017;18(5):e274–83. https://doi.org/10.1016/S1470-2045(17)30229-2.
35. Ward MC, Riaz N, Caudell JJ, et al. Refining patient selection for Reirradiation of head and neck squamous carcinoma in the IMRT era: a multi-institution cohort study by the MIRI collaborative. Int J Radiat Oncol Biol Phys. 2018;100(3):586–94. https://doi.org/10.1016/j.ijrobp.2017.06.012.
36. Iqbal MS, West N, Richmond N, Kovarik J, Gray I, Willis N, Morgan D, Yazici G, Cengiz M, Paleri V, Kelly C. A systematic review and practical considerations of stereotactic body radiotherapy in the treatment of head and neck cancer. Br J Radiol. 2021 Jan 1;94(1117):20200332. https://doi.org/10.1259/bjr.20200332. Epub 2020 Sep 24. PMID: 32960652; PMCID: PMC7774675.
37. Shahid Iqbal M, Kelly C, Kovarik J, et al. Palliative radiotherapy for locally advanced non-metastatic head and neck cancer: a systematic review. Radiother Oncol. 2018;126(3):558–67. https://doi.org/10.1016/j.radonc.2017.12.011.
38. Iqbal MS, Kelly C, Kovarik J, et al. Palliative radiotherapy for locally advanced non-metastatic head and neck cancer: a survey of UK national practice. Radiother Oncol. 2018;126(3):568–9. https://doi.org/10.1016/j.radonc.2017.11.017.
39. Al-Mamgani A, Kessels R, Verhoef C, Navran A, et al. Randomized controlled trial to identify the optimal radiotherapy scheme for palliative treatment of incurable head and neck squamous cell. Radiother Oncol. 2020v;149:181–8. https://doi.org/10.1016/j.radonc.2020.05.020.
40. Iqbal MS, Kovarik J, Kelly C. Challenges in conducting large randomised control trials of palliative radiotherapy in head and neck cancer. Radiother Oncol. 2020;149:246. https://doi.org/10.1016/j.radonc.2020.06.026.
41. Fortin B, Khaouam N, Fillion E, Ngouyen-Tan PF, Bujold A, Lambert L. Palliative radiation therapy for advanced head and neck carcinomas: a phase 2 study. Int J Radiat Oncol Biol Phys. 2016;95:647–53.
42. Gogineni E, Rana ZH, Vempati P, Karten J, Sharma A, Taylor PK, Pereira L, Gabalski E, Paul D, Seetharamu N, Teckie S, Ghaly M. Stereotactic body radiotherapy as primary treatment for medically unfit patients with head and neck cancer. Int J Radiat Oncol Biol Phys. 2019, September 1;105(1):E399–400. https://doi.org/10.1016/j.ijrobp.2019.06.1584.
43. Datema FR, Ferrier MB, van der Schroeff MP, Baatenburg de Jong RJ. Impact of comorbidity on short-term mortality and overall survival of head and neck cancer patients. Head Neck. 2010 Jun;32(6):728–36. https://doi.org/10.1002/hed.21245.
44. Alho OP, Hannula K, Luokkala A, Teppo H, Koivunen P, Kantola S. Differential prognostic impact of comorbidity in head and neck cancer. Head Neck. 2007 Oct;29(10):913–8. https://doi.org/10.1002/hed.20608.
45. Chen AY, Matson LK, Roberts D, Goepfert H. The significance of comorbidity in advanced laryngeal cancer. Head Neck. 2001 Jul;23(7):566–72. https://doi.org/10.1002/hed.1079.
46. Paleri V, Wight RG, Davies GR. Impact of comorbidity on the outcome of laryngeal squamous cancer. Head Neck. 2003 Dec;25(12):1019–26. https://doi.org/10.1002/hed.10333.
47. Paleri V, Wight RG, Silver CE, Haigentz M Jr, Takes RP, Bradley PJ, Rinaldo A, Sanabria A, Bień S, Ferlito A. Comorbidity in head and neck cancer: a critical appraisal

and recommendations for practice. Oral Oncol 2010 Oct;46(10):712–719. https://doi.org/10.1016/j.oraloncology.2010.07.008. Epub 2010 Sep 17.

48. Steinbichler TB, Lichtenecker M, Anegg M, Dejaco D, Kofler B, Schartinger VH, Kasseroler MT, Forthuber B, Posch A, Riechelmann H. Persistent head and neck cancer following first-line treatment. Cancers (Basel) 2018 Nov 3;10(11):421. https://doi.org/10.3390/cancers10110421. PMID: 30400290; PMCID: PMC6265977.
49. Mehanna H, Kong A, Ahmed SK. Recurrent head and neck cancer: United Kingdom National Multidisciplinary Guidelines. J Laryngol Otol 2016 May;130(S2):S181-S190. https://doi.org/10.1017/S002221511600061X. PMID: 27841130; PMCID: PMC4873924.
50. Argiris A, Li Y, Murphy BA, Langer CJ, Forastiere AA. Outcome of elderly patients with recurrent or metastatic head and neck cancer treated with cisplatin-based chemotherapy. J Clin Oncol. 2004 Jan 15;22(2):262–8. https://doi.org/10.1200/JCO.2004.08.039.
51. Vermorken JB, Mesia R, Rivera F, Remenar E, Kawecki A, Rottey S, Erfan J, Zabolotnyy D, Kienzer HR, Cupissol D, Peyrade F, Benasso M, Vynnychenko I, De Raucourt D, Bokemeyer C, Schueler A, Amellal N, Hitt R. Platinum-based chemotherapy plus cetuximab in head and neck cancer. N Engl J Med. 2008 Sep 11;359(11):1116–27. https://doi.org/10.1056/NEJMoa0802656.
52. Vermorken JB, Trigo J, Hitt R, Koralewski P, Diaz-Rubio E, Rolland F, Knecht R, Amellal N, Schueler A, Baselga J. Open-label, uncontrolled, multicenter phase II study to evaluate the efficacy and toxicity of cetuximab as a single agent in patients with recurrent and/or metastatic squamous cell carcinoma of the head and neck who failed to respond to platinum-based therapy. J Clin Oncol. 2007 Jun 1;25(16):2171–7. https://doi.org/10.1200/JCO.2006.06.7447.
53. Baselga J, Trigo JM, Bourhis J, Tortochaux J, Cortés-Funes H, Hitt R, Gascón P, Amellal N, Harstrick A, Eckardt A. Phase II multicenter study of the antiepidermal growth factor receptor monoclonal antibody cetuximab in combination with platinum-based chemotherapy in patients with platinum-refractory metastatic and/or recurrent squamous cell carcinoma of the head and neck. J Clin Oncol 2005 Aug 20;23(24):5568–5577. https://doi.org/10.1200/JCO.2005.07.119. Epub 2005 Jul 11.
54. Fury MG, Sherman E, Lisa D, Agarwal N, Algazy K, Brockstein B, Langer C, Lim D, Mehra R, Rajan SK, Korte S, Lipson B, Yunus F, Tanvetyanon T, Smith-Marrone S, Ng K, Xiao H, Haque S, Pfister DG. A randomized phase II study of cetuximab every 2 weeks at either 500 or 750 mg/m2 for patients with recurrent or metastatic head and neck squamous cell cancer. J Natl Compr Cancer Netw 2012 Nov 1;10(11):1391–1398. https://doi.org/10.6004/jnccn.2012.0144. PMID: 23138167; PMCID: PMC5726232.
55. Wong SJ, Machtay M, Li Y. Locally recurrent, previously irradiated head and neck cancer: concurrent re-irradiation and chemotherapy, or chemotherapy alone? J Clin Oncol. 2006 Jun 10;24(17):2653–8. https://doi.org/10.1200/JCO.2005.05.3850.
56. Ferris RL, Blumenschein G Jr, Fayette J, Guigay J, Colevas AD, Licitra L, Harrington K, Kasper S, Vokes EE, Even C, Worden F, Saba NF, Iglesias Docampo LC, Haddad R, Rordorf T, Kiyota N, Tahara M, Monga M, Lynch M, Geese WJ, Kopit J, Shaw JW, Gillison ML. Nivolumab for recurrent squamous-cell carcinoma of the head and neck. N Engl J Med. 2016 Nov 10;375(19):1856–1867. https://doi.org/10.1056/NEJMoa1602252. Epub 2016 Oct 8. PMID: 27718784; PMCID: PMC5564292.
57. https://clinicaltrials.gov/ct2/show/NCT02823574
58. Burtness B, Harrington KJ, Greil R, Soulières D, Tahara M, de Castro G Jr, Psyrri A, Basté N, Neupane P, Bratland Å, Fuereder T, Hughes BGM, Mesía R, Ngamphaiboon N, Rordorf T, Wan Ishak WZ, Hong RL, González Mendoza R, Roy A, Zhang Y, Gumuscu B, Cheng JD, Jin F, Rischin D; KEYNOTE-048 Investigators. Pembrolizumab alone or with chemotherapy versus cetuximab with chemotherapy for recurrent or metastatic squamous cell carcinoma of the head and neck (KEYNOTE-048): a randomised, open-label, phase 3 study. Lancet. 2019 Nov 23;394(10212):1915–1928. https://doi.org/10.1016/S0140-6736(19)32591-7. Epub 2019 Nov 1. Erratum in: Lancet. 2020 Jan 25;395(10220):272. Erratum in: Lancet. 2020 Feb 22;395(10224):564.

59. https://www.nice.org.uk/guidance/indevelopment/gid-ta10321
60. Kennedy LB, Salama AKS. A review of cancer immunotherapy toxicity. CA Cancer J Clin 2020 Mar;70(2):86–104. https://doi.org/10.3322/caac.21596. Epub 2020 Jan 16.
61. Fayette J. 90TiP FRAIL-IMMUNE: a multicenter, prospective, single arm phase II of the combination of durvalumab with carboplatin and paclitaxel as first-line treatment in patients with recurrent/metastatic squamous cell carcinoma of the head and neck not eligible to standard chemotherapy (GORTEC 2018-03). Ann Oncol 2019; 30, S11, xi32.
62. Laraway DC, Lakshmiah R, Lowe D, Roe B, Rogers SN. Quality of life in older people with oral cancer. Br J Oral Maxillofac Surg 2012 Dec; 50(8):715–720. https://doi.org/10.1016/j.bjoms.2012.01.010. Epub 2012 Feb 11.
63. Maggiore R, Zumsteg ZS, Brintzenhofe Szoc K, Trevino KM, Gajra A, Korc-Grodzicki B, Epstein JB, Bond SM, Parker I, Kish JA, Murphy BA, Vander Walde NA; CARG-HNC Study Group. The older adult with locoregionally advanced head and neck squamous cell carcinoma: knowledge gaps and future direction in assessment and treatment. Int J Radiat Oncol Biol Phys. 2017 Jul 15;98(4):868–883. https://doi.org/10.1016/j.ijrobp.2017.02.022. PMID: 28602414; PMCID: PMC5769962.

Chapter 27
Hematological Cancer in Older Adults with Frailty

Valentin Goede

Introduction

Hematological cancer includes a large number of various diseases such as acute and chronic leukemias, aggressive and indolent lymphomas, multiple myeloma, other myeloproliferative neoplasia, and some myelodysplastic syndromes. While there are remarkable differences among these disorders in terms of their biology, clinical management, and prognosis, most hematological malignancies have in common that disease incidences increase significantly with advancing age. Their median patient age at the time of diagnosis is between 65 and 70 years old [1]. With few exceptions (e.g., acute lymphoblastic leukemia, Hodgkin lymphoma), hematological cancers, therefore, are considered aging-associated diseases (Table 27.1).

Advanced age is not only correlated with increasing susceptibility to develop cancer, but other phenomena such as physiological onset of senescence (resulting, e.g., in the decline of organ function) or pathological occurrence of chronic diseases (e.g., coronary artery disease, chronic obstructive bronchitis, diabetes, osteoarthritis, stroke). Greater vulnerability towards stressors and higher risk of adverse health events arising from these aging-associated phenomena are commonly summarized under the term "frailty." "Frail" patients with hematological cancer thus are older adults diagnosed with one of the above-mentioned blood diseases and concurrently being highly vulnerable to experience further adverse health events. These include morbidity (i.e., toxicity) and early mortality from the hematological treatment, but also onset of intercurrent diseases and geriatric syndromes (e.g., falls, delirium) independent from the blood disease and its therapy.

V. Goede (✉)
Division of Oncogeriatrics, St. Marien Hospital, Cologne, Germany
e-mail: valentin.goede@cellitinnen.de

F. Gomes (ed.), *Frailty in Older Adults with Cancer*,
https://doi.org/10.1007/978-3-030-89162-6_27

Table 27.1 Median age at diagnosis in selected hematological cancers [1]

Hematological cancer	Median age at diagnosis (years)
Leukemia	
Acute myeloid leukemia (AML)	68
Acute lymphoblastic leukemia (ALL)	17
Chronic myeloid leukemia (CML)	65
Chronic lymphocytic leukemia (CLL)	70
Lymphoma	
Hodgkin lymphoma (HL)	40
Follicular non-Hodgkin lymphoma (FL)	63
Diffuse large B-cell non-Hodgkin lymphoma (DLBCL)	66
Multiple myeloma (MM)	69

This chapter will present the tools to identify frailty in patients with hematological cancer, describe the hematological workup and treatment principles in such patients, and provide an overview of their management in the setting of acute myeloid leukemia, chronic myeloid leukemia, chronic lymphocytic leukemia, follicular lymphoma, diffuse large B-cell lymphoma, and multiple myeloma.

Identification of Frailty in Patients with Hematological Cancer

To date, there is no universally accepted clinical procedure or tool to detect and measure frailty in patients with hematological malignancies, with various methods suggested in either routine clinical practice or within clinical trials [2, 3]. However, scientific efforts to build a solid evidence base have remained limited to mostly retrospective studies and small sample sizes.

Frailty Screening in Hematological Cancer

Fried's frailty criteria (phenotype model) and Rockwood's frailty index (deficit accumulation model) are considered academic gold standards to assess frailty in community-dwelling and geriatric settings of care [4, 5], but have only been occasionally studied in hematological cancer patients. In the hematology clinic, these two traditional approaches of frailty assessment, therefore, are hardly applied.

Screening tools that are easier to implement, but similarly to traditional frailty models emerged from outside of the heme-oncological context have been explored in a number of studies with regard to the prevalence and prognostic impact of frailty in patients with hematological malignancies. For instance, frailty as assessed by the

Groningen frailty index (GFI) was found predictive for intolerance of (R)CHOP-based chemotherapy and poor overall survival in older patients with aggressive Non-Hodgkin lymphoma (NHL) [6]. Likewise, the Vulnerable Elders Survey-13 (VES-13) was found predictive for worse outcomes in patients with aggressive NHL when treated with chemoimmunotherapy plus lenalidomide [7]. The Edmonton frailty scale (EFS) was used in an attempt to describe the prevalence of frailty in a cohort of patients with various hematological cancers [8]. Other cancer-unspecific frailty screenings such as the Clinical Frailty Scale (CFS) or the Fatigue, Resistance, Ambulation, Illnesses and Loss of Weight questionnaire (FRAIL) have been proposed for the use in patients with hematological malignancies [3], but specific studies are missing.

Investigations of the more oncology-specific G8 frailty screening [9] within the hematological cancer context were performed in several studies. In a single center study of 108 older patients with various hematological malignancies, abnormal G8 results were predictive of 1-year mortality [10]. However, another single center study in 107 patients with hematological cancers failed to demonstrate prediction of 1-year mortality by the G8 [11]. In other single center studies, G8 was demonstrated to have prognostic value specifically in diffuse large B-cell lymphoma (DLBCL) as well as in acute myeloid leukemia (AML) [12, 13].

Notably, there are no larger prospective studies on G8 or other frailty screenings in hematological cancer so far. As a practical conclusion, such tools might be applied to formally screen for frailty in an older hematological cancer patient, but due to the lack of sound prospective data, treatment decision-making (i.e., deciding for intensive vs. less intensive or no cancer treatment) solely based on frailty screening results is not supported by the currently available data.

Geriatric Assessment in Hematological Cancer

While frailty screenings are limited in guiding treatment decisions in older hematological cancer patients, these tools may help to screen for those patients benefitting from a further geriatric assessment (GA). Having emerged from geriatric medicine, GA meanwhile has been highly propagated as a key approach to identify frail hematological cancer patients [14, 15]. The ability of GA to detect frailty with predicting adverse health outcomes specifically in the hematological cancer context has been examined in greater detail [16, 17]. A recent systematic review reported on 44 GA-studies performed in various malignant hematological disorders including AML, NHL, and multiple myeloma [17]. Of those, 17 studies even made an attempt to identify frail hematological cancer patients based on a summarized GA score. In the majority of studies, single geriatric impairments detected by GA (e.g., comorbidity, impaired activities of daily living, physical capacity or cognition) as well as frailty assigned with summarized GA scores were predictive for shorter survival.

There were also correlations between frailty identified by GA and greater risk of treatment-related toxicity or treatment non-completion. However, GA-studies in hematological malignancies still have remained inconclusive about the ideal composition and practical implementation of GA in a hematology clinic. In particular, the following questions are still unanswered: Which geriatric domains should be assessed by which instrument? What are the cut-offs that could be used to assign frailty in individual hematological cancer patients and allow to calculate risks of particular adverse events?

Recently, a hematology-specific GA tool has been introduced (GAH scale) [18, 19]. Dimensions assessed by this tool are polypharmacy (drugs count), gait speed (measured over 4 m), mood (1 question), activities of daily living (3 questions), subjective health status (1 question), nutrition (4 items from the Mini Nutritional Assessment-short form), mental status (Short Portable Mental Status Questionnaire), and comorbidity (prognostic index). The tool provides detailed instructions on cut-off values to be used for each dimension and can be executed within 10–15 minutes. GAH appears a promising tool to harmonize GA-based assessment of frailty in older patients with hematological malignancies. However, studies on the tool's true prognostic value and its capability to predict adverse health events including calculating risks of treatment toxicity or treatment non-completion are still lacking.

Related to frailty assessment, two chemotoxicity risk calculators which in part are GA-based (CARG score, CRASH score) have become available for the use in older patients with cancers [20, 21]. These tools might be useful to identify frail hematology cancer patients with increased or unacceptable risk of chemotherapy-related adverse events. Unfortunately, there have been no specific studies with CARG or CRASH in specific hematological cancer entities so far and thus uncertainty about the performance of these risk calculators in blood diseases remains high. Moreover, both instruments have not been validated for systemic therapy of hematological malignancies with non-chemotherapeutic drugs which are now part of many contemporary treatment regimens.

Hematological Workup and Treatment Principles

With regard to diagnostic procedures (i.e., cytology, histology, staging), hematological cancer patients with frailty may have a higher procedural risk as compared with patients lacking any frailty features (e.g., increased risk of renal failure during application of contrast media, increased risk of delirium during biopsy takings with short anesthesia). Nevertheless, it is recommended to rather complete than to refrain from performing a standard hematological workup in such patients. Only in very old and severely frail patients (e.g., in subjects with pre-existing confinement to bed or with far advanced dementia) a hematological workup may stop without any further prognostic information or therapeutic consequence and thus left incomplete.

The treatment arsenal for hematological malignancies has undergone fundamental improvements during recent years. Among those were the establishment of dose-reduced chemotherapy regimens as well as the introduction of refined radiation techniques, for instance. Of note, a key development was the advent of novel non-chemotherapeutic drugs such as new monoclonal antibodies, kinase inhibitors, immunomodulators, and growth factors. By combining these agents in a smart way, it has become possible to not just increase therapeutic efficacy, but also to reduce toxicity, thereby opening new avenues for efficacious treatment of older hematological cancer patients with frailty being ineligible for standard therapies due to their vulnerabilities. Drugs that significantly have contributed to novel treatment opportunities in vulnerable patients with hematological malignancies are, for instance, dasatinib, nilotinib, bortezomib, lenalidomide, pomalidomide, obinutuzumab, venetoclax, ibrutinib, idelalisib, and others. It must be noted that such medications can also pose certain risks for patients carrying frailty features. For example, some of these drugs are inhibitors or substrates of the CYP3A4 enzyme and hence could adversely interact with a frail patient's pre-existing polypharmacy. Another example are cognitively impaired frail patients in which oral treatment with such drugs may be unsafe because of low adherence and non-compliance.

Therapeutic management of older hematological cancer patients with frailty may also include targeting frailty itself. Among those vulnerabilities that could be therapeutically targeted are, e.g., fall risk, sarcopenia, malnourishment, delirium, depression, polypharmacy with potentially inappropriate medication, or uncontrolled comorbidities. So far, there have only been very few pilot studies pursuing such approaches [22]. Nevertheless, further trials investigating the benefits of targeting frailty in older patients with hematological malignancies are ongoing [17].

Treatment of Hematological Malignancies

Therapy of older patients with hematological cancer and frailty varies remarkably depending on disease entity. A summary of commonly used treatment regimens in this sub-group of patients is shown in Table 27.2.

Acute Myeloid Leukemia (AML)

In most cases, AML shows an aggressive behavior and without antileukemic treatment results in death after few weeks or months. Almost exclusively and irrespective of whether patients have frailty, their overall prognosis is mainly determined by the hematological cancer. Therefore, control of the leukemia is an important task even in old and frail AML patients. Best supportive care should be an option only in subjects with very severe frailty features (i.e., patients being terminally ill with life expectancy <3–6 months and not due to the leukemia but due to other chronic conditions).

Table 27.2 Treatment regimens for frail patients with hematological cancer (selection)

Hematological cancer	Hematological treatment regimen
Acute myeloid leukemia (AML)	Azacytidine Decitabine Azacytidine/Venetoclax Low-dose Ara-C/Venetoclax
Chronic myeloid leukemia (CML)	Imatinib Dasatinib, Nilotinib
Chronic lymphocytic leukemia (CLL)	Venetoclax/Obinutuzumab (VEN-G) Ibrutinib +/– Obinutuzumab Chlorambucil/ Obinutuzumab (G-CLB) Bendamustine/rituximab (BR)
Hodgkin lymphoma (HL)	Brentuximab vedotin (relapse) Immune-checkpoint inhibitors (relapse)
Follicular non-Hodgkin lymphoma (FL)	Bendamustine/rituximab (BR) Lenalidomide/rituximab (R^2) Idelalisib (relapse)
Diffuse large B-cell non-Hodgkin lymphoma (DLBCL)	R-mini-CHOP Trosphosphamide (relapse)
Multiple myeloma (MM)	Bortezomib/dexamethasone (VD) Lenalidomide/dexamethasone (RD) Bortezomib/Melphalan/prednisolone (VMP) Bortezomib/Lenalidomide/dexamethasone (VdR) Pomalidomide-containing (relapse) Daratumumab-containing (frontline and relapse)

A key decision to be made in newly diagnosed AML is whether a patient is fit enough or too frail for intensive polychemotherapy and eventually hematopoietic stem cell transplant. For routine management of AML, there currently is no other standard than clinical judgement to make such decision. Anyhow, there have been a number of AML-specific studies demonstrating that GA detects patient-inherent vulnerabilities and thereby could support identification of frail AML patients and guide treatment intensity [23–26].

Standard cytarabine- and anthracycline-containing induction and consolidation chemotherapy is difficult to realize in these patients. With such treatment, patients at older age and/or with frailty as assessed by geriatric assessment have substantially higher risks of early death, non-response, and early relapse [24, 25]. Five-year rates of being free of relapse are remarkably low. Chemotherapy-like treatment with the hypomethylating agents azacytidine or decitabine is a valid antileukemic approach for frail AML patients and demonstrated better outcome when compared in several studies with best supportive care or low-dose cytosine-arabinoside (Ara-C) [27]. Very recently, addition of the BCL2-inhibitor venetoclax to low-dose Ara-C or azacytidine resulted in significant and clinically relevant outcome improvements in patients with AML considered too frail and hence ineligible for standard induction chemotherapy [28, 29].

Chronic Myeloid Leukemia (CML)

Treatment of CML is not fundamentally different according to the presence or severity of frailty. In the frontline setting, CML patients with frailty are treated with a tyrosine kinase inhibitor (TKI), which in most cases is imatinib [30]. In case of a non-sufficient response, alternative TKIs are used (e.g., dasatinib, nilotinib). Even in the presence of frailty, these drugs are usually well tolerated. However, slightly increased rates of toxicity and withdrawal from treatment have been observed. Notably, TKI such as imatinib, dasatinib, and nilotinib are CYP3A4 inhibitors; these may increase serum levels of other medications being CYP3A4 substrates and part of a frail patient's polypharmacy. The question, whether long-term therapy with TKI can be stopped at some time point without posing an unacceptable risk of relapse is particularly important in older CML patients with frailty and has been addressed in trials indicating that intermittent treatment is feasible [31].

Chronic Lymphocytic Leukemia (CLL)

Irrespective of a patient's frailty status, treatment of CLL is only indicated if the disease is symptomatic (e.g., presence of B symptoms) or at an advanced stage (Binet C, Rai III-IV). Since the course of the disease is more indolent than in acute leukemia or aggressive lymphoma, competing risks of death by co-existing diseases play a greater role. Until recently, there was a need in such patients to decide whether subjects are fit enough for more intense purine analog-based chemoimmunotherapy or have accumulated frailty features that would make them more suitable for less intense treatment approaches (chemo only, mild chemoimmunotherapy) [32]. The proposed frailty criteria to guide this decision in CLL included both age and co-existing diseases as assessed by specific comorbidity assessment tools (e.g., Cumulative Illness Rating Scale). However, the recent introduction of a number of new and well-tolerated non-chemotherapeutic drugs has started to change this treatment paradigm and identifying of frailty to aid treatment decision has, therefore, become less crucial.

Currently preferred frontline treatments in older patients with CLL and frailty are chemotherapy-free regimens (ibrutinib with or without the addition of obinutuzumab, venetoclax plus obinutuzumab) or mild chemoimmunotherapies (chlorambucil plus obinutuzumab, bendamustine plus rituximab) [33–39]. Chemoimmunotherapy was shown superior to chemotherapy alone with regard to overall survival in this group of patients [39]. Chemotherapy-free ibrutinib- or venetoclax-based approaches have been demonstrated superior to chemoimmunotherapy with regard to progression-free survival [35, 38]. Any of these regimens has specific advantages and disadvantages. In clinical practice, selection is based on disease- and patient-features. Notably, chemoimmunotherapy should only be used in patients without TP53 mutation and without unmutated IGVH status. Patients with frailty carrying these adverse risk factors should receive either ibrutinib- or venetoclax-containing therapy. Notably, venetoclax plus obinutuzumab offers a fixed-duration therapy (12 months) while ibrutinib is an indefinite life-long treatment. Patients with CLL and major impairment of renal function are at risk of tumor lysis during venetoclax therapy. Patients with CLL and cardiac diseases or in need of oral anticoagulation might be less suitable for treatment with ibrutinib because of atrial fibrillation and bleeding events as specific toxicities of this kinase inhibitor. Both drugs are CYP3A4 substrates. Dosing must be done with caution in older patients with frailty who are concomitantly medicated with CYP3A4 inhibitors.

Follicular Lymphoma (FL)

Because of its indolent course, overall prognosis of frail patients with FL is highly determined by other chronic comorbidities. Therapy should only be initiated in symptomatic subjects. Frail patients with FL of limited stage can be safely and effectively treated with local radiation. Patients with mild symptoms may be treated with rituximab only. The standard treatment of frail patients with advanced stage FL is chemoimmunotherapy followed by rituximab maintenance. Most commonly regimens are R-CHOP (rituximab, cyclophosphamide, doxorubicin, vincristine, prednisolone), R-CVP (rituximab, cyclophosphamide, prednisolone), and BR (bendamustine plus rituximab) [40]. A novel regimen that might be offered to FL patients with some frailty is lenalidomide plus rituximab [41]. This regimen is "chemotherapy-free" and appears equally effective when compared with chemoimmunotherapy. However, it is not toxicity-free. While myelosuppression is less frequent with this treatment, cutaneous toxicity is significantly increased. In relapsed patients with frailty, treatment with the TKI idelalisib is an option [42]. This drug has only little risk of myelosuppression. However, autoimmune-mediated diarrhea can occur; older patients with inherent dehydration risk will, therefore, need careful clinical monitoring during this therapy.

Diffuse Large B-Cell Lymphoma (DLBCL)

DLBCL is characterized by an aggressive course. Similar to AML, death usually occurs within weeks or few months if there is no specific therapy. Standard treatment of patients with DLBCL is chemoimmunotherapy with R-CHOP. To ensure a maximal treatment benefit (i.e., cure of the disease) dose reductions are to be avoided whenever possible. However, in older patients with frailty, full-dose administration of R-CHOP could become a significant challenge and often impossible to deliver. For example, chronic heart failure may require modifications including the use of liposomal drug formulations or even omitting of anthracycline dosing. And pre-existing polyneuropathy may require dose modifications for vincristine. A commonly used dose-reduced regimen for older patients with frailty is R-mini-CHOP [43].

Decisions about dosing of R-CHOP in this sub-group of patients are based on clinical judgement with particular look at comorbidities and organ function at baseline (echocardiography, neurography). A supporting role of GA during this decision process has been proposed [44–46], but remains to be further defined. In DLBCL, GA may become particularly helpful to identify those patients who will have minimal chances of cure and in whom therefore no benefit from chemoimmunotherapy is expected compared with best supportive care [47].

Patients with relapsed DLBCL and frailty, after fully-dosed or dose-modified therapy with R-CHOP, are very difficult to re-treat. Due to frailty features, these patients are usually ineligible to autologous transplant. Re-exposure to chemo- or chemoimmunotherapy as well as experimental therapies might be offered, but many of these patients will receive best supportive care.

Multiple Myeloma (MM)

Very similar to CLL, there have been fundamental changes of the treatment landscape of MM during recent years. A plethora of non-chemotherapeutic drugs have become available (e.g., bortezomib, carfilzomib, lenalidomide, pomalidomide, daratumumab). Patients with frailty strongly benefit from these achievements as these patients are usually ineligible for autologous transplant, but thanks to the availability of such drugs can be offered very efficacious chemotherapy-free combination treatments [48, 49].

Frailty assessment by GA is highly recommended in MM [50, 51]. To date, MM is the only hematological cancer for which entity-specific frailty indices have been developed in order to guide treatment decisions. These include the International Myeloma Working Group Frailty Index (IMWG-FI) and the Revised Myeloma Comorbidity Index (R-MCI) [52, 53]. Age, comorbidities, and functional impairments are key variables of both indices. Based on IMWG-FI or R-MCI, older patients with MM can be assigned to the categories "fit," "intermediate," and "frail." Usage of these tools is recommended in several MM guidelines [48].

Despite these efforts to implement GA in the diagnostic workup of MM, selecting the optimal treatment regimen for patients with MM and frailty remains a challenge. Double or triple combinations are recommended. Eventually, these can be combined with antibody (daratumumab). Commonly used regimens in this group of vulnerable patients are, e.g., bortezomib plus dexamethasone (VD), lenalidomide plus dexamethasone (RD), bortezomib plus melphalan and prednisolone (VMP), bortezomib plus lenalidomide and dexamethasone (VdR) [48]. Mild chemotherapy (bendamustine) remains another treatment option in patients with a relapse. Specific toxicities of chemotherapy-free drugs must be taken into consideration when treating chronically ill and patients with frailty (e.g., bortezomib—polyneuropathy, lenalidomide—immunosuppression).

Conclusion

Because hematological malignancies are a heterogenous group of diseases it is unlikely that there will be a universal tool to generally assess frailty in patients with such disorders. Among different approaches, a combination of GAs currently holds the greatest promise to become a method of choice. However, further validation in context of specific hematological cancers and specific treatments are essential. Most importantly, standard cut-offs and summarized GA scores will have to be developed to allow for the calculation of specific risks (e.g., risk of treatment toxicity, risk of treatment non-completion, risk of geriatric syndromes, risk of cancer-unrelated death).

Treatment of patients with hematological malignancies and frailty will be further improved by smart combinations of chemotherapy with non-chemotherapeutic agents or by new chemotherapy-free drug regimens. Next to those agents that have already been established as key treatments for such patients, other drug classes are expected to further broaden the therapeutic spectrum. Among these are immune-checkpoint inhibitors that have been reported to be highly active in some hematological malignancies (e.g., Hodgkin lymphoma) [54, 55] and applicable in patients with frailty features in a more general tumor context [56]. To what extent other fundamental achievements in hematological therapy (e.g., CAR-T cells) will further change the treatment of patients with frailty with hematological cancers remains unclear and will be subject to future clinical trials. Lastly, co-management of vulnerabilities in patients with frailty and hematological cancers may be a promising strategy to improve the overall prognosis of this complex patient population.

References

1. https://seer.cancer.gov/statfacts/html/all.html
2. Abel GA, Klepin HD. Frailty and the management of hematologic malignancies. Blood. 2018;131(5):515–24.
3. Koll TT, Rosko AE. Frailty in hematologic malignancy. Curr Hematol Malig Rep. 2018;13(3):143–54.
4. Fried LP, Tangen CM, Walston J, Newman AB, Hirsch C, Gottdiener J, et al. Frailty in older adults: evidence for a phenotype. J Gerontol A Biol Sci Med Sci. 2001;56(3):M146–56.
5. Mitnitski AB, Mogilner AJ, MacKnight C, Rockwood K. The mortality rate as a function of accumulated deficits in a frailty index. Mech Ageing Dev. 2002;123(11):1457–60.
6. Aaldriks AA, Giltay EJ, Nortier JW, van der Geest LG, Tanis BC, Ypma P, et al. Prognostic significance of geriatric assessment in combination with laboratory parameters in elderly patients with aggressive non-Hodgkin lymphoma. Leuk Lymphoma. 2015;56(4):927–35.
7. Ribi K, Rondeau S, Hitz F, Mey U, Enoiu M, Pabst T, et al. Cancer-specific geriatric assessment and quality of life: important factors in caring for older patients with aggressive B-cell lymphoma. Support Care Cancer. 2017;25(9):2833–42.
8. Atakul E, Akyar I. Frailty prevalence and characteristics in older adults with hematologic cancer: a descriptive study. Asia Pac J Oncol Nurs. 2019;6(1):43–9.

9. Bellera CA, Rainfray M, Mathoulin-Pelissier S, Mertens C, Delva F, Fonck M, et al. Screening older cancer patients: first evaluation of the G-8 geriatric screening tool. Ann Oncol. 2012;23(8):2166–72.
10. Hamaker ME, Mitrovic M, Stauder R. The G8 screening tool detects relevant geriatric impairments and predicts survival in elderly patients with a haematological malignancy. Ann Hematol. 2014;93(6):1031–40.
11. Dubruille S, Libert Y, Roos M, Vandenbossche S, Collard A, Meuleman N, et al. Identification of clinical parameters predictive of one-year survival using two geriatric tools in clinically fit older patients with hematological malignancies: major impact of cognition. J Geriatr Oncol. 2015;6(5):362–9.
12. Sakurai M, Karigane D, Kasahara H, Tanigawa T, Ishida A, Murakami H, et al. Geriatric screening tools predict survival outcomes in older patients with diffuse large B cell lymphoma. Ann Hematol. 2019;98(3):669–78.
13. Umit EG, Baysal M, Demir AM. Frailty in patients with acute myeloid leukaemia, conceptual misapprehension of chronological age. Eur J Cancer Care (Engl). 2018;27(2):e12810.
14. Klepin HD. Ready for prime time: role for geriatric assessment to improve quality of care in hematology practice. Blood. 2019;134(23):2005–12.
15. Goede V, Stauder R. Multidisciplinary care in the hematology clinic: implementation of geriatric oncology. J Geriatr Oncol. 2019;10(3):497–503.
16. Hamaker ME, Prins MC, Stauder R. The relevance of a geriatric assessment for elderly patients with a haematological malignancy--a systematic review. Leuk Res. 2014;38(3):275–83.
17. Scheepers ERM, Vondeling AM, Thielen N, van der Griend R, Stauder R, Hamaker ME. Geriatric assessment in older patients with a hematologic malignancy: a systematic review. Haematologica. 2020;105(6):1484–93.
18. Bonanad S, De la Rubia J, Gironella M, Perez Persona E, Gonzalez B, Fernandez Lago C, et al. Development and psychometric validation of a brief comprehensive health status assessment scale in older patients with hematological malignancies: the GAH scale. J Geriatr Oncol. 2015;6(5):353–61.
19. Cruz-Jentoft AJ, Gonzalez B, de la Rubia J, Hernandez Rivas JA, Soler JA, Fernandez Lago C, et al. Further psychometric validation of the GAH scale: responsiveness and effect size. J Geriatr Oncol. 2017;8(3):211–5.
20. Extermann M, Boler I, Reich RR, Lyman GH, Brown RH, DeFelice J, et al. Predicting the risk of chemotherapy toxicity in older patients: the chemotherapy risk assessment scale for high-age patients (CRASH) score. Cancer. 2012;118(13):3377–86.
21. Hurria A, Togawa K, Mohile SG, Owusu C, Klepin HD, Gross CP, et al. Predicting chemotherapy toxicity in older adults with cancer: a prospective multicenter study. J Clin Oncol. 2011;29(25):3457–65.
22. Klepin HD, Danhauer SC, Tooze JA, Stott K, Daley K, Vishnevsky T, et al. Exercise for older adult inpatients with acute myelogenous leukemia: a pilot study. J Geriatr Oncol. 2011;2(1):11–7.
23. Klepin HD, Geiger AM, Tooze JA, Kritchevsky SB, Williamson JD, Ellis LR, et al. The feasibility of inpatient geriatric assessment for older adults receiving induction chemotherapy for acute myelogenous leukemia. J Am Geriatr Soc. 2011;59(10):1837–46.
24. Klepin HD, Geiger AM, Tooze JA, Kritchevsky SB, Williamson JD, Pardee TS, et al. Geriatric assessment predicts survival for older adults receiving induction chemotherapy for acute myelogenous leukemia. Blood. 2013;121(21):4287–94.
25. Klepin HD, Ritchie E, Major-Elechi B, Le-Rademacher J, Seisler D, Storrick L, et al. Geriatric assessment among older adults receiving intensive therapy for acute myeloid leukemia: report of CALGB 361006 (Alliance). J Geriatr Oncol. 2020;11(1):107–13.
26. Loh KP, Klepin HD. Geriatric assessment in acute myeloid leukemia: current and future landscape. Blood Adv. 2018;2(18):2418.
27. Almeida AM, Ramos F. Acute myeloid leukemia in the older adults. Leuk Res Rep. 2016;6:1–7.

28. DiNardo CD, Jonas BA, Pullarkat V, Thirman MJ, Garcia JS, Wei AH, et al. Azacitidine and Venetoclax in previously untreated acute myeloid leukemia. N Engl J Med. 2020;383(7):617–29.
29. Wei AH, Montesinos P, Ivanov V, DiNardo CD, Novak J, Laribi K, et al. Venetoclax plus LDAC for newly diagnosed AML ineligible for intensive chemotherapy: a phase 3 randomized placebo-controlled trial. Blood. 2020;135(24):2137–45.
30. Gugliotta G, Castagnetti F, Apolinari M, Pirondi S, Cavo M, Baccarani M, et al. First-line treatment of newly diagnosed elderly patients with chronic myeloid leukemia: current and emerging strategies. Drugs. 2014;74(6):627–43.
31. Russo D, Malagola M, Skert C, Cancelli V, Turri D, Pregno P, et al. Managing chronic myeloid leukaemia in the elderly with intermittent imatinib treatment. Blood Cancer J. 2015;5:e347.
32. Stauder R, Eichhorst B, Hamaker ME, Kaplanov K, Morrison VA, Osterborg A, et al. Management of chronic lymphocytic leukemia (CLL) in the elderly: a position paper from an international Society of Geriatric Oncology (SIOG) task force. Ann Oncol. 2017;28(2):218–27.
33. Burger JA, Tedeschi A, Barr PM, Robak T, Owen C, Ghia P, et al. Ibrutinib as initial therapy for patients with chronic lymphocytic leukemia. N Engl J Med. 2015;373(25):2425–37.
34. Eichhorst B, Fink AM, Bahlo J, Busch R, Kovacs G, Maurer C, et al. First-line chemoimmunotherapy with bendamustine and rituximab versus fludarabine, cyclophosphamide, and rituximab in patients with advanced chronic lymphocytic leukaemia (CLL10): an international, open-label, randomised, phase 3, non-inferiority trial. Lancet Oncol. 2016;17(7):928–42.
35. Fischer K, Al-Sawaf O, Bahlo J, Fink AM, Tandon M, Dixon M, et al. Venetoclax and Obinutuzumab in patients with CLL and coexisting conditions. N Engl J Med. 2019;380(23):2225–36.
36. Michallet AS, Aktan M, Hiddemann W, Ilhan O, Johansson P, Laribi K, et al. Rituximab plus bendamustine or chlorambucil for chronic lymphocytic leukemia: primary analysis of the randomized, open-label MABLE study. Haematologica. 2018;103(4):698–706.
37. Moreno C, Greil R, Demirkan F, Tedeschi A, Anz B, Larratt L, et al. Ibrutinib plus obinutuzumab versus chlorambucil plus obinutuzumab in first-line treatment of chronic lymphocytic leukaemia (iLLUMINATE): a multicentre, randomised, open-label, phase 3 trial. Lancet Oncol. 2019;20(1):43–56.
38. Woyach JA, Ruppert AS, Heerema NA, Zhao W, Booth AM, Ding W, et al. Ibrutinib regimens versus Chemoimmunotherapy in older patients with untreated CLL. N Engl J Med. 2018;379(26):2517–28.
39. Goede V, Fischer K, Busch R, Engelke A, Eichhorst B, Wendtner CM, et al. Obinutuzumab plus chlorambucil in patients with CLL and coexisting conditions. N Engl J Med. 2014;370(12):1101–10.
40. Buske C, Hutchings M, Ladetto M, Goede V, Mey U, Soubeyran P, et al. ESMO consensus conference on malignant lymphoma: general perspectives and recommendations for the clinical management of the elderly patient with malignant lymphoma. Ann Oncol. 2018;29(3):544–62.
41. Morschhauser F, Fowler NH, Feugier P, Bouabdallah R, Tilly H, Palomba ML, et al. Rituximab plus Lenalidomide in advanced untreated follicular lymphoma. N Engl J Med. 2018;379(10):934–47.
42. Gopal AK, Kahl BS, de Vos S, Wagner-Johnston ND, Schuster SJ, Jurczak WJ, et al. PI3Kdelta inhibition by idelalisib in patients with relapsed indolent lymphoma. N Engl J Med. 2014;370(11):1008–18.
43. Peyrade F, Jardin F, Thieblemont C, Thyss A, Emile JF, Castaigne S, et al. Attenuated immunochemotherapy regimen (R-miniCHOP) in elderly patients older than 80 years with diffuse large B-cell lymphoma: a multicentre, single-arm, phase 2 trial. Lancet Oncol. 2011;12(5):460–8.
44. Lin RJ, Behera M, Diefenbach CS, Flowers CR. Role of anthracycline and comprehensive geriatric assessment for elderly patients with diffuse large B-cell lymphoma. Blood. 2017;130(20):2180–5.
45. Morrison VA, Hamlin P, Soubeyran P, Stauder R, Wadhwa P, Aapro M, et al. Approach to therapy of diffuse large B-cell lymphoma in the elderly: the International Society of Geriatric Oncology (SIOG) expert position commentary. Ann Oncol. 2015;26(6):1058–68.

46. Soubeyran PL, Cordoba R. Approaches for vulnerable and frail older patients with diffuse large B-cell lymphomas. Curr Opin Oncol. 2019;31(5):369–73.
47. Tucci A, Martelli M, Rigacci L, Riccomagno P, Cabras MG, Salvi F, et al. Comprehensive geriatric assessment is an essential tool to support treatment decisions in elderly patients with diffuse large B-cell lymphoma: a prospective multicenter evaluation in 173 patients by the lymphoma Italian foundation (FIL). Leuk Lymphoma. 2015;56(4):921–6.
48. Larocca A, Dold SM, Zweegman S, Terpos E, Wasch R, D'Agostino M, et al. Patient-centered practice in elderly myeloma patients: an overview and consensus from the European myeloma network (EMN). Leukemia. 2018;32(8):1697–712.
49. Kint N, Delforge M. Concise review - treatment of multiple myeloma in the very elderly: how do novel agents fit in? J Geriatr Oncol. 2016;7(5):383–9.
50. Cook G, Larocca A, Facon T, Zweegman S, Engelhardt M. Defining the vulnerable patient with myeloma-a frailty position paper of the European myeloma network. Leukemia. 2020;34(9):2285–94.
51. Wildes TM, Campagnaro E. Management of multiple myeloma in older adults: gaining ground with geriatric assessment. J Geriatr Oncol. 2017;8(1):1–7.
52. Engelhardt M, Domm AS, Dold SM, Ihorst G, Reinhardt H, Zober A, et al. A concise revised myeloma comorbidity index as a valid prognostic instrument in a large cohort of 801 multiple myeloma patients. Haematologica. 2017;102(5):910–21.
53. Palumbo A, Bringhen S, Mateos MV, Larocca A, Facon T, Kumar SK, et al. Geriatric assessment predicts survival and toxicities in elderly myeloma patients: an international myeloma working group report. Blood. 2015;125(13):2068–74.
54. Kline J, Godfrey J, Ansell SM. The immune landscape and response to immune checkpoint blockade therapy in lymphoma. Blood. 2020;135(8):523–33.
55. Moy RH, Younes A. Immune checkpoint inhibition in Hodgkin lymphoma. Hema. 2018;2(1):e20.
56. Daste A, Domblides C, Gross-Goupil M, Chakiba C, Quivy A, Cochin V, et al. Immune checkpoint inhibitors and elderly people: a review. Eur J Cancer. 2017;82:155–66.

Index

F. Gomes (ed.), *Frailty in Older Adults with Cancer*,
https://doi.org/10.1007/978-3-030-89162-6

D

E

MIX
Papier aus verantwortungsvollen Quellen
Paper from responsible sources
FSC® C105338

If you have any concerns about our products,
you can contact us on
ProductSafety@springernature.com

In case Publisher is established outside the EU,
the EU authorized representative is:
Springer Nature Customer Service Center GmbH
Europaplatz 3, 69115 Heidelberg, Germany

Printed by Libri Plureos GmbH
in Hamburg, Germany